LeBoeuf's
Home
*Health*Care
Handbook

To my wife Donni –
The most caring person
I know.

Eldercare Edition

LeBoeuf's

Home

*Health*Care

Handbook

All you need to become a caregiver in your home

Gene LeBoeuf

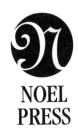

NOEL
PRESS

LeBoeuf's Home Healthcare Handbook
Eldercare Edition

LeBoeuf's Home Healthcare Handbook is designed to provide accurate information with regard
to the subject matter covered. It is distributed and sold with the understanding that the author
and publisher are not engaged in rendering medical, legal, accounting or other professional
services. Whenever possible, patients, caregivers and other readers of this handbook should
first consult a healthcare professional. Furthermore, laws vary from state to state, and if legal
advice, tax advice, or other expert assistance is required, the services of a competent professional should be obtained.

The products, therapies, organizations and associations mentioned in this handbook are for
informational purposes only. Their inclusion in this handbook does not imply their endorse-
ment by the author.

The author and publisher specifically disclaim any liability, damages, loss or risk, personal or
otherwise, which is incurred directly, indirectly, or consequential, resulting from the use and
application of any of the contents of this handbook. Although the publisher accepts no responsibility for inaccuracies or omissions, they are always grateful for suggestions.

Library of Congress Cataloging in Publication Data

Library of Congress Catalog Card Number: 95-94954
Main entry under title:
LeBoeuf's Home Healthcare Handbook: All you need to become a caregiver in your home.

Eldercare Edition.
Includes index.
Editors: Theis, Paul; Miller, Wanda; Herbert, Bruce E.

ISBN 0-9648852-0-4

Manufactured in the United States of America.
The text in this book is printed with soy ink on acid-free paper.

Design, typesetting and art production by Providence Graphics / Clifton, Virginia

Contents

Health Problems, Symptoms & Solutions

Acknowledgments

LeBoeuf & Associates, Inc. is grateful for the assistance of the following individuals, groups, institutions, associations and businesses in compiling this healthcare handbook :

Alzheimer's Association

Alzheimer's Disease and Related Disorders Association, Inc.

American Medical Association

American Association of Retired Persons (AARP)

American Dental Association

American Diabetes Association

American Foundation for the Blind

American Red Cross

Arthritis Foundation

Robert and Gail Breakwell

Crohn's & Colitis Foundation of America, Inc.

Robert G. Donahue, DDS

Fairfax City Police

Robert Flint

Gallaudet University

The George Washington University

Georgetown University

Halt, Jackson & Thrasher

Bruce Herbert

Barbara Holleb

Hospice Association of America

Bradley LeBoeuf

Jim LeBoeuf

Maryland Department of Education, Division of Rehabilitation Services

Massachusetts Department of Public Health, Division of Dental Health

McKesson Drug Company

Wanda Miller

National Institute of Dental Research

National Institute of Disability Rehabilitation Research

National Institute of Health (NIH)

National Institute of Mental Health

National Institute on Aging (NIA)

National Association of the Deaf

Robert Nuttall

Peterson & Basha

Providence Graphics

Karen Rea

Self Help for Hard of Hearing People, Inc. (SHHH)

Sennheiser Electronic Corporation

Bob, Jill and Sean Shaeffer

Hank, Betsy and Andrea Smith

Sunrise Medical

Nancy Theis

U.S. Department of Education (DOE)

U.S. Dept. of Health and Human Services (HHS)

U.S. Dept. of Justice, Office of Juvenile Justice

University of Maryland Medical System, Dental Center for Medically Compromised Patients

Virginia Power

The Visiting Nurses Association of Northern Virginia

Volunteers for Medical Engineering

Carol Wilson

Thelma Zehner

Preface

THIS BOOK never started out to be a book. Rather I intended to help individuals like my mother-in-law Claire learn about the availability of hearing assistive devices. If it were not for my neighbor, Ralph, we never would have learned about a whole world of help for the hearing impaired that would let them once again enjoy television, go to the movies or attend a concert or play. As I was gathering information about some of the hearing assistive devices listed in the product sections of this book, I was told by a variety of people that this kind of information had not been presented in a user friendly format before. While I welcomed their generous words, I found them somewhat surprising as the format seemed quite simple and the most direct way of transferring the information. In the midst of completing this relatively simple project, many of our friends and neighbors were experiencing difficulty in caring for their loved ones who had moved in with them as a result of an incapacitating illness. Time after time in conversation, they told my wife and me of their concerns they had for the level of care that they were able to give their loved one. They expressed real fear that they were not providing the right or adequate care. They felt that they had no one to ask for assistance on a regular basis because they didn't want to bother their doctor with all their questions. For many, it was not until the illness had reached the stage where the Hospice Association would be called to help them through the process of dying that they received outside help.

What they needed was help during the day-to-day care of the patient. What could be done, if anything, to provide additional comfort and care, as well as ease their burden? Where could they go to have reassurance that the level of care they were able to give the patient was more than adequate? Who would answer all the questions they had about the illness as it progressed? How could they strike a balance between the demands of caregiving and their own needs? Who could they turn to when they needed help or a little relief, even for a short time during the day?

No matter how often we assured them, as did their other friends, that they were doing a terrific job of caring for their loved one and to let us know if we could help out, they never felt a level of comfort about what they were doing. This didn't seem right. Why was there no one or anywhere to turn? When we began to help our friends with their care duties, we found out first hand what they were confronting on a regular basis. Information on a range of products, supplies and other helpful devices was not readily available to someone who was not free to spend an inordinate amount of time researching at the library or by telephone. Also, even if they did learn of a product that would afford some comfort, learning how to locate the distributor was another time-consuming ordeal.

It just made perfect sense to me that all this information should be in one place as a resource to save time and ease the burden of the caregiver. To me being a caregiver is God's work and those who choose to keep their loved one at home should be rewarded and helped in every way possible. I saw my friend Erica struggle to find a mail order distributor for her mom's diapers as she was too embarrassed to buy them at the local store. You never saw a happier face than when she told us that they are now being delivered to their home. Many times, despite all the best efforts of her son, Leslie, to provide home care, Polly would be alone and need to get from her bed to the bathroom. A back-up plan for such contingencies as well as a beeper for her son gave them both peace of mind. Monica, whose mother has Alzheimer's disease, readjusted the placement of furniture and breakables to avoid unnecessary accidents so her mother could move about her own home freely. Betsy and Hank showed us how a little ingenuity could turn a dining room into a patient's room on the first floor for her father. None of these individuals were given help to ease their situation. Each learned through just living through tough times and trying to make them better.

This book was written for my friends and all they taught me about the love and endless patience it takes to care for a loved one at home. The rewards are untold in knowing the peace of mind you are giving to them because they are home with their family in familiar surroundings. It is my hope that this book reflects what I learned from them and so much more that I received from the love they gave their parent. I want all the Erica's, Monica's, Leslie's and Betsy and Hank's to know that if you want to care for your loved one at home there are people, organizations and products that can help you every step of the way. They are just a telephone call away. You do not have to feel unsure, you do not have to struggle with a walker, wheelchair, changing a bed or giving a bed bath. The information has been gathered and organized in a manner that makes it easy for the reader to learn what products are available to care for a patient with a certain illness or disability. I pledge to you that if we don't know the answer to a question, we'll tell you, but we will also do our best to locate that information from those who do know it and provide it to you as quickly as possible. Your concerns are our concerns.

Home caregiving is an ever changing and evolving process — those in the business of providing products and services are always making improvements. The seasoned caregiver has much to share with those just embarking on this journey. Like anything else, we can always learn a better way to do something from the person who has been doing it longer and on a more regular basis than anyone else. I hope we can begin a dialogue and exchange ideas through LeBoeuf's and Caregivers, Inc. that will benefit all who take this journey that is filled with untold rewards and acts of love.

Introduction

LeBoeuf's Home Healthcare Handbook will help guide you through the planning process to provide you, your parents or a friend with a comprehensive plan for a successful and rewarding caregiving experience.

HOME HEALTHCARE CAREGIVERS now assist over 10 million Americans with long-term illnesses or disabilities. Although many men are caregivers, three-quarters are women. The average caregiver is 46 years old, married, middle income and employed outside the home. The love and loyalty that radiates from these dedicated people often results in treatment that surpasses anything found in even the very best nursing homes — at a fraction of the cost.

This handbook has been designed to alleviate many of your frustrations and fears. In a simple straightforward manner, it explains numerous methods, products and services that will help you comfort and care for a loved one in the home. However, this unique handbook goes a crucial step further by including sections devoted to products that will assist both the patient and the caregiver.

The product sections contain many items designed for a particular ailment or disease. You will find descriptions of top-notch institutional products never before available to the general public.

Moreover, some products have been broken down into convenient sizes for the first time. After all, few homes could readily accommodate 55-gallon drums of cleaning solutions or gallon sizes of skin care products that make sense for a hospital.

In addition to brands favored by health care professionals but little known to consumers, you will notice plenty of respected names such as Kimberly-Clark, Rubbermaid, Guardian, Detecto, Invacare, Lumex, Bard, Calgon, Johnson & Johnson, etc. Also shown are important items you might not consider otherwise — including bright tape to mark the edges of steps, hot-water sensors, pill counters, handicap signs and much more.

These products have been selected largely because of recommendations from physicians, nurses, hospitals, therapists and other caregivers. The LeBoeuf staff has reviewed every item and has made numerous plant visits to fully understand how each product is made and the quality control that goes into each item. Whenever possible, items included in the product sections are manufactured in the United States. Take advantage of LeBoeuf's "one stop" shopping service — you will gain peace of mind from our guarantee of satisfaction.

In the *Health Problems, Symptoms & Solutions* section, the laymen's description of each ailment has been distilled from some of the most reliable medical references in the world. You will learn about symptoms and what treatments and/or steps to take for appropriate care.

Perhaps more importantly, the handbook shows you where to go and who to call or write for further information and support. For example, someone who discovers that a parent has Alzheimer's Disease may be relieved to discover that the Alzheimer's Association has 220 chapters, 1,800 support groups and 35,000 volunteers throughout the United States. "Nobody can live with Alzheimer's Disease alone," notes the listing for the Alzheimer's Association.

Consider, too, the numerous useful forms and agreements. When hiring help in the home, use our special forms for credit checks and employment histories. Or follow our guide for tracing the family tree, a rewarding activity for both you and the loved one under your care. Note that there are forms for a "family agreement," employment, financial records, document locator and many others that will assist you in staying on top of the information needed. There are also numerous samples of legal documents such as a "Living Will," "Durable Power of Attorney" and others that will help you understand what each document means and help you decide what is best for your situation.

Great care has been taken to make this handbook a useful tool for the home healthcare provider. We hope that you will reach for it whenever questions arise.

If you have comments or suggestions to improve future editions, we would love to hear from you. Your experiences could help us help other people like you.

Naturally, we would also appreciate hearing from anyone who agrees that the handbook enriches the well-being of the patient and eases the daily burden of caregiving. Like you, sometimes our spirits need a boost.

We wish you the best in your home healthcare efforts. Few endeavors are more noble – or more rewarding.

LeBoeuf's
Home Healthcare
Handbook

Caregiving at Home

The Education of the Heart

BY ANNE KEITH

These hands lie heavy
On my knees.
Idled by stiffness,
Stopped by pain.

Once nimble fingers sped,
Obeying every whim.
Wool slid on needles
And warm knitting grew.
String, pulling tight,
Made knots secure and hard.

The tiniest seedling could be lifted
And replanted, sure to grow,
And yet all day strong work
With rake and hoe
Went quite unnoticed
By these hands.

Now knuckles growing into walnuts
Stop the flow.
I sit and look upon this worn-out gift,
These hands.

Thus they become my teachers
In the school of age.
Their lessons are quite clear,
But learning slow.
This is the education of the heart.

Thinking it Through

MOST FAMILIES who are considering bringing an elderly parent, relative or friend into their home for long-term care are uncertain about their duties and responsibilities. LeBoeuf's has developed this Handbook to provide guidance, assistive products and information to help you every step of the way. We at LeBoeuf's will support you in every way we can. We are dedicated to making your caregiving rewarding and as easy as possible. We know and understand the anxiety and pressure you are under and we will work with you on your problems until we find the best solution. You will never be alone in your act of love and kindness.

Nursing home care is expensive, with annual costs frequently exceeding $40,000. Bringing Mom, Dad or another family member into your home is often the best way to handle a very costly and highly emotional situation. Caring for the patient in your home also offers some comfort in knowing the daily condition of the patient, particularly if some warning signs of an emerging disability have been displayed. Other advantages of home care include an opportunity for the caregiver's family to get to know the patient better, maintain the patient's dignity and avoid loneliness. It is a wonderful way to say, "I love you," and a nice way to say, "Thank you for all you have been."

Surveys show that family members provide 80 to 90 percent of the services needed by the elderly whether in their own home or in the home of the caregiver. Services include cleaning, cooking, home maintenance and yard work, driving, banking, feeding, bathing, toileting, shopping, and transferring from bed.

There are more than 18 million elderly in the 65-74 age group, 10 million in the 75-84 age group and over 3 million people in the over 85 age group. About 1.6 million elderly live in nursing homes. Of those older people in the 65-74 age group, only one percent live in nursing homes. The percentage increases to six percent for those in the 75-84 age group. Of those who are over 85, 24 percent live in nursing homes and over 47 percent live alone. It is this age group that is the most vulnerable to health problems. Many receive no help from family or friends and have to rely totally on social services or paid assistance.

Four out five people over 65 have living children. About 66 percent live within 30 minutes of one or more of their children. Nearly 30 percent, or about 9.4 million older persons, live alone. Almost 7.4 million are women and 2.0 million are men. Over half (52 percent) of older Americans live in nine states — California, New York, Florida, Pennsylvania, Texas, Illinois, Ohio, Michigan and New Jersey.

In 1990, about 1.5 million people over 65 had difficulty with daily activities and still lived alone. Of those older persons living with others, 65 percent lived with relatives in his/her home (spouse, child), 18 percent with relatives outside his/her home, and 7 percent lived with friends. The sources of help for the remaining 10 percent are not known.

Becoming a Caregiver is Sometimes an Involuntary Decision

When insurance benefits expire or patients are discharged from a hospital after an unexpected illness, relatives may find themselves suddenly thrust into the role of caregiver. Other times, a caregiver may notice subtle signs of an emerging need for caregiving. A telephone call from a concerned neighbor may alert the relative to the need for intervention. The refrigerator may be empty or filled with spoiled food, utility bills may go unpaid, or noticeable changes in behavior may be symptomatic of the need for outside help.

Persons who may end up as caregivers will have to evaluate not only the particular circumstances of the patient, but themselves, to gauge the extent of their caregiving. The patients' personality, age and illness are all factors which will require treatment tailored to their needs. Persons may be reluctant to become a caregiver because of the uncertainty about their own ability to manage another person's daily life activities. Or caregivers may be physically unable to perform certain tasks, such as moving a bedridden patient. It is important that you and your family carefully discuss the role each will play in the care of the loved one.

One way to determine if you will be able to provide the care needed by your patient is to talk with the patient's doctor and/or physical therapist. They can tell you what you will have to do on a daily basis to care for the patient. If you are not sure that you can perform the necessary tasks and cannot afford to hire the help that would be needed, you may have to look to another family member or a nursing home to care for the patient. It makes no sense to try and do something that you know you cannot do.

Family dynamics are also likely to change. An adult child taking care of an elderly parent will be directing the parent about household rules. Grandmother's pet Schnauzer may no longer have free reign of the house, or her television viewing may be banned during the time set aside for school age children's homework. Both the senior parent *and* the adult child may feel uncomfortable about their role reversals. There have been instances where patients have become so angry with caregivers because of this role reversal that they have removed caregivers from their wills.

Even after committing to being a caregiver, you may have doubts about your decision to become a caregiver instead of hiring someone to help in the patient's home or placing the patient in a nursing home. You may question the quality of care you can provide to a suffering relative. Despite your best efforts at providing treatment, you may be frustrated and disappointed by a patient whose condition does not improve. You may also find your patience severely tested by a patient who is grouchy, irrational and seemingly unappreciative of your efforts and sacrifices. No matter what, you can be assured that LeBoeuf's will be with you every step of the way. We will endeavor to work with you until your problems are solved.

Whatever your emotions and your individual situation, the one prerequisite for caregiving is forgiveness. You, as the caregiver, will have to continually put aside the obstacles between yourself and the patient. The forgiveness that you will offer is very powerful and provides new hope for those for whom you are planning to care. Remember, the patient is most likely in a weakened emotional and physical state and the words and/or actions of the patient will not be typical. You must never act against an unkindness with an unkindness.

Third Party Notice Program

A utility customer may forget to pay the bill, or even pay the same bill twice. One worry for children with elderly parents is whether the bill has been promptly paid. While it may take several weeks of delinquent payments before a utility resorts to terminating service, one simple precaution is to be put on a list of people to be notified in the event a bill goes unpaid. In Virginia, for example, Virginia Power has implemented a **"Third Party Notice Program"** that alerts a designated person if a bill is past-due. The requirements to enroll in the program are simple. The customer signs a form agreeing to allow the electric company to notify a third party, such as a relative, friend, or social service agency if the customer is late making a payment. The third party is not responsible for the paying the delinquent electric bill. Contact your local utility company for a similar **"Third Party Notice Program"** in your area.

Note:
Throughout this book, we refer to all those who are receiving care as "patients." The caregiver can be a spouse, a child, a relative, a friend, a volunteer or an employee. In many cases, there may be more than one caregiver for the patient.

Ten Most Chronic Conditions for People 65 or Older:

As a caregiver, it is possible that you will be coping with one or more of the most chronic conditions for people 65 or older:

CONDITION	Percent of people over 65 who have the condition
Arthritis	48
Hypertension (high blood pressure)	38
Hearing impairment	29
Heart disease	28
Cataracts	16
Deformity or orthopedic impairment	16
Chronic sinusitis	15
Diabetes	9
Vision impairment	8
Varicose veins	8

In addition, mental health problems impact between 15 to 25 percent of older people. Depression, Alzheimer's disease and suicide are the major mental health problems. As people age, the percentage of problems grow until about 50 percent of all people over 85 will exhibit signs of mental illness. (According to the U.S. Department of Health and Human Services, "Aging America, 1991" 47 percent of all people over 85 will exhibit symptoms of Alzheimer's disease.)

Eldercare in the Workplace

For those caregivers who work outside the home, corporate America has come to realize that in addition to childcare, eldercare is an important issue in the workplace. Unlike childcare where its duration is predictable (such as the first five years of a child's life), eldercare may never be required. When eldercare is provided, it may last for many years, even decades. The intensity of care will vary greatly, with some workers only required to perform a minimum of assistance with a patient's daily living activities, while others will find the caregiving demands increasingly consuming more of their non-working hours. Caregivers may find their overnight business trips eliminated or curtailed unless competent substitute help is available. One study among employed caregivers found that nearly 80 percent of workers "were experiencing extreme conflict between the demands of work and the demands of caregiving." Some employers allow "flex time" so the worker can adjust their job hours to the day's particular demands of the patient.

Many companies have set up programs to assist employees who are providing eldercare. The assistance they provide includes:

- Providing information about aging issues and community services
- Making referrals to community agencies and providing consulting services
- Providing services such as adult day-care
- Paying for a portion of the cost associated with eldercare
- Fostering community initiatives to start new service programs

Family and Medical Leave Act of 1993

The purpose of the Act is to entitle employees to take reasonable leave for medical reasons, for the birth or adoption of a child, and for the care of a child, spouse, or parent who has serious health problems.

If your employer has 50 or more employees, you may want to check to see if you are covered under this Act.

An eligible employee who has been employed at least 12 months by the employer or at least 1,250 hours during the previous 12 months shall be entitled to a total of 12 workweeks of leave during any 12-month period for one or more of the following:

(A) Birth of a child.

(B) Placement of child for adoption or foster care.

(C) Care of spouse, child or parent if they have a serious health condition.

(D) Serious health condition that makes the employee unable to perform the functions of the position of the employee.

Stress and Time Management

Caregivers often mention the stress and time commitments required of them when asked about being a caregiver. What may have started as a task requiring only a few hours a week has turned into a full-time activity. It is not uncommon for caregivers to spend 70-80 hours a week helping a disabled person.

The stress and time commitments of being a caregiver can be managed several ways. LeBoeuf's, Caregivers, Inc. and other support groups offer the caregiver a chance to share their experiences, as well as solutions, for coping with difficult patients. Hiring someone to assist with housekeeping, patient sitting, cooking and the patient's personal care, while expensive, can provide much needed relief. Professional nurses working with the caregiver and the patient in the home can assist with the medical aspects of home health care. Adult day care can provide the patient with companionship, exercise and an opportunity for the patient to help others. Community and church groups which offer respite care allow the caregiver a few hours to take care of such personal chores as visiting the dentist or going to the hairdressing salon.

Signs of Approaching Problems with Caregiver Health

You, the caregiver, must pay attention to your own needs. Your own physical and emotional health must be maintained so that you can provide effective care for your patient. Your diet should include adequate amounts of nutritious food and you should allow plenty of time to eat in a relaxed setting. Exercise is also important. You should exercise three to four times a week for a minimum of 30 minutes. If you are over 40, have a doctor give you a physical before beginning any exercise program. Swimming, walking, jogging, bicycling and tennis are all good ways to keep fit. Do not let your emotions get out of hand. Discuss your problems with those involved and attempt to solve them as soon as you can. Always provide time for yourself. You will be needing vacations and long weekends to take a break from your routine. Do not try and carry the whole burden of caregiving on your own shoulders. It will take the support of your family, friends, neighbors and your church to sustain you in this endeavor.

As the caregiver, you should be aware of the signs that indicate that you are in need of more help or some time away from the situation. Do not be afraid to ask for help. We at LeBoeuf's are always there for you (even if it's just to listen). Without your good health, all the effort and sacrifice you have made will be for naught and the person you are caring for will have to be placed where you didn't want him or her to be in the first place. Some of these signs are:

- Anger
- Depression
- Frequent crying
- Inability to sleep or eat, weight loss
- Frequent headaches or stomach aches
- Abuse of alcohol or drugs
- Feeling guilty

Maintaining a sense of humor is very important for both the caregiver's and the patient's emotional health. When the situation becomes outrageously comical, laughing with the patient (not at the patient) may be the best antidote.

Decision Time

LeBoeuf's Home Healthcare Handbook is also designed to help families and friends communicate. Everyone will eventually face the reality that the people they love are getting old. Everyone must plan for the future. If you plan for the worst and nothing happens, nothing is lost. If you do not plan for the future and a crisis develops, the failure to have a plan in place can be frustrating, expensive and may lead to unnecessary stress among family members. By having a plan in place, all parties will have agreed ahead of time exactly what will happen if Mom or Dad can no longer care for themselves. Somehow, some way, someone in the family must take the lead and start the discussion of what can and should be done.

This Handbook will help guide you through the planning process for a successful and rewarding caregiving experience. It tells what you need, when you need it, how it can be done, who should do it, and what products and services are available. By reading and/or completing each section that pertains to your patient — you and the family — as well as the patient, will have a much better understanding of what role each will play in the caregiving plan.

LeBoeuf's Handbook will help you:

- Determine when you must act and what can be done to assist your parent or friend.
- Understand many of the problems patient's may encounter.
- Cope with the patient's physical and mental problems.
- Determine what financial support is available.
- Execute a family agreement and a caregiver agreement.
- Determine what needs to be done to get the patient's room ready.
- Determine what home modifications may be needed.
- Put legal affairs in order.
- Develop a financial plan.
- Locate and inventory all the patient's documents and important papers.
- Develop a family history.
- Find out when and where services, such as nursing, are available.
- Know what products are available to assist with caregiving.
- Cope with death and dying.

Everything you need — from helping with the decision to become a caregiver to saying good-bye — is here. Our goal is to provide you with the latest information, helpful hints, services and products to make your role as a caregiver as easy and rewarding as possible. We at LeBoeuf's will work with you so you can rest assured that you have done all that you could for your loved one and your family.

Activities of Daily Living (ADL)

If the patient is unable to perform any one or more of the following, the caregiver must provide help in the patient's home, bring the patient into the caregivers home, or place the patient in a nursing home. Questions you should ask, and observations you should make, to measure the ability of the patient to cope with the activities of daily living are listed below.

- Can they feed themselves?
- Can they move about or have they had a stroke, surgery or an accident?
- Is the patient suffering from depression or another mental illness?
- Can the patient afford to hire a caregiver to clean house/cook/shop?
- Can they take care of themselves: Dressing, Toileting, Bathing, Grooming
- Does the patient act strange (Alzheimer's)?
- Can the patient manage money or do they have enough money to buy necessities?
- Can the patient manage medications?
- Can the patient see, talk, hear, use the telephone or sense temperature variations?

One of the best ways to determine the patient's medical condition and the ability to cope on their own, is to obtain a complete physical examination and evaluation from the patient's doctor and a physical/occupational therapist. If the examination reveals that the patient should have help, or that the condition will only get worse, the doctor and/or the therapist can work with you to convince the patient of the necessity to make other living arrangements for reasons of health and safety.

The doctor's examination should also include the following:

- Review of patient's sensory systems (i.e. hearing, vision, smell, taste and touch).
- How well the patient manages Activities of Daily Living (ADL) (Bathing, Toileting, Dressing, Grooming, Transferring, Eating, Walking).
- How well patient manages shopping, managing money, transportation, housekeeping, using telephone, managing medications, temperature perception, vibration perception.
- Review of mental status and checks for addiction, mood, memory, perception and judgment.
- A series of tests to determine the patient's range of motion.
- Review the home and neighboring environment.

You will find it next to impossible to obtain the estimated cost of a patient's physical exam over the telephone. Physicals range from about $80 with no lab work to well over $400 if lab work is performed.

Patient Assistive Devices

After the examination and review of the patient's ability to perform activities of daily living, the doctor and/or therapist may recommend assistive devices to help the patient cope. The use of assistive devices is not an end in itself. The idea is to provide the patient with equipment that will allow the maximum amount of independence and support. Some of the general categories of assistive devices are shown below.

- Communication devices
    Computers
    Laryngeal prosthesis
    TTY/TDD
    Large numbers on phone
    Captioning
- Sensory aids
    Braille, large print,
    Alerting devices
    Hearing aids
    Assistive listening devices
    Lighting, low vision aids
- Seating and positioning systems
- Devices to assist or activate the patient's ability to move about.
- Devices for daily activities
    Bathing
    Skin care
    Toileting
    Transfer (beds chairs, transfer boards, etc.)
    Special eating tools, reachers
    Clothing , special dressing sticks, etc.
    Telephones with large numbers, automatic dialing, TDD/TTY, flashing lights, etc.
- Mobility options
    Wheelchair
    Walkers, canes, crutches
    Auto and van adaptations
    Barriers to accessibility such as doors, steps
- Recreation possibilities
    Sports and exercise equipment
    Games, toys
    Computers
    Arts and crafts
- Environmental devices (air purifier, oxygen, etc.)

Assistive products can be evaluated using these criteria:

- *Is it reliable, effective, safe, comfortable and durable?*
- *It is attractive and well designed?*
- *Is the cost of the product and its maintenance affordable?*
- *Is the product easy to store and transport?*
- *Is the product compatible with the patient's other equipment?*

If you need help finding or evaluating assistive products, call LeBoeuf's

☎ 1-800-546-5559

Occupational or Physical Therapists

A physical or occupational therapist has the knowledge, training and experience to evaluate a patient's level of function. The physical and/or occupational therapist can be a big help in working with you to determine what you will have to do to care for the patient. They can also work with you and the doctor to convince the patient that they can no longer live alone. Therapists can also provide you and the patient with information on appropriate assistive devices that can be purchased for use in the home as well as what should be done in the home to accommodate the patient's needs.

What's Next?

Once the decision is made to provide for the patient in the caregiver's home, there are a number of other issues that need to be addressed. While the task may seem overwhelming in the beginning, you will find it easy to follow *the Handbook's* instructions and/or information for performing home modifications, making the home safer, obtaining assistive devices, and completing the legal and financial sections. You should also complete the document locator, medical history, family history and personal sections. Take your time and work with the patient on as many of the sections as you can. You will find that the patient will enjoy talking and reminiscing about many of the things they have accomplished in their life.

The Handbook will also guide you through what may be needed in the home to assist you and the patient. Guiding you in a step-by-step process, we have tried to think of everything you may need. Rely on LeBoeuf's as a source for anything from assistive devices to service providers for you and the patient. We have also tried to provide you with some common sense advice on the timing of when things need to be done for both the caregiver and the patient.

Things to Do

Doorways may have to be widened and ramps built to accommodate a walker or a wheelchair. A den may need to be converted into an extra bedroom. Or a half-bath may need to be expanded to a full bath. Grab bars will need to be installed in the bathroom. Automatic garage doors may need to be installed. Alarm systems and extra telephone lines may be needed. Possible major renovations in the home's structure, such as a room addition, may need to be considered. A section in the *Handbook* will help you through the "what needs to be done to the home" decision making process. We also provide a Home Modification Planning Service to assist you in making your home accessible for the patient.

The *Handbook* includes agreements to outline duties and obligations of all parties. They are designed to facilitate communication between family members who are taking care of an elderly parent and others who live a long distance away. It helps prevent the feeling that the caregiver is unfairly shouldering the major caretaking burden. The "Family Agreement" lists various activities (such as providing transportation, running errands, helping with household chores, financial assistance and respite care) to ease the caregiving burden for the primary caregiver. The agreement is not intended to be legally binding, but merely clarifies the roles for each family member.

LeBoeuf's provides a "Caregiving Agreement" for the caregiver and the patient outlining the obligations of each party. The "Caregiving Agreement" also assists both parties in fully understanding the value of the caregiving service. Many elderly are willing and able to provide financial assistance to the caregiver. The patient may contribute their own resources for paying grocery bills, utility costs, mortgages, rent, and other bills. For many patients, paying their "own way" is a means to maintain some independence. The "Caregiving Agreement" helps to protect both the caregiver and the patient from unreasonable actions by either party.

Using the Handbook

In many cases the patient may have more than one problem. An example would be the patient who has had a *hip replacement,* has a *vision* problem and has become *incontinent.* The caregiver should read the section on hip replacement, the section on vision and the section on incontinence to understand what needs to be done to address all of the patient's problems. In each section there is a listing of what assistive products and services are available to make the caregiver's task easier.

After reading the section(s) relating to the problem(s) of the patient, arranging for services and obtaining the products needed to assist the patient, you can be confident that you will be providing the very best for your patient. You can also be confident that you have made your caregiving task as easy and rewarding as possible.

Teamwork

Whatever your needs may be, LeBoeuf's will be there to help. Caregiving is a team effort. You cannot do everything yourself. All of us have to work together. Caregivers sharing respite care, sharing experiences and knowing what products and services are available will prevent each caregiver from having to "re-invent the wheel." The *Handbook* will assist the caregiver in the who, what, where, when, how and why of caregiving. We are dedicated to make the caregivers task as easy and rewarding as possible. We will endeavor to assist you in this noble task anytime, anyplace.

LeBoeuf's Services

Call **LeBoeuf's** ☎ 1-800-546-5559 for the following services. Please have ready the patient's name, address, zip code, age, telephone number and physical circumstances (Alzheimer's, heart problem, arthritis, etc.) when you call.

- Consulting Service
    - Wheelchairs (design, ultra-light, sports chairs, etc.)
    - Van Conversions
    - Electronics
        - Hearing
        - Vision
        - Security
        - Communication (TTY, Call Buttons, Telephones, etc.)
        - Television, VCR's, Radio, Stereo
        - Computers and Software

- Home Healthcare Workshops

- Caregivers Speakers Bureau

- Incontinent Supply Service

- Respite Network

- Home Modification Planning Service

- Assistive Travel Agency

- Employment Screening Service

- Referral Service for:
    - Hospitals
    - Nursing homes
    - Hospice
    - Visiting nurse associations
    - Adult day care programs
    - Respite care (nursing homes, support groups,)
    - Social services case workers
    - Household help

LeBoeuf's

PHONE **1-800-546-5559**

FAX **1-800-233-9692**

Hearing Impaired with TDD
CALL **1-800-855-2880**

Modifying Your Home and Making It Safer

W HEN TAKING ON THE RESPONSIBILITIES of caregiving, it is important to consider your home and how it can be made to work for both the patient and the caregiver. Some things to consider include:

- Site design and entrances
- Transportation and parking
- Ramps for wheelchairs and walkers
- Bathrooms
- Heating and air conditioning
- Lighting
- Bedrooms
- Closets
- Storage
- Door widths, door handles
- Kitchens
- Windows

When you decide to care for someone in your home, the decision often includes issues related to such practical things as turning a den into a bedroom, making a powder room or half-bath into a full bath and arranging for easy access if the patient uses a walker or a wheelchair.

Stairs probably need to be replaced with ramps or modified for easy access. Smooth hard floors need slip proof coatings or floor coverings. Sometimes it is necessary to change a door so that it swings the opposite way to allow access for a wheelchair. You may even need to enlarge a bedroom window for an emergency exit, if other ways out of the home are blocked. Although this is frequently required by local building codes, it makes sense in any event.

At some point most patients will spend time in a wheelchair or have to use a walker, cane or, possibly, crutches. It makes sense to plan now for accommodating wheelchairs, walkers and other assistive devices so that you can avoid having to perform modifications to the home more than once. The following recommendations can be followed when the home is adapted to provide for the patient. **LeBoeuf's** ☎ **1-800-546-5559** has a Home Modification Planning Service to assist you in deciding what needs to be done to make the home an easy and safe place for the patient to get about.

Obviously, providing a bright and cheerful, yet practical and functional environment is important to both you, the caregiver, and the patient. It will contribute to the patient's overall sense of comfort, privacy and happiness as well as your own peace of mind and a lighter work load. When everyday life runs smoothly, thanks to good planning, you can enjoy more leisure and personal time.

LeBoeuf's ☎ *1-800-546-5559 has a Home Modification Planning Service!*

Ramps

Ramps should be constructed using a fire resistant material (concrete, steel or aluminum), have slip resistant matting or slip resistant surface with a maximum slope of eight degrees so that the patient can use a walker, crutches, cane or wheelchair. Most slip resistant matting comes in three foot widths and is available in lengths up to 75 feet. If the slope exceeds 5 degrees, patients in wheelchairs may have to use handrails on both sides of the ramp to pull themselves up the ramp. Ramps should be protected from weather by canopies or an overhang and have adequate lighting. The minimum width for a ramp is 3 feet 6 inches and the handrail should be between 2 feet 6 inches and 2 feet 8 inches in height. Handrails should have a horizontal bar below to act as a bumper strip. Ideally, the bar should be at the height of the wheelchair foot rests. This will keep the wheelchair from going under the bar and also will prevent those with crutches and canes from placing the tip of their cane or crutch off the ramp surface. The ideal handrail width is 1½ inches. The clearance between the handrail and the wall should be a minimum of 1½ inches.

A 4-inch curb on the sides of the ramp under the handrail is also a good idea to keep the wheelchair from running off the side of the ramp. For long ramps, a level rest platform should be provided every 30 feet. The rest platform should be a minimum of 5 feet by 5 feet so that the wheelchair can be turned if necessary. There are also available a number of portable or semi-permanent ramps made of metal.

Entrances

Entrances should have a level platform to allow patients to maneuver walkers or wheelchairs. The entranceway must be of nonslip material or have a nonslip surface. There should be no obstructions such as door mats or grates. The ideal door width is 36 inches, which is a typical entrance door width for most homes. Thresholds should have a maximum of ¼ inch vertical change or ½ inch with a 45 degree beveled edge. Door locks should be at a convenient height and be easy to open. Door handles should be lever types. It should take no more than five to eight and one-half pounds of pressure to open the door. Add a peep hole viewer at a height that the person in the wheelchair can look through (about 4 feet). You may even want to have two peep holes, one at the normal height and one at the 4-foot height. Avoid storm and screen doors, as two doors are very cumbersome to operate. Doorbells and mailboxes should be mounted at a height of from 3 feet to 3 feet 9 inches. A 12-inch wide shelf for packages is also a good idea.

Carports and Garages

Carports and garages must have a clear area on one side of the car at least five feet wide to enable the patient to maneuver a walker or wheelchair. The minimum width for a one car garage should be 14 feet 6 inches. The minimum length should be 24 feet to allow for a four-foot wide passageway in front or behind the automobile or van. A covered passageway from the garage or carport is a good idea to keep rain and snow off the walk or ramp. Automatic garage doors with lights that will stay on for three to four minutes after the door opens or closes should be incorporated whenever possible. Garage light switches should be easily accessible from within the car or immediately after exiting the automobile. It is also a good idea to have a switch inside the house that will turn the garage lights on and off.

For most wheelchair users, an eight degree slope (even if you have handrails on both sides of the ramp) would be the maximum.

If you are planning on having a van with a lift for a wheelchair or power scooter, be sure to allow enough room for the lift to open inside the garage. You will also need to make sure that the height of the van does not exceed the height of the garage door. If the lift installer says that they will have to raise the roof of the van, make sure that it will still fit in the garage.

Carpeting

Low pile carpeting throughout the house will allow for the use of walkers and wheelchairs and also help cushion accidental falls. Nonslip bathroom rugs, nonslip mats for the bathtub and shower floors are very important to prevent falls. All carpeting must be secured to the floor. Throw rugs, unless secured to the floor so that they do not bunch up or slide, should be removed. Carpeting also reduces sound transmission.

Cotton carpeting or rugs are preferred to reduce the chance of static electricity. This is especially important if the patient is using oxygen.

Doors

Exterior doors should be insulated and weather-stripping provided for all exterior doors and windows. Avoid unnecessary doors, doors in series and doors with conflicting adjacent swings. Doorways should have a minimum of 1 foot 6 inches of clear area on both sides of the door opposite the hinges to allow for positioning the walker or wheelchair when opening the door. The door should open with a single motion and have a minimum of 90 degrees of clear swing. Minimum door opening should be 32-inch wide so hands and elbows will clear. The ideal maneuvering floor area on both sides of the door should be at least 4 feet 6 inches. Door hardware should be of a size that is easily gripped and located at a height of 3 feet to 3 feet 6 inches. A lever-type handle is the best. Kick plates on both sides of the door will prevent damage to the door from the foot rests on the wheelchair and allow the patient to use the footplates on the wheelchair to push against the door. A pull bar on both sides of the door will allow for ease in closing as the patient passes through. Doors to bathrooms or other confined spaces should swing out. Thresholds, divider strips or sliding door tracks should be avoided. Automatic door closers are not recommended. If door closers are used, there must be a minimum time delay of 4 to 6 seconds to allow the patient to clear the doorway. And they must stop automatically if the door encounters an obstruction.

Call LeBoeuf's ☎ 1-800-546-5559 for information and pricing on power door openers, remote controlled switches and electronic voice recognition door openers.

Power door openers can be used when the patient has little or no hand and arm strength. There are many lower cost automatic door openers that can be used in the home situation. Most will work with standard house current and can be installed by the caregiver. Power door openers should open and close the door slowly and stop if anything is in the way. Doors can also be activated by wall and floor switches. There are now electronic voice recognition door openers, electronic locks and remotes that will provide additional convenience and security.

Heating and Air Conditioning

Zone-controlled heating and air conditioning is highly desirable. There are heat/air conditioning units that can be installed in a window or through the wall. Additional heat in the bathroom such as radiant heat is also a good idea. Make sure that the heater has a safety bar or screen to prevent accidental burns. If possible, place the additional heat source high enough so that it cannot be touched accidentally. There a number of heaters that have ground fault interuptors (GFI) to shut off the electricity before someone can be electrocuted. You can also buy plug-in GFI outlets. It is well worth the investment to have an electrician come out and install GFI outlets in the patient's room, kitchen and the bathroom.

Typical charge for installing a GFI outlet by an electrician is $25.00 per outlet.

Windows

Window sills should be a maximum of 2 feet 9 inches above the floor if the windows are intended for viewing by a patient confined to a wheelchair. Window controls should be accessible and easy to operate. If controls are used for opening and closing the windows, the controls should be located at a maximum height of 4 feet 6 inches. Double or triple glazing is recommended, and good weather-stripping required, to avoid discomfort from drafts and extreme temperature variations. Controls for curtains or blinds must be accessible to the wheelchair bound patient. It is much better if the window opening mechanism is located so that the person in the wheelchair can operate the widow from the side of the wheelchair (sitting parallel to the window). Many patients in wheelchairs cannot lean forward far enough to operate the window from the front. If the room for the patient is far from an exit, and the patient is confined to a wheelchair, you may want to consider using the window as an emergency exit (building codes of some jurisdictions require two emergency exits). If you do, the window sill should be no higher than 24 inches (18 inches preferred) above the floor and the window opening should be a minimum of 30 inches wide. Screens should be easily removed.

There are companies that provide for remote operation of windows which can be installed by a local contractor. You can find a contractor by looking in the yellow pages under "window" or by calling **LeBoeuf's** ☎ **1-800-546-5559.**

Call LeBoeuf's ☎ 1-800-546-5559 for information and pricing on illuminated switches, motion sensor switches and remote controlled switches

Wall Switches & Outlets

Wall switches should be placed at a maximum height of 4 feet, with the preferred height being between 3 feet and 3 feet 6 inches. Switches adjacent to doors should be aligned with the door handles for ease in locating the switch. Light switches that are illuminated are a good idea and can be purchased in any hardware store. For wall outlets (be sure the outlets are GFI), the minimum height is 1 foot 6 inches and the maximum height is 4 feet.

There are switches that work by motion as well as a manual on/off capability. There are also wireless switches that can turn on lights up to 150 feet from the switch control.

Telephones

Wall telephones should be mounted at a maximum height of 4 feet. A height of 2 feet 9 inches to 3 feet 3 inches is preferred. Do not mount telephones above counters that restrict access by patients in a wheelchair. Telephone jacks should be provided for bedrooms and bathrooms. Push-button telephones are the easiest to operate.

There are a number of phones that can provide the patient with hands free operation, amplified sound levels, extra loud ringers, text message capability, lighted flashers for the hard of hearing, and many other features to assist the patient to become more independent.

Hallways

Hallways should be a minimum of 3 feet 6 inches in width to allow for easy turning into a door opening of 32 inches. A width of 48 inches or more would be ideal but is not necessary. To protect walls from getting damaged by wheelchair handrims, a nonscuff strip such as a chair rail can be mounted 1 foot up from the floor. Doors to rooms other than the bathroom or other confined rooms should open into the room to allow for unobstructed movement through the hallway.

Stairs

If there are stairs, all risers should be slanted or beveled. Open risers or risers with protrusions or overhanging nosing are not acceptable. A patient wearing leg braces can trip on stairs of this type because they cannot manipulate the toe to clear the nosing. Inclined elevators offer an alternative to climbing the stairs and there are elevators that will accommodate wheelchairs. A good stair lift will cost about $3,000 or more installed.

Bathroom

Information presented here on the size of the bathroom is the ideal. You will find that you can manage with less space in many instances. This is especially true if you or your spouse are strong enough to lift the patient. It is probably a good idea to try out the bathroom as it is before investing in a major remodeling job. However, making the door opening at least 32 inches wide will most likely have to be done. For some reason, the bathroom door is the smallest door in many homes. For added safety and maximum use of available space, you also may want to have the door open out into the hallway rather than opening into the bathroom.

The bathroom presents the most difficult problem in designing a facility that will easily accommodate the patient. Normally, bathrooms are small and do not allow enough space for easy maneuvering to transfer from the wheelchair to the bathtub or the toilet. Ideally, the minimum diameter for a patient in a wheelchair to maneuver in the bathroom is 5 feet. The transfer is easiest if the bathtub and toilet fixtures are about the same height as the wheelchair seat (18-20 inches is the average). Stirrup grabs or suspended hoists aid in the transfer. Grab bars should also be provided for all patients, whether in a wheelchair or not, to prevent falls. Soap dishes, toilet paper holders, towel rods and electrical outlets must be convenient. There are numerous types of transfer benches or seats that help facilitate moving a patient from the wheelchair to the bathtub, shower or toilet. Each patient will develop their own personal transfer technique. Many patients will usually prefer a particular direction of transfer and whenever possible, bathtubs, toilets and shower seats should be located to accommodate that preference.

A clear area 4 feet in length should precede all bathroom fixtures. If the lavatory and the toilet are located on the same wall, enough separation between fixtures must be maintained to accommodate transfer from the wheelchair to the toilet. A minimum of 4 feet must be between the center line of the toilet and the edge of the lavatory. A horizontal grab bar should be mounted at a height of 2 feet 9 inches next to the toilet to aid the patient transferring from the wheelchair. Grab bars should be 1½ inches in diameter and firmly anchored to support the patient's weight. You **must** secure grab bars into the wood stud behind the tile or the drywall. A stud finder that will locate a stud behind the tile on the wall or ceiling is a must when installing grab bars. As a general rule, horizontal grab bars are used for pushing up and vertical grab bars are used for pulling up.

All exposed water supply lines and drains must be insulated to prevent burns. The water spigot should be a minimum of 4 inches clear of any rear obstruction to allow for ease in rinsing. Single lever type temperature controls are recommended. There are electronic systems on the market that will allow for push-button water flow and temperature control. Mirrors should be tilted or lowered to accommodate the person in the wheelchair. The bottom edge should be no higher than 3 feet. Be sure to leave knee space under the lavatory (minimum height of 2 feet 3 inches and a minimum width of 3 feet). The top of the lavatory should not exceed 2 feet 10 inches and not be more than 2 feet 3 inches deep. Faucets should not be more than 1 feet 9 inches from the front edge of the lavatory.

A platform or seat at the end of the bathtub allows the patient easier access to the tub. However, if adding the platform to the end of the tub is not possible or practical, a transfer bench, grab bars, a hoist or a stirrup grip attached to the ceiling can be provided to aid in the transfer. Again, the ideal height of the bathtub would be 18-20 inches. Bathtub controls must be easily accessible before and during immersion. Some patients may prefer side-mounted controls and a remote control drain operation. A hand-held shower with controls on the shower handle and a minimum of 5 feet of hose should be provided. All controls must be carefully located to be accessible from the platform or the tub. Thermostatic controls must be provided to protect the patient against a sudden change in water temperature.

Many wheelchair users prefer showers to baths. To accommodate the patient, there are two types of showers. One is equipped with a seat to which the patient transfers from the wheelchair to the seat built or placed in the shower. The other type of shower is designed to accommodate the patient and a special "shower" wheelchair. The minimum size of any wheelchair shower should be 4 feet square. The minimum shower opening is 3 feet 6 inches, except where a door is provided for a "roll-in" shower. Showers should not have curbs or thresholds which impede access. Nonslip material must be used on the floors. If a bench seat is used, it should be at 18 to 20 inches high. Grab bars should be provided on all three sides of the shower to assist in transfers or to assist in preventing falls. Again, caution must be exercised to insure that the grab bars and hoists are securely fastened. You must have screws long enough to penetrate the tile and drywall and into the wood stud. Use of a stud finder is a must. The shower should be fitted with a flexible hose and shower head. A temperature control must be used to prevent scalding due to sudden changes in water temperature.

Kitchen

Appliances in the kitchen should be carefully selected to meet the patient's needs. Kitchens should provide generous storage space to minimize shopping trips. Sliding cabinet doors and cabinets with pullout shelves are a good idea, as are cabinet and drawer pulls made of rope loops. Storage that is accessible should be within a distance that is 6 inches less than the patient's arm length, seated or standing. If the patient is able to assist in the kitchen, knee space can be provided beneath the sink. Minimum usable shelf height for a person in a wheelchair is 1 foot 6 inches and maximum height is 4 feet 6 inches. The standard counter height in most kitchens is 36 inches, which is 2 to 3 inches higher than the convenient height for someone in a wheelchair. Most wheelchairs can accommodate a tray that fits on the arms of the wheelchair. If you would like the patient in a wheelchair to sit at the kitchen table and eat with the rest of the family, you need a table with at least 31½ inch clearance to enable the wheelchair arms to fit under the table. There are companies that make tables that are adjustable to allow for wheelchairs.

Microwaves and ovens should have a landing area for placing food hot out of the oven. For patients in a wheelchair, knee space to one side or the other of the oven will allow the patient to get close enough to reach into the oven or microwave.

Washers and dryers should be front-loading.

When designing a shower for a patient who will be using a special "shower" wheelchair, be sure you check the size of the chair. Call LeBoeuf's and we will contact the wheelchair manufacturer to give you or your contractor the recommended dimensions of the shower stall.

Emergency Warning Systems

Smoke detectors in good working order should be installed on each floor of the home. Change the batteries at least once a year. There are smoke detectors that will flash a bright light for patients who are hard of hearing and smoke detectors that will send a message to a vibrator for those who are hard of hearing and asleep in bed. In addition to smoke detectors, there are special safety lights that go on when the power fails, carbon monoxide testers, microwave testers and water quality testers.

An emergency warning signal that alerts neighbors to an emergency within the house is a good idea. This is especially true if the patient is wheelchair bound. All warning systems such as smoke alarms must be compatible with the patient's sensory disabilities (deafness, blindness, etc.). All doors to any confined space should swing out. In-swinging doors pose a potential danger should the patient fall and block the door.

Computer controlled television monitoring of the interior and exterior of the home is now available and can be installed fairly easily. Many systems are able to respond to voice commands. Remote controlled lighting can be installed that allows all the lighting to be controlled remotely from a bed, chair or wheelchair. There are now sensors available that will turn the lights on and off whenever anyone enters or leaves a room.

Bedroom and Sitting Room

A well thought out bedroom/sitting room for the patient is important to both the patient and the caregiver. Access to doors, windows, closets, dressers and other furnishing should be carefully considered. Obviously, a first floor room would be ideal for both the patient and the caregiver. This is especially true if you are caring for a patient who has to be in a wheelchair or use a walker.

For those patients who are in wheelchairs or need to use a walker, the ideal size for a bedroom would allow three feet on each side of the bed (3 feet 6 inches would be better) to maneuver a wheelchair or walker and assist in making the bed and at least 4 to 5 feet at the end of the bed. A room 12 feet by 12 feet or bigger, not including the closets, would be ideal. Most hospital beds are about 86 inches long with headboard and 40 inches wide with side rails. A five foot area would ideally be in front of the closets. A clear area of at least 3 feet must be provided on one side of the bed. This will allow for transfer from the wheelchair to the bed and back to the wheelchair.

A passageway of at least 3 feet, but preferably 3 feet 6 inches or 4 feet, should be provided between the end of the bed and the wall or closet. A night stand and/or dresser can be put up near the head of the bed. For any furnishing, you must allow at least 3 feet in front for the patient in a wheelchair to have access. Remember, if the patient is unable to bathe, perform toilet, change clothes or eat, you will need space to perform baths, change bed linens and room for an over-the-bed table for food and a night stand. For the patient to turn around in a wheelchair, you will need a 5 foot diameter circle or 3 foot by 5 foot T-shaped space to allow for a three point turn. This "T" space could include the knee space under a desk if it is at least 36 inches wide and 27 inches high.

The room should be uncluttered and, if possible, divided to provide for a bedroom and a sitting room. Even if the room is small, a simple curtain hung between the bed and the rest of the room will provide for privacy. If at all possible, a sitting room for the patient and visitors adjacent to the bedroom would give the patient a feeling of privacy and independence. The sit-

If you are using a bedboard to firm up the mattress, you will need at least a 3/4-inch thick sheet of plywood. The bedboard should be large enough to fit over the springs and prevent the mattress from sagging. Most lumber yards will make at least two saw cuts free of charge. Not only will they be able to cut the plywood straighter, the finished bedboard should easily fit in the trunk of your auto.

A comfortable chair in the room will encourage guests and family members to visit with the patient.

ting room could be as small as 10 × 8 feet. All you need is room for a couch and/or a couple of chairs, a table or desk, lamp, and a wardrobe or dresser. Cotton rugs are probably best because they do not create static electricity. This is especially important when using oxygen.

A dresser with pull out drawers should not be over 3 feet 6 inches above the floor or the wheelchair bound patient won't be able to see into the top drawer. Wire baskets, or drawers with perforations in the sides, allow the patient to see the contents without having to open the drawer.

Closets

Closet door openings should be a minimum of 32 inches wide to allow the patient in a wheelchair to reach the closet contents. Closets should have clothes hanger rods between 3 feet 6 inches and 4 feet from the floor. This is adequate for most clothing and in easy reach of a person in a wheelchair. Shelves should be mounted at a maximum height of 4 feet 6 inches and the shelf depth should not exceed 1 foot 4 inches. If sliding doors are used, floor mounted tracks or guides must not obstruct the wheelchair user. Bifold or pocket doors give easier access to the entire closet. There are a number of closet organizer systems available that will allow you to configure any closet to the patient's needs. Remember, within easy reach means 6 inches less than arms' length either standing or sitting. If you are using patient lifts, care should be taken to allow for wide enough doors so that storage of the lift in a closet is possible. Any "walk-in" closet should have a minimum of a 5 foot diameter clear turn around space. You can include in this 5 foot space, 1 foot under the clothes.

LeBoeuf Home Modification Planning Service

To help you plan for all of this, we have developed a unique reasonably priced step-by-step program. You may use our guide to figure out for yourself what you need to do and approximate the cost, or complete the check list and send it along with your drawing to LeBoeuf's and we will make suggestions and create a cost estimate to guide you as you make preparations.

The program has three parts:

First, we need to know about the physical condition of your patient — a list of simple questions follows.

Second, we need a sketch of each room that will be used. Just follow the example given.

Third, fill out a separate check list for each room so that we don't forget anything.

If you would like us to provide you with a cost estimate, make a copy of your work sheets and mail them along with your payment of $65.00 to :

LeBoeuf and Associates, Inc.
768 Walker Road, Suite 266
Great Falls, VA 22066

Give us a week or two and we will mail back a detailed estimate that you may use as a guide whether you do the work yourself or hire a contractor. Just completing the forms and drawing out your plan will help you to better visualize the tasks ahead. Call **LeBoeuf's** ☎ 1-800-546-5559 if you have questions about our Home Modification Planning Service.

Home Modification Planning Guide

Patient's Physical Condition

Patient's Name _____

☐ Male   ☐ Female   Date of Birth _____   Relationship _____

Eyesight: ☐ Good   ☐ Fair   ☐ Poor   (check one)

Hearing: ☐ Good   ☐ Fair   ☐ Poor   (check one)

Ambulatory: ☐ Good   ☐ Fair   ☐ Poor   (check one)

Disability _____

_____

Does patient use: ☐ walker   ☐ wheelchair   ☐ scooter   ☐ crutches   ☐ cane

Is the patient incontinent?   ☐ Yes   ☐ No   ☐ Occasionally

Does the patient need help eating meals?   ☐ Yes   ☐ No

General strength: ☐ Good   ☐ Fair   ☐ Poor

Special Care Requirements

Full electric bed _____

Oxygen _____

Special monitors _____

Physical therapy _____

Amount of assistance patient is currently receiving in hours.

   Your time _____

   Other family members _____

Anticipated needs _____

_____

Special Considerations — patient _____

_____

Special Considerations — yours _____

_____

Instructions for Preparing Your Sketch

Use the check list below to help you draw your layout. Make your drawing on a copy of the grid on page 26, or use your own graph paper. You do not have to make the drawing to scale as long as you put dimensions on it. The purpose here is to be sure that as many needs, both current and future, are met to ensure the safety, convenience and comfort of the patient and the caregiver.

1. Label as much of the drawing as possible.

2. Show the locations of heating and air conditioning vents, even if they are in the ceiling.

3. Note the location of all electrical outlets, switches and lights.

4. Show which way the doors swing.

5. Show the size and shape of any rooms next to a half bath that needs to be enlarged to a full bath.

6. Use a separate drawing, if necessary, to show the outside entrance and steps so we can figure the type and size ramp you may need.

7. Note which floor(s) of your home will be used by the patient.

8. You may also show us where you think the bed and other furniture will go, if you like.

9. What floor is the patient's bedroom on and what are the room dimensions?

10. Size of closet(s)

11. Width of all doors and type of door (sliding, bifold, pocket, swinging, etc.).

12. What type of floor covering? Carpet, vinyl, etc. Is floor wood, concrete, hardwood, plywood, etc.?

13. Is there a full floor below, a crawl space or a concrete slab?

14. What are the window dimensions?

15. How far off the floor is the window sill and how far is it to the ground outside the window?

16. What kind of window, double hung, casement (crank out to side), awning (crank up), sliding, etc.

17. What type of frame do the windows have? Steel, aluminum, wood, vinyl or other.

18. What kind of exterior surface is around the windows? Brick, wood siding, vinyl siding, aluminum siding, stucco or other.

19. How wide is the hallway?

20. Show size of the bathroom (including location and measurements of fixtures such as tub, shower, etc.)

21. Width of bathroom door and which way it swings.

22. Exterior door width.

23. Is there a storm door?

24. How many steps to enter house, size of landing or porch and height of each step. Sketch the general layout showing paths, sidewalks, type of material such as brick, flagstone, concrete, gravel, etc. Show distances in feet and inches.

25. Note any special problems such as curved or straight steps, wood, concrete, brick, etc. Are there lift systems in place?

26. What kind of heat? Are there ducts? Does current system maintain heat between 68 and 74 degrees?

27. Air conditioning type (whole house, window, etc.)

28. Kitchen cabinet heights, counter height and height of tables (show distance from floor to first obstruction of a wheelchair arm).

29. Washer and dryer. Indicate whether they are top load or front load.

30. Show any ramps or other features that are now in place to assist the patient.

31. If the patient has a manual or power wheelchair and/or a power scooter please provide the make, model and year of each unit.

Sample Plans

Make a separate sketch for each room or area in your home that needs to be modified. Label each room clearly. Include sketches of exterior entrances and all interior hallways and rooms that will be used by patient.

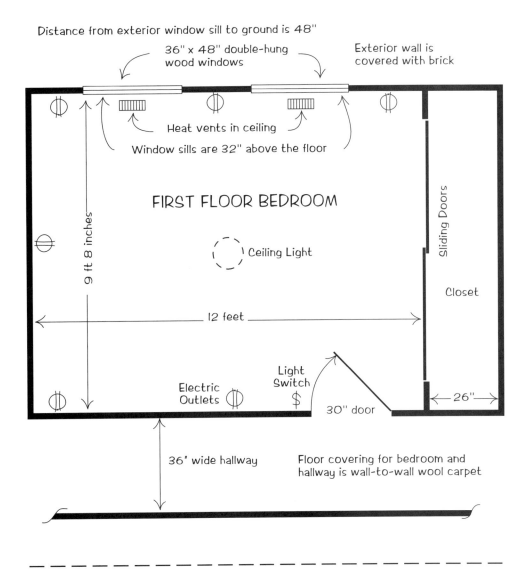

Distance from exterior window sill to ground is 48"

36" x 48" double-hung wood windows

Exterior wall is covered with brick

Heat vents in ceiling

Window sills are 32" above the floor

FIRST FLOOR BEDROOM

Ceiling Light

9 ft 8 inches

12 feet

Sliding Doors

Closet

Electric Outlets

Light Switch

30" door

26"

36' wide hallway

Floor covering for bedroom and hallway is wall-to-wall wool carpet

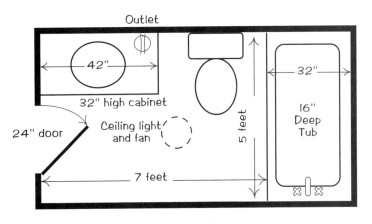

Outlet

42"

32" high cabinet

24" door

Ceiling light and fan

5 feet

7 feet

32"

16" Deep Tub

BATHROOM

Make a separate sketch for each room or area that needs to be modified.
Be sure that you label each room.   Make copies of this page or use your own graph paper.

Hiring the Home Remodeler

If you must have extensive work done in your home to accommodate the patient, and will have to hire outside labor to perform the work, the following procedure should be followed:

- Make a list of areas that you want to modify before talking to the contractor to insure that all contractors are bidding on the same job requirements. Explain the situation to the contractors. They may have some good ideas that could improve safety and reduce your costs.

- Get at least three bids in writing.

- Obtain, in writing, the amount of time the contractor will take to complete the job.

- Obtain, in writing, the start and completion dates.

- Tell the contractor that you will hold him responsible for completing the job on time. You may be able to work out a reward/penalty arrangement with the contractor to give him an incentive to finish on time. You have to be careful with any penalties. If the the contractor knows that the job will not be done on time and the penalties are too severe, he may just walk away. A little common sense rather than a "hard-nosed" attitude may be needed in some situations.

- Do not pay for the whole job up front. Pay as the work is completed. The usual arrangement is 30 percent when the job starts, 30 percent upon substantial completion of the job and 40 percent upon completion of the total job.

- Ask the contractor for at least three references. After you have selected the best bid, talk to all the references. Ask each reference if the job was completed on time, if the bid amount was the amount that was finally billed, if the workers were good craftsmen, and if the contractor worked well with them (reference). Ask the reference if it would be possible to come over and look at the work that was done.

Some examples of home remodeling project costs are shown below. These costs are contractor costs. If you are handy with tools, the cost can be reduced substantially. Whatever you do to change the home to accommodate the patient, be sure you keep careful records of the costs for tax purposes.

- Change door size from 30 to 36 inches — $300.00

- Install handrail — $20.00 to $30.00 per linear foot

- Install concrete ramp (outside) — $28.00 square yard

- Install 4-inch curb on ramp — $10.00 per linear foot

- Doorbell with one remote signaler with light flashing in two rooms of the home — $150.00. Additional remote signalers (light flashing) — $44.95 each

Call LeBoeuf's ☎ 1-800-546-5559 or the Home Builders Association in your area for the names of contractors to remodel your home. There are over 850 Home Builders Association chapters throughout the United States.

Film and Batteries

Item Number	Item Description	Size	Price
Film			
Le 131-9920	Kodak Gold Super 200 GB110	24 exp	$4.35
Le 143-2327	Kodak Gold Super 200 GB135	24 exp	$5.65
Le 143-2343	Kodak Gold Super 200 GB135	36 exp	$7.35
Le 143-2418	Kodak Gold Ultra 400 GC135.	24 exp	$6.25
Le 143-2210	Kodak Film Gold+ 100 GA135	24 exp	$5.45
Le 184-7458	Polar Film 600+ 1pk 604447.	10 exp	$12.95
LE 246-3065	Polar Film Spectra 2pk 610022	20 exp	$23.95
Batteries			
Le 133-4176	Alka Dura MN2400B2	AAA	$2.45
Le 185-3928	Alka Dura MN1500B2	AA	$2.75
Le 249-8848	Alka Dura MN1500B4	AA	$4.35
Le 185-3910	Alka Dura MN1400B2	C	$3.65
Le 133-3848	Alka Dura MN1300B2	D	$3.95
Le 133-3954	Alka Dura MN1604B	9V	$3.95
Le 149-7924	Ener Ever E92BP-2	AAA	$2.75
Le 275-2962	Ener Ever E92BP-4	AAA	$4.85
Le 229-4361	Ener Ever E91BP-2	AA	$2.95
Le 149-7916	Ener Ever E91BP-4	AA	$5.25
Le 149-7890	Ener Ever E95BP-2	D	$4.45
Le 121-7199	Ener Ever 522BP	9V	$4.45
Le 180-6496	H/D Ever 1215BP-4	AA	$2.45
Le 170-4071	H/D Ever 1215BP-2	AA	$1.45
Le 170-4063	H/D Ever 1235BP-2	C	$1.85
Le 170-4055	H/D Ever 1250BP-2	D	$1.85
Le 168-9868	BH/D Ever 1222BP	9V	$2.10
Le 166-2139	G/P Ever 1015BP-4.	AA	$1.95

TO ORDER CALL TOLL FREE

LeBoeuf's

PHONE 1-800-546-5559

FAX 1-800-233-9692

Hearing Impaired with TDD
CALL **1-800-855-2880**

*Replace the batteries
in your smoke detectors
at least once a year.*

Accident Prevention

AS PART OF THE THOUGHT PROCESS of determining what is needed when making modifications to the home, you need to look at the safety needs and requirements of you and your patient. Listed below are some guidelines and hints that will reduce the likelihood of accidents.

Accidents seldom "just happen," and most can be prevented. There are simple steps that can be taken to make your home safer and reduce the likelihood of serious injury. The leading type of accident in the home is falls, with burns second. Approximately 85 percent of all stair related deaths occur in people over age 65. Cooking, smoking, careless use of matches and bathing are the greatest reasons for burns in the older population. About one in ten older burn victims are burned from bathing in water that is too hot.

As people age, eyesight, coordination, muscle strength, reflexes, hearing, balance and medication all can contribute to injury from falls (the most common cause of fatal injury in older people), burns and auto accidents (whether in an auto or as a pedestrian). Older people are more likely to have treatable disorders — including diabetes or conditions of the heart, nervous system and thyroid. In addition, older people take more drugs that may cause dizziness or lightheadedness.

It is estimated that about one out of three elderly people will have a fall serious enough to restrict their mobility. Many times patients will restrict their activities after a fall because of fear and anxiety, regardless of the extent of the injury.

Preventing falls is especially important for people who have osteoporosis, a condition in which bone mass decreases so that bones are more fragile and break easily. Osteoporosis is a major cause of bone fractures in women after menopause, and older persons in general. Although all bones are affected, fractures of the spine, wrist and hip are the most common.

Here are some guidelines to help prevent falls and fractures:

- Have the patient's vision and hearing tested regularly and properly corrected.

- Talk to the doctor or pharmacist about the side effects of the patient's medicine and whether the medicines affect his/her coordination or balance.

- Have the patient reduce or eliminate the use of alcohol. Even a small amount can affect balance and reflexes.

- Have the patient use caution and not get up too quickly after eating, lying down or resting. Low blood pressure may cause dizziness at these times.

- Make sure the nighttime temperature in the home is at least 65 degrees (most older people are most comfortable at about 74 degrees). Prolonged exposure to cold temperatures may cause a drop in body temperature, which in turn may lead to dizziness and falling.

Studies have shown that there is no way to identify a person or a group as "accident-prone." Studies also have shown that emotional stress appears to be the main contributing factor to accidents.

- Have the patient use a cane, walking stick or walker to help maintain balance on uneven or unfamiliar ground if the patient feels dizzy. Use special caution in walking outdoors on wet or icy pavement.
- The patient should wear supportive rubber-soled or low-heeled shoes if the shoes will not impede walking (it is not recommended that Parkinson's patients wear rubber or crepe soled shoes as they can cause a stumble or fall.). Avoid wearing smooth soled slippers or only socks on stairs and waxed floors.
- Maintain a regular exercise program to improve strength and muscle tone.

Home Safety:

- Light all stairways; have light switches at the top and bottom of stairs.
- Put bright colored tape on the top and bottom step.
- Put a hand rail on *both* sides of the stairway.
- Ramps and steps should have non-slip mats or surface
- Tack down carpeting and use nonskid adhesive carpet tape or rubber matting.
- Do not use throw rugs that tend to slide or bunch up.
- Arrange furniture so it does not create an obstacle course.
- Provide bedside remote-control light switches or night lights.
- Don't let the patient smoke in bed.
- Make sure the telephone is easy to reach from the bed.
- Use bed stabilizers to keep the bed from rolling.
- Install GFI electrical outlets in bathroom, bedroom and outdoors.
- Use a non-skid mat in the tub and shower.
- Use grab bars in bathrooms.
- Do not have the patient go out in icy weather if at all possible. Walking on bare floors that are wet is also very risky. Why take the chance?
- Don't let the patient wear loose fitting clothing when cooking.
- Set water heater temperature so water will not scald the skin. The U.S. Product Safety Commission states that a temperature above 120 degrees can cause scalds.
- Make sure the smoke detectors are working and that they meet the patient's sensory requirements.
- Have an escape plan and a where-to-meet-outside-the-house plan so you know everyone has escaped; practice the plan.
- Insulate radiators and hot pipes.

The number one cause of accidental death in the 65 to 74 age group is motor vehicle accidents. The number two cause is falls and the number three cause is fires.

In the 75 and over age group, the number one cause of accidental death is falls. The number two cause is motor vehicle accidents and the number three cause is choking.

More than one-third of falls in the elderly (over 74) result in fracture of the spine, hip (femur) or wrist. Death often follows complications associated with the accident. It pays to do all you can to prevent falls.

Six Ways to Sleep Safely:

- Install smoke detectors on every floor.
- Keep portable heaters at least 3 feet from beds or other flammable materials.
- Do not smoke in bed.
- Buy a new mattress if yours or the patients was made before 1972.
- Keep matches out of children's reach.
- Make sure electric blankets are UL approved.

Oxygen Safety:

- Do not smoke.
- Use non-smoking sections in restaurants.
- Do not use flammable products such as aerosols, paint thinners or oil based lubricants.
- Keep an all-purpose fire extinguisher on hand.
- Install a smoke detector.
- Secure oxygen cylinders to a fixed object to prevent them from being knocked over and taking off like a rocket.
- Inform the electric company if your patient is using an oxygen concentrator — you will be given priority to have the electric service restored.
- Alert visitors so they will not trip over tubes from the oxygen concentrator, PCA units or feeding units.

Attention to safety can prevent accidents. Encourage the patient to slow down and take it easy.

Home Modification and Safety Products

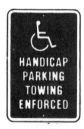 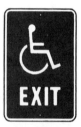
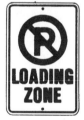 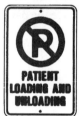

Be 20

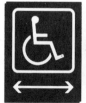 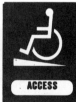
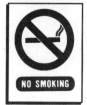 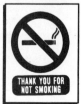

Be 19

Stair Lifts

There are stair lifts that will assist wheelchair bound patients with a wheelchair platform or a chair seat. There is even one that can be used in a standing position. There are both exterior and interior stair lifts. Stair lifts can be installed on about any type of stairway design. Currently, there are no standards by which stair lifts can be rated. Once you find a dealer who will install a lift, obtain the names of other buyers and, if at all possible, visit the location to check the lift system out. LeBoeuf's ☎ 1-800-546-5559 can provide you with a listing of companies that install stair lifts in your area.

Bruno Electra-Ride Stairway Elevator. The Electra-Ride was designed to be easy to use. The padded seat swivels smoothly to make the patient's entry and exit as convenient as possible. The seat and footrest folds up out of the way when not in use. With the press of a button, the patient is whisked up or down with battery powered safety. Batteries are charged continuously by a charger that plugs into any 110v household outlet. Works even when the power goes off. Installation by the dealer, if needed, is extra.

Br SRE-1500	16′ feet of rail	$3,140

Traffic Signs

Best Screen-Printed Signs. Made of heavy gauge bonderized steel or .063″ aluminum. Handicap signs are blue with white symbol. For signs with arrows, specify left or right. Informational signs are black and/or red screen printing. "Stop," "Yield" and "Do Not Enter" signs are red. Custom signs may be made to order. Carriage bolts and nuts included.

Be 20	12″ x 18″ 18 ga. bonderized steel	$40.95
Be 20	18″ x 24″ 18 ga. bonderized steel	$67.95
Be 20	12″ x 18″ .063 aluminum	$30.95
Be 20	12″ x 24″ .063 aluminum	$50.95
Be 20	Bead reflectorized add for each sign	$12.95
Be 20	U-channel powder coated green steel posts, 8 foot	$28.95

Best Word & Picture Signs. Available in plastic (self extinguishing), satin finish brass, bronze, stainless steel, fiberglass for exterior use. All signs are 6″ × 7¾″ and are ⅛″ thick.

Be 19	Plastic	$38.95
Be 19	Satin finish brass or bronze	$62.95
Be 19	Satin finish stainless steel	$60.95
Be 19	Polished finish brass or bronze	$68.95

Custom order Best signs are also available. Best has about any sign that you can think of. Call LeBoeuf's for a full color catalog.

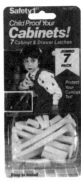

Sa 11617

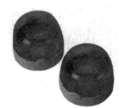

Sa 242

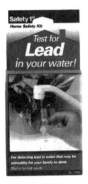

Sa 7601

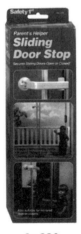

Sa 220

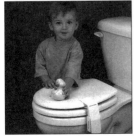

SA 11251

We have carefully chosen the following products to assist you in making your home as safe as it can be. For those patients who have special needs, you may also want to look at the products shown in the preparing the patient's room(p. 43), hearing assistive devices(p. 285), and vision aids(p. 403), ambulatory aids(p. 301) and the bath and toilet aids (p. 435) sections. If you require a special product and we don't have the product in the *Handbook*, call us and we will help you locate what you need.

Safety Locks and Testing Kits

Safety 1st Cabinet and Drawer Latches and Locks. Cabinet and drawer latches to keep your patient out of cabinets and drawers.

Sa 116	4 Cabinet and drawer latches		$1.95
Sa 11617	7 Cabinet and drawer latches		$2.95
Sa 516	3 Pack of spring latches		$2.95
Sa 115	Double locks catch automatically when opening or closing.	3 per pack	$3.95
Sa 110	Cabinet slide lock	Each	$1.95
Sa 11002	2 Cabinet slide locks		$3.95
Sa 510	Cabinet flex lock, triple touch release lock	Each	$2.95

Safety 1st Stove Knob Covers. Safety covers to prevent your patient from turning on the stove.

Sa 242	Package of 4 knob covers	$4.95

Safety 1st Appliance Locks. Lock the refrigerator, microwave and oven. Zip to open and press to close.

Sa 121	Appliance lock	Each	$2.95

Safety 1st Oven Lock. Locks oven and microwave door. Easy to install.

Sa 241	Oven lock	Each	$2.95

Safety 1st Testing Kits.

Sa 7601	Lead testing for paint, ceramics, glass, soil	$6.95
Sa 7603	Carbon Monoxide, 3 pack	$12.95
Sa 7602	Radon Testing	$14.95
Sa 7605	Test for lead in water	$3.95
Sa 7604	Microwave radiation tester	$8.95
Sa 7606	Water testing kit, pack of 8 tests	$9.95

Safety 1st Door Knob Covers. Grip and squeeze.

Sa 518	Door knob covers	Package of 3	$2.95

Safety 1st Sliding Door Stop. Secures sliding doors open or closed.

Sa 220	Sliding door stop	Each	$3.95

Safety 1st Window locks. Keeps windows locked open.

Sa 140	Window locks	Package of 2	$2.95

Safety 1st Corner Cushions. Protect your patient from sharp corners with soft and cushy corner covers.

Sa 111	Corner cushions	Package of 4	$1.95

Safety 1st Toilet Lock. Keeps patient from opening toilet.

Sa 11251	Toilet lock	Each	$6.95

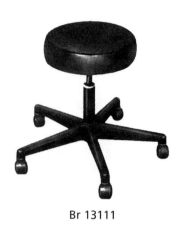

Br 13111

We can also supply rolls of indoor/outdoor polypropylene and vinyl base mats, vinyl and rubber matting for walks, ramps and decks. Our matting provides for surer footing and noise control. Sizes up to 75 feet in length and 6 feet in width. Please call for pricing.

First Watch Door Viewer. Solid brass. Fits doors 1⅜″ to 2″ thick. Easy to install. You will need a ½ ″ drill bit to drill a ½ ″ hole in the door.

| Ho 154-261 | 160 degree view | $4.95 |
| Ho 154-288 | 190 degree view | $8.95 |

Brandt Revolving Stools. Professional quality. 14-inch round upholstered seats. Backrests are 13 inches wide and 9½ inches high. Five legs provide better stability when rolling about. Composite base. Height adjustable.

Br 13111	17½″ to 23″ height adjustment	$145.95
Br 13112	17½″ to 23″ height adjustment, 2 position backrest	$202.95
Br 13131	20½″ to 28″ height adjustment	$155.95
Br 13132	20½″ to 28″ height adjustment, 2 position backrest	$215.95

Floor, Bath and Stair Safety Products

3M Scotchlite Reflective Tape. Provides the highest nighttime reflective brightness. Ideal for doors, steps, signs, etc. Apply to clean smooth surfaces.

| Fa 86-0160-1 | 1″ × 40″ roll | $2.95 |

3M Scotch Clear Tub and Shower Strips. For use in tub and shower.

| Fa 86-0370-6 | 1″ × 180″ roll | $9.95 |
| Fa 86-0371-4 | 2″ × 180″ roll | $11.95 |

Magic Safety Treads. For shower, tub, ladders and stairs. Will not crack or discolor. Self adhesive and waterproof. White.

| Ho 465-291 | 7/8″ × 80″ roll | $6.55 |

3M Home and Recreation Safety Tread. Gray color. For use on steps and walkways.

| Fa 86-0377-1 | 2″ × 180″ roll | $11.95 |

3M Heavy Duty Anti-Slip Tape. Durable mineral surface with adhesive backing. Black. Great for steps and ramps.

| Fa 86-0332-6 | 2″ × 60′ (720″) | $51.95 |
| Fa 86-0333-4 | 4″ × 60′ (720″) | $101.95 |

3M Scotch Brand Anti-Slip Tape. Provides a fast economical way to reduce hazards of slippery areas. For stairs, ladders, decks, etc.

| Fa 86-0161-9 | 1″ × 96″ roll | $5.95 |

3M Scotch Brand Rug-N-Carpet Tape. For safely securing rugs and carpets to floors.

| Fa 86-0142-9 | 1¼″ × 150″ roll | $3.55 |

Tools

Zircon "Pro" Stud Finder. Finds wooden studs through tile and dry wall.

| Ho 197-275 | Stud finder | $26.95 |

Buck Brothers Miter Box with Saw. Miter box is 12″ long and 4″ inside width. 45 and 90 degree cuts.

| Ho 972-442 | Miter box with saw | $14.95 |

Empire Level Set. 3-piece set includes pocket level, torpedo level and 2 foot level. Plastic.

| Ho 757-944 | 3-piece level set | $8.95 |

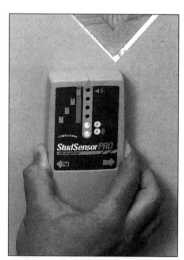

Ho 197-275

Empire 2 foot Metal Level

Ho 714-826   Metal level $7.95

Empire 4 foot Level. Made in the USA. Plastic.

Ho 177-107   Plastic level $9.95

Stanley Tool Box Saw. 15″ crosscut. Cuts wood 50 percent faster than conventional saws.

Ho 524-340   Box saw $19.95

Plumb 16 oz. Claw Hammer. Fiberglass handle with rubber grip.

Ho 842-127   Claw hammer $12.95

Empire 5 oz. Plumb Bob. Steel.

Ho 678-503   Plumb bob $4.95

Skill Cordless Drill. Variable speed, reversible. Removable battery. 9.6 volt.

Ho 318-720   Cordless drill $75.95

Black & Decker Cordless Drill. Variable speed, reversible. 8.4 volt

Ho 450-367   Cordless drill $63.95

Stanley Hand Drill. Perfect drill for those little jobs.

Ho 184-497   Hand drill $21.95

Black & Decker Glass/Tile Bit. Bit sizes are ⅛″, ³⁄₁₆″ and ¼″. For drilling through tile in the bath or kitchen. These bits will get through the tile clean and neat. You will also need a longer drill bit to drill on into the stud.

Ho 797-677   1/8″ bit $6.95
Ho 797-685   3/16″ bit $7.55
Ho 797-693   1/4″ bit $7.95

Vermont American High Speed Drill Bit Set. 10-piece set from ¹⁄₁₆″ to and including ¼″. For metal, plastic and wood.

Ho 771-687   Drill bit set $12.55

Buck Brothers Screwdriver Set. 14-piece set includes both straight and Phillips head screwdrivers.

Ho 437-424   Screwdriver set $18.95

Stanley Screwdriver Set. 6-piece set includes both straight and Phillips head screwdrivers.

Ho 186-171   Screwdriver set $5.55

Stanley Handyman 16′ Steel Tape Measure. Comes with Power Lock.

Ho 263-329   Tape measure $10.95

Stanley 33′ Tape Measure.

Ho 839-971   Tape measure $12.95

W-D 40. For stopping squeaks, cleaning tools. Protects against rust, loosens metal parts. In spray can.

Ho 953-563   2 oz. can $1.35
Ho 273-022   12 oz. can $2.55

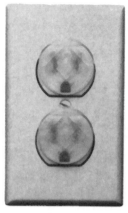

Sa 117

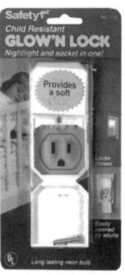

Sa 112

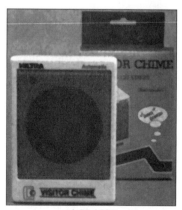

Li 834625

Electrical Products

Safety 1st Safety Outlet Plug Covers and Switch Locks. Outlet plug covers and dual outlet covers. Switch locks are suitable for all switches. A must for disposals.

Sa 117	Packs of 12 single outlet	$1.95
Sa 11721	Packs of 24 single outlet	$2.95
Sa 517	Pack of 4 protects eight sockets (can be used as single)	$1.95
Sa 10401	Automatically swivels to close outlet when not in use	$1.95
Sa 128	2 Switch locks	$1.95

Safety 1st Cord Short'ner. Neatly winds up electrical cords. Helps prevent patient from tripping over cords.

Sa 114	Cord shortener	$2.95

Safety 1st Glow'N Lock. Nightlight and socket cover in one. Long lasting neon bulb.

Sa 112	Nightlight	$2.95

LILA Power Failure Emergency Light. If power fails, the light automatically goes on and lasts for about 4 hours. Unit stays plugged in when not being used and is constantly recharging. Can be detached from the wall and used as a flashlight.

Li 628439	Buy one for each hallway, bedroom and stairway	$13.95

LILA Visitor Motion Sensor Chime. Senses when someone passes in front up to 23 feet away. Pleasant "ding-dong" chime can be set to different volume levels or turned off. Alerts you when the patient leaves a room or the house. Battery operated and be placed or hung anywhere. Batteries included.

Li 834625	4½ × 3½ × 2½ inches	$19.95

Abco Smart Bulb Signal Flasher. Recommended by firefighters, emergency crews and police. Easy to use. All you have to do is turn the light on and off twice and the computer in the base will flash the light for 2 hours. Can also be used to alert the neighbors that help is needed.

Ho 747-747	Signal flasher	$6.95

Levitron Single Pole Illuminated Toggle Switch. Silent operation. Replaces any standard switch.

Fa 62-5138-3	Illuminated toggle switch	$7.95

Levitron Illuminated Rocker Switch. Replaces any standard switch. Smooth and quiet operation.

Fa 62-5515-2	Illuminated rocker switch	$9.95

Mason Shock Protection Kit. Built-in shock protection when using electricity outdoors.

Fa 61-1299-9	Shock protection kit	$31.95

Levitron Shock Saver Plug-In (GFCI). Portable. Plugs into any single gang outlet. No wiring required. Ivory.

Fa 62-5168-0	Portable GFCI plug-in	$22.95

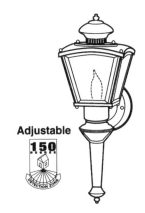

Adjustable

Kr SL-4150

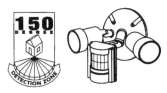

Kr SL-5411

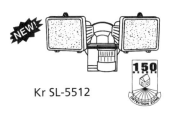

Kr SL-5512

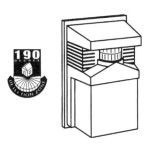

Kr SL-5630

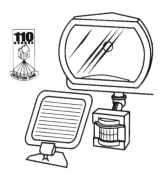

Li 690705

Heath Zenith Decorative Motion Sensing Lantern. Daylight shut-off. Detects motion at 30 feet. Comes with manual override. Selectable shut-off delay for 1, 5 or 10 minutes. Available in Polished Brass, Antique Brass, Black, White or Verde. Solid Brass

| Kr SL-4150 | Takes up to a 100 watt bulb | $29.95 |

Heath™ Zenith Decorative Motion Sensing Lantern. Daylight shut-off. 30 foot range. Off, 3 hour, 6 hour or Dusk to Dawn selectable Dual Brite™ Timer. Available in Black, White or Verde. Die cast aluminum.

| Kr SL 4192 | Takes up to a 100 watt bulb | $33.95 |

Heath™Zenith Decorative Motion Sensing Lantern. Daylight shut-off. Manual override. Off, 3 hour, 6 hour or Dusk to Dawn selectable Dual Brite™ timer. Cast Aluminum. Available in Black, White or Verde.

| Kr SL-4196 | Takes up to a 100 watt bulb | $45.95 |

Heath™ Zenith Motion Sensing Floodlight. 6,400 square foot sensor coverage. 70 foot sensor range. Durable metal fixtures. Daylight shut-off. Selectable shut-off delay for 1, 5 or 10 minutes. Available in Gray or White.

| Kr SL-5411 | Takes up to two 150 watt flood lights | $19.95 |

Heath™Zenith Motion Sensor Light Control with Protective Metal Bell Fixtures. Daylight shut-off. 70 foot sensor range. Manual override. Available in Bronze and White.

| Kr SL-5412 | Takes up to two 150 watt flood lights | $25.95 |

Heath™ Zenith Dual Brite™ Motion Sensing Twin Halogen. Daylight shut-off. Manual override. 70 foot sensor range. Heavy duty die cast metal fixtures. Dual Brite™ 2 level lighting. Off, 3 hour, 6 hour or Dusk to Dawn timer. Two 150 watt Quartz Halogen bulbs included. Available in Bronze and White

| Kr SL-5512 | Wall or eave mountable | $33.95 |

Heath™ Zenith Professional Wide Angle 500 Watt Quartz Light. Daylight shut-off. Selectable shut-off delay for 1, 5, or 20 minutes. Manual override. Durable metal fixtures, Tempered glass. Selectable range or 70 or 100 feet. 500 watt Halogen bulb included. Available in Bronze.

| Kr SL-5311 | Wall mount | $33.95 |

Heath™ Zenith Dual Brite™ Security Lite. Daylight shut-off. Selectable shut-off delay for 1, 5 or 20 minutes. 1,500 square foot sensor coverage. 30 foot sensor range. 100 watts of Halogen lighting. Instant-on. Available in Bronze.

| Kr SL-5630 | Wall mount | $45.95 |

Heath™ Zenith Entryway Motion Sensor Light Control. Daylight shut-off. Manual override. Selectable shut-off delay for 1, 5, or 10 minutes. 30 foot range. Available in Bronze finish non-metallic fixture with glass cylinder.

| Kr SL-5610 | Takes a 60 watt bulb | $25.95 |
| Kr SL-5615 | Takes a 60 watt bulb | $25.95 |

Heath™ Zenith Solar Powered Motion Sensor Floodlight. Daylight shut-off. 30 second shut off delay. 50 foot sensor range. Operates up to 15 days without sunlight. Available in White.

| Kr SL-7001 | Brightest light output available | $79.95 |

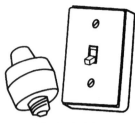

Kr. SL-6138

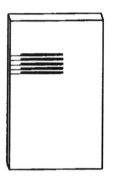

Kr. SL-6195

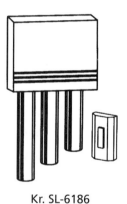

Kr. SL-6186

Heath™ Zenith Motion Sensing Wall Switch. On, Off or Automatic motion sensing. Adjustable daylight shut-off. 500 watts incandescent lighting or 400 watts fluorescent lighting. Fits standard electric switch boxes. Variable shut-off delay of 12 seconds to 30 minutes. Available in White or Ivory.

| Kr SL-6109 | LED indicates current operation mode | $23.95 |

Heath™ Zenith Wireless Light Switch. 100 foot transmission range. Screw-in lamp module.

| Kr. SL-6138 | Can handle up to150 watts of lighting | $25.95 |

Heath™ Zenith Wireless Switched Outlet. 100 foot transmission range. Can handle up to 500 watts of incandescent lighting, 300 watts of fluorescent lighting, appliances up to 400 watts and motors up to 1/3 HP. Available in White or Ivory.

| Kr SL-6136 | Add switch control to an outlet | $25.95 |

Heath™ Zenith Wireless Doorbell. Push button battery included. Single door application. Up to 150 foot range. 3 year battery life. Ding Dong or Westminster Chime sound. Available in White.

| Kr SL-6195 | Volume control, 32 selectable codes | $19.95 |

Heath™ Zenith Wireless Plug-In Doorbell. Push button battery included. Volume control. Up to 100 foot range. Single door application. Plugs into standard wall socket. Available in Designer White.

| Kr SL- 6166 | Single transmitter | $29.95 |

Heath™ Zenith Decorative Wireless Westminster Chimes. Single door application. Volume control. Up to 150 foot range. 3 year battery life. 128 selectable codes. Available in Solid Oak or Solid Cherry finish with satin chime tubes.

| Kr SL-6186 | Push button battery included | $55.95 |

Fire Safety Equipment

Kidde Fire Extinguisher. ABC for all fires. Dry Chemical. A must to have in the home and garage.

Ho 185-156	Industrial strength	$41.95
Ho 547-476		$27.95
Ho 547-514		$13.95

First Alert Smoke Alarm. 9 Volt battery included.

| Ho 586-706 | | $9.25 |
| Ho 998-621 | With light | $20.95 |

ResQLadder Life Ladder. All steel construction. Tested to 1000 pounds. Easy to install.

| Ho 544-905 | For a 2 story home | $39.95 |
| Ho 721-704 | For a 3 story home | $49.95 |

Mag-Lite Flashlight. Water and shock resistant flashlight. Takes three D cell batteries (not included). Spare Krypton lamp inside tail cap. Rugged aluminum construction.

| Ho 122-998 | Flashlight | $24.95 |

Preparing the Patient's Room

A WELL THOUGHT OUT bedroom/sitting room for the patient is important to both the patient and the caregiver. Access to doors, windows, closets, bathrooms, dressers, the bed and other furnishings should be carefully considered. If at all possible, a first floor room that is sunny and airy would be ideal for both the patient and the caregiver — especially if you are caring for a patient who is now, or may eventually be, in a wheelchair or using a walker. We will work with you to come up with some ideas for modifying your home to insure the patient's comfort and safety while providing you with the most efficient and least intrusive configuration possible.

Bedroom Size

For those patients who are in wheelchairs or need to use a walker, the ideal size for a bedroom would be three feet on each side of the bed (3 feet 6 inches would be better) for maneuvering a wheelchair or walker and for making the bed (a 12′ × 12′ room or bigger, not including the closets, would be great). At least 4 to 5 feet of clear space should be at the end of the bed. Most hospital beds are about 86 inches long with headboards and 40 inches wide with side rails. If there is not enough room for a clear area of at least 3 feet on both sides of the bed, 3 feet must be obtainable on one side of the bed. This will allow for transferring the patient from the wheelchair to the bed and back to the wheelchair. A passageway of at least 3 feet (3.5 feet or 4 feet would be best) should be provided between the end of the bed and the wall or closet. A night stand and/or dresser can be put at the head of the bed. For any furnishing (such as a dresser), you must allow for at least 3 feet of clearance in front to allow for the patient in a wheelchair to have access.

Remember, if the patient is unable to bathe, perform toilet, change clothes or feed themselves, you will need space to perform baths, change bed linens and stand or sit while feeding. You will also need room for an over-the-bed table for food and a night stand. For the patient to turn around in a wheelchair, you will need a 5 foot diameter circle or 3 foot by 5 foot T-shaped space to allow for a three point turn. This "T" space could include the knee space under a desk if it is at least 36 inches wide and 27 inches high.

Hospital Bed

If you are using a regular bed, it is a good idea to remove the casters.

A hospital bed that raises and lowers is very helpful but in many cases is not necessary. Standard hospital beds are usually 26 inches high. For patients who are nonambulatory, beds that will lower mechanically are available for ease of transfer from the bed to the wheelchair. Some hospital beds will lower to 13 inches (with the mattress at about 17-18 inches) to ease patient transfers. You can raise a bed in a number of ways such as placing on blocks, chairs, and even an extra box spring. If the patient will not need a hospital bed for an extended period of time, there are companies that will rent beds. In some areas of the United States there are service organizations that loan equipment at no charge. You can also watch the classified ads for hospital beds and other home care equipment such as wheelchairs, portable ramps, etc.

A clever way to provide for side rails and to raise the bed is to place the bed on four straight high-backed chairs and tie the bed to the chairs. This raises the bed and provides for side rails at the same time. The only problem is that you cannot lower the rails when attending to the patient. Or if the patient is in a wheelchair, it will be difficult, if not impossible, to transfer the patient.

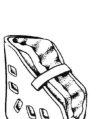

Foot Support

Footboards are used to provide support and maintain natural foot position (toes pointed straight up toward ceiling; not toward foot of bed) and keep the bed covers off the patient's feet. If a patient is confined to bed, a footboard will help prevent the patient's muscles and tendons at the back of the legs from shortening. When the muscles and tendons shorten, the patient will have a hard time walking and will be unable to stand flatfooted. To keep the patient's feet in the correct position, you can use pillows or blankets to fill the space between the patient's feet and the footboard. There are products that can be purchased which fit on the patient's feet that will also prevent foot drop (see left).

Most hospital beds will also have controls to raise the bed at the head or at the feet. Some will raise in the middle and the ends. You can get just about any configuration in a hospital bed that you can imagine. Your doctor or nurse can provide you with information on the type of bed that would best suit the patient's needs. For little added cost, a full electric bed is probably the best way to go. A full electric bed allows the patient to change positions with the push of a button. Saving one or two trips a day to the patient's room to change the bed's position will more than pay for the difference in price. The patient will also appreciate the convenience. Be sure that the patient doesn't elevate the head section over 30 degrees and leave it in that position for any extended period of time unless the doctor or nurse tell you differently. If you leave the bed in the over 30 degree position, additional pressure to the lower back and buttocks will occur and could cause bed sores.

Full electric hospital beds rent in the range of $235 or so a month. If you will be needing a bed for over eight months, it will pay you to buy instead of renting. Used hospital beds are like cars in that they depreciate quickly. If you are able to locate a hospital bed in the classifieds, do not use the mattress. Buy a new one. Always check with the doctor, therapist or nurse on how to use the hospital bed's controls and how to position the patient in the bed for eating, bathing, changing linen, reading, etc.

If you are able to buy a used hospital bed, make sure that you obtain the instructions that came with the bed and make sure you have the cranks and pendant control for adjusting the bed. Ask the seller for a demonstration of the bed's features and what, if any, problems they had with the bed. Wipe the bed down with disinfectant before taking it into your home. If parts of the bed are missing or broken, we will help you find the missing pieces and/or repair parts.

Closets

Closet door openings should be a minimum of 32 inches to allow the patient who is in a wheelchair reach the contents of the closet. Closets should have clothes hanger rods between 3 feet 6 inches and 4 feet from the floor. This is adequate for most clothing and in easy reach of the person in a wheelchair. Maximum rod height should be 4 feet 6 inches. Shelves should be mounted at a maximum height of 4 feet 6 inches and the shelf depth should not exceed 1 foot 4 inches. If sliding doors are used, floor mounted tracks or guides must

Partitioning a Room:

Building a wall to partition off part of a room is relatively simple. Tools needed include: handsaw, framing square, chalk line, plumb bob, hammer, pencil, tape measure, stud locator, sanding block, drywall knife and joint compound broad knives. Be sure to allow for door openings of at least 32 inches. Door openings of 36 inches are best.

Materials for the wall should include 2 × 4 lumber, 8d and 16d common nails, wood shims, metal connectors, sand paper, paint, half-inch drywall, drywall nails or screws, joint compound and joint tape.

not obstruct the wheelchair user. Bifold or pocket doors give easier access to the entire closet. There are a number of closet organizer systems available that will allow you to configure any closet to the patient's needs. Remember, "within easy reach" means 6 inches less than arms length, either standing or sitting. If you are using patient lifts, care should be taken to allow for wide enough doors so that storage of the lift in a closet is possible. Any "walk-in" closet should have a minimum 5 foot diameter clear turn around space. You can include in this 5 foot space one foot under the hanging clothes.

A dresser with pull out drawers should not be over 3 feet 6 inches above the floor or the wheelchair bound patient will not be able to see into the drawer. Wire baskets or drawers with perforations in the sides allow the patient to see the contents without having to open the drawer. Remember, you must have at least 3 feet of clear space in front of the dresser or other furnishing for a patient in a wheelchair to have access.

Sitting Room

If at all possible, a sitting room for the patient and visitors adjacent to the bedroom (could be same room with a curtain capable of being drawn across the room to separate the bed area from the seating area) would give the patient a feeling of privacy and independence. The sitting room could be as small as 10 × 8 feet. All you need is space for a couch and/or a couple of chairs, a table or desk, lamp, wardrobe or dresser.

Lighting

Lighting for the patient's room should include a light at the head of the bed with a flexible neck. An overhead light with a switch as you enter the room is also a good idea. You will need good lighting to check the patient's skin condition, read medication instructions and read the results of various diagnostic equipment. A signal light or an intercom the patient can use to call for assistance is also a good idea. Keep a flashlight available for both the patient and yourself in the event the power goes off.

Basic needs for furnishing a patient's room include:

EQUIPMENT:
- Bed with a good firm mattress
- Cotton and/or cotton/polyester permanent press sheets
- Waterproof mattress covers
- Waterproof sheeting (disposable waterproof underpads, bed pads)
- 4 pillows
- Blankets (should be washable)
- Dresser
- Good lighting and a good reading light
- Chair
- Night stand
- Water pitcher (insulated)
- Commode

Bed Making Guidelines:

- *Never shake soiled linen in the air.*

- *Strip and make one side of the bed completely before going to the other side.*

- *Change bedding after any soiling (urine or feces).*

- *Always remove waterproof pad if the sheets have been soiled. If disposable, discard. If you use a waterproof pad, wash it with the sheets.*

- *Always check to see if the blankets have been soiled. If they have been, wash them.*

- *Change bedding at least once a week. Use softener in your washer or dryer.*

- *Apply a thin layer of cornstarch to the bedsheet to reduce friction (reduces chance of patient getting bed sores).*

- Curtains for windows that can block out light and, if possible, cubicle curtains for privacy.
- Cotton floor covering (Floor covering should be made of cotton because it does not create static electricity. This is especially important when using oxygen.)
- Good ventilation.
- Adequate heat (most elderly patients are more comfortable in a room that is about 74 degrees; never let temperature get below 65 degrees).
- Air conditioning.
- Bed safety rails.
- Scale.
- Blanket support (keeps blanket off the feet) or bed with footboard.
- Electric outlets (make sure you have enough, convert them to ground fault interrupter (GFI) and test monthly)
- Over-the-bed table.
- Bedpans.
- Remote controlled TV, radio, stereo and VCR.
- Fire and smoke detector.
- Fire extinguisher.
- Phone.
- Intercom.
- Notebook (*LeBoeuf's Handbook*).
- Footstool.
- Clock or watch with second hand.
- Wastebasket (use liners).
- Diaper pail.

SUPPLIES:

- Thermometer.
- Heating pad.
- Humidifier or vaporizer.
- Night gowns and bathrobe.
- Wash cloths.
- Towels.
- Litter bags.
- Sweaters.
- Toothbrush and other personal items (brush, comb, hairdryer, etc).
- Blood pressure kit (optional).
- Heart rate monitor (optional).
- Skin care products.

For those patients with special needs such as oxygen concentrators, air purifiers, special testing equipment for diabetics, patient lifts, portable baths, IV stands and many others, we either have the product or if the product is still manufactured, we will find it for you.

Currently, full electric hospital beds rent in the range of $235 per month. If the patient will be needing a hospital bed for more than eight months, it will pay to purchase a bed instead of renting one.

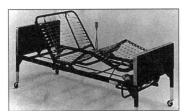

Mc 220-3818

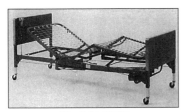

Mc 147-6985

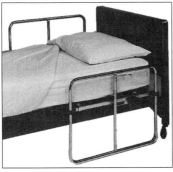

AC 112 L

Setting Goals

Planning the patient's room with the patient can be an enjoyable experience. Setting up a schedule of things that need to be done and developing a routine is very important for both the caregiver and the patient. The schedule gives organization and structure to the daily needs of the caregiver and the patient. Developing a check list for medications, nutritional requirements, obtaining furnishings, exercise plans, doctor and visiting nurse appointments, etc. allows both parties to be in control and to know that they have done all that can be done when it should have been done. Setting goals and accomplishing them is important. Don't try and set goals that are unrealistic or you and the patient will become frustrated and discouraged. If you feel that things are not going as you think they should, call us and we can help you think through what is happening and why, and/or provide you with information on people and services that are available in your area to help solve the problem.

Beds and Bed Accessories

Invacare Full Electric Homecare Bed. Six-position pendant control adjusts bed height and upper body and knee sections. Motorized pull-tube assembly allows easy adjustment of frame/spring angle for greater back comfort. Bed height adjustment controlled spring-loaded drive shaft. Two-piece frame/spring. 450 pound weight capacity.

Le 220-3818	36″ × 88″	$1,880.95

Invacare Semi-Electric Single Crank Hi-Lo Bed. Four position pendant control adjusts knee and head sections. Bed height adjusted by hi-lo crank attached to foot of bed; crank folds away for storage. Two-piece frame/spring. 450 pound weight capacity.

Le 220-2711	37″ × 88″	$1,519.95

Smith & Davis Full Electric 3-Motor Bed. Synchronized motor system eliminates "out of timing." UL listed. 6 button hand control pendant. Heavy-duty frames. Adjusts from a low of 13″ to a high of 22″. 600 pound capacity.

Le 147-6985	36″ × 88″	$1,825.95

Invacare Manual Single Crank Hi-Lo Bed. Quick set up and minimum effort in operation. Hi-low crank is at foot of bed. Head and foot spring assemblies operated by pull-tube cranks: cranks are permanently attached and fold away for storage. 450 pound weight capacity.

Le 220-3495	36″ × 88″	$939.95

Activeaid Sturdi-Sides™ Bed Rails. Quickly and easily installed on any size home bed including king size. May be lowered below mattress level for clear patient access to and from bed. Attaches to bed frame for maximum strength. Raises and lowers to three positions.

AC 112	For regular and queen size beds	$368.95
AC 112 L	Adapter for king size bed	$ 27.00

Activeaid Sturdi-Sides™ Hospital Bed Rails. Chrome finish. Can be lowered below mattress level. Easily installed. Designed to move with bed frame on adjustable head end of bed. Adjustable to three positions.

AC 110	Hospital bed rails	$285.95

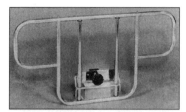

Mc 220-6126

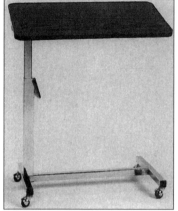

Mc 220-0327

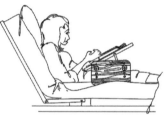

Co 8.4

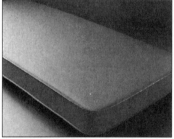

Mc 5085

SunMark Half Length Bed Rails. Fit all hospital beds. Easily attached without tools.

| Le 220-6126 | 37″ | $147.95 |

Futuro Hospital Bed Side Rail, Telescoping. Plated steel tubing. No tools necessary for installation. Rails telescope lengthwise from 51″ to 77″.

| Le 110-4108 | Side rail, per pair | $332.95 |

SunMark Overbed Table. One-piece top of oak laminate. Adjustable height side release 25¾ inches to 39 inches. Adjustable tilt, 45 degrees in both directions. ¾-inch raised T-molded plastic edge. 1½-inch hooded ball casters. Chrome plated welded steel construction.

| Le 220-0327 | Top measures 30″ × 15″ | $159.95 |

Invacare Overbed Table. Walnut wood-grain laminate top with ¾-inch flush-mounted T-molded edge. Height adjusts from 28″ to 45″ with spring loaded, locking handle. Column and "U" base are chrome plated welded steel; support bracket is stamped steel. Hooded 1½-inch ball casters.

| Le 111-5997 | Top measures 30″ × 15″ | $191.95 |

Consumer Care Products Bed Desk. For those patients who need or want to read and write in the bed. Provides stable and yet easy to store work surface. Adjustable. Solid maple with a pencil edge.

| Co 8.4 | 14″ deep × 26″ wide | $109.95 |

SunMark Footstool. Sturdy and tip-proof. Chrome plated, heavy steel tubing legs, reinforced rubber tips. Rugged 1-inch top. 9 inches high.

| Le 220-0681 | Top measures 10″ × 14″ | $32.95 |

Tubular Fabricators Foot Stool with Hand Rail. Width of top of stool is 14 inches and depth is 10 inches. Stool height is 9 inches. 1-inch aluminum legs and hand rail. Grip height is 33½ inches.

| Tu 6351/2 | Weight capacity of 250 pounds | $62.95 |

Bedding, Pillows and Blankets

Invacare Deluxe Mattress. Fluids will not penetrate acid-resistant surface. High-quality innerspring for firm support. Premium grade cotton felt and high-density urethane foam upholstery. Flame retardant—meets federal requirements.

| Le 5085 | 35″ × 80″ | Call for pricing |

SunMark Deluxe Mattress Cover. Zipper style. Waterproof vinyl/plastic.

| Le 220-1614 | Fits hospital size mattress | $11.95 |
| Le 220-2810 | Economy slip-on style fits hospital size mattress | $10.95 |

SunMark Waterproof Sheeting. Moisture-proof. Washable and reversible. 100% vinyl.

| Le 186-0600 | 36″ × 54″ | Fits single bed | $7.95 |
| Le 186-0618 | 36″ × 66″ | Fits double bed | $8.95 |

Salk Carefor Flannel-Rubber Sheet. Reusable and economical; helps protect environment. Completely washable. Combines absorbent cotton flannel with waterproof Butyl rubber for moisture protection.

| Le 132-5265 | 36″ × 54″ | $17.95 |

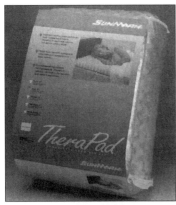

Mc 270-2389

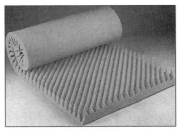

He CP5200

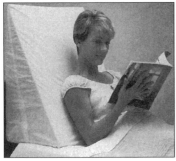

Mc 123-9300

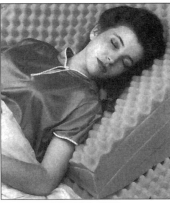

Mc 194-1350

SunMark Therapad Bed Pads. Therapad Egg-crate® design helps distribute body weight for improved comfort. Therapad design also allows for improved air circulation — cooler in summer and warmer in winter. Helps prevent bed sores.

Le 270-2389	2″ depth	Fits twin bed	$19.95
Le 270-2801	2″ depth	Fits full size bed	$25.95
Le 270-6729	2″ depth	Fits queen size bed	$28.95
Le 270-4237	2″ depth	Fits California king size bed	$38.95

SunMark Therapad Bed Pads also come in 3″ and 4″ depths. Call for pricing.

SunMark Easy-Fit Contour Fitted Sheet. Extra long. Fits all hospital beds. Easy to put on. Permanent press 50% cotton, 50% polyester.

Le 220-2059	36″ × 80″	$16.95

Hermell Hospital Sheets and Pillow Cases. 120 thread count. White polycotton. High quality and designed specifically for the hospital bed. Washable.

He CS 3680	36″ × 80″	Contour fitted sheet	each	$15.95
He CS 3685	66″ × 104″	Flat sheet	each	$20.95
He CS 3690	30″ × 20″	Pillow case	each	$ 5.95
He CS 3695	Set of 1 each of the above			$38.95

Hermell Convoluted Pad. Prevention and management of decubitus ulcers (bed sores), tissue trauma and other related problems. Reduces pressure points over bony prominences while gently massaging with each body movement. Flame retardant, single layer construction.

He CP5200	4″ thick × 36″ × 80″	Twin	$44.95
He CP 5201	4″ thick × 54″ × 80″	Double	$62.95
He CP 5202	4″ thick × 60″ × 80″	Queen	$69.95
He CP 5203	4″ thick × 76″ × 80″	King	$85.95

SunMark Bed Wedges. Ideal for foot, head, leg elevation. Cover removes easily for washing.

Le 123-8568	7″ high	$28.95
Le 123-9110	10″ high	$34.95
Le 123-9300	12″ high	$36.95

RoLoKe Good' N Bed® Adjustable Wedge. 3 wedges in 1. Removable wedges in center allow height adjustments of 8″, 12″ or 16″. Choice of positions, semi-reclined or sitting up with torso cradled. Cover included.

Le 194-1350	Fingers of foam provide comfortable support	$65.95

Rothco Blankets. 60% virgin wool, U.S. made. 62″ × 82″

Ro 9082	White USN	$22.95
Ro 10231	Blue USN	$22.95
Ro 9082	Olive Drab U.S.M.C	$22.95
Ro 9084	Olive Drab U.S. Army	$22.95
Ro 10249	Grey	$22.95

Burney Products Pillows. Cotton Polyester ticking. Polyester fiberfill (siliconized fiber blend). Machine washable.

Bu 235-C2127	21″ × 27″	$7.95
Bu 235-C1824	18″ × 24″	$7.55

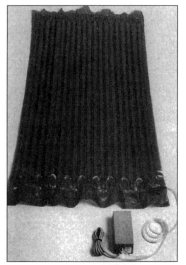

Mc 221-1456

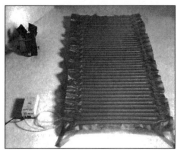

Mc 127-6260

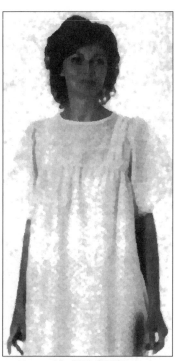

Mc 271-8153

Burney Products Disposable Pillows. Blue nonwoven ticking. Polyester fiberfill (siliconized fiber blend). Disposable pillows reduce cross contamination and eliminates laundering.

Bu 235-D2127	21″ × 27″		$5.95
Bu 2335-Y1824	18″ × 24″	Yellow isolation pillow	$6.95

Burney Products Chemtick Soft Pillows. Laminated white vinyl ticking. Anti-bacterial and non-allergenic. Polyester fiberfill (siliconized fiber blend) Wipes clean and there is no laundering.

Bu 235-S2127	21″ × 27″	$9.95
Bu 235-S1824	18″ × 24″	$8.95

Grant Dyna-Care System Pressure Relief Pads and Pumps. Alternating air pressure relief prevents pressure sores (bed sores) by constantly massaging body tissue. No vibration or noise in pad; quiet controls. Pad constructed of tough long lasting vinyl. Comes with pump. The patient's doctor or nurse can provide you and the patient with information on how to properly use this equipment.

Le 221-1456	32″ × 72″ when inflated	$165.95

Bio Clinic Bio Flote Control Unit and Pad. Alternating air pressure massages and stimulates inactive tissue. Horizontal cell design of pad increases pressure changes and provides better lift and support for heels. Universal straps on all four corners of pad for secure fit. Simple, quiet operation. Always ask the doctor how to properly use the equipment.

Le 127-6260	32″ × 70″ inflated	$187.95

Patient Gowns & Stockings

SunMark Convalescent Gown. Machine washable cotton, no ironing. Large sleeves, reinforced neck, two ties in the back. One size fits all. White

Le 186-0527	38″ long	$15.95

Salk Ladylace Fashion Gown. Easy care 50% cotton, 50% polyester. Wraparound design provides full body coverage. Fastens with easy to reach snaps on the shoulder. Lace on yolk and sleeves. Shirred bustline and shoulder, short sleeves. Yellow print and one size fits all.

Le 271-8153	36″ long	$16.95

Burney Products Dignity Tie-Top Stockings. Designed to stay up on the thigh without the use of elastic bands or Velcro. Two soft, narrow fabric ties attached just below the top hem of the stocking are tied together to form a bow and the hem is rolled over the bow. Alternatively, the ties may be fastened to the underwear.

Bu 630-001	Beige	Pack of 12	$21.95
Bu 630-002	Taupe	Pack of 12	$21.95

Salk Men's Patient Gown. Easy care fabric 50% cotton, 50% polyester. Wraparound design provides full body coverage. Fastens with easy to reach snaps on the shoulder. One size fits all. Fleur-de-lis print.

Le 271-7692	36″ long	$16.95

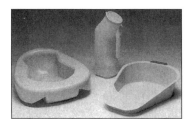

Mc 130-7693   Mc 130-7701

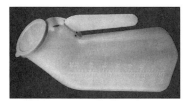

Vi 221000

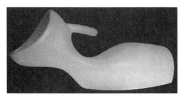

Vi 201000

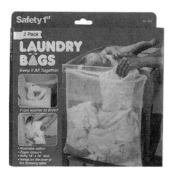

Sa 252

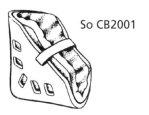

So CB2001

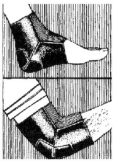

So HL/EL 401

Miscellaneous Necessities

SunMark Standard Adult Bedpans. Made of molded, polyethylene plastic. Easy grip handle on front and both sides. (Bedpan on left)

Le 130-7693	14¼″ × 11¼″	$9.95

Viscot Industries Male Urinal. Balanced design with a wide base that resists tipping when on its side or standing. Includes cap that fits tightly to stop odors and leakage.

Vi 221000	32 oz. capacity	$7.95

Viscot Industries Female Urinal. Unique anatomically correct design for the female patient. Patient may use unassisted on her back without spilling. Easy to use and comfortable.

Vi 201000	Has graduated measurement scale	$9.95

SunMark Fracture Bedpan. Easy-grip loop handle. For use with immobile or fracture patients. (Shown in picture above on right)

Le 130-7701	Can also be used a female urinal	$8.95

Viscot Industries 24 Hour Specimen Collection Container. Wide mouth opening. 3000 ML capacity. Leakproof screwcap top. Carrying handle.

Vi 2400A	Amber color	$2.95

Uniflex Bedside Litter Bag. Safe and convenient way to dispose of patient waste. Medium weight polyethylene with full width adhesive tape for secure attachment to bed or night table.

Un LD 811	8½″ wide × 11″ high	Box of 250	$33.95

Safety 1st Laundry Bags. Keep all your patient's washables together. Cotton with zipper closure. 18″ × 18″ size. Goes from washer to dryer. Hangs on dressing table or door.

Sa 252	Package of 2	$7.95

Safety 1st Odor-Less Diaper Pail System. Simply seals in dirty diaper odor with a quick turn of the top. Uses regular kitchen garbage bags. Top springs open with the touch of the button.

Sa 41681	Diaper pail system	Each	$24.95

SunMark Kodel Bed Pads. 100% Kodel polyester pile. Machine washable

Le 186-0535	24″ × 30″ regular pad	$12.95
Le 277-7183	30″ × 40″ large pad	$23.95

Southwest Technologies Foot Protectors. Protects the entire foot and ankle. Reduces pressure and distributes weight. Prevents irritation from shearing and friction. Helps prevent foot drop. Washable and re-usable. Inexpensive replaceable foam liners.

So CB2001	Hook and loop closures on boot	per pair	$35.95
So PL 1001	Foam liners	per pair	$7.95

Southwest Technologies Gel Sleeves. Combines the soft pliable Elasto-Gel™ with a nylon fabric to produce an exceptionally comfortable and effective elbow and heel protector.

So HL/EL 401	Heel/Elbow Gel Sleeve	Small	each	$18.95
So HL/EL 402	Heel/Elbow Gel Sleeve	Medium	each	$19.95
So HL/EL 403	Heel/Elbow Gel Sleeve	Large	each	$20.95
So HL/EL 404	Heel/Elbow Gel Sleeve	X-Large	each	$22.95

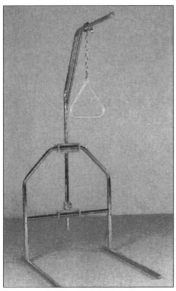

Mc 123-8039

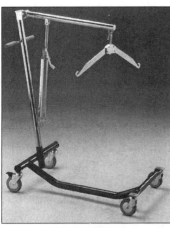

Mc 135-9413

Patient Lifters

There are many styles of patient lifters. Before purchasing a patient lifter, check with the doctor and/or therapist to be sure you are buying a lifter that will work for you. These items are prescription items. Make sure that the lifter will go through the doorways, fit in the bathroom, maneuver out to the car, etc. It's probably a good idea to have the therapist come to your home and see what is the best course of action before you purchase a patient lifter. Otherwise, you may waste a lot of money. It may be that a patient lift will not do what you need or want it to do without a lot of costly modifications to the home. Prior to using the lift, have the therapist and/or nurse show you how to operate the equipment safely.

Invacare Trapeze Bar. Helps patient change position in bed or move to commode or wheelchair. Attaches easily to head of hospital bed or stands free with accessory floor base. Adjustable height vertical bar for best positioning. Plastic coated brackets protect bed finish. Be careful that you follow installation instructions carefully. Some headboards may not be suitable for the trapeze bar. If in doubt about the strength of the headboard, purchase the floor stand. Let the therapist or nurse show you how to position the bar for the patient and instruct the patient how to use it.

Le 123-8039	Trapeze bar	$213.95
Le 123-8385	Trapeze bar floor stand	$190.95

SunMark Transfer Board. Molded high-impact, heavy duty plastic. Contoured design facilitates patient transfer from bed or wheelchair. 250 pound weight capacity. *Make sure you have been trained on how to use this product.* Most caregiver back injuries are caused by trying to move a patient. It takes just a few minutes of instruction by the nurse or therapist to show you how to do it right and prevent you from hurting your back. If the patient is coming out of the hospital, let the hospital personnel show you how to correctly move the patient from the bed to the wheelchair and back to the bed. The hospital personnel should also show you how to perform baths, use patient lifts and change bed linens with the patient in the bed.

Le 220-7298	8¼″ x 28¼″	$39.95

Invacare Portable Patient Lift with "C" Base. Offset mast centers patient over base; minimizes swaying. Shorter wheel base improves maneuverability. Offset mast provides clear lift path; no need to turn patient. 450 pound lifting capacity. You will need to purchase the lift, a sling and either a sling strap assembly or a sling chain assembly to have a complete lift. It is very important that you are trained by the nurse or therapist on how to use this equipment. It only takes a few minutes of instruction. Make sure that they show you how to place the patient in the sling and how to maneuver the lift from room to room. They should also show you how to place the patient in the tub, toileting, chair, commode, car, wheelchair, etc.

Le 135-9413	Base width 25⅓″; length 47¾″	$1,095.95
Le 137-8256	Canvas sling	$96.95
Le 186-6441	Canvas sling with headrest	$146.95
Le 186-6698	Canvas sling with commode opening	$155.95
Le 137-8199	Nylon mesh sling	$86.95
Le 186-6565	Sling strap assembly kit	$47.95
Le 137-8439	Sling chain assembly kit	$42.95

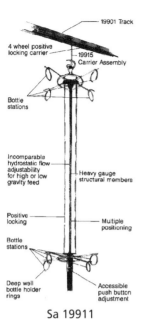

Sa 19911

Sa 19901—Track

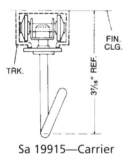

Sa 19915—Carrier

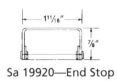

Sa 19920—End Stop

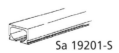

Sa 19201-S

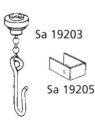

Sa 19203

Sa 19205

Accessories

Lumex Hi-Lo I.V. Stand. Anodized aluminum tubing with stable cast-iron base. Ram's horn hook design for security.

Le 220-0202	Adjusts 49½" to 87"	$131.95

Salsbury Industries I.V. Holder. Ceiling mounted track to allow for moving the I.V. Holder is adjustable to multiple high or low gravity positions. Adjustment control is always in convenient reach, yet off the floor and out of the way. Unique eight hook unit locks securely at required hydrostatic flow point. All rods, tubing and internal operating parts are of stainless steel. Length of unit is 32" retracted, 54" extended. When grounded, this system will eliminate the danger of static electricity.

Sa 19911	For ceiling heights *under* 9 feet	$230.95
Sa 19912	For ceiling heights *over* 9 feet	$280.95

Salsbury Industries Tracks, Carriers and End Stops for the I.V. Holder. Anodized aluminum track . Stainless steel and aluminum carrier assembly.

Sa 19901	8 foot I.V. Channel track designed to be jam proof ($3.50 ft.)	$28.95
Sa 19920	2 End stop fittings	$12.95
Sa 19915	4 wheel carrier assembly with locking device	$40.95

Cubicle Curtains

Salsbury Industries Cubicle and Shower Curtains. The perfect way to provide privacy to the patient. Cubicle privacy curtains and shower curtains of institutional quality are now available for the home. Cubicle curtains are flame retardant and come in up to 14 different colors. Shower curtains are available in a variety of fabrics including 8 oz. white duck. Available in widths from 3 feet to 24 feet and heights from 5 feet to 9 feet. Recommended cubicle curtain height from floor is 12 to 18 inches. When measuring for width, order 10 percent wider than track to allow for fullness and loss of goods due to seaming of panels and side hems. Curtains are flame retardant, washable and some are anti-bacterial and anti-static. All cubicle curtain track and hardware allow for quiet curtain movement. Samples of the curtain material are available from LeBoeuf's and we will assist you with ordering. Please allow two weeks for delivery as all orders are custom made. Easy to install.

Typical bill of materials:

Sa Curtains	7 foot height and 12 foot length	$224.95
Sa 19201-S	7 foot straight track	$19.95
Sa 19201-C	4 foot curved track (2′ × 2′, 90 degree bend)	$17.95
Sa 19203	Carriers (2.2 per foot of track)	$23.95
Sa 19205	2 End stop fittings	$1.95

You will need to purchase screws for installing the track. Use your stud finder. Instructions for installation will come with the order.

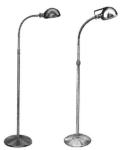

Br 41013   Br 41123

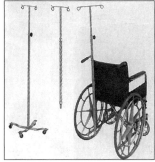

Br 35700, Br 35702,
                            Br 35707

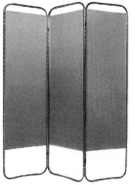

Br 70000

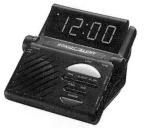

So SB1000

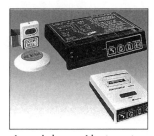

Ameriphone Alertmaster

Brandt Examining Lamps. High performance and long life. Professional quality at a reasonable price. 12-inch flexible arm. Stationary base. Chrome steel shade. Great reading lamp too.

Br 41013	Height adjusts from 36 inch to 64 inch	$79.95
Br 41123	Same as above but with a safety handle for easy lamp movement	$89.95
Br 032	Protective wire guard (if required)	$8.95

Brandt Infusion Stands. Low center of gravity bases are mounted on 2-inch twin disc casters for ease of movement and balance. Ram's horn hooks permit simultaneous application of intravenous containers.

Br 35700	Height adjusts from 40" to 77"	$113.95
Br 35702	1/2" bed insert adjusts from 22 1/2" to 43 1/2"	$75.95
Br 35707	Wheelchair IV holder. Adjusts from 40" to 77"	$79.95

Brandt Folding Screens. Hospital quality ¾-inch diameter anodized aluminum frames with stainless steel hinges. Panels are 6 mil, flame retardant bacteriostatic vinyl. Height 68 inches. White

Br 70000	Standard screen, 3 panels extended length 48 inches	$129.95
Br 70001	King size screen, 3 panels extended length 85 inches	$159.95
Br 70002	Standard screen, 4 panels extended length 62 inches	$159.95

Brandt Deluxe Supply/Service Carts. Perfect for storage of monitors and other diagnostic devices. Has adjustable middle shelf. Textured gray plastic shelves will not chip, peel, or dent. Chrome Plated support posts. 4-inch casters. 400 pound capacity.

Br 31801	28" wide × 18" deep × 33" high	$189.95

Communications, Monitoring and Warning Systems

Sonic Alert Boom Alarm Clock. Wakes the heaviest sleepers by audio alarm, flashing lights or shaking bed (bed vibrator sold separately). Adjustable volume control. Large bright green LED display. Time display is adjustable. Battery back up.

So SB1000	Snooze control	$49.95
So SS12V	Bed shaker vibrator	$29.95

Ameriphone Alertmaster AM-6000. Alertmaster alerts you to all the activities around the home. Telephone ringing, knocking at the front door, alarm clock/timer, sound monitoring, motion sensor, remote receivers, bed shaker and personal signaler that will signal you up to 80 feet from the patient's room if the patient needs anything. Wireless system is easy to set up, just plug it in.

Am 01866	Console, wireless doorbell, remote receiver and bed shaker	$209.95
Am 01871	Baby monitor (Use as a sound monitor in patient's room)	$49.95
Am AM-PXB	Light weight signaler you wear on your belt	$89.95
Am AM-SX	Motion sensor	$69.95
Am AM-100	Phone/Door notification signaler	$79.95

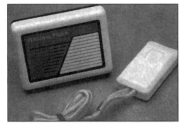

Li 657829

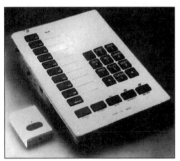

Am 68268

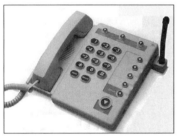

Ho 2X Mainstreet

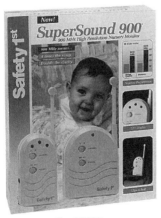

Sa 49001

LILA Wireless Personal Pager. Effective up 100 feet. Patient can use intercom button on the transmitter (12V battery included) to call for assistance. Receiver chimes and can be carried clipped to your belt or set on the counter. Uses 2 AA batteries (not included).

Li 657829	Chimes	$42.95
Li 757842	Vibrates for the hard of hearing	$76.95

Firex Smoke Alarm. 85 decibel electronic alarm with an automatic flashing yellow safety light designed to penetrate dense smoke to help guide you and the patient to safety. LED indicator to show full power or to indicate the need to replace batteries.

Po Firex	Mounting hardware and batteries included	$29.95

Ameriphone Visual Smoke Detector. Super bright strobe, polarized lens and a solid state 90 decibel horn. Great for taking on trips or at home.

Am 00472	Portable. Just plug it in	$169.95

Ameriphone NCI VR-4000 and NCI VR-100 Decoder for TV Sets. For TV's without built-in decoder or cable. Displays dialogue and sound effects as subtitles on the TV screen. Easy to install.

Am 76802	For regular TV's	$185.95
Am 76801	For cable reception box	$135.95

Ameriphone Remote Control Speaker Phone. Pressing the on/off button or the remote control automatically dials the operator or whatever telephone number is stored in the first memory location. Hands free communication up to 15 feet away through a highly sensitive built-in microphone and loud speaker. Incoming calls can be answered by pressing the remote button. External assistive devices such as pillow switch, puff-and-sip switch, headset and lapel microphone are available. 18 number memory for one touch dialing.

Am 68268	Model RC-3000	$499.95
Am 68245	Lapel microphone Model M-100	$49.95
Am 61561	Pillow switch	$39.95
Am 61562	Sip and puff switch with mounting clamp	$89.95

Mainstreet Messenger®. Personal emergency response system. Whenever the cordless pendant is pressed or the activity alarm is activated, the Mainstreet Messenger will automatically dial pre-programmed numbers such as 911, a neighbor, friend or relative. The speakerphone allows for hands-free two way voice communication. Each time phone is used, an internal activity monitor is reset for a period of 12, 18 or 24 hours. If the telephone is not used again within the pre-set time, the emergency help numbers will be activated to alert someone to check on the patient's situation.

Ho 2X Mainstreet	Alert button and single button dialing	$595.95
Ho Smoke	Smoke detector	$249.95

Safety 1st 900 MHz Super Sound Monitor. For the clearest and longest transmission available. The contemporary design is complimented by an LED light display, 2 channel option and volume control. Each unit also comes with an AC adapter to help save on batteries. Caregiver's unit comes with a convenient belt clip and 9 volt battery for easy portability.

Sa 49001	Sound Monitor	Each set	$69.95

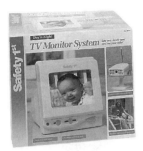

Sa 48010

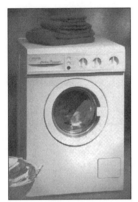

Eq EZ1000

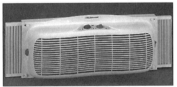

La LPRW-1

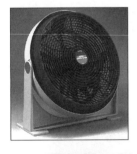

La 007

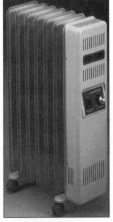

La 7000/A

Safety 1st 900 MHz TV Monitor System. The latest state of the art electronic technology for you to keep an eye on the patient. Features a 5½-inch black and white TV monitor with 2 channels. Has an adapter for the VCR for taping. Camera has wide angle lens and infrared light source for night vision. Can be mounted on a standard tripod or on the wall. Both units come with LED power lights and volume control. Monitor uses C batteries or an AC adapter with 6 foot cord. Camera uses AC adapter with 10 foot cord.

Sa 48010   TV monitor system   Each system $285.95

Washers, Fans and Heaters

Equator Corporation Clothes Processor. Washes and dries in one unit. Simple, one step operation with on/off switch. No special installation required. Uses 110 volt outlet. Can be hooked to a single faucet with only cold water. Front loading with easy to reach controls. 3 wash cycle settings. Two dryer heat settings.

Eq EZ1000   33" high × 23½" wide × 20½" deep   Delivered price $895.95

Lakewood Reversible Window Fan. Dual blower control. Can be either intake or exhaust air flow. Variable speed control with thermostatically controlled on/off temperature setting. Quiet operation. Cabinet is high impact plastic.

La LPRW-1   10" high, 8" deep, adjusts from 24 to 40" wide $49.95

Lakewood Kool Operator®. High, medium and low speeds. Adjusts to any air stream in a 180 degree arc. Moves 25 percent more air than a 20-inch box fan. High impact plastic construction.

La 007   7-wing propeller blade $34.95

Lakewood Oil-Filled Radiator Heater. No fumes, no flames, no fuels required. UL approved. Three settings—600, 900 and 1500 watts. Thermostatic control with numbered dial maintains constant temperature. Automatic on/off cycles. Easy rolling casters. Enclosed heating element-oil is safely heated internally. Perfect for the bathroom and bedroom.

La 7000/A   Seven fin design. Unit weighs 28 pounds $69.95

Hiring Outside Help

WHEN IT BECOMES APPARENT that additional help is needed with general housekeeping chores, cooking, laundry and patient care — and the cost of employing someone from an agency is too great — the caregiver will need to advertise to obtain help. One of the best ways to find reliable help is through friends and the church. If there is no one available, you will need to advertise in the newspaper classified ads. If you have a neighborhood paper, it is probably best to advertise there to reduce the number of calls from people who may live too far away. The problem of commuting for prospective employees is critical if you rely on them to show up every day so that you can go to your employment. Of course, if you intend to have the help live in, it probably won't matter where you advertise.

When you place your ad, include the following essential information:

- Type of work (i.e., housekeeping, cooking, elder care, child care, or combinations, etc.).
- Hours of work, if not live-in.
- Days per week they will work (M-F, M-Sat, etc.).
- When they will start, if hired.
- Requirement for driver's license.
- Your phone number (*never* put your name or address in an ad!). Use the newspaper's box service if you want applicants to mail a resume.
- General location (i.e., north side of Chicago, name of area such as Great Falls, etc.).
- Hours you will answer the phone (i.e., call between 6 and 9 p.m., afternoon calls only please, etc.).
- Type of experience needed and/or required.
- References required.
- Required credit check.
- Drug screening. (you do not have to list the drugs that will be checked. The five drugs that are included in a drug screening are marijuana, cocaine, opiates, amphetamines, and PCP.)

Leave out discussion about wages and how often you will pay.

Checking Out the Applicants

After the prospective employees call and appear to be qualified, send them applications along with preaddressed stamped envelopes (use return address labels to save addressing time). All applicants must fill out an employment application form.

Ask the newspaper in what section of the "help wanted" your ad should be placed. Some newspapers have special sections and may feature certain types of jobs on a particular day.

Sample of a classified ad:
ELDER CARE. Mon-Fri, 7 a.m. to 6 p.m. Great Falls area. Needed immediately. Must have exp. with patient transfers, bathing and feeding. Driver's license, credit history, previous employment and criminal record will be checked. Drug test required. Call (000) 000-0000 7 to 9 p.m. only, please.

Typically, non-medical home care will cost between $280 and $300 for a 40-hour week. In addition, you need to add about $50 a week for your portion of Social Security and unemployment taxes.

No applicant should have a driver's license for more than one state. If the applicant has just moved to your state, insist upon a new driver's license. The complete record will be transferred.

Do not let anyone drive your auto until you have checked for a clear driving record. Do not let anyone drive your auto who has a DUI (Driving Under the Influence) violation. Some states have DWI (Driving While Intoxicated). If you are in doubt about what is on the report, call the state motor vehicle department. A ticket for reckless driving may also indicate a problem with drinking.

Most states will provide a copy of the applicant's driving record for a fee of from $1.00 to $5.00. It normally takes 7 to 10 days by mail. Some states will provide the information at a branch office while you wait.

Remember, you can't ask the prospective employee about on-the-job-injuries or workmen's compensation claims until you have made a conditional offer of employment.

While we recommend that you take the time to carefully check the background of potential employees before bringing them into the home, we know that this is a time-consuming task. LeBoeuf's offers you an applicant background search service at a nominal fee.

Once you have received an application, check out the information provided or have LeBoeuf's do the checking for you — *before* you schedule an interview. Even if you are desperate for help, you **must** check the people out. Never hire anyone until you have checked all references, verified employment dates, verified education, performed a driver's license check, a credit check and a criminal check if your state has an "open record" policy. Do not use the telephone numbers on the applicant's resume or application. Look up the numbers in the telephone directory's white pages or call 411 for local numbers and 1-area code-555-1212 for numbers outside your area. If you or the operator cannot find the number, or the number is not the one listed for the reference, you need to be very cautious about the applicant.

Compare the dates of employment written on the application with dates reported by previous employers and make sure that all dates match. Investigate all gaps in time, regardless of length. Insist that previous employment references provide you with *written* confirmation of employment dates on their company letterhead. Never rely entirely on telephone reference checks!

If a previous employer will not provide a reference in writing, explain to the applicant that you cannot hire them until the employer does so — no exceptions! Many companies will not give a recommendation one way or another about an employee, but will provide you with a certificate that states the dates the applicant worked at their place of business. Remember to look in the phone book for the employer's address and phone number. *References provided by the applicant,* even if on a company's letterhead, are not worth the paper they are written on.

You can, if you wish, require drug screening. Even if you have to pay for the test, it is strongly recommended if the applicant is going to be left alone with the patient or will be driving. Drug testing can be done in two to four days. One way to find out the cost and how long a drug test will take is to call a trucking company in your area. All truck drivers must take a drug test before they are hired. Normally, a drug test will cost between $50 and $100. Shop around for the best price. Call LeBoeuf's ☎ 1-800-546-5559 for a list of drug screening labs or blood drawing collection services in your area. You can require that prospective employees pay for the tests and reimburse them if they pass. Tell the applicant what drug screening lab to go to so you can call to find out if they showed up.

Our experience has shown that only one in ten applicants who agree to drug screening will show up for the test. It is a good idea to mention that you will require drug screening (testing) in your classified ad. Try and work out an arrangement with the drug screening company so that you will not be charged for "no shows." Many drug screening companies do not require appointments, so check around. Alcohol testing can also be done, but it is largely ineffective because a person can stop drinking for three hours or more and alcohol will not show up in the test.

If you want high school transcripts, the applicant will have to obtain them for you.

If the process of screening an employee seems overwhelming to you, we have a two phase pre-employment check designed to save you time and money. Call **LeBoeuf's** ☎ **1-800-546-5559** and our associates will perform a pre-employment check for you. Before we can begin the process, you need to furnish copies of the signed application and signed affidavits for the credit check and driver's license checks. For the driver's license check, you need to obtain the applicant's driver license number. For the criminal check, you will need to furnish the applicant's date of birth, Social Security number and, in some cases, the applicant's place of birth.

LeBoeuf's Employment Screening Service pricing:

Phase I — $55.00 per applicant
Pre-employment investigation includes:

- Consumer credit report
- Social Security number verification
- Address verification
- Employment date verification only(not history)
- College education verification

Usually, LeBoeuf's can provide the pre-employment Phase I check in three days or less.

Phase II — $65.00 per applicant
Pre-employment investigation includes:

- Motor vehicle record check
- Criminal history record search
  (one county search felony and misdemeanor through county court; no state repository information).
  Additional criminal searches—$25.00 per county.
- Workmen's compensation, where allowed.
- Employment history verification.

One way to tell if applicants will treat your possessions with care and have good housekeeping habits is to look inside their automobiles. If they are full of food wrappers, pop and beer cans and other junk, you can be reasonably sure that they will treat your possessions in the same manner. You can walk the applicants out to their autos when the interviews are completed.

If the applicant passes the Phase I pre-employment investigation, we strongly recommend that you also perform the Phase II pre-employment investigation. The Phase II investigation can take up to three weeks or so. The amount of time it will take is dependent upon the states. Some states are very responsive while others take two to three weeks to respond to a request for information. Before ordering the Phase II investigation, *you must provide a conditional offer of employment in writing* so we can check out the workmen's compensation history in those states that allow such a check (38 states).

Some do's and don'ts of interviewing include:

- *Do* check and review all information on the application prior to the interview.
- *Do* have a list of your requirements and the patient's requirements that you can give to the applicant. Always list the most important and end with "other tasks as assigned."
- *Do* be objective (a person may not look the part, but may be a gem).
- *Do* make sure that all qualifications are job related.
- *Do* choose a quiet and private setting for the interview.
- *Do* explain in detail what you expect and what the patient's needs are.
- *Do* thank the applicant for coming to the interview.
- *Do* ask for transcripts from high school, college or trade school.
- *Do* encourage applicants to talk about themselves, their experiences and their families.
- *Do* let neighbors know that you will be interviewing applicants and have them call you during the interview to "borrow" something. Tell neighbors that it will be okay for them to come over in 20 minutes (or when you think you will be finished with the interview). If the applicant disturbs or frightens you, have the neighbor come right over. This lets the neighbor know that you are uncomfortable with the applicant. If you do not answer the phone, the neighbor is to call 911 immediately.
- *Do* have patients, if able, sit in on the interview (patients should be told to listen but not interrupt unless you want them to ask questions). Agree ahead of time who will ask what questions.
- *Do* make the job offer for the position in writing stating wages, schedule, starting date and any other special arrangements such as providing bus transportation, lunch, etc.
- *Don't* interview the applicant in the presence of people outside the family.
- *Don't* rush the interview.
- *Don't* repeat the same question unless you explain why you are doing so.
- *Don't* ask questions related to workmen's compensation prior to making a conditional offer of employment.
- *Don't* ask questions about on-the-job injuries until a conditional offer of employment has been made
- *Don't* make promises you will be unable to keep.
- *Don't* knock previous employees.

The "Application for Employment" form shown can be copied or you can buy similar application forms at any office supply store. You should also make copies of the request for a driver's license check, credit check and drug testing. Forms for a criminal history record check should be obtained from your state or local police. Applicants must sign all forms. If they will not sign the forms, do not hire them.

Application for Employment

NAME (Last name first):	Telephone number

Present Address: (City/State/Zip Code)

Permanent Address: (City/State/Zip Code)

Referred by: (newspaper ad/friend)

Are you currently employed? ☐ Yes ☐ No   May we inquire of your present employer? ☐ Yes ☐ No

FORMER EMPLOYMENT: (Last employer first)

Dates (Month/Year)	Name and Address of Employer	Wage	Position	Reason for Leaving
From				
To				
From				
To				
From				
To				
From				
To				

REFERENCES: (Names and addresses of three persons not related to you who have known you for at least one year.)

Name	Address	Years Known	Phone

EDUCATION/TRAINING:

School	Years Attended	Graduation Date	Subjects Studied

MILITARY SERVICE: ☐ Yes ☐ No   Rank _____   *(application form continued)*

(application form continued)

AUTHORIZATION

"I hereby certify that the facts contained in this application are true and complete to the best of my knowledge and understand that, if employed, falsified statements on this application shall be grounds for dismissal.

I authorize investigation of all statements contained herein and the educational institutions, references and employers listed to give you any and all information concerning my education/training, previous employment and any other information pertinent to this application they may have, personal or otherwise. I hereby release the educational institution and employer from all liability for any damage that may result from utilization of such information.

I also understand and agree that there is no agreement for employment for any specified period of time unless it is in writing and signed by the employer."

DATE _____   SIGNATURE _____

This application is for general use throughout the United States. LeBoeuf & Associates, Inc. assumes no responsibility and hereby disclaims any liability for the inclusion in this form of any questions or requests for information upon which a violation of local, state and/or federal law may be based. It is the user's responsibility to insure that the form's use complies with applicable laws, which change from time to time.

Affidavit for Release of Driver's License Information:

I hereby give consent and authorize _____ to request a copy of my driving record from the State(s) of _____.

DATE _____   SIGNATURE _____

Affidavit for Release of Drug Screening Results:

I hereby give consent and authorize _____ to provide the results of my drug screening to _____.

DATE _____   SIGNATURE _____

Credit Investigation in Conjunction with Job Application:

Applicant understands that, as part of the application process for the position applied for with Employer, a credit investigation may be undertaken. Applicant grants Employer permission to obtain a credit report concerning the applicant. Applicant understands that Employer agrees to hold all information received from a credit reporting agency in strict confidence and for the exclusive use of employment purposes. Employer and Applicant agree that the information obtained from any credit reporting agency concerning Applicant will be used for the purposes permitted by Section 604 of the Fair Credit Reporting Act, as such act may be amended from time to time, and for no other purposes.

DATE _____   SIGNATURE _____

Criminal History Record Request Form

Each state that has an "open records" policy has its own criminal history record request form. Some states will allow you to check on criminal records and some will not. You need to check with the state police in your state to see if you can obtain records. Normally, it takes from 10 to 14 days to receive a record, if there is one. Some states are looking into an electronic interface so that certain agencies such as the Visiting Nurses, Hospice and others can hook into state criminal records via a personal computer and modem. There is no national records check available to persons other than law enforcement officials.

SP-167 (Revised 7-1-94)

CRIMINAL HISTORY RECORD REQUEST

A Certified Check/Money Order Or Company Check Made Payable to "VIRGINIA STATE POLICE" For $15.00 Must Accompany This Request Before A File Check Will Be Initiated.
* **Personal Checks Not Accepted*** (See Instructions On Reverse Side)

MAIL REQUEST TO: VIRGINIA STATE POLICE, RECORDS MANAGEMENT DIVISION, CENTRAL CRIMINAL RECORDS EXCHANGE, P. O. BOX C-85076, RICHMOND, VIRGINIA 23261-5076

OFFICE USE ONLY: ☐ CHARGE ☐ PAID ☐ VISA ☐ INT. ADOPTION ☐ ADOPTION

1. **PERSON NAMED IN RECORD**

LAST NAME - PRINT ONLY | FIRST | MIDDLE | MAIDEN | SEX | RACE | DATE OF BIRTH / /

PLACE OF BIRTH - County or City | PLACE OF BIRTH - State or Country | SOCIAL SECURITY NUMBER — —

AFFIDAVIT FOR RELEASE OF INFORMATION

I hereby give consent and authorize the Virginia State Police to search the files of the Central Criminal Records Exchange for any criminal history record and report the results of such search to the agent or individual authorized in this document to receive same.

Signature of Person Named in Record

State of ________; County/City of ________, to wit:
Subscribed and sworn to before me this ____ day of ________, 19__. My commission expires ________, 19__.

Signature of Notary Public

2. **AGENCY, INDIVIDUAL OR AUTHORIZED AGENT MAKING REQUEST**

MAIL REPLY TO: Agency, Individual or Authorized Agent

NAME
STREET\RFD
CITY STATE ZIPCODE

ACCOUNT NUMBER

As provided for in Section 19.2 - 389, Code of Virginia, I hereby request the criminal history record of the individual named in Section 1 above and swear or affirm that I have the consent of the person to obtain his/her record and will not further disseminate the information received, except as provided by law.

Signature of Person Making Request

State of ________; County/City of ________, to wit:
Subscribed and sworn to before me this ____ day of ________, 19__. My commission expires ________, 19__.

Signature of Notary Public

☐ Check here if additional copy of record is to be provided to the individual named in the record and attach a separate check or money order in the amount of $5.00.

NOTICE

Response based on comparison of information about person named in request against a master name index contained in the files of the Virginia State Police Central Criminal Records Exchange only.
☐ No Conviction Data - Does Not Preclude the Existence of an Arrest Record. ☐ No Criminal Record - Name Search Only
☐ No Criminal Record - Fingerprint Search

Department of State Police, Central Criminal Records Exchange

Date ________ By ________

Please fold reply at marks indicated

DATA GRAPHICS, INC. 06759

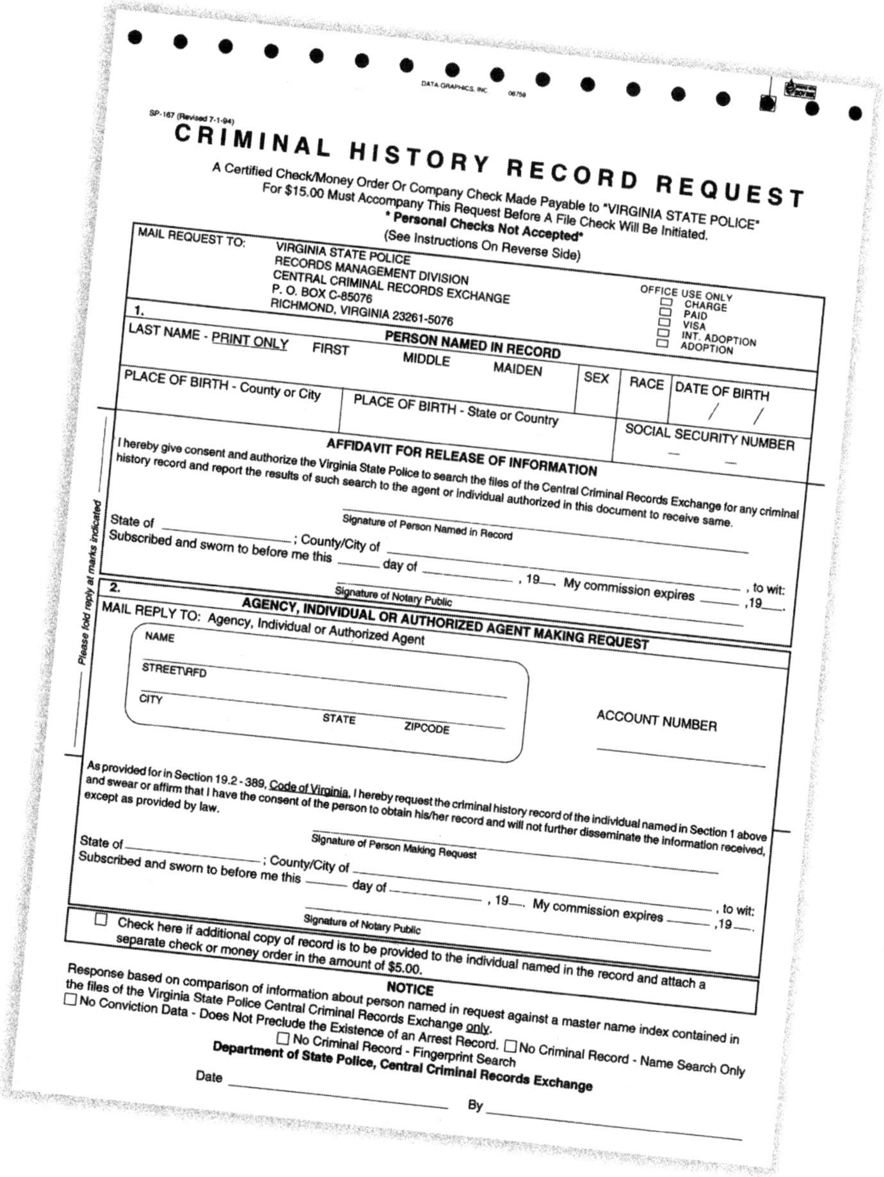

Virginia's form is shown at left. Basically, the only information you need is the applicant's name, date of birth, place of birth and Social Security number. The only problem logistically is getting a Notary Public to witness the signatures for you and the applicant. The same Notary Public does not have to witness both signatures. You could take a number of the forms to a Notary Public and have them witness your signature and sign off on all the forms at one time. It is a good idea to send the prospective employee to your Notary Public. Tell applicants that you will pay the Notary fee only if they use your Notary. That way you can call to see if they showed up. If they didn't — forget about them.

A copy of the following form should be sent to each of the applicant's previous employers and references. Applicant's original signature is required on each copy.

Authorization to Release Information

Caregiver Name: _____

Address: _____

_____

Telephone number: _____   Fax number: _____

To whom it may concern:

The prospective employee shown below has made application for a position to assist in the care of a patient in my home. Any information you wish to provide is welcomed. We are especially interested in employment dates and/or if the applicant's conduct or actions may have established a reasonable basis for suspecting physical, psychological or sexual misconduct with others.

Regarding:

Applicant's name: _____

Current address: _____

_____

Applicant's Social Security Number _____

I, the undersigned, authorize and consent to any person, firm, organization or corporation provided a copy (including photocopy or facsimile copy) of this Authorization to Release Information by the employer named above to release and disclose to such employer any and all information or records requested regarding me including, but not necessarily limited to my employment records, volunteer experience, military records, criminal information records (if any), and background. I have authorized this information to be released, either in writing or via telephone, in connection with my application for employment.

Any person, firm, organization, or corporation providing information or records in accordance with the Authorization is released from any and all claims or liability for compliance. Such information will be held in strict confidence by the Employer.

This authorization expires on: _____

Date _____   Signature of Applicant _____

Date _____   Signature of Witness _____

Failure to provide information requested may result in automatic disqualification of the applicant.

Employment Forms and Taxes

Information on Federal employment taxes for household help can be found in IRS Publication 926. You can obtain it by visiting your local IRS office, order the publication from an IRS Forms Distribution Center or you can photocopy forms and publications from reproducible copies kept at participating public libraries.

Employment taxes for household employers beginning in 1995 will be reported and paid on your annual Form 1040 — not Forms 942 and 940. Also beginning in 1995, you must verify that the employee is eligible for employment (not an illegal immigrant) and keep a record of the name and social security number. Social Security and Medicare taxes apply only if you pay a household employee wages of $1,000 or more in 1995. This applies separately to each household employee. If you pay an employee more than $1000 in a calender year, you will need to fill out and attach Schedule H to your Form 1040.

The IRS usually uses the following to determine if the person hired is an independent contractor or an employee. The two usual characteristics of an employer/employee relationship are that you, the employer:

- Can fire the employee, and
- Give the employee tools and a place to work.

For independent contractors, the general rule is that workers who perform services subject to your right to control or direct only the result of the work and not the means and methods of accomplishing the result, are not household employees and can be considered independent contractors. In plain English, what they are saying is — if you can tell the worker what you want done but not give the worker the tools or tell the worker how to do the job, it is likely that the IRS will consider the worker to be an independent contractor. It is all very confusing and you have to be careful if you want the worker to be considered an independent contractor. The IRS can be capricious and rarely, if ever, sides with the employer (you). To be sure that you are following the current IRS rules on independent contractors, you should check with an accountant.

Wages subject to income tax withholding include:

- Salaries.
- Bonuses.
- Vacation allowances.
- Meals (unless provided at your home for your convenience).
- Lodging (unless provided at your home for your convenience and as a condition of employment).
- Clothing and other noncash items.

The combined Social Security rate is 12.4% (6.2% employer share and 6.2% employee share). The combined Medicare tax rate is 2.9% (1.45% employer share and 1.45% employee share).

You do not have to withhold federal income tax from your household employee's wages unless the employee asks you to withhold taxes and you agree. An employee who wants you to withhold federal income tax must give you a completed form W-4.

If you wish to pay the employee's share of the Social Security and Medicare tax, you do not have to withhold from the employee's pay. However, you must pay all the tax — 12.4% for social security and 2.9% for Medicare. The portion of taxes you pay for the employee will count as additional income to the employee.

You will also have to pay Federal Unemployment Tax (FUTA). This tax rate is 6.2% of the first $7,000 of cash wages you pay in 1995 for each of the household employees earning $1,000 or more for the year. However, if you pay state unemployment taxes, you may be able to take a credit of up to 5.4% against the FUTA tax.

In addition, you will most likely have to pay state unemployment taxes and you may have to withhold state and local income tax. Each state and locality has different requirements and you will need to check with the state and local agencies dealing with employment taxes. In addition, you should ask about worker's compensation obligations.

Payroll records should be kept for every day an employee works. You can find payroll record forms at any office supply store. Some of the forms come with duplicate copies so that you do not have to make a separate statement to go along with the paycheck. There are also a number of inexpensive bookkeeping and payroll programs for computers which are easy to operate. Have the employee sign the payroll record (your copy) for each payroll period. Your bank also has payroll checks that have space for all the taxes and other withholding if you want to keep a separate checking account for payroll. Always pay by check. Show on the check stub the amount withheld for FICA, Medicare, state withholding, and other taxes if you have the room. It will make life much easier should you ever have an audit.

Information on employees that you should retain:

- Employee name.
- Address.
- Social Security Number.
- Hours worked each day.
- Dates of each pay period and length of employment.
- Rate of pay.
- Type of work.
- Amount of other pay (room, board, etc.).
- If withholding Federal Income Tax, the number of exemptions.
- State income tax.
- Medicare tax.
- Social Security tax.
- Local withholding tax.
- Cash advances.
- Other withholding (bonds, merchandise, etc.).
- Employee's signature on your payroll record for each period.

All the above may seem like a lot of work — and it is. You can count on spending at least one hour a week to prepare payroll and at least two or more hours every month/quarter for all the state and federal reports. Most of the states and localities will help you work through what is needed, or you can call an accountant for advice and assistance.

Transportation and Travel

FOR MANY PATIENTS, finally getting outdoors after several days in a hospital or being confined to a bed is an exciting event. Pond fishing may seem like a roller coaster ride after staring at the ceiling for a week. This section of the handbook provides some hints and suggestions on how to make traveling easier. You should not dread traveling with a handicapped or sick patient. Most, if not all, companies providing service to the traveling public are able and willing to provide assistance to you and your patient. The most important thing you can do is to let the company know what the problem is ahead of time and they will work with you to minimize delays and smooth the way. In 1991 more than 13 percent of all travelers had some kind of handicap. You will not be alone and you will find that most people will go out of their way to assist you.

The key to traveling successfully is to plan ahead and allow plenty of time. There are a number of companies and organizations that provide travel plans and services for the disabled. You can call **LeBoeuf's** ☎ **1-800-546-5559** to make arrangements for all travel services. These services range from arranging for transportation to and from dialysis (the cost of which may be covered under the patient's insurance, Medicare or Medicaid) to arranging special vacation trips and tours for the elderly and/or handicapped.

In recent years, the passage of the Americans With Disabilities Act (ADA) has made it easier for the elderly and disabled to use public facilities and public transportation. Doorways have been widened, wheelchair ramps installed, pay telephones lowered and bathrooms have been modified to allow easy access for patients in wheelchairs. In addition, special assistive equipment must be made available for the visually and hearing impaired at all hotels, motels and hospitals.

Restaurants, theaters, shopping centers and malls, retail stores, museums, libraries, parks, private schools, day care centers and other similar types of facilities open to the public may not discriminate on the basis of someone's disability. Before you take the patient out, it is important to call ahead and explain what your patient's needs are. Tell the establishment that your patient is confined to a wheelchair, needs to use a walker, is hard of hearing or visually impaired, etc., and the establishment will let you know if there will be problems accommodating the patient. Taking the patient to a restaurant, shopping mall, etc., can be an enjoyable experience if you plan ahead and use some common sense.

When you are scheduling doctor, dentist, therapist, and other appointments for the patient, it is important to let them know what the patient's circumstances are. If your patient is in a wheelchair, be sure to ask the doctor, dentist, therapist, etc. if the patient will be able to get to their office. Always ask the doctor or his/her staff how they work with patients in a wheelchair. Many doctors and dentists can and will work on the patient while he/she remains in the wheelchair.

Put all medications and other items that might spill or break in unbreakable containers or reclosable plastic bags. Roll up clothing like a newspaper to lessen wrinkling.

Airlines have braille safety cards for passengers who read braille. In 1992, American Airlines worked with wheelchair manufacturers to develop a special wheelchair that will fit in the aisle of an airplane. Check with your airline to see if they have these smaller wheelchairs.

If the patient does not understand the safety message provided by the airline crew, they can ask for an individual safety briefing. As always—if in doubt, ask.

Most patients confined to a wheelchair prefer "bulkhead" or First Class seats on the airplane.

Travel light to reduce the need for assistance and for easier trips through train or bus stations and airport terminals. Take the time to make a list prior to packing everything you and the patient want to take and check off each item as it is packed. Keep jewelry, keys, wallet, medications, prescriptions, eyeglasses, tickets, money, passport, camera and other valuables in your carry-on luggage. Put all medications and other items that might spill or break in unbreakable containers or reclosable plastic bags. Roll up clothing like a newspaper to lessen wrinkling. Don't overpack and lock your luggage before checking it in. If the patient is diabetic and needs to carry needles, the doctor's prescription should be in their possession to avoid problems at airport security. Make sure that you receive a separate claim check for each piece of luggage and that the city shown is the one to which you are traveling. If in doubt about the destination code shown on the baggage tags, ask the attendant or Red Cap to be sure the bags are going where you are going.

Any time you travel with the patient, you must allow for the patient's early morning stiffness, medication requirements, mealtime schedules, rest periods and special seating or transportation arrangements. Ideal travel time for most patients would be from late morning to early afternoon. Make sure there is plenty of time between airline flights, train and bus connections. You should allow at least 30 minutes, but an hour is preferable. In many airports, such as Atlanta, it can take 10 to 15 minutes for a person without handicaps to go from gate to gate.

When you are making reservations for an airline flight, try and obtain a non-stop flight if at all possible — or at least a flight that does not require the patient to change planes. Try and give the airlines at least two weeks notice so the airline can check with the patient's doctor to be sure the airline can meet the patient's needs (have the doctor's name and telephone number ready when talking with the airline). The airline will call you back and let you know what services they can provide and let you know what you and/or the patient need to do.

For those patients using oxygen, always ask what the extra charge for oxygen will be and what extra charge will be levied each time the patient changes planes. Prices for oxygen can range from $50 to $250 or more. It is a good idea to arrive early and let the patient board the plane ahead of the other passengers to get hooked up to the oxygen cylinder without interfering with other passengers (airlines usually put oxygen cylinder in the overhead rack).

You can make arrangements for an electric cart with a driver, or a wheelchair with an attendant, if your patient needs assistance with walking. Also, an hour before landing, remind the stewardess that a wheelchair or an electric cart has been requested when the plane arrives. Make sure that you tell the travel agent or the airline what special needs (food, seating, etc.) your patient may have. You will find the airlines to be very accommodating and most, if not all, of your needs can and will be met. The person taking the reservation will not know all the services the airline can provide and, while they will make every effort to find the information, it is better to wait until the special assistance people from the airline call you back.

If you are traveling with an electric wheelchair or scooter, allow at least one hour if disassembly is needed. If traveling by air, the airlines will want to know what type of battery the wheelchair or scooter has. You should also take along the assembly instructions that came with the wheelchair or scooter to speed assembly and delivery time when you arrive at your destination. If the patient uses an animal trained for aiding the hearing or vision impaired, let the transportation company know ahead of time. All airlines, and other transportation companies can accommodate the animal. However, guide dogs, hearing dogs or other service animals are not allowed in Hawaii or in many of the island nations such as Australia, Great Britain and New Zealand without a long quarantine (can be as long as 40 days or more). Be sure to ask the airline what restrictions the country you are traveling to has on service animals.

Currently, Greyhound Lines, Inc., the only nationwide bus company, does not have any lift equipped buses. Structural changes in over-the-road buses to provide access for wheelchair or scooter users are not required until July 26, 1996 (or a year later for small bus companies). Any newly manufactured commercial for-hire and public over-the-road passenger buses must be accessible to the disabled. The date to convert existing buses may be extended for an extra year after the completion of a study. We are in touch with the Greyhound people and we can assist you with the most current status of Greyhound's ability to accommodate patients in wheelchairs or scooters. Greyhound will provide free transportation to a person who needs to help the handicapped patient.

Passenger railroads such as AMTRAK, and light rail such as subways, are usually accessible to the handicapped. Even so, getting on and off the train can be a problem at many stations. There are some stations without platforms that require passengers to use stairs or step stools to get on and off the train. You need to check with the railroad or subway company to be sure that the stations you will be using are set up to provide easy access to the train car for the patient. If the railway company does not have handicapped access at the station you want to use, ask whether the station before or after the preferred station has handicapped access. It may be that a short cab ride will solve the access problem.

Hotels and hospitals must have available for use, free of charge, special equipment and services for the hearing impaired and blind, such as an interpreter, TTY/TDD device, doorbell signaler, or a smoke detector with a bright strobe light and noise alert. Ask the hotel management or your travel agent whether the room is equipped (or can be readily equipped) with such auxiliary aids and services. While the hotel must have equipment available, they may not have enough equipment to meet the needs of all their guests. Be sure you call ahead to reserve assistive equipment. For those staying in private homes, or other places that are not required to follow ADA guidelines, you may want to bring your own equipment. Assistive devices can easily be carried in a small suitcase. By Federal law, all hotels with more than 100 units must include such features as grab rails, non-slip tubs, higher sinks and access to public facilities.

Always call ahead to the hotel to see if they have features such as grab rails, non-slip tubs and doors wide enough for wheelchairs especially the bathrooms. Check to see if the hotel has ramps and access to all public facilities, including recreational areas such as the swimming pool.

The American Automobile Association (AAA) TourBook guides are a good source for hotels and other lodging that are accessible to wheelchair users. You can call **LeBoeuf's** ☎ 1-800-546-5559 for the number of the nearest AAA office, or you can use **LeBoeuf's Special Assistance Travel Agency** to make all the transportation and lodging reservations as well as arrange for any other special assistance the patient may require.

The ADA Accessibility Guidelines require that hotels and hospitals must provide:

- Text Telephones (TTY/TDD-TDD)
- Notification systems (door knocking, bed shaker, special alarm clocks, etc.)
- Telephone amplifier
- TV Closed-Caption Decoder
- Visual Smoke Detector

LeBoeuf's ☎ 1-800-546-5559 is a dealer for the major manufacturers of assistive equipment required for hotels and hospitals.

Telephone companies must provide Telecommunications Relay Services (TRS) for hearing-impaired and speech-impaired persons 24 hours a day. Many public telephones now have an adjustment on the receiver to allow the patient to adjust both the volume and the tone quality. In addition, most hotels and many travel agencies have TTY/TDD-TDD (text telephone) service for their hearing impaired customers.

When the Patient Can't or Shouldn't Drive

For many elderly persons, possessing a valid driver's license is a sign that they are still in control. They believe that their car and driver's license allows them to have some independence. Most caregivers will have a very difficult time convincing a patient to sell the car and not continue to drive. While state driving tests help screen out the most impaired and hazardous of the elderly drivers, many senior citizens are reluctant to voluntarily restrict their driving habits. However, after a series of collisions or near misses, they may be too scared to continue driving. Many may restrict their driving to daylight hours, non-rush hour traffic, good weather, short distances and familiar routes. They may avoid freeways and roads with high-speed traffic.

Telling the patient not to drive is a two-edged sword. Once the patient has agreed to no longer drive, you will now become the chauffeur. If you have taxi service in your area, it may be worth your while to work with the taxi company and let them assist with the patient's chauffeuring. It may cost a little more, but the convenience is well worth the money.

In most areas, public transportation will not be the answer. If you live in a rural area, there is little or no public transportation. And if you live in an urban area, public transportation for the elderly or handicapped may be unreliable and/or too dangerous.

Public transportation often does not reach the preferred destination of the patient. Freedom of movement is limited by the routes of buses, subways and train cars. Appointments with doctors and therapists need to be adjusted to fit bus schedules. Some patients may even need to change doctors because of the difficulty in reaching a physician's office. Missing a doctor's appointment can seriously impair a patient's treatment schedule.

Wheelchair and Scooter Van Lifts and Auto Lifts and Holders

The caregiver for a wheelchair-bound patient may need to make some minor alterations to their car to accommodate a wheelchair. There are a number of lifts and holders that can accommodate a wheelchair for transport in or on a car. The lifts and holders are operated by simple devices that attach to a car's bumper or trailer hitch. Lift devices are usually manually operated, but there are battery-powered wheelchair lifts available as well. Electric lifts are useful when the caregiver is unable to lift the wheelchair. (Wheelchair weights vary widely. Attendant-propelled wheelchairs range from about 30 to 60 pounds. Motorized (battery operated) wheelchairs weigh about 110 to 180 pounds.)

There are also van lifts which allow patients to remain in their wheelchair and eliminate difficult and awkward transfers of the patient and the wheelchair into the vehicle. There are no universal standards for van lifts and you must be certain that the lift will fit your vehicle. If you live in a snowy or very hot region, you need to check out the capabilities of the van lift for reliability. Ask the van lift dealer for the names of purchasers of van lifts in your area and check out the reliability of the lift. If you live in an area that has heavy snows, you **must** check the references. Some lifts do not work well in the snow.

Another item to consider is the patient's existing wheelchair. Some wheelchairs have a wheelbase that is too long for a lift. This is especially true if the patient uses a scooter. You should also make sure there is a manual emergency back-up system on the lift. There are a number of tie-down systems for the patient and the wheelchair. Be sure to ask to see what the dealer has. Some of the wheelchair tie-downs are simple to operate while others require that you have a special fixture installed in the vehicle. In addition to the wheelchair tie-down, the patient must have available — and use — a regular seat belt. Because there are so many different types of van lifts, it is impossible to list them all. To find out who the dealers are in your area, call LeBoeuf's ☎ 1-800-546-5559.

You and the patient should work with the doctor and the physical or occupational therapist to determine the most suitable assistive equipment that will enable the patient who has special needs to continue driving. Special assistive equipment includes a left-footed accelerator, steering knobs, hand throttle, hand brake control, turn signals on the right side, etc. There are also a number of driver education companies qualified to teach the disabled. Insurance can also be a problem — it pays to shop around for the best coverage and price. You can call us for a list of manufacturers of adaptive equipment and, if you are having trouble obtaining insurance for the patient, the number of your state's insurance commissioner's office.

Shopping can be an unpleasant ordeal for many patients. (Just try lugging a gallon bottle of bleach or a twelve-pack of soda home. Even for the healthy, a three block walk carrying these heavy items can quickly become laborious.) Some packaging is obviously made for lifting products from the grocery shelf into the cart, but not from the check-out line to the home a half-mile away. Wagons, knapsacks, bicycles (or tricycles), baskets on the walker or wheelchair, and wheeled walkers with a basket can immensely ease the burden of transporting groceries. A little common sense and a small expenditure goes a long way toward helping the patient cope with shopping.

Caregivers who transport patients by auto should make sure their vehicle is in good working order. Back-up plans should be in place for alternative transportation in the event the car is unavailable or out of service. Arrangements made with a neighbor for substitute transportation will lessen the panicked nature of some incidents such as when the car won't start on a cold winter day, a flat tire is found, or when the only available car at the home is being used elsewhere. Joining a car club or an automobile association is well worth the money. Many gasoline companies as well as the American Automobile Association (AAA) offer good service for a reasonable annual fee. It may also be a good idea to have a cellular phone in the car. Some auto companies will provide a cellular phone as part of their service when you purchase a specially equipped vehicle for a disabled patient. The base cost of a cellular phone is normally less than $30 a month plus charges for usage.

What to do:

Contact the American Automobile Association's Traffic Safety and Engineering Disabled Driver Program. They are located at 1000 AAA Drive, Heathrow, Florida 32746. You can also call any of the AAA locations throughout the United States for information. It does not cost much to join the AAA. The AAA does a very good job of staying on top of what is available for their disabled customers. Knowing that help from AAA is but a phone call away is well worth the cost of membership.

Chrysler's Automobility Program — 1-800-255-9877 or you can write to them at P.O. Box 3124, Bloomfield Hills, MI 48302-3124. Chrysler offers reimbursements for adaptive equipment conversion costs for certain vehicles purchased or leased from a Chrysler dealer.

Ford Motor Company's Ford Mobility Motoring — 1-800-952-2248 or you can write Ford's Lance Worden at P.O. Box 529, Bloomfield Hills, MI 48303. Ford offers financial assistance, a Ford cellular telephone and roadside assistance to eligible customers.

General Motors Corp.'s GM Mobility Assistance Center — 1-800-833-9935 or you can write GM at P.O. Box 9011, Detroit, MI 48202. GM offers reimbursements for adaptive equipment conversion costs and financing assistance on new vehicle purchases or leases. GM will reimburse conversion costs up to $1000.

National Mobility Equipment Dealers Association (NMEDA) — 1-800-833-0427 or you can write NMEDA c/o Becky Plank, Executive Director, 909 East Skagway Avenue, Tampa, FL 33613. NMEDA works to insure safer conversion of vehicles, provides a network for dealers/manufacturers concerned with quality and helps consumers solve problems.

Contact Greyhound Lines, Inc. — 1-800-231-2222 if the patient needs to be assisted and 1-800-752-4841 if no special assistance is required. Call 48 hours before departure. For TTY/TDD service, call 1-800-345-3109.

Contact AMTRAK — 1-800-USA-RAIL (872-7245) for information on what stations are not accessible to the handicapped. Call 1-800-523-6590 for TTY/TDD service.

Contact the Society for the Advancement of Travel for the Handicapped (SATH) — It is located at 347 Fifth Avenue, Suite 610, New York, NY 10016. It has been serving the handicapped traveling public since 1975. It has a travel magazine (Access Magazine) and is very active in improving conditions for disabled travelers. You can become a member for $45 a year or subscribe to their magazine for $13 a year.

LeBoeuf's Services

Call **LeBoeuf's** ☎ 1-800-546-5559 for the following services. Please have ready the patient's name, address, zip code, age, telephone number and physical circumstances (Alzheimer's, heart problem, arthritis, etc.) when you call.

- Consulting Service
     Wheelchairs (design, ultra-light, sports chairs, etc.)
     Van Conversions
     Electronics
          Hearing
          Vision
          Security
          Communication (TTY, Call Buttons,
               Telephones, etc.)
          Television, VCR's, Radio, Stereo
          Computers and Software

- Home Healthcare Workshops

- Caregivers Speakers Bureau

- Incontinent Supply Service

- Respite Network

- Home Modification Planning Service

- Assistive Travel Agency

- Employment Screening Service

- Referral Service for:
     Hospitals
     Nursing homes
     Hospice
     Visiting nurse associations
     Adult day care programs
     Respite care (nursing homes, support groups,)
     Social services case workers
     Household help

LeBoeuf's

PHONE **1-800-546-5559**

FAX **1-800-233-9692**

Hearing Impaired with TDD
CALL **1-800-855-2880**

LeBoeuf's
Home Healthcare
Handbook

Family
& Friends

Friends

BY ANNE KEITH

What can I say of friends?
Without them I run down
Like the tall clock
In the hall.

When my weights
Touch bottom,
They wind me up
To tick and tock
And ring my special bell of hours.

Scheduling Visitors

Family and visitors should always be cheerful when visiting with the patient.

VISITORS TO A HOUSEHOLD with an infirm patient should be informed of the patient's schedule. A phone call placed in advance of the visit is recommended. Phone calls will help select an appropriate time for a visit. The caregiver can then inform the visitor whether the patient is having a "good day," or if any sudden mood flare-ups or infections have recently appeared. Of course, some patients are still capable of scheduling their own visitors.

The distress of an ill person is frequently difficult to comprehend for someone who has never been sick, incapacitated, or exposed to an ailing person. Visitors who are overly chatty may bore the patient. Three half-hour visits a week may be more welcome than a single hour and a half long sitting. Similarly, a roomful of visitors may tire the patient. Visits may need to be limited to one or two people at a time. The personal health of the visitor is also a consideration. Contagious ailments such as a cold, flu or hepatitis may pose unacceptable risks to an already ill person.

Trusted visitors can also provide respite help. This will allow the caregiver time to run errands, attend a meeting, or gain the opportunity to take a much-needed nap.

It is not a good idea to allow drinking of alcoholic beverages by either the guest or the patient during visits. Guests should not be allowed to invite other guests unless they clear it with the caregiver first. To break up a visit that seems to be going in the wrong direction and/or is agitating the patient, you can break in and say that the discussion should be continued some other time. A good guest arrives on time and knows when to leave. A small gift is always welcome.

Children in the household pose their own unique visitation concerns. Certain play activities may be disruptive and disturbing to the patient. A roomful of boisterous grandchildren excited at seeing Grandmother again after a long trip may be overwhelming for the bed-ridden. Loud music and television viewing may need to be moderated by the use of headphones or special equipment to reduce the noise (and stress) level.

Some children may be embarrassed by the condition of the patient. The children, who were fond of entertaining their friends at home, may become embarrassed about Grandpa's wandering spells or incoherent ranting and no longer want to play a game of checkers with their friends. Some children are reluctant to have guests over until the patient has recovered.

The caregiver and patient should also consider being visitors themselves. Being cooped up in a room or house for days on end can be excruciatingly boring. Even a short trip to the park, a garden or museum will ease the monotony. Friends who are also incapacitated could benefit from a visit by the patient.

Parents Who Live Away

I F YOUR PARENT LIVES A LONG DISTANCE AWAY, you must have a plan in place to insure that communications can be made with either your parent or someone who lives close by, such as a neighbor or a friend. With a little planning, you can reduce much of the stress and anxiety that results from not knowing what is happening. A little planning will also reduce or eliminate unnecessary and costly trips to check on your parent.

While there are no set number of times you should visit a parent, it pays to use a little common sense. Remember, your parents have taken care of themselves for many years and, unless they are ill or have a serious handicap, they can usually manage to fend for themselves. If you are employed, let your employer know what is going on with your parent and be sure that you plan days off for travel. Most employers will understand and work with you to arrange time off that is convenient for both parties. Start a travel fund and make arrangements for child-care, if necessary, ahead of time.

Find a neighbor or a friend close to your parents who can keep a key to their home. Introduce yourself and get to know the neighbor(s) who have agreed to keep a key and act as your eyes and ears. Most neighbors will be more than happy to help and will provide you with information on the condition of your parent whenever you call. Many will call to let you know when something does not seem right (i.e., an abrupt physical change, a car accident, lots of repair people coming and going, etc.). It is a good idea to call the neighbor once in awhile to let them know how much you appreciate what they are doing. A nice note or card from time to time will also let the neighbor know that you appreciate their kindness.

When you are concerned about your parents, call the neighbor(s) who have a key first. Second best is to call a friend of your parents who can check on them. The friend should live within a reasonable distance, have transportation and possess a key to your parents' home.

Most police departments will respond to a call from a concerned family member and dispatch an officer to check on parents. However, some police departments will request that you go to your local police station and fill out a missing persons report. Be sure that you check on what your parents' police department will require *before* an emergency. Your local police department will then wire (Fax) the report to the police department in your parents' area. This all can be done in a matter of minutes. The reason for filing the missing persons report is to protect the police from a lawsuit if they have to force entry into your parents' home.

Always call the police first. They will call for Fire and Rescue or other support. Always take *LeBoeuf's Handbook* with you if you have to go to the police station. If your parents are on any special medication, you should be able to tell the police what it is and the dosage. You should also inform the police if one of your parents is blind, hard of hearing, bedridden or any other information that will assist them in helping.

Make copies of the form on the following pages and ask your parents to fill out the information and return the form to you. Your parents should provide you with at least two names of their neighbors and/or friends. Make sure that they have completed all sections and ask them to call you if they make any changes. It is a good idea to fill out the form in pencil so you can easily make changes. Copies of the completed form should also be made available to other children in the family.

Information About Your Parents

Parent(s) Full Name(s): _____

Address: _____

Parents' Local Police Telephone Number (Not 911): _____

Parents' Local Fire and Rescue number (Call Police First): _____

Doctor: _____ Telephone _____

Pharmacist: _____ Telephone _____

Lawyer: _____ Telephone _____

NEIGHBORS

Name _____ Telephone _____

Address _____

Have key? Yes ☐ No ☐   Hours normally at home _____

Name _____ Telephone _____

Address _____

Have key? Yes ☐ No ☐   Hours normally at home _____

FRIENDS:

Name _____ Telephone _____

Address _____

Have key? Yes ☐ No ☐   Transportation: Yes ☐ No ☐

Hours normally at home _____

Name _____ Telephone _____

Address _____

Have key? Yes ☐ No ☐   Transportation: Yes ☐ No ☐

Hours normally at home _____

SPECIAL MEDICINES:

Yes ☐ No ☐

Make sure that you inform the people attending to the parent who gets what medicine

Brand Name _____ Dosage _____

_____

_____

_____

SPECIAL NEEDS:

_____

_____

_____

_____

REMARKS:

_____

_____

_____

*Information About
Your Spouse's Parents*

Parent(s) Full Name(s): _____

Address: _____

Parents' Local Police Telephone Number (Not 911): _____

Parents' Local Fire and Rescue number (Call Police First): _____

Doctor: _____ Telephone _____

Pharmacist: _____ Telephone _____

Lawyer: _____ Telephone _____

NEIGHBORS

Name _____ Telephone _____

Address _____

Have key? Yes ☐ No ☐   Hours normally at home _____

Name _____ Telephone _____

Address _____

Have key? Yes ☐ No ☐   Hours normally at home _____

FRIENDS:

Name _____ Telephone _____

Address _____

Have key? Yes ☐ No ☐   Transportation: Yes ☐ No ☐

Hours normally at home _____

Name _____ Telephone _____

Address _____

Have key? Yes ☐ No ☐   Transportation: Yes ☐ No ☐

Hours normally at home _____

SPECIAL MEDICINES:

Yes ☐ No ☐

Make sure that you inform the people attending to the parent who gets what medicine

Brand Name _____ Dosage _____

_____

_____

_____

SPECIAL NEEDS:

_____

_____

_____

_____

_____

REMARKS:

_____

_____

_____

Family Caregiving Agreement

IT IS A GOOD IDEA to prepare an agreement outlining the responsibilities of all the parties involved in the task of caregiving. An agreement is especially necessary when you have members of the family living far apart. While the family agreement is strictly voluntary, it provides an outline of things that need to be considered by the primary caregiver and other family members. Family members must be made aware of the time, financial and physical requirements that the primary caregiver will be expending, and the need for help, especially respite care. Many situations in caregiving require more than one person to help with the patient and, if hiring help is not feasible, the caregiver must be able to rely on help from other family members. Nobody can do it alone.

Be as specific as you can about the assignment of responsibilities. For example, you must be specific on the definition of yard chores. In other words yard chores should be defined in detail. Mowing, trimming, sweeping the walks and raking the leaves are what is meant by yard chores. How often? Once a week? Once every two weeks? Who will do the work? One of the grandchildren or the parent? What or whose equipment will they use? In other words, try to get everything on the table at the beginning to avoid problems and the potential for hurt feelings and major frustration later. The same goes for all activities pertaining to the patient that you can think of. You know that you have everything covered for each task if you can answer who, what, where, when, and how for each.

All seems easy in the beginning. But, after months of caregiving, you will realize that you have undertaken a monumental task. It is much better to lay all the cards on the table and try not to be a hero. Do not take on all the responsibility for caregiving by yourself. You will be needing help and if you do not plan for other family members to help, you may find that other family members do not understand your needs or are reluctant to help after they have seen the problems you have faced and will continue to face.

Make as many copies of the following agreement as there are primary and secondary caregivers. Remember, each secondary caregiver may not be able to perform the same tasks or provide the same support.

It is a good idea to give all parties a complete Family Caregiving Agreement package showing what task or support each family member has committed to perform or provide.

Some tasks or situations that you may want to address in the agreement:
- Running errands
- Banking and handling the patient's money
- Shopping
- Financial support
- Illness or accident to primary caregiver
- Transportation to church, doctor, therapy, movie, etc.
- Minimum days of respite care
- Visitation by friends and family members

Make copies of the following form, add all the items that you can think of that would help you in the task of caregiving, and give each family member a signed and dated copy of what they have agreed to do. Make sure that all family members understand that the items listed in the agreement are the minimums and that extra help is not only appreciated, but may be necessary later on. As conditions change, you may want to call another meeting and change the caregiving agreement to reflect the current state of affairs.

FAMILY CAREGIVING AGREEMENT

This Family Caregiving Agreement is made between the Primary Caregiver(s) _____
_____ and the

Secondary Caregiver(s), _____
_____.

The Caregivers seek to list their responsibilities and duties for the caretaking of the Patient, _____
_____.

The Caregivers understand that this agreement is wholly voluntary. It is not intended to be legally binding. This agreement is intended to help clarify the respective roles of the Caregivers and to settle questions relating to the care of the Patient.

The Caregivers have made known to each other the obligations, needs and financial commitments for the care of the Patient. However, the Caregivers recognize that the health and particular needs of the Patient will eventually change and that it is not practical to have rigid, specific details for taking care of the Patient.

They agree to confer with each other on all important matters pertaining to the Patient's health and welfare with a view to arriving at a harmonious policy to promote the Patient's best interests.

The Caregivers are aware that the Primary Caregiver may be required to spend significant amounts of time, energy and financial resources for the caretaking of the Patient. They agree that the welfare of the Patient is the paramount consideration for each of them.

In recognition of the efforts made by the Primary Caregiver in taking care of the Patient, the Secondary Caregiver agrees to:

1) Telephone the Patient regularly, at least _____ times per _____ (week, month).

2) Visit the Patient at the Primary Caregiver's residence at least _____ times per _____ (week, month). The dates and times of the visit should be arranged in advance for the mutual convenience of the Caregivers and the Patient.

3) Offer respite care for the Primary Caregiver. The respite care may be from the Secondary Caregiver or such other person(s) as mutually agreed upon. The duration of the respite care shall be for _____ (hours, days, weeks) per month/year _____

4) The Secondary Caregiver also agrees to host Patient visits at the Secondary Caregiver's home. The duration of the visits shall be for _____ (hours, days, weeks) per _____ (month/year).

5) Contribute at least $_____ per month to help defray the extra costs incurred by the Primary Caregiver for taking care of the Patient.

6) List of additional activities such as providing transportation, running errands, performing yard chores, etc. (Be specific and as inclusive as you can. Remember to answer who, what, where, when and how for each activity.):

_____
_____
_____
_____
_____
_____
_____

AGREED TO, THIS _____ DAY OF _____, _____ BY:

_____   _____
Primary Caregiver   Secondary Caregiver

_____   _____
Primary Caregiver   Secondary Caregiver

NOTE: The various Secondary Caregivers may offer their help in ways different from those listed above. Not all Secondary Caregivers may be able to perform all of the items mentioned in this agreement. *Make a separate agreement for each Secondary Caregiver and make sure that they take a copy with them.*

Legal Guidelines

Sister Talk

BY ANNE KEITH

Now that our winter's come
We light the fire of our memories
With words.
Good words, dry words
That flare and crackle,
Bringing warmth and light
To our own childhoods
And our children's years.

Outside the darkness grows
And war winds whistle in the trees,
But all in this small room
Seems snug.
We rest here for awhile,
Protected as we were
By parents' love
And our own innocence.

Caregiver Contract

BECAUSE OF THE ROLE REVERSAL that often occurs when an adult child (caregiver) begins to instruct a parent as to when they can watch TV, eat, and set other rules, some patients become resentful and very upset with the primary caregiver. Many times, the patient will become so upset that they change their will or trust and disinherit the caregiver. To help protect the caregiver against unreasonable actions by the patient, we had our legal department develop a "Caregiving Agreement."

"Caregiving Agreements" between caregivers and patients define the duties and obligations of each party. Subjects such as food, lodging, utilities, medical costs, fees and other items are defined and agreed to in writing in order to avoid problems or misunderstandings later on.

"Caregiving Agreements" also help all parties involved fully understand the value of the agreed upon caregiving service. There are many costs associated with providing care in the home and, if a patient has the income to help with expenses, they should do so. Patients may contribute their own resources to help with grocery bills, utility costs, mortgages, rent, and other bills. For many patients, paying their "own way" is a means of maintaining a degree of independence.

If the parent is unable to provide much or any support to the cost of their care, a "Caregiving Agreement" provides a means for the caregiver to protect against disinheritance by establishing an amount that would be due the caregiver upon the death of the patient. If, for some reason the caregiver is left out of the patient's will or trust, the cost of services they have provided to the patient can be recouped if there is any money in the estate.

The best way to establish the value of the lodging and services that you will be providing to the patient is to obtain quotes and/or fee schedules from home care nursing providers (Visiting Nurses, Hospice, etc.), cleaning services, temporary help agencies and nursing homes in your area. The quotes and/or fee schedules can be used to establish the value of housing, food, nursing care, homemaking assistance and other services that you, as the caregiver, will be providing to the patient. Keep a record of the quotes and information you received and make sure that the material is dated. Attach the quotes and fee schedules to the Caregiver Contract.

AGREEMENT FOR CAREGIVER SERVICES

NOTE: This Agreement is intended only as a guideline. Consult an attorney for tax and/or legal issues that may apply to your specific caregiving situation.)

This Agreement for Caregiver Services is made between the Caregiver(s) _____

_____ ,

residing at _____ ,

City of _____ , County of _____ , State of _____

(hereinafter called "Home" or "Residence"), and the Patient, _____ .

Section 1. OBLIGATIONS OF CAREGIVER

Caregiver agrees to furnish Patient board, room, lodging care and services at the Home as listed in this Agreement for the period of time indicated or the remainder of the natural life of Patient.

Section 2. BOARD

Caregiver will provide Patient a minimum of two nutritionally well-balanced meals each day. Special diets may be provided but only upon the express written order of the Patient's physician.

Section 3. LIVING ACCOMMODATIONS

A. Caregiver shall furnish to Patient a [room/apartment] in the Home.
B. Caregiver [allows/does not allow] smoking in the Home.
C. Caregiver [allows/does not allow] use of alcohol in the Home.

Section 4. FURNITURE

The [room/apartment] occupied by Patient at the Home will be furnished by [Patient/Caregiver].

Section 5. UTILITIES

Caregiver shall furnish to Patient all utilities reasonably required in connection with the occupancy of Patient's living accommodations. These utilities are to include water, electricity, heat, and trash removal. Patient [is/is not] responsible for costs

for telephone service and long distance calls, except for those calls _____

_____ .

Section 6. PERSONAL ASSISTANCE

A. Caregiver shall furnish such personal assistance as needed and requested by Patient. These activities of daily living include (circle those presently required):

1. Walking
2. Bathing, shaving, brushing teeth, combing hair
3. Dressing
4. Eating
5. Getting in and out of bed
6. Laundry
7. Cleaning room/apartment
8. Managing money
9. Shopping
10. Using local transportation
11. Writing letters
12. Making telephone calls
13. Setting appointments
14. Arranging transportation for appointments
15. Self-administration of medication
16. Recreational and leisure activities

In addition to the items mentioned above, Caregiver will provide: _____

_____

_____

_____

B. Caregiver shall provide assistance to Patient to carry out the instructions of physicians and attending professional nurses (RN's).

C. Caregiver will generally keep aware of Patient's whereabouts. Caregiver shall not restrict Patient's individual movement and will not be responsible for any harm resulting from the voluntary absence of Patient from the Home.

D. Caregiver will attempt to monitor the activities of Patient to ensure the Patient's health, safety and well-being. Caregiver shall notify _____

_____

_____

of any significant changes in circumstances noted by Caregiver.

Section 7. MEDICAL COSTS

A. Patient [shall / shall not] be responsible for the payment of the costs of drugs, vitamins, glasses, medicines, treatment of mental illness, or of any ailment existing at the time of residing with Caregiver.

B. Patient shall, from time to time as appropriate, sign forms as are reasonably necessary to secure payment to any hospital, extended care facility, doctor, Caregiver, or any other parties who provide services rendered to Patient and for which benefits are available.

C. Any benefits paid under this Section shall be excluded from the services provided by the Caregiver or any other agreement with Patient.

Section 8. FEES

A. Patient agrees to pay Caregiver the sum of

$_____ (_____ Dollars) upon signing this Agreement.

B. Patient shall pay to Caregiver the sum of

$_____ (_____ Dollars) per [week / month],

payable [weekly/monthly] in advance, subject to adjustment as noted in Section 9 of this Agreement.

Section 9. ADJUSTMENT IN FEES

Caregiver shall endeavor to maintain its [weekly / monthly] fees at the lowest possible rate consistent with the operation on a sound financial basis and maintenance of the quality of services. Patient shall be given at least sixty (60) days notice of any adjustment to the fee charged by the Caregiver for the care of Patient.

Section 10. TRANSFER OF PATIENT

In the event Patient becomes so ill or disabled as to require special attention, becomes infected with a contagious or dangerous disease, or becomes mentally ill to such a degree that [his/her] presence in the Residence shall be deemed detrimental to the health, safety or well being of other residents of the Home, Caregiver shall have the authority to transfer Patient to another facility suitable for such instances.

Section 11. INJURY OR DAMAGE BY PATIENT

Patient agrees to reimburse Caregiver for any loss or damage suffered by Caregiver as a result of the carelessness or negligence of Patient, except any insured loss or damages by Caregiver.

Section 12. LIEN FOR MEDICAL CARE WHERE PATIENT IS INJURED BY THIRD PARTY

A. Patient may, on request, receive care in situations where Patient is injured as the result of the fault, negligence, or carelessness of a third party where such third party's responsibility may exist. In the event Caregiver provides such care, Patient assigns to Caregiver a lien against any recovery that Patient may obtain from any third party or parties compensating Patient for injuries sustained by Patient. The lien shall secure reimbursement to Caregiver for the cost of the care furnished to Patient by Caregiver because of the injuries to Patient for which Patient is compensated by any third party. The lien shall be enforceable by Caregiver against the property of Patient, the estate of Patient after death, or the property held by the heirs or assigns of Patient.

B. Patient (or the legal representative of Patient) shall have the duty to diligently pursue any claim for compensation due from any third party for injury to Patient and to cooperate with Caregiver in collecting such compensation and reimbursing Caregiver for the cost of the care furnished to Patient.

Section 13. TERMINATION DURING PROBATIONARY TERM

There shall be a probationary term of _____ days during which this Agreement may be canceled by either party without advance notice and regardless of the health of Patient. Upon cancellation of this Agreement, Caregiver shall refund to Patient the difference between any amounts paid and the daily cost of services. Caregiver and Patient have determined by mutual consent that the daily cost for Caregiver to provide the services to Patient under this Agreement **during the probationary** term is $ _____ per day.

Section 14. AGREEMENT TERMINATION BY PATIENT

This Agreement may be terminated by Patient at any time after the probationary terms by giving Caregiver _____ days written notice. Caregiver and Patient may also by mutual agreement terminate this Agreement on a specific date, regardless of the notice requirement in this Section.

Section 15. DEATH OF PATIENT

Upon the death of Patient, this Agreement shall automatically be terminated. All payments made by Patient to Caregiver shall remain the property of Caregiver and shall not be transferable by the will of Patient or subject to claim by Patient's estate or heirs.

IN WITNESS WHEREOF, the parties have executed this agreement at _____

on this _____ day of _____, 19_____.

_____
Caregiver

_____
Caregiver

_____
Caregiver

_____
Patient

Legal Documents

IN THIS SECTION are samples of a living will, durable power of attorney for healthcare, will, codicil to will and a living trust. It is probably a good idea to work with a lawyer on these — especially the living trust. You can count on a lawyer billing you two to three hours for both the living will and a durable power of attorney for health care. Depending on the size of the estate, setting up a will or a living trust can require many hours and the costs can vary widely. You must ask in advance what the lawyer charges per hour. Legal fees vary from $65 per hour in some areas to more than $250 per hour in others. Sometimes you can negotiate a flat fee. It does not hurt to shop for a lawyer and negotiate a price. It is possible to obtain the forms for the living will and durable power of attorney for healthcare from your state and local social agencies, hospital or from an office supply store. It is strongly suggested that you invest in a lawyer's advice and let the lawyer prepare and file the documents with the appropriate authorities (if necessary) and instruct you on who should also have copies of the documents.

State laws vary on the particular requirements to execute a valid will, living trust, power of attorney, power of attorney for healthcare and other legal documents. Some states have specific filing requirements in order for the document to have full force and effect.

In 1990, Congress passed the Patient Self-Determination Act. The Act requires health care institutions to tell patients their rights about their medical care. These rights include the right to accept or refuse care and the right to make advance directives about their care.

When the patient receives information from a doctor and agrees to the recommended treatment, the patient has given informed consent. The patient has the right to refuse the recommended treatment. The patient can make recommendations and choices of medical treatment in advance in writing and/or name someone they trust to make the decisions for them if they are unable to tell the doctor what treatment they want. These documents are known as *advance directives*. Anyone 18 years old or older can sign an advance directive.

Most states have laws that allow the patient to make advance directives. You and/or the patient need to check with your state and find out what is allowed. Most states will allow either a living will (Natural Death Act declaration) or a durable power of attorney for health care. Massachusetts, Michigan and New York do not have a living will statute. However, patients in these states can complete a living will. Case law and the U.S. Constitution support the patient's right to do so.

Most states will allow the patient to sign a living will that will tell doctors and others who will be caring for the patient how to care for them if they have a terminal illness and are unable to make the decisions themselves. Terminal illness is an incurable condition in which death is imminent. It can also mean a persistent vegetative state (permanent coma). In either case, the doctor has determined that there is no hope for recovery. Living wills only apply when a person has a terminal condition.

When the patient receives information from a doctor and agrees to the recommended treatment, the patient has given his/her informed consent.

75% of Americans agree that advance directives are something they should have. However, less than 20% have signed an advance directive.

Terminal illness is an incurable condition in which death is imminent.

*Life prolonging procedures
do not include treatments
needed to make the patient
comfortable or to relieve pain.
The patient will automatically
be provided treatment or
drugs to relieve pain and make
the patient comfortable unless
the patient has stated in the
living will that such
ministrations are not wanted.*

*The death of a patient who
refuses life-prolonging
treatment will not be
considered a suicide under
the Natural Death Act.*

There are two basic types of living wills:
- The patient decides in advance what procedures the doctors should perform or not perform and puts those decisions in writing.
- The patient names someone they can trust to decide whether life prolonging procedures should be performed.

Life prolonging procedures do not include treatments needed to make the patient comfortable or to relieve pain. The patient will automatically be provided treatment or drugs to relieve pain and make the patient comfortable, unless the patient has stated in their living will that such ministrations are not wanted. Usually, most people will want to have all life-prolonging procedures except food and water withdrawn when a cure is not possible and continued care will only prolong dying.

If the patient does not have a living will and has a terminal illness, the desired treatment may be specified in front of witnesses. The death of a patient who refuses life-prolonging treatment will not be considered a suicide under the Natural Death Act.

Advance Directives: Living Will and Durable Power of Attorney for Healthcare

A durable power of attorney for healthcare does not replace a will and automatically terminates upon the death of the declarant. A will is used for handling the affairs of the patient after the patient dies.

A durable power of attorney for health care can be separate from or combined with a living will. It is a written document that appoints someone the patient trusts to act as agent on health care in the event of incapacitation. Decisions by the person the patient has chosen to act as agent are not limited to end-of-life decisions, but can include decisions on medication, surgery or other procedures. The law prevents the person the patient has chosen to make decisions which do not meet with the patient's religious beliefs, basic values and stated preferences.

While a lawyer is helpful, the patient does not have to have a lawyer prepare either a living will or a durable power of attorney for healthcare. These advance directives may be available from the hospital, state medical societies, the patient's doctor or from the patient's insurance company. If the patient is retired military, forms may be obtained from the legal offices at the closest base. If the patient revokes or makes changes in either the living will or the durable power of attorney for health care, be sure the old one is destroyed.

The advance directive should be signed and dated in front of at least two adult witnesses (over 18 years old) who are not relatives or possible heirs to the patient's estate. The witnesses also cannot be paying for the patient's medical care. Make sure that all issues such as the patient's religious beliefs on nutrition and tube feeding are clear. Also, you and the patient should notify the person or persons who have been named as the patient's healthcare agent and make sure that the wishes of the patient are fully understood. (You as the caregiver should also prepare an advance directive.) If you and/or the patient have a home in another state (summer home) and spend any amount of time there, make sure that you and the patient have an advance directive for each state.

Make sure that the family and the doctor have copies of the advance directive. Otherwise, nobody will know what the patient's wishes are for medical treatment. However, do not give the advance directive to the doctor until the patient is under the doctor's care; you do not want to influence the doctor's diagnosis. The hospital and the nursing home must ask the patient if they have an advance directive and you should make sure that the patient's medical records show that the patient has one.

Make sure that you know where the patient's living will or durable power of attorney for healthcare is located. Have the patient carry a card in their wallet or purse that provides the location of these papers. It is also a good idea to review the advance directives when the patient has moved from one state to another state, medical condition changes, marital status changes or there are drastic changes in the patient's financial status.

Many states have developed model documents that may or may not be recognized by other states. All states except Alabama and Alaska have durable power of attorney for healthcare statutes.

A sample "Durable Power of Attorney for Healthcare" approved for use in Virginia is shown on the following page.

Sample:

Durable Power of Attorney for Healthcare

I, _____, willfully and voluntarily make known this _____ day of _____ 19____, this Durable Power of Attorney and declare as follows:

I hereby appoint the following as my primary agent to make health care decisions on my behalf as authorized in this document:

_____ (_____) _____
Primary Agent   Phone Number

_____
Street Address   City   State   Zip Code

If the above named Primary Agent is not reasonably available or is unable or unwilling to act as my agent, I then appoint the following as a successor agent to serve in that capacity:

_____ (_____) _____
Successor Agent   Phone Number

_____
Street Address   City   State   Zip Code

I hereby grant to my agent named above, full power and authority to make healthcare decisions on my behalf as described below whenever I have been determined to be incapable of making an informed decision without providing, withholding or withdrawing medical treatment. The phrase "incapable of making an informed decision" means unable to understand the nature, extent and probable consequences of a proposed medical decision or unable to make a rational evaluation of the risks and benefits of a proposed medical decision as compared with the risks and benefits of alternatives to that decision, or unable to communicate such understanding in any way. My agent's authority hereunder is effective as long as I am incapable of making an informed decision.

The determination that I am incapable of making an informed decision shall be made by my attending physician and a second physician or licensed clinical psychologist after a personal examination of me and shall be certified in writing. Such certification shall be required before treatment is withheld or withdrawn, and before, or as soon as reasonably practicable after, treatment is provided, and every 180 days thereafter while the treatment continues.

In exercising the power to make healthcare decisions on my behalf, my agent shall follow my desires and preferences as stated in this document or as otherwise known to my agent. My agent shall be guided by my medical diagnosis and prognosis and any information provided by my physicians as to the intrusiveness, pain, risks, and side effects associated with treatment or nontreatment. My agent shall not authorize a course of treatment which he knows, or upon reasonable inquiry out to know, is contrary to my religious beliefs or my basic value, whether expressed orally or in writing. If my agent cannot determine what treatment choice I would have made on my own behalf, then my agent shall make a choice for me based upon what he believes to be in my best interest.

Further, my agent shall not be liable for the costs of treatment pursuant to his/her authorization based solely on that authorization.

Powers of my agent *(Optional. Cross through any language that you do not want and add any language you do want.)*

The powers of my agent shall include the following:

1. To consent to or refuse or withdraw consent to any type of medical care, treatment, surgical procedure, diagnostic procedure, medication and the use of mechanical or other procedures that affect any bodily function, including but not limited to artificial respiration, artificially administered nutrition and hydration, and cardiopulmonary resuscitation. This authorization specifically includes the power to consent to the administration of dosages of pain-relieving medication in excess of standard dosages in an amount sufficient to relieve pain, even if such medication carries the risk of addiction or inadvertently hastens my death;

2. To request, receive and review any information, verbal or written, regarding my physical or mental health, including but not limited to medical and hospital records, and to consent to the disclosure of this information;

3. To employ and discharge my healthcare providers;

4. To authorize my admission to or discharge (including transfer to another facility) from any hospital, hospice, nursing home, adult home or other medical care facility; and

5. To take any lawful means that may be necessary to carry out these decisions, including the granting of releases of liability to medical providers.

This advance directive shall not terminate in the event of my disability. By signing below, I indicate that I am emotionally and mentally competent to make this advance directive and that I understand the purpose and effect of this document.

_____ _____
Date   Signature of Declarant

The declarant signed the foregoing Durable Power of Attorney in my presence. I am not the spouse or a blood relative of the declarant.

_____ _____ _____ _____
Witness   Date   Witness   Date

Living Will

A living will is a written statement from the patient to the doctor instructing the doctor on the desires of what is to be done related to life-sustaining procedures in the event of terminal illness, unconsciousness or if the patient becomes comatose and is unable to tell the doctor what is desired for continued treatment. For the living will to be valid, it must be written while the patient is of sound mind.

Some lawyers suggest that the living will not be given to the doctor or let it become part of the medical records until it needs to be used. The concern is that the doctor, hospital or others would misapply the living will and not provide the necessary and proper medical care.

A living will is in force only if the patient is terminally ill or near death and cannot make competent decisions. Each state has their own definition of terminally ill or near death.

A sample of a "Living Will" is shown on the next page.

Sample:

Natural Death Act Declaration
"LIVING WILL" DECLARATION

In accordance with the Virginia Natural Death Act, the Declaration was made on Month _____ Date _____ Year _____.
I, _____, willfully and voluntarily make known my desire to do hereby and declare:

(Choose one, and only one, paragraph shown below)

☐ PARAGRAPH ONE:

If at any time I should have a terminal condition and I am comatose, incompetent or otherwise mentally or physically incapable of communication, I designate _____ to make decisions on my behalf as to whether life-prolonging procedures shall be withheld or withdrawn. In the event that my designee decides that such procedures should be withheld or withdrawn, I wish to be permitted to die naturally with only the administration of medication or the performance of any medical procedure deemed necessary to provide me with comfort care or to alleviate pain. (OPTION: I specifically direct that the following procedures or treatments be provided to me:

_____
_____)

OR

☐ PARAGRAPH TWO:

If at any time I should have a terminal condition where the application of life-prolonging procedures would serve only to artificially prolong the dying process, I direct that such procedure be withheld or withdrawn and that I be permitted to die naturally with only the administration of medication or the performance of any medical procedure deemed necessary to provide me with comfort care or to alleviate pain. (OPTION: I specifically direct that the following procedures or treatments be provided to me:

_____
_____)

In the absence of my ability to give directions regarding the use of such life-prolonging procedures, it is my intention that this declaration shall be honored by my family and physician as the final expression of my legal right to refuse medical or surgical treatment and accept the consequences of such refusal.

I understand the full import of the declaration and I am emotionally and mentally competent to make this declaration.

_____
Signature

_____
Social Security Number

The declarant is known to me and I believe him/her to be of sound mind.

_____
Signature of Witness   Date

_____
Signature of Witness   Date

Note: Spouse or blood relative may not serve as witness.

Complete the following if you selected Paragraph One of this form: Name, address and telephone number of person designated to serve as substitute decision-maker:

_____
Name

_____
Street Address

_____
City/State/Zip

_____
Work Phone   Home Phone

Living Trust

If your patient has a large estate and does not have a living trust, you should encourage the preparation of one.

A living trust is a legal document that allows an individual to transfer ownership of titled and personal property to an entity called a "trust." You can think of the "trust" as a company that now owns everything the patient has and the patient owns and controls the company. This is the only way to avoid probate if the patient owns anything. A living trust allows the patient to "own" nothing in their own name; yet control everything just like before.

Living trusts are not just a way to beat taxes. Living trusts have been used for centuries. The living trust is created while an individual is alive and can be revoked or changed at any time. It is similar to a will and distributes property as desired but it does not go through probate.

A living trust does not eliminate the need for a will. You will need to have the patient prepare a will called a pour-over will. The pour-over will is needed to cover those assets that for some reason or another have not been transferred to the trust. The grantor should leave the residue of the estate to the living trust. Like everything else to do with legal affairs, it is strongly recommended that a lawyer assist you and the patient in preparing all the required documents.

When the patient sets up a living trust, a trustee is named who will control the trust. The patient will most likely want to be trustee in order to personally conduct affairs as long a possible. If the patient is married, the spouse is usually named as joint trustee. If one dies, the other instantly has control over all the property in the trust without going to court. It is also a good idea to name a back-up trustee in case something happens to both. The back-up trustee will need a copy of the death certificate (or a letter from a doctor if the patient is disabled or incompetent), a copy of the trust document and personal identification. Death certificates are usually obtained from the funeral home. The back-up trustee can be required to keep beneficiaries informed of all actions.

A good back-up trustee is a bank. The bank will charge a very reasonable fee. The fee is published and will only be charged when it actually takes over. Annual fees charged by banks to handle trusts range from about 1% to 2% of the value of the trust. Banks usually set a minimum size for a trust and if the patient's estate is less than $250,000, most banks will not agree to act as a trustee.

When the patient dies, the back-up trustee acts just like an executor would if the patient had a will but does not have to go through the courts. The trustee duties may go on for a lifetime or even several lifetimes. If the patient becomes disabled or incompetent, the back-up trustee will be able to write checks, apply for disability benefits, pay bills, and in general keep the financial and personal affairs in good order.

If the patient has minor children, they have to set up a children's trust within your living trust to prevent the court from taking control of your property. The property in the trust goes to the children's trust, not to them individually and they will avoid probate.

Although there are standardized trust forms, an attorney is needed to make sure the living trust is prepared properly and to make any modifications to handle the patient's specific situation. Normally, a lawyer will charge somewhere between $500 and $1,000 to set up a living trust depending on the value of your property, special provisions and lawyer fees where you live. If your estate is worth more than $600,000 the patient will also need to talk with the lawyer about setting up a "common" trust to pass on up to $1.2 million tax free to their children.

Lawyers do not like living trusts because they cut off one of their most lucrative pieces of business—fees to the lawyer for probate. The patient can avoid all that expense with a living trust and the estate will save thousands of dollars.

It is not uncommon to have more than one living trust in a family. Each spouse may have a living trust for property owned before the marriage and a joint living trust for property acquired during the marriage. It can be an effective pre-nuptial agreement.

The patient would continue to file the same personal tax returns and does not need a separate tax identification number. The same Social Security number is used and there is no requirement to file a return on the living trust. The patient should change the beneficiaries on all life insurance to the trust.

Living trusts can be contested, but not as easily as a will. To contest a trust, the heirs must hire a lawyer and file civil suit. Because the property is not frozen, the trustee can distribute the property to the beneficiaries, thereby forcing the left out heirs to file suit against every beneficiary.

Decisions the patient will have to make:

- Who will take care of them if they become disabled.?
- Does the patient have special requests for medical care?
- Who does the patient want to give their property to when they die?
- How does the patient want children and step-children to share in their inheritance?
- Does the patient want to disinherit anyone?
- If the patient has minor children, who will manage their inheritance?
- Who shall be the children's guardian?
- When does the patient want the children to receive the inheritance?
- If everyone in the family dies, to whom does the patient want their property to go?
- If the patient has pets, who will take care of them?

A living trust takes effect as soon as it is established. Once the trust has been established, it is critical that all the assets are transferred to the trust or the work and cost of setting up the trust will be for nothing. There are a number of lawyers who specialize in trusts and will assist in the appropriate transfer of assets. Correctly transferring the assets can be a very time consuming and costly job for someone who has a large estate. Many lawyers can provide the asset transfer service and the cost of this service may well be worth it. It pays to check it out with the lawyer and try to get a complete package deal. Make sure that a written estimate of the cost is provided and insist that any changes to the estimate are to be made in writing.

A sample "Living Trust" is shown on the following two pages. We did not attach a sample of a Schedule A as it is only a listing of the property (assets) that the Grantor wants to put into the trust. Property would include such items as coin collections, automobiles, real estate, stocks, bonds, etc.

Sample

IRREVOCABLE LIVING TRUST
Joint Trustees (Husband & Wife)
for Benefit of their Adult Children
NOTE: This Agreement is intended only as a guideline. Consult an attorney for tax and/or legal issues that may apply to your specific caregiving situation.)

I, _____, as "Grantor" residing at _____,
City of _____, County of _____,
State of _____make this Living Trust Agreement with _____ and
_____ as "Trustees" dated this _____day of _____, 19_____.

1. **TRUST PROPERTY.** The Grantor, desiring to create trusts for the benefit of his adult children and for other good and valuable consideration, irrevocably assigns to the Trustees the property described in Schedule A, in trust, for the purposes and the conditions stated in this Agreement. (Schedule A is attached hereto.)

2. **BENEFICIARIES.** The Beneficiaries of the Trust are my two children, _____ and _____. The Trustees shall divide the trust property equally into two separate trust funds: the " _____ Trust" and the " _____ Trust." The Trustees shall hold, manage, and invest the trust property, and shall collect and receive the income thereof. The Trustees shall deduct all necessary expenses incident to the administration of these trusts and shall dispose of the corpus and income of the trusts as described in this Trust.

3. **TRUST UNTIL SPECIFIED AGE.**
   A. Until the Beneficiary reaches the age of _____ the Trustees shall pay the net income to or for the benefit of the Beneficiary at least annually.
   B. The Trustees may also pay to or for the benefit of the Beneficiary as much of the principal as the Trustees consider appropriate for any purpose.

4. **TERMINATION OF TRUST.** When the Beneficiary reaches the age of _____, the Trustees shall distribute the trust assets (including any undistributed income) to the Beneficiary.

5. **LIMITED POWER OF APPOINTMENT.** If the Beneficiary dies before reaching the age of _____, the trust for his or her benefit shall cease. The corpus, including any undistributed income, shall be paid to the Beneficiary's then living descendants, in equal share, per stirpes. If there are no descendants of the Beneficiary then living, the Trustees shall distribute the unappointed assets to the other Beneficiary, in trust, or if the Beneficiary has not attained the age of _____, to be added to, held, administered and distributed as part of the trust set apart for the other Beneficiary. If such other Beneficiary is not living, then to the living issue of such other Beneficiary in equal shares, per stirpes. If there is not such issue, then to the estate of the Beneficiary for who such trust was being held originally.

6. **PAYMENT TO PERSONS UNDER AGE 21.** If a Beneficiary (other than the Beneficiaries named in Section 2) entitled to receive any assets under this Agreement is under the age of 21, the Trustees may retain the assets in a separate trust. The Trustees may pay to or for the benefit of the beneficiary as much of the net income or principal as the Trustees see appropriate for any purpose. When the Beneficiary reaches age 21, the Trustees shall distribute the trust assets to the beneficiary. If the Beneficiary dies before reaching that age, the Trustees shall distribute the trust assets to the Beneficiary's estate.

7. **TRUSTEE PROVISIONS.**
A. *Trustees' Powers*
   In the administration of the trusts, the Trustees shall have the following powers, in addition to all other powers granted by law, all of which shall be exercised in a fiduciary capacity, primarily in the interest of the Beneficiaries:
   1. To hold as an investment the property received hereunder, and any additional property which may be received by them, so long as they deem proper, and to invest and reinvest in any securities or property, whether or not income-producing, deemed by them to be for the best interest of the trusts and the Beneficiaries.
   2. The Trustees shall not exercise any power that would cause trust income to be taxable to the Grantor or the trust assets to be taxable in my estate.
   3. The Trustees may borrow money for any purposes of the trusts that the Trustees consider to be in the best interests of the trusts and the beneficiaries. The Trustees may secure such borrowings with any assets of the trusts.
   4. Pay the ordinary and necessary expenses of administration, including (but not limited to) attorneys' fees, accountants' fees, and investment counselors' fees.
   5. To rent or lease any property of the trusts for such time and upon such terms as they deem just and proper and for the best interest of the trusts and beneficiaries hereunder, irrespective of any statute or the termination of any trust.
   6. To sell and convey any of the property of the trusts or any interest therein, or to exchange the same for other property, for such price and upon such terms as they deem in their discretion in the best interest of the trusts and the beneficiaries hereunder, and to execute and deliver any deed(s), receipts, releases, contracts or other instruments necessary in connection therewith.

7. To pay all taxes, insurance premiums and other legal charges that may be due by the trusts.

8. To vote, hold, redeem, sell or otherwise dispose of any securities belonging to the trusts, and to become a party to any stockholders' agreements deemed advisable by them in connection with such securities.

9. To consent to the reorganization, consolidation, merger, liquidation, readjustment of, or any other change in any business entity or association and any other act that may be permitted by any person owning similar property.

10. To settle, arbitrate or defend any claim or demand in favor of or against the trusts.

11. The powers granted in this Agreement to the Trustees shall be deemed supplementary to and not exclusive of the general powers of trustees pursuant to law, and shall include all powers necessary to carry this Agreement into effect.

8. SUCCESSOR TRUSTEES

A. Each of the Trustees shall have the power to appoint his or her successor Trustee. If either of the Trustees shall die, resign, become incapacitated, or refuse to act further as Trustee, without having appointed a successor Trustee, the other Trustee may, but is not required, appoint a successor Trustee. Any successor Trustee shall have all the duties and powers of the Trustees as specified in this Agreement, including the power in any successor trustee to appoint his or her own successor. The appointment of a successor Trustee shall be made, in writing, and delivered to the primary beneficiaries and to the remaining Trustee, if any. The appointment shall become effective upon the successor Trustee's written acceptance.

B. No Trustee serving under this Agreement shall be responsible for or required to inquire into any acts or omissions of a prior Trustee.

9. **COMPENSATION OF TRUSTEES.** The trustees waive the payment of any compensation for their services. However, this waiver shall not apply to any successor Trustee who qualifies and acts under this Agreement.

10. **IRREVOCABLE TRUST.** The trust shall be irrevocable. The Grantor expressly waives all rights and powers to alter, amend, revoke or terminate the trust, or any of the terms of this Agreement.

11. **ADDITIONAL CONTRIBUTIONS.** The Grantor reserves the right to himself and any other person, by deed or will, to add to the corpus of either or both of the trusts herein created. Any contributions so added shall be held, administered, and distributed as part of such trust(s).

12. **PROTECTION FROM CLAIMS.** To the extent permitted by law, the principal and income of any trust shall not be liable for the debts of any Beneficiary or subject to alienation or anticipation by a Beneficiary, except as otherwise noted.

13. **ADOPTION.** A person related by or through adoption shall take under this Agreement as if related by or through birth.

14. **GOVERNING LAW.** This Living Trust Agreement shall be governed by the laws of _____.

In witness whereof, the Grantor and the Trustees accept and execute this Irrevocable Living Trust Agreement in triplicate.

_____
Grantor and Trustee

_____
Trustee

State of _____)

_____) ss.

_____ of _____)

The foregoing instrument was acknowledged before me this _____ day of _____, 19_____

by _____ and _____.

                                                    _____
                                                    Notary Public

(SEAL)

My commission expires: _____, 19_____.

Will and Codicil to Will

A will is a legal document that states a person's wishes about the disposal of property after death. Wills have to be probated and probate costs usually run from 5% to 15% of the gross value of the estate. Probate is the process that determines if the will is valid in court and the process can be slow and expensive. Probate fees vary from state to state. Wills are not private because probate proceedings are a matter of public record.

When the patient creates a will, an executor must be appointed. Executors are sometimes called a "personal representative." The person the patient chooses should have some financial knowledge, understand bookkeeping, know how to keep records and be aware of the needs of the beneficiaries. The executor should also agree to perform the necessary duties. It is a good idea to name a back-up executor in case the original choice is incapacitated and unable to perform the needed tasks. The executor does not have to be a lawyer. The executor is allowed to charge a fee based upon the value of the estate. The amount the executor is allowed to charge varies from state to state.

The executor's duties can require a lot of time and if the estate is complex, it may be wise to hire a probate lawyer. The executor will need to:

- Take control of the assets that belonged to the decedent
- Protect the property against loss and harm
- Prepares and files the estate and income tax returns
- Present the will to the appropriate court
- Notify the beneficiaries
- Notify Social Security, pension plan, insurance company, banks, stock brokers
- Arrange for an appraisal of the assets
- Pay bills and collect any amounts due to the estate
- Distribute the estate's property to the heirs

A sample will and a sample codicil to will is shown on the next three pages. A codicil to will is a way to change the will without having to prepare a new one.

The will shown is intended for use by a married couple with children. In this sample will, the spouse distributes the estate to the other spouse, with the children named as alternate beneficiaries. It is best to consult a lawyer for the drafting of a will that will be best for your particular circumstances.

Power of Attorney

The power of attorney *does not* replace a will. The power of attorney automatically terminates upon the death of the declarant. A will is used for handling the affairs of the patient after the patient dies.

Power of Attorney is a document that authorizes another person to act as your agent or attorney. An example would be to give your accountant your power of attorney to negotiate with the IRS on a tax matter.

Sample

WILL

I, _____, of _____, State of _____,
(Name of Testator/Testatrix)   *(City or County Name)*

make this will and revoke all my earlier wills and codicils.

My spouse is _____. I have _____ children living on the date of this will.
Their names are _____

_____

_____.

Article I
DISTRIBUTION OF ESTATE

A. *Tangible Personal Property.* I give my household furnishings, personal effects, automobiles, and all other tangible personal property to my spouse, if he/she survives me. If my spouse does not survive me, I give this property in equal shares to my children who survive me and the descendants who survive me, per stirpes, of my children who do not survive me.

B. *Remaining Estate.* I give the residue of my real and personal estate to my spouse, if he/she survives me. If my spouse does not survive me, I give the residue in equal shares to my children who survive me and the descendants who survive me, per stirpes, of my children who do not survive me.

Article II
TRUST FOR A BENEFICIARY UNDER AGE

If a beneficiary entitled to receive any assets of my estate is under the age of _____, my Executor may transfer the assets to my Trustee to be held in a separate trust. My Trustee may pay to or for the benefit of the beneficiary as much of the net income or principal as my Trustee considers appropriate for any purpose. When the beneficiary reaches the age of _____, my Trustee
(Insert Same Age as Above)
shall distribute the trust assets to the beneficiary. If the beneficiary dies before reaching that age, my Trustee shall distribute the trust assets to the beneficiary's estate.

Article III
PAYMENT OF DEBTS AND EXPENSES

A. *Debts and Funeral Expenses.* My Executor shall pay or arrange for the payment of my legally enforceable debts, my charitable pledges, and the expenses of my funeral and burial (including any headstone or marker). My Executor shall not seek contribution from my spouse toward the payment of our joint debts. If my spouse wishes to retain any residence or other real property subject to a mortgage or similar indebtedness and so advises my Executor in writing within three months after my death, my Executor may elect not to pay the indebtedness.

B. *Taxes.* My Executor shall pay or arrange for the payment of all estate, inheritance, and similar taxes payable by reason of my death as a cost of administering my estate without apportionment. This includes taxes on assets not passing undue this will and interest on taxes.

Article IV
EXECUTOR AND TRUSTEE

A. *Executor and Trustee.* I nominate and appoint the _____ Bank, of _____, State of _____ as Executor and Trustee and request that no bond or security be required. The _____ Bank shall receive for its services the compensation specified in its published fee schedule in effect at the time it renders it services, and its compensation may vary from time to time based on that schedule.

B. *Executors and Trustee's Management Power.* My Executor and Trustee may borrow money for any purpose that my Executor or Trustee considers to be in the best interests of my estate or any trust. My Executor or Trustee may secure such borrowings with assets of my estate or trust.

C. *Certain Investments.* I may hold assets at my death that would not meet the standard in the State of _____ as suitable investments to be held by my Executor or Trustee. My Executor and Trustee may nevertheless retain the assets for as long as my Executor or Trustee considers appropriate even if the assets represent an over concentration or do not meet the standard of prudence. My Executor or Trustee may invest the assets of my estate or any trust in money market funds or other mutual funds affiliated with my Executor or Trustee. The compensation of my Executor or its affiliate from the fund shall not reduce the compensation of my Executor or Trustee under this will.

Article V
GUARDIANS

If my spouse cannot serve, I name _____, or either of them, to be guardians of

(Names of Guardians)

the person of my minor children. If they both fail or cease to serve, I name _____,

(Names of Successor Guardians)

or either of them, to be guardians of the person of my minor children. I request that no security be required of any guardian.

Article VI
MISCELLANEOUS PROVISIONS

A. *Protection from Claims.* To the extent permitted by law, the principal and income of any trust shall not be liable for the debts of any beneficiary or subject to alienation or anticipation by a beneficiary, except as otherwise provided.

B. *Adoption.* A person related by or through adoption shall take under my will as if related by or through birth.

C. *Consolidation of Trusts.* My Trustee may consolidate for administrative purposes any trust with any other trust having the same trustee and substantially the same dispositive provisions.

I have signed and sealed my will consisting of _____ typewritten pages on this _____ day of _____, 19_____.

_____

(Name of Testator)

The testator signed, published and declared this as the testator's will in our presence on the date shown above. At the testator's request, and in the presence of the testator and each other, we have signed our names as witnesses.

_____   Address: _____
Witness   _____
                                                                    _____

_____   Address: _____
Witness   _____
                                                                    _____

_____   Address: _____
Witness   _____
                                                                    _____

Sample

CODICIL TO WILL

I, _____, of _____,
(Name of Testator/Testatrix)   *(City or County Name)*

State of _____ this codicil to my will that was signed on _____, 19_____.

1. _____

_____

_____

2. Except as changed by this codicil, I confirm, ratify, and republish my will and all prior codicils. *(Note: if this is the first codicil to the will and there are no other previous codicils, delete the phrase "all prior codicils.")*

I have signed and sealed this codicil to my will consisting of _____ typewritten pages on this _____ day of _____, 19_____.

_____
(Name of Testator/Testatrix)

The testator/testatrix signed, published and declared this as a codicil to the will in our presence on the date shown above. At the testator's/testatrix's request, and in the presence of the testator/testatrix and each other, we have signed our names as witnesses.

_____ Address: _____
Witness   _____
                                            _____

_____ Address: _____
Witness   _____
                                            _____

_____ Address: _____
Witness   _____
                                            _____

LeBoeuf's
Home Healthcare
Handbook

Personal & Family Information

The New Baby

BY ANNE KEITH

We must collect, remember, put away
   The precious things,
The words that turn a picture on,
The sights that must be fashioned
   Into words,
The smells that tantalize
   with hints of a forgotten day.
Remember now, before she grows
How small and warm the row of toes
   Felt in the hand
And her hands folded
   With a dancer's grace.
Remember too the curve of brow
   To tiny nose
And sleek warm cap of hair.
The first words too
From that short time
Before our language is imposed.
Holding our breath, we watch her grow,
Remembering to remember
   What we can.

Personal Information

HAVING THE PATIENT'S PERSONAL PAPERS IN ORDER will save much time and aggravation. It can be exasperating and expensive to obtain a court order to handle the patient's personal affairs when advance planning can avoid time-consuming, frustrating and expensive legal intervention.

The following personal information forms should be filled out as soon as possible after your loved one has moved in with you.

Personal Data

FULL LEGAL NAME

Current Address:

Legal Address:

Home Telephone: Work Telephone: Fax Number: E-Mail Address:

Occupation:

Business Name

Business Address

Business Tax ID Number: Federal   State

Social Security Number: Date of Birth: Place of Birth

Veterans Administration Number: Military Service Number:

FATHER'S NAME: Father's Date of Birth: Father's Place of Birth:

Father's Current Address:

Home Telephone: Work Telephone: Fax Number: E-Mail Address:

MOTHER'S NAME: Mother's Date of Birth: Mother's Place of Birth:

Mother's Current Address:

Home Telephone: Work Telephone: Fax Number: E-Mail Address:

SPOUSE'S NAME: Maiden Name (if applicable)   Spouse's Date of Birth: Spouse's Place of Birth:

Spouse's Occupation: Employer:

Name Spouse's Father: Name Spouse's Mother:

DATE AND PLACE OF MARRIAGE:

Married By:

Prior Marriages: Name of Spouse   Date of Divorce:

                         Name of Spouse: Date of Divorce

Education:

Elementary School:	Years Attended	City/State
Elementary School:	Years Attended:	City/State
High School:	Graduation Date:	City/State
High School:	Graduation Date:	City/State
College:	Degree	City/State
College:	Degree	City/State
College:	Degree	City/State

Religion:

| Religious Affiliation: | Name of Church or Synagogue: |
| Names of Clergy: | Telephone: |

Memberships:

Organization:	Telephone:
Organization:	Telephone:
Organization:	Telephone:
Organization:	Telephone:
Organization:	Telephone:
Organization:	Telephone:
Organization:	Telephone:

Awards and Special Recognition:

Children:

CHILD'S NAME: | Date of Birth: | Place of Birth

Current Address:

Home Telephone: | Work Telephone: | Fax Number: | E-Mail Address:

CHILD'S NAME: | Date of Birth: | Place of Birth

Current Address:

Home Telephone: | Work Telephone: | Fax Number: | E-Mail Address:

CHILD'S NAME: | Date of Birth: | Place of Birth

Current Address:

Home Telephone: | Work Telephone: | Fax Number: | E-Mail Address:

CHILD'S NAME: | Date of Birth: | Place of Birth

Current Address:

Home Telephone: | Work Telephone: | Fax Number: | E-Mail Address:

CHILD'S NAME: | Date of Birth: | Place of Birth

Current Address:

Home Telephone: | Work Telephone: | Fax Number: | E-Mail Address:

CHILD'S NAME: | Date of Birth: | Place of Birth

Current Address:

Home Telephone: | Work Telephone: | Fax Number: | E-Mail Address:

CHILD'S NAME: | Date of Birth: | Place of Birth

Current Address:

Home Telephone: | Work Telephone: | Fax Number: | E-Mail Address:

CHILD'S NAME: | Date of Birth: | Place of Birth

Current Address:

Home Telephone: | Work Telephone: | Fax Number: | E-Mail Address:

CHILD'S NAME: | Date of Birth: | Place of Birth

Current Address:

Home Telephone: | Work Telephone: | Fax Number: | E-Mail Address:

Other Next of Kin:

NAME:	Date of Birth:	Relationship:

Current Address:

Home Telephone:	Work Telephone:	Fax Number:	E-Mail Address:

NAME:	Date of Birth:	Relationship:

Current Address:

Home Telephone:	Work Telephone:	Fax Number:	E-Mail Address:

NAME:	Date of Birth:	Relationship:

Current Address:

Home Telephone:	Work Telephone:	Fax Number:	E-Mail Address:

NAME:	Date of Birth:	Relationship:

Current Address:

Home Telephone:	Work Telephone:	Fax Number:	E-Mail Address:

NAME:	Date of Birth:	Relationship:

Current Address:

Home Telephone:	Work Telephone:	Fax Number:	E-Mail Address:

NAME:	Date of Birth:	Relationship:

Current Address:

Home Telephone:	Work Telephone:	Fax Number:	E-Mail Address:

NAME:	Date of Birth:	Relationship:

Current Address:

Home Telephone:	Work Telephone:	Fax Number:	E-Mail Address:

NAME:	Date of Birth:	Relationship:

Current Address:

Home Telephone:	Work Telephone:	Fax Number:	E-Mail Address:

NAME:	Date of Birth:	Relationship:

Current Address:

Home Telephone:	Work Telephone:	Fax Number:	E-Mail Address:

Document Locator

It is important that all documents, keys and other information is accounted for. If you are unable to locate any of the papers or keys, mark the list and plan on researching or replacing the documents and keys as soon as you can. It may take you weeks, if not months, to locate everything, but if you work at it, the task will eventually be completed. As you find the documents, it will prove most helpful to read them. Have them revised if they are out of date. If documents are stored at a bank, you must obtain a signature card so that you can get to the documents. If the documents are stored in the home, it is a good idea to buy a fire resistant lock box or fire resistant safe for the most important documents. Take some of the document folders (not the documents) with you when you buy a lock box or safe to be sure the documents will fit inside. Make sure that you know where the key is located or the combination of the safe or both. Obviously, if the patient does not have a living will, durable power of attorney or a living trust, you must convince the patient that this should be done right away.

If you have any questions, please do not hesitate to call **LeBoeuf's** at ☎ 1-800-546-5559.

Document	*Location*
Abstracts	
Adoption Papers	
Automobile Titles and Registrations	
Awards	
Baptismal Certificate	
Bills of Sale	
Birth Certificate	
Bonds	
Burial Instructions	
Certificates of Deposit	
Citizenship Papers	
Collections:	
Stamp	
Coin	
Other	
Deed to Burial Plot	
Deeds to Real Property	
Diplomas (Transcripts)	
Divorce Papers	
Durable Power of Attorney	
Employment Records	
Financial Records	
Health Care Power of Attorney	
Income Tax Returns	
Insurance Policies	
Disability	
Health	
Home	
Life	
Long-Term Care	
Liability	
Auto	
IRA's	

Document	Location
Keys:	
House	_____
Auto	_____
Rental Properties	_____
Summer Home	_____
Other	_____
Leases:	
Auto	_____
Equipment	_____
Real Estate	_____
Legal Agreements	_____
Living Trust	_____
Living Will	_____
Marriage Certificate	_____
Medical Records	_____
Medicare Card	_____
Medicaid Card	_____
Military Discharge Papers	_____
Mutual Fund Records	_____
Notes Due to Others	_____
Notes Due to You	_____
Naturalization Papers	_____
Other Tax Records	_____
Passport	_____
Pension Records	_____
Personal Property Inventory	_____
Pre-Nuptial Agreement	_____
Property Tax Receipts	_____
Rental Agreements	_____
Safe Deposit Boxes (Number)	_____
Where keys are kept	_____
Name of authorized user (telephone)	_____
Social Security Records	_____
Stock Certificates	_____
Title Policies	_____
Trust Documents	_____
Unclaimed Lottery Tickets	_____
Will (Spouse)	_____
Will (Yours)	_____
Will (Patient)	_____

While it is not necessary that the caregiver be in possession of all these documents, they should be easily located and safely stored.

Medical Information

PATIENT'S NAME: _____ | Blood Type: _____

Medical Conditions:

_____

_____

_____

_____

_____

_____

_____

_____

_____

_____

_____

_____

_____

_____

_____

_____

_____

_____

_____

_____

_____

_____

_____

_____

PRESCRIPTION MEDICINES

■ PRESCRIPTION NAME | Prescription Number

Doctor's Name & Telephone Number | Pharmacy Name & Telephone Number

Special Instructions

■ PRESCRIPTION NAME | Prescription Number

Doctor's Name & Telephone Number | Pharmacy Name & Telephone Number

Special Instructions

■ PRESCRIPTION NAME | Prescription Number

Doctor's Name & Telephone Number | Pharmacy Name & Telephone Number

Special Instructions

■ PRESCRIPTION NAME | Prescription Number

Doctor's Name & Telephone Number | Pharmacy Name & Telephone Number

Special Instructions

■ PRESCRIPTION NAME | Prescription Number

Doctor's Name & Telephone Number | Pharmacy Name & Telephone Number

Special Instructions

■ PRESCRIPTION NAME | Prescription Number

Doctor's Name & Telephone Number | Pharmacy Name & Telephone Number

Special Instructions

■ PRESCRIPTION NAME | Prescription Number

Doctor's Name & Telephone Number | Pharmacy Name & Telephone Number

Special Instructions

HEALTH CARE PROVIDERS

▶ PRIMARY CARE PHYSICIAN | Telephone

Address

▶ SPECIALIST | Telephone

Address

▶ SPECIALIST | Telephone

Address

▶ SPECIALIST | Telephone

Address

▶ ALLERGIST | Telephone

Address

▶ CHIROPRACTOR | Telephone

Address

▶ DENTIST | Telephone

Address

▶ DERMATOLOGIST | Telephone

Address

▶ DIALYSIS | Telephone

Address

▶ EYE DOCTOR | Telephone

Address

▶ PHYSICAL THERAPIST | Telephone

Address

▶ SURGEON | Telephone

Address

▶ VISITING NURSE | Telephone

Address

▶ NURSE'S AIDE | Telephone

Address

▶ HOSPICE NURSE | Telephone

Address

▶ OTHER HEALTH CARE PROFESSIONAL | Telephone

Address

▶ OTHER HEALTH CARE PROFESSIONAL | Telephone

HEALTH CARE FACILITIES

▶ HOSPITAL | Telephone

Address

▶ CLINIC | Telephone

Address

HEALTH CARE INSURANCE

▶ INSURANCE COMPANY & AGENT | Telephone

Address

▶ INSURANCE COMPANY & AGENT | Telephone

Address

TRANSPORTATION SERVICES

▶ PRIVATE AMBULANCE | Telephone

Address

▶ TAXI | Telephone

Address

Keep a list of doctor visits, hospitalizations, dentist and eye exams and the information on each visit.

Date	Doctor's Name	Reason for Visit	Diagnosis	Treatment	Prescription	Instructions for Patient Care and Medication Schedules

Family History

And above all things have fervent charity among yourselves: for charity shall cover the multitude of sins.

1 Peter 4:8

Love (God's love in us) takes no account of the evil done to it – pays not attention to a suffered wrong.

1 Cor 13:5

God grant me the serenity to accept the things I cannot change, the courage to change the things I can, and the wisdom to know the difference.

Serenity Prayer

As a way to preserve the history of the family the following questionnaire has been prepared. It will take a bit of effort and time but it is an opportunity for the family to share in the good times as well as the bad times. You and the patient will find that talking about the history of the family will provide an outlet for any repressed anger, generate an understanding of the depth of their relationships with other family members and allow all family members a chance to understand why events happened as they did.

Time does not heal all wounds. In many families there are unresolved conflicts that have divided family members for years. Talking about the problems can lead to reconciliation. Sometimes you only have to say, "I'm sorry."

There is tremendous power in the forgiveness you and the patient can share. You need to open up and reveal feelings, problems and misunderstandings. If you communicate acceptance, the patient will respond. In the long run, acceptance does not mean that you approve of the actions, it means that you accept them in spite of their faults. To be successful in reaching out, you must learn to listen. Listen carefully and do not be quick to speak. Only by listening to the whole story will you be able to understand what the patient is trying to communicate.

By learning what organizations were important to the patient during their healthy active years, the caregiver and the family will be able to discuss with the patient the possibility of reestablishing contacts. It may be that some of the organizations have programs for older members that will provide some respite care for the caregiver or activities that the patient would enjoy.

Information can also be used to provide additional outreach to those family members who have not been in contact for many years. Sometimes all it takes is a call or a letter.

Personal Data

FULL LEGAL NAME

Current Address:

Legal Address:

| Home Telephone: | Work Telephone: | Fax Number: | E-Mail Address: |

Occupation:

Business Name

Business Address

| Business Tax ID Number: | Federal | State |

| Social Security Number: | Date of Birth: | Place of Birth |

| Veterans Administration Number: | Military Service Number: |

| FATHER'S NAME: | Father's Date of Birth: | Father's Place of Birth: |

Father's Current Address:

| IIome Telephone: | Work Telephone: | Fax Number: | E-Mail Address: |

| MOTHER'S NAME: | Mother's Date of Birth: | Mother's Place of Birth: |

Mother's Current Address:

| Home Telephone: | Work Telephone: | Fax Number: | E-Mail Address: |

| SPOUSE'S NAME: | Maiden Name (if applicable) | Spouse's Date of Birth: | Spouse's Place of Birth: |

| Spouse's Occupation: | Employer: |

| Name Spouse's Father: | Name Spouse's Mother: |

DATE AND PLACE OF MARRIAGE:

Married By:

| Prior Marriages: | Name of Spouse | Date of Divorce: |
| | Name of Spouse: | Date of Divorce |

Places Lived

ADDRESS:

City/State/Zip   Years:

ADDRESS:

City/State/Zip   Years:

ADDRESS:

City/State/Zip   Years:

ADDRESS:

City/State/Zip   Years:

ADDRESS:

City/State/Zip   Years:

ADDRESS:

City/State/Zip   Years:

Places Worked:

BUSINESS NAME & ADDRESS: Years

Occupation: Position:

BUSINESS NAME & ADDRESS: Years

Occupation: Position:

BUSINESS NAME & ADDRESS: Years

Occupation: Position:

BUSINESS NAME & ADDRESS: Years

Occupation: Position:

BUSINESS NAME & ADDRESS: Years

Occupation: Position:

BUSINESS NAME & ADDRESS: Years

Occupation: Position:

BUSINESS NAME & ADDRESS: Years

Occupation: Position:

Husband's Side of the Family:

HUSBAND'S FATHER:	Birth Date:	Place of Birth
Address:		Telephone
Husband's Paternal Grandfather:	Birth Date:	Place of Birth
Address:		Telephone
Husband's Paternal Grandmother (Maiden Name):	Birth Date:	Place of Birth
Address:		Telephone
HUSBAND'S MOTHER (Maiden Name):	Birth Date:	Place of Birth
Address:		Telephone
Husband's Maternal Grandfather:	Birth Date:	Place of Birth
Address:		Telephone
Husband's Maternal Grandmother (Maiden Name):	Birth Date:	Place of Birth
Address:		Telephone

Wife's Side of the Family:

WIFE'S FATHER:	Birth Date:	Place of Birth
Address:		Telephone
Wife's Paternal Grandfather:	Birth Date:	Place of Birth
Address:		Telephone
Wife's Paternal Grandmother (Maiden Name):	Birth Date:	Place of Birth
WIFE'S MOTHER (Maiden Name):	Birth Date:	Place of Birth
Address:		Telephone
Wife's Maternal Grandfather:	Birth Date:	Place of Birth
Address:		Telephone
Wife's Maternal Grandmother (Maiden Name):	Birth Date:	Place of Birth
Address:		Telephone

Children:

CHILD'S NAME:	Birth Date:	Place of Birth
Address:		Telephone
Spouse's Name:	Birth Date:	Place of Birth:
Grandchild's Name:	Birth Date:	Place of Birth:
Grandchild's Name:	Birth Date:	Place of Birth:
Grandchild's Name:	Birth Date:	Place of Birth:
CHILD'S NAME:	Birth Date:	Place of Birth
Address:		Telephone
Spouse's Name:	Birth Date:	Place of Birth:
Grandchild's Name:	Birth Date:	Place of Birth:
Grandchild's Name:	Birth Date:	Place of Birth:
Grandchild's Name:	Birth Date:	Place of Birth:
CHILD'S NAME:	Birth Date:	Place of Birth
Address:		Telephone
Spouse's Name:	Birth Date:	Place of Birth:
Grandchild's Name:	Birth Date:	Place of Birth:
Grandchild's Name:	Birth Date:	Place of Birth:
Grandchild's Name:	Birth Date:	Place of Birth:
CHILD'S NAME:	Birth Date:	Place of Birth
Address:		Telephone
Spouse's Name:	Birth Date:	Place of Birth:
Grandchild's Name:	Birth Date:	Place of Birth:
Grandchild's Name:	Birth Date:	Place of Birth:
Grandchild's Name:	Birth Date:	Place of Birth:

LeBoeuf's
Home Healthcare
Handbook

Healthcare Services & Providers

The Acorn Grinders

BY ANNE KEITH

We stood in spring grass
Round the rock's great face,
Four solemn moderns
Trying to evoke the past,
Gazing intently
At those cups worn smooth
Like dimples in the stone's hard skin.
But then you laughed and said,
"Oh, how they must have gossiped here!"

That did the trick.

My mind fell backward.
Knocked off balance by your words,
It tumbled to another age.
I saw the seven women grinding meal.
The bride was silent at her smaller cup.
The older women, laughing,
      rocked with life,
Their legs sprawled outward
      on the sun-warmed rock,
Some squatting like brown frogs
      to do their work.
So for a spark of time
I lived and saw those women
      from another age.
The veil was torn,
And for an instant I was one of them.

Home Healthcare Agencies

THERE ARE APPROXIMATELY 12,000 home healthcare agencies in the United States providing services for patients in the home. Approximately 7,800 of the agencies are certified to provide Medicare and Medicaid services. However, just because a home health care agency is not certified by Medicare does not mean that it cannot provide services. Some states will pay less than Medicare or Medicaid rates for unlicensed or uncertified providers. In many cases, the services provided by the unlicensed or uncertified providers are no different from those provided by licensed agencies.

Services provided by most home healthcare agencies include:

- Private duty nursing
- Nutrition counseling
- Infusion therapy
- Physical therapy
- Diabetic care
- AIDS care
- Speech therapy
- Post medical and surgery care
- Pain management
- Psychiatric care
- Bereavement counseling
- Enterostomal therapy
- General health education
- Cardiopulmonary care
- Home health aides
- Homemaker services
- Pharmaceuticals
- Durable medical equipment
- Social workers

Interestingly, in a recent study the conclusion was reached that home care patients have fewer hospital and nursing home admissions, shorter lengths of stay, fewer outpatient visits, more positive attitudes and more satisfaction with respect to their perceived health. It was also found that home healthcare was less expensive, even with intensive home nursing services for those who were seriously ill. Patient satisfaction was higher for those being cared for in the home than those patients being treated in a hospital.

Each home healthcare agency survives and continues in business only by providing good care. It is in the best interest of the healthcare agency to continually stress quality and continuing education to keep up with, or stay ahead of, their competition. Each agency competes with other agencies for patients. However, costs for providing services can be high and without Medicare or Medicaid, most families cannot afford the service.

Almost all Medicare certified home healthcare agencies provide skilled nursing care by a registered nurse (RN). There are also licensed practical nurses (LPN's), licensed vocational nurses (LVN's), nurses aides (NA's) and home health care aides (HHA's).

The minimum standards established by the Omnibus Budget Reconciliation Act of 1987 (P.L. 100-203) established the following requirements for home healthcare certification by Medicare:

- Patient "Bill of Rights" to know and understand all procedures, charges, services, etc. supplied by the provider
- Established minimum training requirements for home health care aides
- Random oversight of each provider program by Medicare (at least once every 15 months)
- Stronger enforcement tools
- Hotline for making complaints

Home healthcare agencies can only be reimbursed by Medicare for services provided by home healthcare aides who have received formal training. Under Medicare, the aides can perform personal care such as bathing, feeding, simple treatments, planning and preparing meals and assisting with self-administered medications. Agencies will not be reimbursed for homemaking services such as cooking, cleaning, running errands, baby-sitting, etc.

Over 39 states have licensing programs for home healthcare agencies and there is a great deal of pressure to have the remaining states establish similar licensing requirements. State or federal licensing does not necessarily assure quality of service; it merely determines if the agencies and their staff meet minimum training requirements.

It is important to make sure that the agency providing services in the home is qualified, certified, trustworthy and registered with either Medicare and/or the state. Registration serves two primary purposes:

- Reimbursement, if covered, by Medicare or Medicaid for services provided by the agency
- Assurance that the person providing the service is appropriately trained

If an agency is not certified by Medicare, ask if the state will pay for the healthcare service under a state plan. Some states have their own Medicare/Medicaid type healthcare program and will pay for the services of a non-certified (Medicare, Medicaid) healthcare provider.

You and the patient are not required to have any one healthcare agency. You and the patient can find out about the various agencies by asking the doctor, the staff at the hospital, other patients, friends, social agencies or LeBoeuf's. Most home healthcare agencies offer their services 24 hours a day, seven days a week.

LeBoeuf's ☎ 1-800-546-5559 can provide you with a listing of all home healthcare agencies in your area that meet the "Conditions of Participation" for certification by Medicare.

Make copies of the check list and use one for each agency interviewed.

Name of Agency:

_____

Telephone number:

_____

Address:

_____

_____

Date evaluated:

_____

Person interviewed:

_____

Notes:

_____

_____

_____

_____

_____

_____

_____

_____

_____

_____

Home Healthcare Agency Evaluation Check List

- Are they certified by Medicare?
- Are they licensed by the state?
- Do they have written personalized care plan for the patient?
- Do they have written financial arrangements with all parties?
- 24 hour/7 days a week support and supervision?
- What type of training does the agency provide for their employees?
- Are the employees certified or do they have minimum experience requirements?
- What quality control checks are in place?
- Does the doctor know and recommend the agency?
- How long has the agency been in business?
- Does the agency respect confidentiality?
- Does the agency provide written and oral information with respect to services provided and the amount you will have to pay?
- Does the agency publish a fee schedule?
- Is there a clear understanding of who will provide what services? For example: a Home Health Aide may be all that is needed to provide the care and the rate is about half the skilled nursing rate.
- Does the Better Business Bureau have any complaints about the agency?
- Does the agency check employee backgrounds (credit, previous employment and criminal records)?
- Are your questions answered in a professional and respectful manner?
- Will the agency provide insurance services with respect to billings, questions and concerns?
- Does the agency have written, video and/or audio materials to help train the caregiver?
- Does the agency have insurance (malpractice and workmen's compensation)?
- Does the agency have a written personnel policy?
- What emergency plans does the agency have?
- Is there free in-home consultation before the start of services?
- Does training of personnel cover the situation with which you are faced— such as Alzheimer's disease?
- Do the employees have reliable transportation?
- Are personnel files updated annually?
- Is there a list of references available? (Be sure to check them out!!)
- Are the employees bonded and insured?
- Does the agency have emergency prescription service? Will they deliver?

Nursing Care

Almost all Medicare-certified home health care agencies provide skilled nursing care by a registered nurse (RN). There are also licensed practical nurses (LPNs), licensed vocational nurses (LVNs), nurses aides (NAs), certified nurses aids (CNAs) and home health care aides (HHAs).

The nurse's role in home health care is that of a leader, manager, researcher, record keeper and friend to both the caregiver and the patient. In many home care situations, the nurse becomes part of the family. Nurses respect the dignity of the patient and the caregiver and do everything they can to enhance self-esteem. Probably the best phrase that will describe the nurses role in making the patient and caregiver feel good about themselves is, "Never a discouraging word."

Every patient is different and every situation is different. The nurse will develop a strategy to ensure that the patient is involved, preserve the patient's natural defenses, prevent complications such as pressure ulcers, provide for patient comfort and support, and make sure that all nursing activities are carefully implemented.

In addition, the nurse is the primary:

Communicator

The nurse communicates with other health care personnel, including doctors, and is the primary link between the caregiver, the patient and the doctor. Based upon the care plan developed by the patient's doctor, nurse, patient and caregiver, the nurse will write the procedures and record the results and status of the patient. The nurse is the main communicator between the patient and other health care personnel in most home care situations. The nurse will also be the patient's guardian by questioning any procedures and medications that appear to be ambiguous and a departure from acceptable practice.

Teacher

The nurse will be the primary person who helps both the patient and the caregiver learn what the care objectives are and how to perform the tasks necessary to ensure successful caregiving.

Counselor

The nurse will help the patient and the caregiver to recognize and cope with the stress of caregiving. The nurse will provide emotional support and show how to develop a sense of control over the situation to both the patient and the caregiver.

Advocate

The nurse will help the patient and the caregiver by calling on any and all assistance they believe necessary to protect the patient's health. The nurse will recognize the effect that changes in the patient's condition will have on others and balance that recognition with what the patient actually requires.

In the initial interview, the nurse will spend time with both the caregiver and the patient to gather data. The nurse will ask for the patient's name, birth date, height, weight, allergies, previous health problems and:

- Patient's understanding of the care plan
- Nutrition
- Bowel, bladder and skin problems
- Exercise
- Hearing, sight and other sensory problems
- Sleep patterns
- State of patient and caregiver with respect to stress, relationships (especially family) and actual physical ability of the caregiver and patient to cope with the situation.
- Sexuality
- Values, including spiritual

The nurse will help the caregiver make a list of the equipment and supplies that will be needed to assist and support the patient in the caregiver's home.

Certified Nursing Assistants

Most home care agencies can provide certified nursing assistants (CNAs) to help with the patient's personal needs. Most states will *not* allow CNAs to:

- Cut hair, but may shampoo
- Clip fingernails or toenails
- Give an enema or suppository
- Pour or take medications out of a bottle and give to the patient. If you need to leave the house, pour or take the medication out and leave it for the CNA to hand to the patient.
- Give an injection
- Change settings on oxygen equipment
- Insert or irrigate a urinary catheter
- Change any sterile dressing
- Suction the patient.

If the above tasks are needed, the nurse will teach you how to do it. It is a good idea to have more than one person in the family learn to perform those tasks that need to be attended to every day. In other words, train some backup. If you have to hire help, they should also be trained to assist the patient.

Nursing Homes

Nursing homes are divided into two kinds:

- *Skilled Nursing Care facilities are for those patients who need around-the-clock nursing care by a registered nurse, doctor and/or therapy.*

- *Nursing Facility Care is for those patients who need around-the-clock supervision and direction by registered nurses and/or doctors but do not need the care on a daily basis.*

THERE ARE ABOUT 1.5 MILLION PEOPLE in nursing homes in the United States — about five percent of the older population. Over two-thirds of the patients in nursing homes are women. About 30 percent of all people can expect to spend some time in a nursing home. There are about 25,000 nursing homes in the United States.

The level of care is determined by the doctor. Many states also require pre-screening by a social agency to determine the type of care needed by the patient. Check with the nursing home, or with the local social service agency, to determine whether or not your state has this requirement.

Today's nursing homes are greatly improved and more accommodating to the needs of patients than in the past. However, most people still prefer to remain in their own homes as long as possible. There are a wide variety of choices available in the types of nursing homes. From facilities that provide day care programs and respite care to nursing homes that provide around-the-clock nursing care.

When home care is no longer feasible in order to provide the best physical and emotional care without undue stress, nursing homes remain the best alternative. Nursing homes offer much more than just nursing. Most nursing homes today offer medical, pharmacy, recreation, dietary and social services. In addition, many also offer rehabilitation, occupational and physical therapy and speech therapy.

Each state has an ombudsman with the Office on Aging. They act as referee when there are complaints from patients or their families about a nursing home. If you are having a problem with a nursing home, contact us for the telephone number and address of your state's Long Term Care Ombudsman Office.

The Social Security Administration is also a good source of information about nursing homes and has information on all nursing homes licensed by Medicare. Ask to look at the state survey that all nursing homes participating in the Medicare program must complete each year.

Nursing homes can also be grouped as follows:

- **Residential Care Facilities** provide room and board and may offer social, recreational and spiritual programs.

- **Continuing Care Facilities**, a new concept that insures all needs of the patient are met — including health care, room and board and social activities.

- **Assisted Living Facilities** are probably the best choice if the patient is generally ambulatory and include retirement homes as well as board and care homes. Services can include meals, recreation, security, assistance with walking, bathing and dressing.

- **Skilled Nursing Facilities** are the best choice for those patients who require 24-hour medical care and supervision. Emphasis is on medical care and rehabilitative therapy to improve or maintain abilities.

Make copies of the check list and use one for each nursing home checked.

Name of Nursing Home:

_____

Telephone number:

_____

Address:

_____

_____

Date evaluated:

_____

Person interviewed:

_____

Notes:

_____
_____
_____
_____
_____
_____
_____
_____
_____
_____
_____

Selecting the Right Nursing Home

Before placing a patient in a nursing home, you must first assess the level of care that the patient will require. Normally, the doctor, the nurse, and possibly a social worker, form a team to provide the caregiver with support and guidance in finding the right nursing home for the patient. The transition from a home setting to a nursing home takes time to adjust to and can be very difficult for both the patient and the caregiver.

Choosing the right nursing home includes checking the following:

Nursing Home Credentials

- Look in the yellow pages, talk with friends and family, with your doctor or a social services agency. Hospitals and state departments of health are good sources as well.
- Visit the home with the patient and, if at all possible, visit several times during different shifts. Talk with other families visiting the home and find out if they have had any problems with the staff or the facilities.
- Make sure the home has a current state license.
- Is the nursing home certified for Medicare and Medicaid programs?

Resident Care

- Are the current residents of the nursing home well cared for and content?
- Are most of the patients out of bed and dressed?
- Can patients wear their own clothes and have some of their own furniture in their room?
- Is there a statement of patient's rights posted?
- Will the nursing home provide special care for Alzheimer's patients?
- Will the patient receive mail unopened?
- What is the noise level?
- Will the nursing home allow the patient to be treated by a doctor of their choice?

Facility Amenities

- Is the atmosphere warm and pleasant?
- Is the nursing home accessible to family and friends?
- Do rooms provide privacy? Is there a locker or a drawer that can be locked in each room?
- Is there an activity room?
- Is the nursing home clean, orderly and free of unpleasant odors?
- Are toilet and bathing facilities accessible to disabled patients?
- Are there grab rails, handrails and call buttons in the rooms and halls?
- Is the nursing home equipped with smoke detectors, sprinkler systems and emergency lighting? Does the home hold regular fire drills?

The National Institute for Nursing Research states that the most common cause of death in nursing homes is infection. It would be prudent to ask the nursing home what infection control programs are in place to reduce institution-acquired infections. Because of the frequent movement of patients between hospitals, nursing homes and home, a good infection control program is essential.

- Does the home have a security system to keep patients from wandering out of the building?
- Are there phones in the patient's rooms? If not, are there telephones that the patient can use privately?
- What is the nursing home's policy on using physical and chemical restraints?
- What is the nursing home's bedsore incident rate?
- What is the staff's reaction to a patient with toilet distress? How long before they help the patient?
- Can the room be reserved if the patient is transferred to a hospital? If so, for how long?
- What type of laundry service does the nursing home provide? Ask residents about the service and lost or ruined clothes.
- Is the lighting adequate? Does the home provide assistive devices for the hard of hearing and sight impaired?
- Does each room open onto a hallway?

Nursing Home Staff

- Is the staff polite to visitors and residents?
- Does the staff respect the privacy of the patient? Will the staff knock on the door and wait for the patient to answer?
- How long does it take for the staff to answer the call bell?
- Is the staff watching television?
- Determine levels of staffing for each shift and each day.
- What is the average length of time staff have worked in the home?
- Does the staff treat patients with dignity and respect?
- Does the home have arrangements with a hospital in case of an emergency?
- Are pharmaceutical services available and supervised by a qualified pharmacist?
- Does the nursing home offer physical therapy and other rehabilitative services?
- Are there field trips and other activities for the patients?
- Are arrangements made for patients to go to church?
- Are there activities for patient and family?

Diet & Nutrition

- Is there a weekly menu? Will the staff help the patient to the dining area or will the patient have to eat in his or her room?
- Are the dining room and kitchen clean? Will the kitchen provide food other than at mealtime?
- Eat a meal at the home to see if the food is good. Are the servings adequate? Does the meal served match what is on the menu?
- Will the staff assist patients who cannot feed themselves?
- Are there special diets for patients with health, religious or ethnic preferences?
- Are the chairs the right size for each patient? Can patients choose where they can sit?

Plan of Care

- Does the nursing home have a plan of care for each individual patient?
- How often are plan of care conferences held and who participates in the conference?
- How often are plans of care evaluated (at least every three months)?
- Does the nursing home include the family in the development of the care plan? (They should)

Cost Considerations

- Compare the cost with other homes.
- Is there a contract that spells out the financial terms?
- Do patients' assets remain in their control, or that of their families?

What to do:

Contact the National Citizens Coalition for Nursing Home Reform — Call 1-202-332-2275 or write to them at 1424 16th Street, NW, Suite 202, Washington, DC 20036. The Coalition helps protect the rights of nursing home residents and their families. If you have not been able to obtain help with a nursing home problem from the local authorities you and/or the patient may want to call them.

Contact the American Association of Retired Persons (AARP) — 1-202-434-2277 or write to them at AARP Fulfillment, 601 E Street, N.W., Washington, DC 20049. They can provide you with many good publications on long-term care. One of the best is *Nursing Home Life.*

Contact the Alzheimer's Association — Contact your local chapter. It will have information on homes for adults, nursing homes and other facilities.

Contact the National Council of Senior Citizens. 1-202-347-8800. You can write it at National Council of Senior Citizens, Nursing Home Information Service, National Senior Citizens Education and Research Center, Inc., 1331 F Street, N.W., Washington, DC 20004. It has information on nursing homes and has a free guide on how to select a nursing home.

Contact local social services organizations — There are many agencies that will provide information and listings of nursing homes available in your area. Agencies such as the offices on aging, local health agencies as well as religious-affiliated service groups provide information and support. There are also associations and companies that provide care management services to serve as the link between you and community-based services. They charge for their services, so be sure you understand what it will cost to have them provide assistance. You can also call us ☎ 1-800-546-5559 and we will put you in touch with the organizations in your area.

During the evaluation process, make at least one unannounced visit to the nursing home.

Working with Doctors

CHOOSING A DOCTOR becomes more difficult as you grow older. It may take some time to find a doctor who will meet what you believe are your patient's healthcare needs. Finding a doctor who will take new patients who are on Medicare or who will accept the patient's insurance plan is especially difficult. A good place to start is the state or local agency on aging, medical schools, hospitals and special services in many of the larger metropolitan areas that help screen patients and match doctors to the needs of the patient. None of these organizations charge for their services.

Many older people tend to under-report health problems and think that symptoms are "old age" rather than disease. Older persons need doctors who are aware of their special health needs and problems. A good doctor will treat each patient with respect and maintain an open line of communication. The doctor should allow the patient to play an active role in deciding when to seek medical attention, when to accept the doctor's advice and when to seek a second opinion from another doctor. Never be reluctant to ask questions of the doctor if you or the patient do not understand what needs to be done. Otherwise, the doctor will assume that everything is okay.

Communicating with Doctors

Good health care is a team effort. The doctor, pharmacist nurse, dentist, therapist, you and the patient must all work and communicate together to promote good health.

One of the most serious and disconcerting problems is the specialization of doctors and the lack of communication between them. There are doctors for the heart, doctors for the kidneys, doctors for the colon; a specialist for every part of the body. No one seems to be coordinating all the information and communicating the diagnosis from each specialist about tests, surgery, etc. You and the patient must insist that your questions and concerns be addressed — especially when you receive conflicting reports. Insist that the prognosis and proposed treatment be a coordinated effort between all the doctors, the nurses, the hospital, the patient and yourself. While it may be impossible to have all the doctors meet at the same time and put everything on the table, it is possible to write out a list of questions and expect answers.

Examples of questions to ask your team of doctors:
- Explain the illness and treatment choices
- If surgery is recommended, what is the operation?
- What are chances of survival without the operation?
- How will the operation affect the patient's lifestyle and health?
- What will the patient not be able to do after the surgery?
- What are the risks of surgery?
- How long will the recovery period be?
- What will the operation and/or treatment cost?
- What is the success rate of this type of surgery (percentage)? For how many years?
- Who will administer the anesthesia?
- Is the surgeon board certified?

- Is the doctor a Fellow of the American College of Surgeons?
- Does the surgeon do this operation on a regular basis (several times a week)?
- How many times a week is this type of operation performed in the hospital?

These are but a sample of the questions you should be asking. Always ask for a second opinion and maybe even a third. The doctor should not have a problem forwarding the patient's medical records to another doctor. If you get mixed messages, let your family doctor sort it out and explain the whys and wherefores of the differences between surgeons. You and the patient must feel assured that the decision to have surgery is the right one. Never feel embarrassed. Asking for a second opinion is just a way to ensure that you have made the right decision after weighing all the factors.

Selecting a Family Doctor

Before your first visit with a family doctor, be prepared so you can get the most out of the visit and demonstrate that you want a good business-like relationship. Getting off on the right foot will help develop mutual respect and allow for open communication. One good way to find out if the doctor is good is to chat with the nurse or receptionist. You can quickly get a feel for whether or not the staff thinks highly of the doctor. Good doctors usually have a staff that practically worships them.

When selecting a family doctor the following should be considered:

- Does the doctor's personality match yours? Are you comfortable with the doctor?
- Is the doctor's office conveniently located?
- How many patients does the doctor see every day?
- Where did the doctor study medicine?
- How long has the doctor been in practice?
- Has the doctor ever lost hospital privileges?
- At what hospital(s) does the doctor have admitting privileges?
- Is the hospital close to your home and does it have a good reputation for good service and/or special services?
- Does the doctor belong to an HMO?
- How are payments handled?
- Will the doctor accept Medicare and/or Medicaid patients?
- Has the doctor ever had malpractice insurance canceled?
- Does the doctor have many older patients?
- Will the doctor honor living wills and durable powers of attorney for health care?
- If you are worried about costs, be sure to let the doctor know your concerns.
- In what field does the doctor specialize? What experience does the doctor have with the problem that you have?
- Is the doctor board-certified? (Board-certified means that the doctor has passed a special examination in the area of specialization.)

- Does the doctor have good communication skills?
- Will the doctor take new patients?
- What are the office hours?
- What is the doctor's availability on weekends?
- What days does the doctor see patients?
- Will the doctor make house calls?
- How fast can the doctor be seen in an emergency?
- How far in advance should appointments be made?
- How long is an average visit?
- How long is the average waiting time?
- If the doctor has a solo practice, who will handle your health needs when the doctor is away?
- If the doctor is in a group practice, what arrangements can be made to have continuing care from the doctor with whom you feel most comfortable?

Take *LeBoeuf's Handbook* with you to the doctor. If you have filled out all the sections, you should be able to have the following information ready to give to the doctor:

- Insurance card (number) and/or Medicare card (number).
- What the patient needs (flu shot, pneumonia vaccine, etc.).
- Illnesses that have occurred in the family such as cancer, heart disease, stroke, arthritis, diabetes, high blood pressure, etc.
- Personal health habits of the patient (smoking, drinking, exercise, etc.).
- Childhood diseases.
- Dates of last shots and what they were.
- Allergies or reactions to drugs.
- Medications being taken now and in the past (it may be a good idea to take all the current medications with you).
- What illnesses or health problems has the patient had?
- What surgery or hospitalizations and approximate dates? Doctors' names and phone numbers will be helpful if a recent surgery has occurred.
- Any significant changes in health during the past year.
- Describe the current problem and how long the patient has had the problem.
- What symptoms does the patient have?

Be honest with the doctor. Encourage the patient to talk to the doctor about sensitive subjects such as incontinence, sexuality, depression, memory problems, and other personal problems. None of these conditions are a normal part of aging. They need be made known to the doctor so they can be addressed and corrected. Doctors are used to talking with people about personal problems and they will try to make the discussion as comfortable as possible.

Take Careful Notes

Before leaving the doctor's office, you and the patient should learn as much as possible. Make sure you are in the room with the doctor when the discussion of what, when and how takes place. Take notes. Insist that you be part of the conversation on what needs to be done because, as caregiver, you have the responsibility and the need to know. Get as much in writing from the doctor as you can and as much information on the disease or problem as possible (brochures, video's, books, etc.).

Find out the following:

- What is the diagnosis and treatment?
- How long will treatment last?
- What risks are associated with the treatment?
- Will further tests be required?
- When will the results from tests be available?
- Are there alternatives to the medical treatment?
- What is the medication for?
- Are there any side effects from the medication?
- What should I do if there are side effects from the medication?
- What information will I be able to give to the visiting nurse to assist the patient?
- If either you or the patient is hard of hearing or is sight impaired, let the doctor know so he can be sure you have all the information you need and that you understand the information and directions.

Do not leave the doctor's office until you have a complete understanding of what needs to be done. If the doctor rushes you, you may want to think about finding another doctor. Remember, the doctor only sees the patient for a couple of hours a month. You must attend to the patient 24 hours a day, 7 days a week. You should be able to leave the doctor's office with the confidence that you and/or the patient can perform all the necessary health care procedures correctly.

Evaluate Your Experience

After you have chosen a doctor and had a couple of appointments, you may want to evaluate your experience:

- Do you and the patient feel comfortable with the doctor?
- Does the doctor rush through the appointment?
- Does the doctor communicate well?
- Does the doctor make an effort to understand how to move the patient to the examination table if the patient has a problem with mobility?
- Will the doctor work with you on the cost of the health care?
- Do you feel the doctor will stand by the patient no matter how difficult the situation is or may become?
- Does the doctor listen and answer specific questions about the causes and treatment?
- Does the doctor allow time for questions?
- Does the doctor seem to prescribe drugs automatically rather than deal with the real medical problem?
- Does the doctor attribute the patient's problems to "old age?"
- Does the doctor take a thorough history and ask questions about past physical and emotional problems, drugs that the patient is taking, family medical history?

What to do:

Check credentials in American Board of Medical Specialties Directory. 1-800-776-2378. Being Board Certified means the doctor has completed a residency program and has passed a rigorous exam. The Directory also provides information about where the doctor went to medical school and where the doctor trained. It is available in many public libraries.

Contact the American Medical Association. 1-312-464-5000 or write them at 515 North State Street, Chicago, IL 60610. The association can provide you with numerous books and information on doctors, emergency care, drugs and other medical issues. Most of these books are also available at your local library or are for sale at most book stores.

Contact the American Geriatrics Society. It is located at 770 Lexington Avenue, Suite 300, New York, NY 10021. They can help you locate a doctor who has a special interest in treating older people.

Contact Second Surgical Opinion Hotline. 1-800-638-6833. If in Maryland, call 1-800-492-6603. They can help you find a specialist in your area who can give you a second opinion.

In a 1994 report prepared by the Medical Board of California, 69 doctors were disciplined since 1991 for gross negligence that resulted in a patient's death or other serious violations. All but one of the doctors were not board certified.

The AMA can provide, for $60, biographical information on as many as four doctors

Surgeons who belong to the American College of Surgeons (FACS), have to be board certified in the specialty he or she is practicing, must have practiced in one location for at least two years and must have a hospital appointment in good standing.

LeBoeuf's Services

Call **LeBoeuf's** ☎ 1-800-546-5559 for the following services. Please have ready the patient's name, address, zip code, age, telephone number and physical circumstances (Alzheimer's, heart problem, arthritis, etc.) when you call.

- Consulting Service
  - Wheelchairs (design, ultra-light, sports chairs, etc.)
  - Van Conversions
  - Electronics
    - Hearing
    - Vision
    - Security
    - Communication (TTY, Call Buttons, Telephones, etc.)
    - Television, VCR's, Radio, Stereo
    - Computers and Software

- Home Healthcare Workshops

- Caregivers Speakers Bureau

- Incontinent Supply Service

- Respite Network

- Home Modification Planning Service

- Assistive Travel Agency

- Employment Screening Service

- Referral Service for:
  - Hospitals
  - Nursing homes
  - Hospice
  - Visiting nurse associations
  - Adult day care programs
  - Respite care (nursing homes, support groups,)
  - Social services case workers
  - Household help

LeBoeuf's

PHONE 1-800-546-5559

FAX 1-800-233-9692

Hearing Impaired with TDD
CALL 1-800-855-2880

Easing Hospital Stress

When choosing a hospital (non-emergency), you and the patient should consider the location, credentials, state license, accreditation by the Joint Commission on Accreditation of Healthcare Organizations and whether or not the hospital is certified for Medicare and Medicaid. Ask the hospital about their mortality rate for the same treatment the patient is scheduled to undergo. Does the hospital provide private and/or semi-private rooms? Are visiting hours strictly limited? Can only family members visit?

Either by choice or in an emergency, entering a hospital can be a frightening experience. With all the strange sounds and smells, everyone worries about what may happen. To make the experience less stressful, the following information will help the patient to cope.

What to bring (put the patient's name on everything with indelible ink or sew on name tags):

- Nightclothes, bathrobe and sturdy slippers (the patient's own as long as they do not interfere with treatment)
- Clothes to wear home
- Toothbrush, toothpaste, shampoo, comb & brush, deodorant and fully-charged cordless razor (do not bring an electric razor that is not cordless — they might not be grounded properly)
- List of medicines patient has been taking (include all prescription and nonprescription medicines)
- History of past illnesses, surgeries and any allergies
- Insurance/Medicare card
- List of names and telephone numbers of family and/or friends to contact in case of an emergency
- Money to buy newspapers, books, magazines, etc. from gift shop (about $10-$20 should be enough)
- A friend or family member. It is now recommended that everyone entering a hospital have someone at their bedside every minute of every day.
- *LeBoeuf's Handbook* (Information on insurance, medications, past illnesses, surgeries, allergies, telephone numbers of friends and family will be readily available if the patient and caregiver have completed the entries)

What *not* to bring

- Jewelry, cash over $20, watches, wedding rings
- Credit cards
- Checkbook
- Hair dryers and curling irons

The Admittance Process

Whether a planned visit or an emergency (unless very serious), the first stop should be the admitting office. The patient or a family member will be given papers to sign that allows the hospital staff to provide treatment and release medical information to the insurance company. Those who do not have insurance will be provided information about other financial arrangements. Almost all hospitals will accept credit cards and will work with the patient to come up with a satisfactory method of payment. Make sure that you and the patient are informed by the hospital admitting office about what is covered by your insurance and/or Medicare. Most insurance policies and Medicare will not cover telephone charges, television rentals and private room charges.

The hospital will provide information on financial aid such as Medicare and Medicaid. Be sure the patient is given "An Important Message from Medicare" which informs patients about their rights to medical care and how to use the Peer Review Organization (PRO) which monitors the quality of services provided by the hospital for Medicare patients.

Under Medicare, the patient has the right to receive all of the hospital care that is necessary and appropriate for the proper diagnosis of the illness or injury. The discharge date should be determined by the patient's medical needs. The patient also has the right to be fully informed about decisions affecting Medicare payments or coverage for the hospital stay. The patient has the right to request a review, a reconsideration or, ultimately, an appeal of any written notices that Medicare will no longer pay for the patient's hospital stay.

Each state has a PRO. If the hospital sends, with your doctor's agreement, a written notice of noncoverage stating that the patient no longer needs hospital care, the patient will have to pay beginning the third calendar day after receiving the notice. If you and/or the patient disagree with that finding, you must:

- Request an immediate review by calling the PRO by noon of the next workday after receiving the notice.
- The PRO must solicit your views before making its decision.
- The PRO must send you, the doctor and the hospital its decision within the next full workday after receiving your request and the hospital records.
- If the PRO agrees with you, Medicare will continue to pay for the hospital stay.
- If the PRO agrees with the doctor and the hospital, the patient will be charged beginning noon of the calendar day after you receive the PRO decision.

Getting Comfortable

Once admitted, patients will be assigned a room. If not happy with a roommate, they have the right to insist on being transferred to another room. The patient's medical information is confidential and medical personnel are not permitted to discuss it openly. Every patient has an attending physician who is in charge of the overall patient care while at the hospital. The attending physician can be the patient's regular doctor, a member of the hospital staff who has been referred, or a specialist such as a surgeon. The attending physician directs the nursing staff at the hospital. In a teaching hospital, the patient may undergo a number of exams by student doctors. However, patients have the right to refuse to see interns, family, friends or anyone else not connected with their care in the hospital. In a non-teaching hospital, only the attending physician will treat patients.

Most hospital patients are under a great deal of stress — even if they don't show it — and are in need of spiritual help. It is very important to know and understand the patient's religious beliefs. The patient may have religious beliefs that can hinder recovery or believe that medical therapy is not allowed. If you are uncomfortable talking with the patient about religious beliefs, contact the hospital clergy. Every hospital has clergy on call for almost every religion. Meditation and prayer also help to reduce stress. Do not criticize the patient's religious beliefs. The patient wants to feel comfortable with you and prayer is probably the best way to for both you and the patient to develop a sense of "we are in this together."

Nursing Care and Therapy

In the average hospital, 70 percent of all nurses are RN's. The most ideal patient-to-RN ratio is one for every one or two patients in intensive care and one RN for every six patients in other areas of the hospital.

Registered nurses, practical nurses, nurse's aides, and nursing students will provide many services such as taking the patient's blood pressure, temperature, pulse, give medications as directed by the doctor, bathe the patient, and teach the patient how to care for themselves. There is normally a head nurse who coordinates nursing care for each patient. As nurses are the major caregivers in the hospital, it is a good idea to ask the hospital how many patients each nurse sees per shift. You and the patient will then have some indication about what quality of service to expect.

The nurses will try to minimize the patient's concerns and see to their comfort and safety. They list and protect the patient's personal property. Nurses will also see that all equipment needed for the patient's needs is in place, e.g. intravenous pole, oxygen equipment, urinal, call signal, TV remote control, bed controls, etc. The nurse will also orient the patient as to how the call system works, where the bathroom and showers are, where the patient's locker is located, show how to work the lights and how to work any equipment that the patient needs to operate.

Physical and occupational therapists provide help in teaching the patient how to build muscles and improve coordination. The therapists will use exercise, heat, cold and water therapy to assist the patient in the ability to perform daily tasks such as cooking, eating, bathing, walking, and dressing. They will also teach the patient how to use crutches, canes, wheelchairs and other assistive equipment. Make sure that you and the patient understand how to use the equipment before leaving the hospital.

Staffing at the Hospital

Respiratory therapists prevent and treat breathing problems. Normal breathing is inhaling about 1 to 1.5 seconds and exhaling 2 to 3 seconds. Respiratory therapists teach patients various exercises after surgery to prevent lung infections (often, after surgery, patients breath shallowly and are afraid to cough because of the pain — causing a buildup of secretions that can lead to the collapse of part of the lung). Techniques for controlling the rate and depth of breathing aid in relaxing the patient.

X-ray technicians and laboratory technicians perform a variety of tests such as blood and urine tests.

Dietitians teach patients how to plan well balanced diets.

On average, hospital patients receive 10 different drugs.

Pharmacists prepare medications used in the hospital

Social workers provide patients with support and details about what social services are available after leaving the hospital, what financial aid programs are available and other home-care services.

Safety Tips

While in the hospital it is a good idea for you and the patient, as well as friends and other family who are helping, to follow these safety tips:

Make sure that the wrist band the hospital provides matches your patient's name and indicates any of the patient's drug allergies. Make sure the nurse checks the band each time drugs are given to the patient.

If the patient is receiving solid foods and drinking fluids and is still on an IV, check with the nurse and/or doctor. The doctor or nurse may have forgotten to change from an IV to an oral medication.

- The patient should have someone at bedside at all times (family or friend). That person should know why the patient is in the hospital and should listen carefully to the doctors and nurses to know what is going on with the patient. If the nurse, doctor or other hospital staff change any procedure, they should question why. If the nurse, doctor or staff change what has been said previously, find out why. Question any turning off of equipment. Keep notes (in a notebook) by shift and date and be sure to give the notebook to the next shift. Review medications every 72 hours.
- Know how to use the call bell.
- Lower the bed before getting in or out.
- Do not trip over any of the wires or tubes around the bed.
- Keep things the patient needs in easy reach.
- Take only medicines prescribed by the doctor.
- Do not allow the patient to take over-the-counter drugs without the doctor's permission.
- Be sure that the patient is careful getting in and out of bathtubs or showers.
- Always instruct the patient to use the handrails in hallways or stairways.
- Do not smoke around oxygen.

Leaving the Hospital

When the patient is ready to leave the hospital, the doctor will have to prepare discharge orders. You and/or the patient will also have to obtain a release form from the hospital business office. Discharge planning is offered so that when the patient arrives home there will be support (c.f., meals-on-wheels, visiting nurses, hospice, social workers and housekeeping help, etc.).

Do not try to do too much when the patient first arrives home from the hospital. It is much better to have assistance with cooking, housekeeping and other chores as well as moving the patient until you feel comfortable that you can do what needs to be done. If you have any questions on the best way to care for the patient, ask them before leaving the hospital. You will know that you have all the information needed to assist the patient if you can answer who, what, when, where and how to all of your questions on patient care.

Emergencies

If an emergency arises because of illness or accident, and it is vital that the patient seek medical help right away, call 911 or the telephone operator. Make sure that you describe the type of emergency and give your location (when you dial 911, most systems (if enhanced) will tell the operator where the call is coming from). In most cases, help will arrive in minutes. If you are transporting the patient to the emergency room, drive safely and do not panic. There will be signs at the hospital to tell you where the emergency entrance is located. It is a good idea to scout out the emergency entrance of the hospital closest to your home, and the hours they are staffed, prior to an emergency.

If the injury or illness is not severe, call the doctor or a nearby clinic instead of going to the emergency room at a hospital. If the doctor thinks that you should go to the emergency room at the hospital, they will call ahead and let the hospital know you are on your way. The doctor will, in most cases, try and meet you there.

If there is time, try to bring the following items with you:

- Health insurance card or name of insurance company and policy number
- Doctor's name and telephone number
- List of medications currently being taken (include prescription and nonprescription medications)
- List of any other medical problems such as asthma, diabetes, allergies, etc.
- Names and telephone numbers of close family members
- *LeBoeuf's Handbook* which will have all the information the hospital will need if the sections on the patient's personal history, medical history, financial planning and the legal section have been completed.

If at all possible, have a relative or friend go with you and the patient to the hospital. If the patient is going by ambulance, find out if you can ride along. If not, ask which hospital they will be taking the patient to and get there as soon as you can with the information listed above.

Outpatient Visits

If the patient is going to the hospital for an outpatient visit, try and arrange to take all the tests in the doctor's office before going. In many hospitals, you can take care of pre-admission testing and paperwork three to 14 days before a scheduled visit. Bring a friend or relative with you to help take the patient home. If the patient will have any anesthesia other than a local, they are not permitted to take public transportation. The patient cannot take a taxi unless accompanied by another adult. Take any needed assistive devices with you on the day of the visit (crutches, canes, etc.). Make sure that you have arranged to have someone help out at home while you are at the hospital and for a couple of days afterward.

A good hospital in an urban area will have at least 80 percent of the staff doctors board certified. The smaller hospitals will generally have fewer board certified doctors.

What to do:

Contact the Joint Commission on Accreditation of Health Care Organizations (JCAHO) — 1-708-916-5800. You can write it at One Renaissance Boulevard, Oakbrook Terrace, Illinois 60181. They will provide you and the patient with the hospital's accreditation rating.

Contact local social services organizations — There are many agencies that will provide information and listings of hospitals available in your area. Agencies such as the offices on aging, local health agencies as well as religious-affiliated service groups provide information and support. There are also associations and companies that provide care management services to serve as the link between you and community-based services. They charge for their services — so be sure you understand what it will cost to have them provide assistance.

Hospice Care

THE AMERICAN HOSPICE MOVEMENT began in the 1960s and credit for starting the movement can be attributed to Dame Cicely Saunders of London, England. The first hospice in this country began home service in March of 1974 and was funded by the National Cancer Institute. Hospice care is provided by a team of professionals and volunteers to support the terminally ill as well as the patient's family. Hospice care is primarily based in the home — allowing families to remain together in peace, comfort and dignity. A recent Gallup Poll found that 9 out of 10 Americans would prefer to be cared for at home if they were diagnosed with a terminal illness. Today there are more than 2,500 certified hospice programs in the United States. Over seventy percent of all hospice patients are over 65. Approximately seventy-eight percent of hospice patients are cancer patients, ten percent are heart-related patients, four percent are AIDS patients, one percent Alzheimer's and seven percent are "other."

Hospice care under Medicare is available if the following conditions are met:

- Patient has a terminal disease and life expectancy is no more than six months of life-limiting progressive illness.
- Patient no longer seeks a cure.
- Patient has a family member, friend or other appropriate person(s) to share in the care and decision making.
- Patient has a personal physician (the patient can use the hospice physician(s))

Dr. Elisabeth Kubler-Ross, author of *On Death and Dying,* identified the five stages through which many terminally ill patients progress.

- Denial
- Anger
- Bargaining
- Depression
- Acceptance

Dr. Kubler-Ross is in favor of home care instead of institutional care, arguing that patients should have a choice and the ability to participate in the decisions that affect them. She felt that home care and the support of trained nurses and other competent and trained personnel would provide the best spiritual, emotional and financial help for the patient.

Hospice treats the patient, not the disease. The focus is on the family, not the individual, with emphasis on the quality of life rather than the duration. It is not a way of dying, but a way of living. Hospice also helps patients find a sense of peace and dignity.

Under the hospice program the following services are available:

- Nursing care by registered nurses
- 24-hour on-call services
- Pain control and symptom management for maximizing comfort and activity levels (about 70 percent of hospice patients are cancer patients)
- Nutrition counseling
- Social workers provide advice and counseling to the patient and family. The social workers also provide information on community resources.
- Patient's physician provides and/or approves the plan of care with the hospice team.
- Clergy and other counselors are available to visit and provide spiritual support.
- Certified nursing aides (CNAs) help with bathing, shaving and other personal needs of the patient.
- Homemakers, in some areas, are available to assist with light housekeeping and cooking.
- Therapists assist patients in developing new ways of coping.
- Hospice can make arrangements for extended care facilities outside the home and continue to provide care for the patient at the facility.
- To provide respite relief for families, hospice may arrange a brief period of in-patient care (care outside the home). This respite care is covered under Medicare hospice benefits.
- Bereavement support. This support continues for 13 months after death at no cost.

Since 1983, Medicare has included coverage for hospice care. To qualify for Medicare benefits, a physician must certify that the patient has less than six months to live if the disease runs its normal course. The physician must recertify the patient at the beginning of each benefit period (two periods of 90 days each, one of 30 days, and an indefinite fourth period).

In addition, the patient signs an elective statement indicating an understanding of the nature of the illness and of hospice care. By signing the statement, the patient surrenders rights to other Medicare benefits related to terminal illness. This means that Medicare will pay for such things as a hospital bed, wheelchair, oxygen and other medications and treatments associated with the disease to relieve pain and suffering. Be sure to check with the physician and/or the hospice to make sure that the services and equipment the patient will be needing are covered by Medicare (a family member may sign the election statement if the patient is unable to do so, or if the patient has a durable power of attorney for health care).

In all states, the state health department certifies hospices. Only certified hospices are eligible for Medicare and, in some states, Medicaid hospice services.

Hospice volunteers vary in age and background and are the backbone of hospice. Volunteers offer help with patients, special services (lawyers, barbers, etc.), administrative support and bereavement. Hospice volunteers for patient care and bereavement service participate in intensive volunteer training programs. The volunteers receive supervised training programs for approximately 20 hours. After training, volunteers provide support for both the patient and the family.

Hospices are required to maintain a volunteer staff large enough to provide administrative or direct patient care equal to at least 5 percent of the total patient care hours of all paid hospice employees and contract staff. Failure to meet this volunteer participation requirement can result in the hospice program being decertified. Normally, Medicare certified hospices have one volunteer for every two paid staff.

What to do:

Contact the Hospice Association of America — 1-800-658-8898 which is the Hospice Hotline to obtain the telephone number of the hospice closest to you anywhere in the United States and to obtain information on the hospice program. You can write it at 519 C Street NE, Washington, DC 20002-5809.

Contact the Hospice Alliance — 1-800-545-0522 to obtain the telephone number of the hospice closest to you in Virginia, Maryland and the District of Columbia. You can write it at 6400 Arlington Blvd, Suite 1000, Falls Church, VA 22042.

Contact the National Hospice Organization — 1-800-658-8898 which is the Hospice Helpline. You can write it at 1901 N Moore Street, Suite 901, Arlington, VA 22209. The National Hospice Organization provides materials and information about hospice care.

Eldercare Locator Service

THE ELDERCARE LOCATOR provides information and references for a number of services. The Locator provides resource referrals for home-delivered meals, transportation, legal assistance, housing options, adult day care, social and recreational activities, senior center programs and nursing home ombudsmen.

This program is sponsored by the Administration on Aging, the National Association of Area Agencies on Aging (NAAAA) and the National Association of State Units on Aging (NASUA).

The toll free number is: 1-800-677-1116

Office hours are between 9:00 a.m. and 5:00 p.m. Eastern Standard Time.

When you call the following information will be requested:

- Name, address and zip code
- Brief description of the problem or type of assistance needed

Because they use the postal zip code to identify what is available in your area, be sure that you have the number handy to help speed up the process.

Paying for Healthcare

Vision

BY ANNE KEITH

When out of the shining heart of God
Love sweeps to startle our dull minds,
It is magnificent as rivers made of light
Coming to glorify each littleness,
To magnify the dust from ferns
And pollen drifting from the pines
Until each grain glows separately
And every person naked stands, precious,
Important as a new-born star.
Then we will swing into the current,
Join the dance.
It is forever—this enormous love.

Financial Planning

FINANCIAL RECORDS are necessary for every family. You will need to prepare or have knowledge of the following:

- Budget — a plan describing expected activities in dollars and cents for a specific period of time.
- Social Security and Medicare information
- Income — retirement, interest from bonds, stocks and property rents
- Insurance information
- Bank accounts — checking, savings, CDs, credit union
- Assets and liabilities — what you own and what you owe
- Credit card register
- Taxes
- Location of all personal items of value such as jewelry, heirlooms, boats, furniture, etc.

The first thing to be done is to make sure that there is a line of succession for control over the estate of the patient. If there is no durable power of attorney, living will or living trust that provides for someone other than the patient to handle personal and financial affairs, consult with an attorney and put at least a living trust in place. Having the caregiver as one of the trustees in a living trust would be beneficial. To have someone other than the caregiver, unless it is the spouse of the patient, be the trustee will most likely result in an unworkable situation.

Budgeting, while time consuming, is extremely important. Budgeting will:

- Improve communication between all parties
- Provide a guideline for determining costs
- Make all parties aware of the costs and understand the limits everyone will have to abide by
- Help develop a way to measure success
- Help all parties direct their activities toward a goal

Developing a realistic budget requires that a budget plan be developed for at least a year. The budget plan should be broken down by month to allow for tracking and measurement of whether or not you are living within your budget. You will probably be revising and making adjustments to the budget frequently during the year. It is not unusual to revise a budget a number of times due to changes in circumstances — you should not avoid or resist making changes to the budget. Your budget is a tool that allows you to get a better picture of your financial situation and what any changes will mean to you and your patient. Your budget should not be used as a hammer and needs to remain flexible. However, a disciplined approach is appropriate. If everyone participates in the process, they will understand the limits. The patient must be included in this process and should be making a financial contribution if there is retirement income or income-producing assets.

Make at least fourteen copies of the budget forms that follow. One for each month, one to summarize the complete year and one to use as a worksheet. Buy a calculator that has a paper tape, counts the items, shows minus numbers in red and has typewriter-size keys. To try and add columns of figures without a tape is very hard to do correctly.

If income is all salary and wages, social security and/or pension, the previous year's totals will be a good starting point (use after tax amounts, or what you received that you could spend). Divide by twelve. Be realistic about your income. You can't spend promises or wishes. Once you have completed one month, it is easy to transfer the numbers to the next month. Other income items should be estimated on the conservative side. If the patient and the family receive dividends, interest payments, rents, etc. and taxes are not withheld, allow for payment of the tax and count only what you will have to spend *after* paying the tax.

For expenses, use last year's expenses as a good starting point. This will be especially true of such things as mortgage/rent, utilities, property taxes, auto expense, tuition, tithing, life and auto insurance, vacation and recreation. Expense items that will probably change or will be added, will be medical expense, clothing, housekeeping, telephone, travel, medical insurance, respite care, adult day care, nursing supplies and food.

Remember, you should revisit the budget every month or so to record all the income and expense items. Try to review and post income and expense items at least every couple of months. Otherwise, the amount of data to enter can become overwhelming. If you don't keep fairly current, all the work putting the budget together will be for nothing. Use your checkbook as your expense ledger and transfer the totals from your checkbook to the budget at least once a month. Write checks for everything you can and make sure you identify in the checkbook what the check was for. (Do not write a check to the grocery store and add $50 for pocket money without an entry in the checkbook reminding you that the $50 was for pocket money and not food.) If you see that your expenses are running over budget, you should call a family meeting and discuss how to make adjustments to bring the budget into line. If you are running under budget, put the money in an interest bearing account (savings account). Do not spend the overage right away. See how the budget goes for three or four months (sometimes you will receive five paychecks in one month, but the following month you will only receive four).

Family Budget for the month/year of _____

Show income of all members of the family contributing to the family budget, including the patient:

(round up figures to the nearest dollar)	Budgeted Amount	Actual Amount	Over (Short)	Year to Date Over (Short)
Salary	$_____	$_____	$_____	$_____
Wages	_____	_____	_____	_____
Interest	_____	_____	_____	_____
Dividends	_____	_____	_____	_____
Social security	_____	_____	_____	_____
Retirement Income	_____	_____	_____	_____
Insurance Income	_____	_____	_____	_____
Sale of investments	_____	_____	_____	_____
Rents	_____	_____	_____	_____
Medicare	_____	_____	_____	_____
Other	_____	_____	_____	_____
TOTALS	$_____	$_____	$_____	$_____

Show estimated expenses, including the patient's:

(round up figures to the nearest dollar)	Budgeted Amount	Actual Amount	Over (Short)	Year to Date Over (Short)
Savings account	$_____	$_____	$_____	$_____
Income taxes (State, local and federal) . .	_____	_____	_____	_____
Property taxes	_____	_____	_____	_____
Insurance				
Auto	_____	_____	_____	_____
Health	_____	_____	_____	_____
Home	_____	_____	_____	_____
Life	_____	_____	_____	_____
Disability	_____	_____	_____	_____
Liability	_____	_____	_____	_____
Long term care	_____	_____	_____	_____
Mortgage/rent (principle and interest) . .	_____	_____	_____	_____
Electric	_____	_____	_____	_____
Heat	_____	_____	_____	_____
Garbage collection	_____	_____	_____	_____
Telephone	_____	_____	_____	_____
Auto payments/leases	_____	_____	_____	_____
Auto payments/leases	_____	_____	_____	_____
Food	_____	_____	_____	_____
Entertainment	_____	_____	_____	_____
Expenses sub-total	$_____	$_____	$_____	$_____

Estimated expenses — *continued*

(round up figures to the nearest dollar)

	Budgeted Amount	Actual Amount	Over (Short)	Year to Date Over (Short)
Expense sub-total carryover ...	$_____	$_____	$_____	$_____
Personal (hair cuts, beauty shop, etc.) ...				
Vacation				
Hobbies				
Gifts				
Tithe				
Education				
Clothing				
Medical				
Doctor				
Nurses				
Nurses aide				
Hospital				
Nursing home				
Respite care				
Therapy				
Housekeeper				
Adult day care				
Home improvements				
Travel costs				
Nursing				
Incontinent supplies				
Gloves, gowns, etc.				
Bathing				
Skin care				
Oxygen				
Medicines				
Ostomy				
Wound dressings				
Medical Equipment				
Bed				
Wheelchair				
Lift				
Furniture				
Other				
TOTAL EXPENSES	$_____	$_____	$_____	$_____

Amount over (short) $_____ for the month of _____

Amount over (short) $_____ for the year _____

Pension Benefits:

Name of employer _____

Pension Plan number _____ Amount of pension $_____

Employer address _____

Employer telephone (_____) _____–_____

Name of pension plan administrator _____

Administrator address _____

Administrator telephone (_____) _____–_____

Cost-of living?   Yes ☐   No ☐

Medical insurance?   Yes ☐   No ☐

Does pension cover spouse if person dies?   Yes ☐   No ☐

Does medical insurance cover spouse if person dies?   Yes ☐   No ☐

Insurance Policies

Health Company _____ Policy No. _____

Address _____

Agent's name _____ Telephone (_____) _____–_____

Medicare _____ Policy No. _____

Address _____

Agent's name _____ Telephone (_____) _____–_____

Medigap _____ Policy No. _____

Address _____

Agent's name _____ Telephone (_____) _____–_____

Disability _____ Policy No. _____

Address _____

Agent's name _____ Telephone (_____) _____–_____

Life _____ Policy No. _____

Address _____

Agent's name _____ Telephone (_____) _____–_____
Cash surrender value:

Life _____ Policy No. _____

Address _____

Agent's name _____ Telephone (_____) _____–_____
Cash surrender value: $_____

Other _____ Policy No. _____

Address _____

Agent's name _____ Telephone (_____) _____–_____

Bank Accounts

NAME ON BANK ACCOUNT _____

Name of Bank _____

Address _____

	Account Number	Contact person	Telephone
Checking			
Saving			
Trust			
Other			

NAME ON BANK ACCOUNT _____

Name of Bank _____

Address _____

	Account Number	Contact person	Telephone
Checking			
Saving			
Trust			
Other			

Certificates of Deposit

ACCOUNT IN NAME OF _____

Deposit Date _____   Amount deposited $_____

Certificate Number _____   Maturity Date _____   Interest Rate _____

Name of Bank or Credit Union _____

Address _____

Contact _____   Telephone _____

ACCOUNT IN NAME OF _____

Deposit Date _____   Amount deposited $_____

Certificate Number _____   Maturity Date _____   Interest Rate _____

Name of Bank or Credit Union _____

Address _____

Contact _____   Telephone _____

ACCOUNT IN NAME OF _____

Deposit Date _____   Amount deposited $_____

Certificate Number _____   Maturity Date _____   Interest Rate _____

Name of Bank or Credit Union _____

Address _____

Contact _____   Telephone _____

Stocks, Bonds & Mutual Funds

BROKERAGE COMPANY _____ Account Number _____

Contact Name _____ Phone Number _____

Name of Stock or Fund	Date Purchased	Number of shares	Price of each share	Total Purchase Price
_____	_____	_____	$_____	$_____
_____	_____	_____	$_____	$_____
_____	_____	_____	$_____	$_____
_____	_____	_____	$_____	$_____
_____	_____	_____	$_____	$_____
_____	_____	_____	$_____	$_____
_____	_____	_____	$_____	$_____
_____	_____	_____	$_____	$_____
_____	_____	_____	$_____	$_____
_____	_____	_____	$_____	$_____
_____	_____	_____	$_____	$_____
_____	_____	_____	$_____	$_____
_____	_____	_____	$_____	$_____
_____	_____	_____	$_____	$_____

BROKERAGE COMPANY _____ Account Number _____

Contact Name _____ Phone Number _____

Name of Stock or Fund	Date Purchased	Number of shares	Price of each share	Total Purchase Price
_____	_____	_____	$_____	$_____
_____	_____	_____	$_____	$_____
_____	_____	_____	$_____	$_____
_____	_____	_____	$_____	$_____
_____	_____	_____	$_____	$_____
_____	_____	_____	$_____	$_____
_____	_____	_____	$_____	$_____
_____	_____	_____	$_____	$_____
_____	_____	_____	$_____	$_____
_____	_____	_____	$_____	$_____
_____	_____	_____	$_____	$_____
_____	_____	_____	$_____	$_____
_____	_____	_____	$_____	$_____
_____	_____	_____	$_____	$_____

Individual Retirement Accounts

Name on account _____ Account Number _____
NAME OF FINANCIAL INSTITUTION _____
Address _____
Contact person _____ Telephone _____
Initial amount deposited: $_____ Date _____ Interest rate _____
Current value: $_____ Date _____

Name on account _____ Account Number _____
NAME OF FINANCIAL INSTITUTION _____
Address _____
Contact person _____ Telephone _____
Initial amount deposited: $_____ Date _____ Interest rate _____
Current value: $_____ Date _____

Name on account _____ Account Number _____
NAME OF FINANCIAL INSTITUTION _____
Address _____
Contact person _____ Telephone _____
Initial amount deposited: $_____ Date _____ Interest rate _____
Current value: $_____ Date _____

Name on account _____ Account Number _____
NAME OF FINANCIAL INSTITUTION _____
Address _____
Contact person _____ Telephone _____
Initial amount deposited: $_____ Date _____ Interest rate _____
Current value: $_____ Date _____

Name on account _____ Account Number _____
NAME OF FINANCIAL INSTITUTION _____
Address _____
Contact person _____ Telephone _____
Initial amount deposited: $_____ Date _____ Interest rate _____
Current value: $_____ Date _____

Name on account _____ Account Number _____
NAME OF FINANCIAL INSTITUTION _____
Address _____
Contact person _____ Telephone _____
Initial amount deposited: $_____ Date _____ Interest rate _____
Current value: $_____ Date _____

Credit Card Information:

COMPANY NAME _____ Contact _____
Address _____
Telephone _____ Account Number _____ Expiration Date _____

COMPANY NAME _____ Contact _____
Address _____
Telephone _____ Account Number _____ Expiration Date _____

COMPANY NAME _____ Contact _____
Address _____
Telephone _____ Account Number _____ Expiration Date _____

COMPANY NAME _____ Contact _____
Address _____
Telephone _____ Account Number _____ Expiration Date _____

COMPANY NAME _____ Contact _____
Address _____
Telephone _____ Account Number _____ Expiration Date _____

COMPANY NAME _____ Contact _____
Address _____
Telephone _____ Account Number _____ Expiration Date _____

COMPANY NAME _____ Contact _____
Address _____
Telephone _____ Account Number _____ Expiration Date _____

COMPANY NAME _____ Contact _____
Address _____
Telephone _____ Account Number _____ Expiration Date _____

COMPANY NAME _____ Contact _____
Address _____
Telephone _____ Account Number _____ Expiration Date _____

COMPANY NAME _____ Contact _____
Address _____
Telephone _____ Account Number _____ Expiration Date _____

COMPANY NAME _____ Contact _____
Address _____
Telephone _____ Account Number _____ Expiration Date _____

COMPANY NAME _____ Contact _____
Address _____
Telephone _____ Account Number _____ Expiration Date _____

What are you worth?

For net amounts due on mortgages, notes or loans you can call the financial institution or mortgage company and ask for an amortization schedule. This schedule will show you the amount you still owe by month on principal and interest until all the money borrowed is repaid.

ASSETS (What you have)   **Amount**

Cash .... $_____

Saving Accounts .... _____

Checking Account .... _____

Certificates of Deposit .... _____

IRA's .... _____

Money Market Funds .... _____

Stocks .... _____

Bonds .... _____

Mutual Funds .... _____

Annuities .... _____

Pension .... _____

Cash Value of Life Insurance .... _____

Value of Business (net) .... _____

Home (current value) .... _____

Vacation Home .... _____

Motor Home .... _____

Autos (Blue Book) .... _____

Personal Property

    Collections .... _____

    Jewelry .... _____

    Boats .... _____

Other .... _____

    Total Assets .... $_____

LIABILITIES (What you owe)   **Amount**

Credit Cards .... $_____

Auto Loans .... _____

Business Loans .... _____

Personal Loans .... _____

Mortgage Principal (not interest) .... _____

Second Mortgage Note .... _____

Taxes .... _____

Other .... _____

    Total Liabilities .... $_____

Subtract liabilities from assets and you have your net worth.
If you come up with a negative number, you owe more than you own.   **Total Net Worth** $_____

Medicare & Medicaid

Over 95% of the elderly not living in nursing homes are covered by Medicare hospital and doctor insurance.

MEDICARE is a health insurance program available to people over 65. Some people under 65 are eligible for Medicare if they have permanent kidney failure or are permanently disabled, and are entitled to Social Security benefits. If the patient is already receiving Social Security or Railroad Retirement benefits, they will automatically receive a Medicare card in the mail when they turn 65. The patient is automatically enrolled in Part B when entitled to Part A. However, because the patient has to pay a monthly premium to enroll in Part B, the patient has the option of declining Part B. If the patient has been a disability patient under Social Security or Railroad Retirement for 24 months, the patient will automatically receive a Medicare card in the mail.

The patient does not have to be eligible for Social Security benefits to be eligible for Medicare. If the patient is 65 or older or has Part B, but does not have enough Social Security work credits for premium-free Part A, the patient can pay a monthly premium to obtain Part A coverage. The premium ranges from $183 per month to $261 per month, depending on the number of quarters of Social Security work credits the patient may have.

If the Medicare card does not come in the mail automatically, the patient must apply for Medicare benefits:

- The patient should apply during the seven month period that starts three months before their 65th birthday.
- The patient should file the application during the initial enrollment period to avoid late enrollment surcharges under Medicare Part B.
- If the patient does not sign up for Medicare during the first three months of the initial enrollment period, there will be a delay in Part B coverage. The patient's coverage could be delayed from one to three months after enrollment.
- If the patient does not enroll in Medicare Part B at any time during the initial enrollment period, the patient will not have another chance to enroll until the next general enrollment period which is held each year from January 1 through March 31. If the patient enrolls during this period, Medicare Part B benefits will not begin until July of that year.

The Medicare card shows the patient's health insurance claim number. The claim number usually has nine digits and one or two letters. The full claim number must be included on all Medicare claims and correspondence. The patient and spouse each receive a separate card and claim number. Make sure that the exact name and claim number shown on the card is used. Keep the card handy and have the patient carry it when away from home. If the card is lost, call the Social Security office immediately. Never let anyone other than the patient use the card.

Medicare comes in two parts:

Part A covers:

- Inpatient care in a hospital, some skilled nursing facilities, some home healthcare services and hospice care
- Semiprivate room (two to four beds)
- All meals, including special diets
- Regular nursing services
- Costs of special care units, such as intensive care or coronary care units
- Drugs furnished by the hospital during the patient's stay
- Blood transfusions furnished by the hospital
- Lab tests in the hospital bill
- X-rays and other radiology services
- Medical supplies such as casts, surgical dressings
- Use of assistive devices such as a wheelchair
- Operating room and recovery room costs
- Rehabilitation services such as physical therapy

Part B covers:

- Doctor care
- Outpatient hospital services
- Durable medical equipment (bath transfer benches, wheelchairs, walkers, etc.)
- Diagnostic tests
- Ambulance services
- Other services and supplies not covered under Part A

Medicare pays under Part A:

Hospitalization:

First 60 days, all but $716.
61st to 90th day, all but $179 a day.
91st to 150th day, all but $358 a day.
Beyond 150 days, Medicare pays nothing.

Skilled Nursing Facility:

First 20 days Medicare pays 100%
if approved amount.
Additional 80 days all but $89.50 per day.
Beyond 100 days Medicare pays nothing.

Visiting Nurses:

For as long as doctor certifies need.
Medicare pays for outpatient drugs and
inpatient respite care.

Hospice Care:

For as long as doctor certifies need.
Medicare pays for outpatient drugs and
inpatient respite care.

The Medicare home health benefit has experienced rapid growth. In 1989, spending was $2.7 billion. By 1994, spending increased to about $12.7 billion.

GAO – March, 1996

In 1989, 1.7 million Medicare beneficiaries received home health services. By 1993, this number increased to 2.8 million.

Home health claim volume increased from 5.5 million in 1989 to 16.6 million in 1994.

Blood:	Unlimited for all but first 3 pints per calendar year.
Home Healthcare	Full cost of medically necessary services. 80 percent of approved amount for durable medical equipment.

Medicare pays under Part B:

Part B is purchased separately for a monthly premium that for 1995 is $46.10 per month. Congress is taking a hard look at Medicare and changes are likely. To find out what changes may have been made, call **LeBoeuf's** ☎ **1-800-546-5559** or Social Security 1-800-772-1213.

Under Part B, after the patient pays the first $100 in approved charges for covered medical expenses in a calendar year, the annual deductible is fulfilled regardless of the number of times the patient enters the hospital. In other words, the patient will only have to pay a total deductible of $100 in any one calendar year (January 1 to and including December 31) regardless of the number of times the patient incurs charges.

Co-insurance after paying the annual deductible is normally 20 percent of the Medicare approved amount. If the patient's services were provided on assignment (service provider agrees to be paid by Medicare), the patient only pays the coinsurance. If the services were not on assignment, the patient will have to pay the doctor the full amount and submit a claim to Medicare for payment. If the patient's services were not provided on assignment and the charges for the patient's services were more than the Medicare approved amount, the patient will owe the Medicare coinsurance (20%) plus charges above the Medicare amount. The most that the doctor can charge is 115 percent of what Medicare approves for that service. Doctors who charge more than this limit can be fined. In almost all cases, doctors, suppliers and other providers of Part B services must file the Medicare claim for the patient. Make sure that the person or agency from whom the patient is receiving services will file the claim and ask that a copy of the claim submitted to Medicare be sent to you and/or the patient. Check the billing being sent to Medicare to be sure that the patient will receive the amount covered.

Medigap Insurance

Medigap insurance is purchased to cover the cost of healthcare not covered by Medicare. The patient only needs one Medigap policy. There are 10 standardized plans of benefits. All insurance companies must have the same standardized plans. If the patient is eligible for Medicaid, Medigap insurance is not needed. There are many plans available, and it is against the law for an insurance agent to sell you a policy if the patient already has one — unless the patient wants to replace the insurance policy already owned.

Basic Benefits in all 10 Medigap Insurance Plans

Part A — Pays patient's co-payment for hospital stays 61 to 90 days, co-payment for hospital stays 91 to 150 days, and 100% of up to 365 additional days per lifetime.

Part B — Pays patient's 20% co-payment of Medicare's allowed amount for doctor charges and the first three pints of blood.

There are nine other plans that provide additional coverage and the patient should contact the insurance agent to determine whether or not your state allows the plan to be sold.

Some advice on buying Medigap insurance that is best for the patient:

- Watch the cost. The patient does not need to buy all that can be afforded. Costs of insurance plans are heading up and if the patient buys the maximum now, the policy premiums may increase to such an extent that the policy will be too expensive for the patient to maintain.

- Take advantage of the open enrollment period (period when a person is 65 or older and is first entitled to enroll in Medicare Part B). The Medigap open enrollment period is a one time opportunity. After the six month period ends, you may not be able to buy the insurance policy of the patient's choice at the best price. The insurance company cannot refuse to cover the patient because of health condition. However, there may still be a period of time before the patient will be covered for health costs related to pre-existing conditions. Be sure that you and the patient understand what the coverage is and get it in writing from the insurance company. Also, managed care plans are not Medigap insurance and you must be very careful to be sure that the patient is not giving up Medigap coverage.

- Compare premiums between insurance companies over the past three to four years. Make sure the patient understands "Attained Age" and "Issue Age." Attained age premiums increase each year as the patient gets older. Issue Age premiums do not go up as the patient gets older.

- Check out the insurance company to be sure it can pay the claims. The best place to find out the company's rating is to go to the library and look at the A. M. Best Company rating. The Best Company ranks insurance companies from A+ = superior to C- = fair.

- Don't let the Part B deductible of $100 be a big concern. You may find that a policy that covers the $100 deductible may end up costing well over $100 or more extra per year. Remember, the patient only pays the $100 deductible once in a calender year.

- Obtain a policy that has provision for preventive health care. Be sure to check the cost because the premium may be more than it would cost to go to the doctor and pay for the exam.

- Do not buy "dread disease" (cancer, AIDS, etc.) insurance until you are convinced that the benefits gained will equal or exceed the extra cost. Medigap and Medicare cover most medical care for these diseases.

Home Healthcare Under Medicare:

Medicare will pay for home healthcare services only if all four of the following conditions are met.

- Care the patient needs includes intermittent skilled nursing care, physical therapy or speech therapy (intermittent means less than eight hours per day).
- Patient is confined at home (patient is considered homebound if leaving home requires a considerable and taxing effort).
- The patient is under the care of a doctor who determines that the patient needs home healthcare and sets up a home healthcare plan for the patient with a home healthcare agency.
- Home healthcare agency providing services participates in Medicare.

Medicare covers these services:

- Part time or intermittent skilled nursing care.
- Physical therapy.
- Speech therapy.
- Occupational therapy.
- Medical social services.
- Medically necessary supplies.
- Durable medical equipment.
- Home health aides.

Medicare will not pay for:

- 24-hour a day nursing care in the home.
- Drugs and biologicals.
- Meals delivered to the home.
- Homemaker services such as housekeeping and cooking.
- Blood transfusions.
- Comfort items such as diapers, gloves, etc.

Hiring a geriatric care manager will normally cost between $200 and $350 for the initial evaluation. It will cost between $40 and $150 per hour for follow-up services. This cost is not covered by Medicare or Medicaid. Always be sure to check what fees will be charged and what services will be included in the fee. Get it in writing!

To determine if the patient is eligible for home healthcare services, ask a home healthcare agency such as visiting nurses or hospice to evaluate the case and determine whether or not the requirements for Medicare coverage are met. The home healthcare agency should not charge for this evaluation.

If the patient is eligible for coverage under Medicare, Medicare will pay the full approved costs of all covered home visits. However, Medicare pays only 80% of durable medical equipment (co-insurance). The patient is responsible for paying the other 20%. Only the doctor should prescribe durable medical equipment for the patient. To be considered durable medical equipment, the equipment must be able to withstand repeated use, primarily serve a medical purpose and be appropriate for use in the home. LeBoeuf's is a supplier of durable medical equipment and an approved Medicare supplier.

If you are purchasing durable medical equipment for the patient, and want Medicare to reimburse you for the cost, you must be sure the doctor has prescribed the equipment, know why the patient needs the equipment and know how long the equipment will be needed. We will complete form HCFA-1500 and send it to you to approve and sign. We do not accept assignments. There is no charge for this service. While the process is relatively painless, your reimbursement from Medicare may take awhile. If your claim for durable medical equipment is denied, you normally have six months to appeal.

Medicaid Coverage

Medicaid is healthcare coverage for very low income people of any age. If a person is eligible for Medicaid, no other health insurance will be required or needed. Although the federal government sets the guidelines for Medicaid, each state has its own eligibility requirements and each state has different services covered. Not all doctors accept Medicaid patients. You and/or the patient must be sure that the doctor accepts Medicaid before making an appointment. You can apply for Medicaid at the local welfare office. To find out if the patient is eligible and what services are covered, you can contact **LeBoeuf's ☎ 1-800-546-5559** for the name of a lawyer or professional geriatric care manager in your area. You can also contact the local state health and/or social services department in the state where the patient resides.

Medicaid covers:

- In-patient and out-patient hospital care from hospitals that accept Medicaid patients.
- Doctors, nurses.
- Tests ordered by a doctor.
- Home care services ordered by a doctor.
- Nursing home care if ordered by a doctor.
- Transportation to and from healthcare providers.
- In some states: chiropractic care, dental care, prescription drugs, etc. You need to check with the local welfare office to find out what is covered as each state has different coverage under Medicaid.

Medicaid is the main provider of long-term care for older Americans. Over 50 percent of nursing home income is from Medicaid. Almost 70 percent of nursing home patients rely on Medicaid to pay or help pay their bills. Because of the cost, the government is looking to reduce expenditures for this program and the elderly are likely to be impacted. The impact of the changes in Medicaid will certainly result in more families having to care for their loved ones in the home.

To apply for Medicaid:

- Complete a form supplied by a local welfare, public health or Social Security office.
- Show proof of age, income, assets, citizenship, residency, disability and medical expenses for the patient.
- Set up an appointment for an interview.
- Take proof of the information asked for on the form to the interview.

Medicaid decisions on eligibility will usually be made within 45 to 60 days. Each state has a time limit for the decision making process.

If the patient is denied coverage, appeal immediately. Medicaid must provide a form for the appeal and will help the patient fill it out. Do not delay the appeal or the patient may lose their right to appeal (most states have an appeal window of from 10 to 90 days).

If the patient must enter a nursing home and has no or few assets, Medicaid could be the answer to nursing home costs. To qualify, the patient must:

- Be at least 65, blind or disabled as defined by the state in which the patient lives.
- Need the care provided by the nursing home.
- Meet income limitation test.

The rules to qualify for Medicaid and the rules concerning the patient's assets are very complex. It is important to start planning early to prevent financial tragedy.

Social Security

To obtain the most accurate and timely information on the patient's Social Security benefits call 1-800-772-1213 and ask for a statement of the benefits the patient has earned or is entitled. They will send you the form within two weeks to be filled out by either the patient or the caregiver. While you are at it, ask for a form for each family member. It is a good idea to check on everyone in the family who is over 50 to see if proper account credit has been made over the years.

The nine digit Social Security number is divided into three parts. The first three numbers generally indicate the state of residence at the time a person first applies for a Social Security card. The lowest numbers were originally assigned in the New England states. The middle two digits have no special significance. The last four characters represent a straight numerical progression of assigned numbers. So far, about 365 million Social Security numbers have been issued.

The current form for requesting an earnings and benefit estimate statement is very simple to fill out. There are only ten questions:

1. Name as shown on Social Security card
2. Social Security number as shown on the card
3. Date of birth
4. Other Social Security numbers that patient may have used
5. Sex
6. Other names the patient may have used.
7. a. Actual earnings for last year (do not include earnings not covered by Social Security)
   b. The current year's estimated earnings
8. Age patient stopped working or will stop working (show only one)
9. Average yearly amount patient would earn between now and when the patient expects to stop working.
10. Address where statement should be sent.

Sign the form, put a stamp on the envelope and mail it. The statement should be back in six weeks or less.

You can call LeBoeuf's or go to your Social Security office to get a Factsheet that will tell you how to figure your retirement benefit. While there are only five steps, it can become quite involved and we strongly suggest that you or the patient fill out the benefit and earning statement. Most people don't have a clue as to how much they have earned each year for the last 35 years.

Sources of income for older Americans in 1988:

38%	*Social Security*
25%	*Savings, rents and selling assets*
18%	*Pensions*
17%	*Wages*
3%	*Other (children, church, friends, etc.)*

Nine out ten elderly receive some income from Social Security. Three out of ten rely on Social Security for 80% or more of his/her income.

As a result of the aging population, researchers predict that the number of elderly needing long-term care may double in the next 25 years. In the year 2020 the number of people needing long term care will be between 10 and 14 million. This is compared with the 7 million today.

"Disabled" means that the patient has a physical or mental condition that prevents working for at least a year, or is expected to end in death.

For the patient's records you need to have the following information:

Name _____

Social Security Number _____ - _____ - _____

Amount of retirement benefits $_____

Disability Payments: ☐ Yes ☐ No   Amount $_____

Survivor's Benefits: ☐ Yes ☐ No   Amount $_____

Supplemental Security Income (SSI)

Call 1-800-772-1213 for information on this program. Again this is part of the Social Security program, but SSI is funded by the general fund and not the Social Security Trust Fund.

SSI is a federal program that provides income assistance for people who are blind or disabled, 65 or older, have assets totaling no more than $2,000 except for a house, household goods and a car that has no more than $4,500 in value, and who do not have an income of more than $953 a month. The requirements under this law are in constant flux and the information presented here may have changed since this writing. It is important for you and the patient to call the 800 number and ask for the latest information on benefits and what the current eligibility requirements are. "Disabled" means that the patient has a physical or mental condition that prevents working for at least a year, or is expected to end in death.

If you are having problems obtaining information or answers from the Social Security office, the most effective way to get timely assistance is to call your Congressman or Senator. All Representatives work with the Social Security House Liaison Office to answer constituent questions and you will find that your questions will be addressed quickly. Telephone numbers for your Representative or Senator are in the phone book under Federal Government, Congress of the United States.

Long-Term Care Insurance

Insurance for long-term healthcare has rapidly grown to be one of the fastest growing segments of the insurance industry. One of the most noticeable shifts in long term healthcare policies has been the increase in benefits for services in the policyholder's home.

Long-term care policies normally apply to long-term chronic conditions that private health insurance and Medicare benefits do not cover. The most reputable long-term care policies cover all types of care in the home. The best policies will cover doctor care, nursing and custodial care to perform such duties such as bathing and feeding

Coverage under most of the insurance policies will take place when the doctor determines that the patient is unable to perform Activities of Daily Living (ADL's). Activities of daily living include: eating, toileting, dressing, transferring from bed to wheelchair and personal grooming. Usually, benefits will be paid when the patient is unable to do two or more of the ADL's.

Insurance polices that focus on home care can be designed to pay for many services in addition to the physical care of the patient. Cooking, laundry, shopping, babysitting, running errands and general housekeeping can also be covered under some policies. For an insurance policy to provide these types of services, the insurance company will usually use a "pool of money" concept. The "pool of money" concept usually means that there is a fixed dollar amount of benefits that can be used for expenses. An example would be if an insured has a "pool of money" that equals $140,000, and the benefit that is paid out equals $100 per day, the "pool of money" will last about four years. If the patient uses only $50 per day, the "pool of money" would last about eight years.

Long term inflation protection is available, but is also expensive. Premiums rise at a dramatic pace as the insured ages. Most premiums will triple between the ages of 50 and 70. Another factor to consider is the health of the insured. If the insured waits too long and a serious health problem is evident, the cost of insurance would most likely be prohibitive.

Example of current costs for a long-term healthcare policy at age 57 for $120 per day of benefits for 4 years with a 5 percent compounded inflation option and a 20 day waiting period: The annual premium would be $1,884 for $175,000 of coverage. In 25 years — with the 5 percent compounded inflation option — the total amount of benefits available would be $592,612 which could be paid out at a rate of $406 per day for four years.

Shoppers' Guide to Long-Term Care Insurance

The National Association of Insurance Commissioners (NAIC), whose members are the chief insurance regulators in all 50 states, has developed *A Shoppers' Guide to Long-Term Care Insurance*. The guide includes insurance for nursing homes and other long-term facilities.

The guide has three sections for you to fill out. Section 1 asks you to fill in information about the availability and cost of long-term care in the patient's area. Section 2 asks you to fill in information about companies that are selling long-term insurance. Section 3 asks you to fill in information about various long-term care insurance policies.

Some of the information that the guide will ask you to obtain includes: Levels of care the policy covers, such as skilled nursing care. Whether or not the insurance policy covers care by home health aides and adult day care centers. Does the policy cover the cost of adult day care centers or other community centers? The guide asks what the limits are on payment to home care, nursing home care or combinations. There are many other questions and, if you are looking into buying long-term care insurance, this is one way to be sure that you have covered all the bases.

You can call **LeBoeuf's** ☎ **1-800-546-5559** and we will send you NAIC's *A Shopper's Guide to Long-Term Care Insurance* at no cost.

Health Problems, Symptoms & Solutions

Grace Notes

BY ANNE KEITH

These grace notes
Decorate the darkness of today.
Like sparks they shine
Against the winter's lingering—
Pink tongues of peony
Pushing through damp earth,
And sparrows, freshly striped with white.
The sudden flocks of juncos come to feed.
Bold squirrels ride the branch tips
Till they bend and sway
To eat precariously of maple buds.
These give me hope
With promises that spring
Is riding in on this high wind.

Acquired Immune Deficiency Syndrome (AIDS)

PEOPLE WHO ARE DIAGNOSED as having AIDS have become infected by the Human Immunodeficiency Virus (HIV). HIV kills certain cells of the body, particularly those that protect from disease. A person with HIV can develop rare illnesses that healthy people do not get. It is estimated that 50 percent of all AIDS patients experience dementia in the later stages of the disease.

Testing positive for HIV does not necessarily mean a person has AIDS. AIDS symptoms may lie dormant for several years after a person has been diagnosed with HIV. The National Institutes of Health has reported that slightly over 10 percent of new AIDS cases are being reported for those age 50 and older.

At the present time there are no proven treatments and no vaccines for AIDS. Presently, no cure exists for AIDS. However, many symptoms of the disease respond to antibiotics, radiation therapy, some anticancer drugs and some antiviral drugs. Research is on-going and, while many drugs have shown promise, clinical trials have failed or have shown serious side effects.

Unsafe sex practices (such as anal sex and sex without contraceptive devices) increase the risk of becoming infected with HIV. Reducing the risk of infection can be accomplished by reducing the number of sex partners, knowing the sex history of the partner, not sharing needles and stopping oral sex. Breastfeeding can transmit the virus to a baby. Unfortunately, some have been infected with HIV through blood transfusions. All donated blood, organs and semen are now checked for HIV antibodies. The HIV-positive individual should not donate blood.

The National Institutes of Health has reported that slightly over 10 percent of new AIDS cases are being reported for those age 50 and older.

Symptoms:

- Persistent fever or sweating at night.
- Swollen lymph nodes in neck, armpits or groin that last more than 2 months .
- Profound and persistent fatigue.
- Weight loss of more than 10 pounds in less than 2 months.
- Persistent and unexplained diarrhea.
- White coating or spots on tongue or throat.
- Blurred vision.
- Persistent and severe headaches.
- Rash or skin discoloration that persists or spreads.
- Bleeding or bruises that are unexplainable.

The Caregiver Role

The caregiver should make sure the patient gets adequate sleep and rests often during the day. Encourage the patient to eat good, nutritious meals regularly, even if the appetite has been lost. Have the patient avoid crowds as much as possible to reduce the possibility of contracting a cold and/or the flu.

One advantage of home healthcare for AIDS patients is the opportunity for caregivers to observe the day-to-day condition of their patients. Changes in the patient's health, such as a fever, persistent cough, weight loss, fatigue, numbness, blurred vision, stomach pain or diarrhea are signals to seek professional medical treatment.

The AIDS caregiver can take several precautions to help control the spread of the disease:

- Cover any open sores, cuts, or breaks on open skin with a bandage.
- Use an electric razor to shave an AIDS patient. Do not use a razor blade because of the chance of cuts.
- Wear protective gloves when attending to a patient's open sores, vomit or when attending to a patient's toilet.
- Wear a full plastic face mask, or a mask and goggles, to prevent the patient's bodily fluids from entering the eyes or mouth of the caregiver.
- If large amounts of blood, vomit or fecal material are present, wear a waterproof apron or smock to prevent infection and your own clothes from being stained.
- Wash your hands after attending to the patient's needs.

Household Cleaning

The Centers for Disease Control and Prevention has stated that cleaning kitchen utensils and clothes used by someone with AIDS does not require any special procedures. Unless there is blood on their clothing, it is not necessary to use bleach to wash clothing worn by a person with AIDS.

Waste Handling and Disposal

Always wear protective gloves if you will have contact with blood or other body fluids of an AIDS patient. Protection from body fluids includes reducing exposure to urine, feces and vomit. Wash your hands after any contact with body fluids — before and after removing your gloves.

Two types of protective gloves are recommended. Disposable gloves are used for nursing the HIV patient. For household chores, heavy duty rubber gloves may be used. Rubber gloves should be discarded if they become cracked or punctured.

Liquid wastes may be flushed down the toilet. Items that should not be flushed include paper towels, sanitary pads, needles, and wound dressings. Used bandages should be placed in a plastic bag and closed securely. Needles should never be reused or shared. It is not necessary to replace the cap on the needle or break the tip after use. Used needles should be placed in a puncture-proof container such as a metal coffee can. Some areas have special waste handling requirements for medical waste, so check with the doctor, nurse or local health department for proper disposal methods.

Health of the Caregiver

The personal health of the caregiver has some important applications. Some caregivers may be the sex partner of the AIDS patient. Continued sexual activity by an HIV-positive patient should be modified to avoid transmitting the disease to an uninfected person. The caregiver should also consider being tested for signs of HIV. For those concerned about the privacy of HIV test results, contact the clinic to see if anyone but you can learn the test results.

Special precautions are needed when a household member has contagious infections such as chickenpox, measles, hepatitis or shingles (herpes zoster). Contact your doctor or nurse for specific instructions and medications when afflicted. For caregivers who are ill, and caretaking of the AIDS patient is unavoidable, it is suggested that the caregiver wear a surgical mask, glasses and gloves. Caregivers (and patients) who have diarrhea due to an infection should not prepare foods for others.

Household pets also pose infection problems for the HIV patient. Animals carry their own disease sources that may adversely affect the patient. The patient's hands should always be washed after handling a pet. Litter boxes should be emptied daily. Sick pets and their litter should not be handled by the AIDS patient.

What to do:

Contact the doctor — Make sure the patient keeps the appointment. There are many experimental treatments undergoing study for the treatment of HIV complications. The patient's medical records are private.

Contact the Centers for Disease Control and Prevention National AIDS Clearinghouse — 1-800-458-5231, P.O. Box 6003, Rockville, MD 20849-6003. 1-800-342-AIDS (English Hotline), 1-800-344-SIDA (Spanish Hotline) 1-800-243-7012 (TTY/TDD) Provides AIDS prevention and education materials, programs, services, funding and information about HIV-related upcoming events. Brochures, posters, reports and videotapes are available.

Contact the NAMES Project Foundation — (415) 882-5500, 310 Townsend Street, Suite 310, San Francisco, CA 94107. The NAMES Project AIDS Memorial Quilt is a giant quilt with thousands of names of AIDS victims. Traveling exhibits of the quilt are periodically displayed around the country.

Contact the National Gay and Lesbian Task Force — (202) 332-6483 or (202) 332-6219 (TTY/TDD). You can write them at 1734 14th Street, N.W., Washington, D.C. 20009. The task force has four main departments: lobbying, organizing, education and action.

Contact the National Native American AIDS Prevention Center — Call (510) 444-2051 or 1-800-283-2437 (American Indian specific). You can write them at 3515 Grand Avenue, Suite 100, Oakland, CA 94610 The center provides AIDS-related information for American Indians, Hawaiian natives and Alaskan natives. The toll-free line is for American Indian related questions.

LeBoeuf's Services

Call **LeBoeuf's** ☎ **1-800-546-5559** for the following services. Please have ready the patient's name, address, zip code, age, telephone number and physical circumstances (Alzheimer's, heart problem, arthritis, etc.) when you call.

- Consulting Service
    - Wheelchairs (design, ultra-light, sports chairs, etc.)
    - Van Conversions
    - Electronics
        - Hearing
        - Vision
        - Security
        - Communication (TTY, Call Buttons, Telephones, etc.)
        - Television, VCR's, Radio, Stereo
        - Computers and Software

- Home Healthcare Workshops

- Caregivers Speakers Bureau

- Incontinent Supply Service

- Respite Network

- Home Modification Planning Service

- Assistive Travel Agency

- Employment Screening Service

- Referral Service for:
    - Hospitals
    - Nursing homes
    - Hospice
    - Visiting nurse associations
    - Adult day care programs
    - Respite care (nursing homes, support groups,)
    - Social services case workers
    - Household help

LeBoeuf's

PHONE **1-800-546-5559**

FAX **1-800-233-9692**

Hearing Impaired with TDD
CALL **1-800-855-2880**

Infection Control

ANYONE WHO WORKS CLOSELY with a patient who has a contagious disease runs the risk of self-infection. Infection transmissions can originate from direct contact with the infected person, indirect contact (through equipment, bedding and clothing etc.), or contact with airborne particles.

The most common way infectious diseases are transmitted is through body fluids originating from skin, eyes, nose, mouth, mucous membranes, and skin punctures. Transmission of disease often occurs by sneezing, coughing or even speaking.

To reduce the chance of infection, keep everything the infected person comes in contact with as clean as possible. Take these precautions when taking caring for a patient who is infected:

- Use personal protective equipment.
- Use cleaning and disinfecting solutions to decontaminate equipment, beds, mattresses, floors, carpeting and walls.
- Reduce the possibility of air contamination by using air cleaners.
- Dispose of waste carefully.
- Wash hands, face and all exposed skin areas with soap and water or antimicrobial wipes after removing and disposing gloves.

Infection Control Products

Burney Products Open-Back Protective Gown. Large-cut, long sleeve gown made from white polyethylene-coated spunbound polypropylene nonwoven fabric. Offers full frontal protection from all liquids. Elastic cuffs, neck ties, and wrap-around belt. Disposable.

Bu 125-715	Open-back protective gown	Each	$2.95

Burney Products Full Closed-Back Protective Gown. Large cut, long sleeve, full closed back made from the same fabric as the open back gown. Elastic cuffs, neck ties, and wrap-around belt.

Bu 125-716	Closed-back protective gown	Each	$2.95

Burney Products Laboratory Coats. White coated nonwoven coat designed for comfortable all-day wear. Made with two pockets. Comes with open cuffs, elastic cuffs or knit cuffs. Just like the doctor wears.

Bu Special	Small, medium, large or extra large	Each	$4.95

Burney Products Disposable Coveralls. Zippered front.

Bu 120-805	Medium	Each	$5.95
Bu 120-806	Large	Each	$5.95
Bu 120-807	Extra Large	Each	$5.95
Bu 120-807x	Extra Extra Large	Each	$6.95

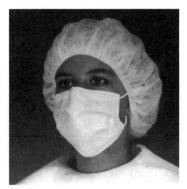

Al N 831

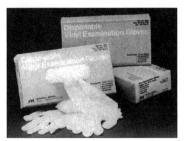

Le 146-0328 / Le 146-1623 /
Le 146-2266

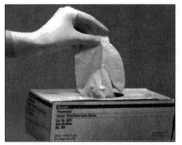

Bu 125-715

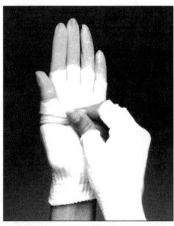

Al Ag 5305

Burney Products Surgeon's Hood. Legionnaire's style. Disposable

Bu 100-201	Pack of 10	$5.95

Alliance Supply Bouffante Caps. 21″ and 24″. White. Lightweight. Non-woven polypropylene. Disposable.

Al N 831	21″ Bag of 100	$16.95
Al N 831	24″ Bag of 100	$17.95

Alliance Supply Shoe Covers. Protects shoes from contaminants and spillages. Non-Skid.

Al 803	Universal size	Case of 100	$18.95

Burney Products Stainless Steel Step-On Hamper. Contains no springs. 3″ locking ball bearing casters. Uses 33-gallon plastic bag. Unique bag clips don't slip.

Bu BP 1000	Hamper 12″ × 18″ × 36″ high	$240.95

Burney Heavy Duty Latex Gloves. Choose unlined or flock-lined gloves. Fingertips are pebbled for non-slip grip.

Bu 160-VML		Case of 10 pair $9.95

Marshall Disposable Latex Gloves. Secure economical protection without sacrificing sense of touch. Lightly powdered, ambidextrous. Rolled cuff for easy application. Non-sterile.

Le 146-0328	Small	Box of 50	$8.95
Le 146-1623	Medium	Box of 50	$8.95
Le 146-2266	Large	Box of 50	$8.95

Marshall Disposable Vinyl Gloves. Secure economical protection. Lightly powdered, ambidextrous. Rolled cuff for easy application. Non-sterile

Le 146-2373	Small	Box of 50	$7.95
Le 146-2662`	Medium	Box of 50	$7.95
Le 146-2894	Large	Box of 50	$7.95

Baxter Flexam Sterile Latex Exam Gloves. Durable, ambidextrous design offers protection for sterile procedures. High quality latex with ribbed, tapered cuffs.

Le 220-6456	Small	Box of 100	$48.95
Le 220-6530	Medium	Box of 100	$48.95
Le 214-0002	Large	Box of 100	$48.95

Alliance Absorbie Glove Liners. Glove liners to absorb perspiration when worn under exam gloves. Liners may be washed and reused. Nylon full and partial finger liners are also available as well as heavy knit cotton liners for those who may have to work outside.

Al Ag 24	100% Cotton Available in S, M, L	Pack of 50	$17.95
Al Ag 5305	100% Nylon Partial Finger (fits all)	Pack of 20	$28.95
Al Ag 5306	100% Nylon Full Finger (fits all)	Pack of 20	$26.95
Al Ag 5308	100% Cotton, Heavy Knit (fits all)	Pack of 50	$18.95

Alliance Chin Length Face Shield. Plastic full face shield.

Al F S01		Box of 20 $60.95

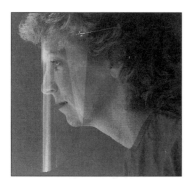

Bu 105-441

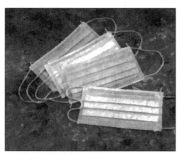

Le 118-8515

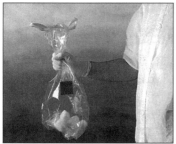

Un ED 1020

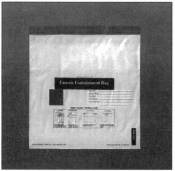

Un EM 1010

Steridyne Zero-G®, Face Guard. Mylar face shields with elastic band. Lightweight mask protects eyes, nose and mouth from sprayed contaminated fluids. Glare free.

St F-100   Pack of 10 $7.95

Burney Products Plastic Goggles. Clear lens, clear body. To wear when attending to infectious patient. Use with surgical type face mask.

Bu 105-441 $6.95

Burney Product Plastic Goggles for Visitors. Less expensive goggles to provide to visitors. Should be worn along with surgical type face mask.

Bu 105-461   Box of 12 $37.95

3M™ Earloop Face Mask. Fluid resistant. Greater than 99% bacterial filtration efficiency. Folded type expands for full coverage, nosepiece molds for snug fit. Easy to put on, no strings to tie. Lightweight, breathable.

Le 118-8515   Box of 20 $17.95

Baxter InstaGard, Earloop Style Masks. Soft stretchable earloops. Odorless, glass free, blue, nonwoven fabric is nonirritating. High bacterial filtration efficiency.

Le 176-4083   Box of 50 $14.95

Johnson & Johnson Germ Filter Mask. Protects against inhaling irritants like dust and pollen. One size fits all. Allows normal breathing and talking.

Le 321-3055   Box of 5 $4.95

3M™ Air Warming Mask. White, non-woven molded fiber mask. Warms and moistens inhaled air. Helps protect against breathing dry, cold air. Allows easier breathing for people with certain respiratory conditions.

3M 2644   Box of 3 $5.95

Uniflex Arm-Shield™ Collection Bag. Heavyweight arm-length bag protects exposed skin from items being collected that may be contaminated with blood and other possibly infectious body fluids. Easy to use. Hand is placed in bag and object is grasped through the bag. The bag is then inverted down the arm which places the object in the bag. The built-in cord is then used to tie the bag for disposal. Bag is transparent so you can see what you are doing. Great for picking up bandages and soiled disposable incontinent products.

Un ED 1020   10″ wide × 20″ high   Box of 50 $15.95

Uniflex Emesis (Vomiting) Containment Bag. Liquid-tight. Press and Close, safety seal. Extra-wide opening is designed for ease of use. Hands slip under flaps on each side to protect against splatter. After use, pull away strip over adhesive and press to close. 100% disposable and recyclable. Can be used for disposal of other infectious bodily fluids such as urine and feces.

Un EM 1010   10″ wide × 10″ high   Box of 100 $18.95

White Cross HemaGuard™ Stat Protection Kit. Helps limit the exposure to blood and other infectious materials. Compact size fits in pocket or purse. Ideal for traveling. Contents include Stat Strip™ pull open adhesive bandages, antiseptic hand wipes, latex gloves, paper towel, biohazard waste disposal bag.

Wh 09230   Each $3.95

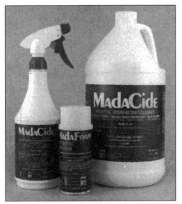

Wh 09234

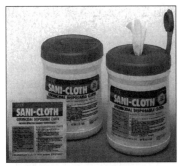

Le 148-8584 / Le 240-6452 /
Le 198-0598

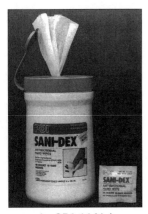

Le 354-1141 /
Le 354-1208

TO ORDER CALL TOLL FREE

LeBoeuf's

PHONE 1-800-546-5559
FAX 1-800-233-9692

Hearing Impaired with TDD
CALL 1-800-855-2880

White Cross HemaGuard™ C.P.R. Protection Kit. Administer C.P.R. without fear of contamination from the patient. Contents include 2 latex gloves, 1 adult C.P.R. valve mask, 2 antimicrobial hand wipes, 1 red biohazard waste disposal bag.

Wh 09234	$13.95

MadaCide Hospital Disinfectant/Cleaner. Ready-to-use, multipurpose, broad spectrum disinfectant/cleaner for infection control on surfaces and instruments. Bactericidal, virucidal, fungicidal, and tuberculocidal. Biodegradable detergent, non-corrosive, non-staining, non-toxic.

Le 379-1035	24 oz spray bottle	$9.95
Le 379-1100	1 gallon bottle	$25.95

MadaFoam Antiseptic Skin Foam. Multipurpose, antimicrobial skin foam cleanses and moisturizes contaminated hands without water. High level of antibacterial and antifungal action.

Le 379-1175	6 oz can	$10.95

PDI Sani-Cloth, Germicidal Disposable Cloth. Premoistened, disposable cloth for disinfection of hard, nonporous surfaces. Effective against gram positive and gram negative bacteria, fungi and yeast. Kills viruses such as influenza, A2 and HIV-1.

Le 148-8584	Large 6″ × 6¾″	160 per canister	$8.95
Le 240-6452	Extra large 11″ × 12″	60 per canister	$10.95
Le 198-0598	Individual packets, 11½″ × 11¾″	Box of 50	$32.95

PDI Sani-Dex™ Antimicrobial Hand Wipes. Effective against gram positive and gram negative bacteria, fungi and yeast. Reduces the risk of cross contamination. Friction removes transient and resident microorganisms. Gentle, contains aloe vera.

Le 354-1141	Regular	135 per canister	$7.95
Le 354-1208	Individual packets	100 per box	$6.95

ConvaTec Alcare, Foamed Hand Degermer. For use with routine and high-risk patient care. Effective against Herpes Simplex Type 2 Virus, Influenza A2. Leaves hands soft. Will not stain clothing or linen. Requires no water.

Co 6395-57	7 oz	$8.95

Alcoholism

Alcohol abuse or dependence among older men and women is a more serious problem than most people realize. It is estimated that there are approximately five million alcohol-dependent people and about seven million people who have trouble controlling their consumption of alcohol in the United States. Until recently, older problem drinkers tended to be ignored by both health professionals and the general public. Few older people were identified as alcoholics — chronic problem drinkers often died before old age — and because they were retired or had fewer social contacts, older people were often able to hide drinking problems.

A sure sign of an alcoholic is drinking alcohol in the morning to relieve the withdrawal symptoms from the previous night's drinking.

The physical effects of alcohol include the slowing down of brain activity, thereby impairing mental alertness, judgment and physical coordination. Heavy drinking also increases the risk of falls and accidents.

The toxic ingredient in alcoholic beverages is ethanol. Ethanol slows down the activities of the central nervous system (brain and spinal cord). It can impair reasoning and for many persons, removes inhibitions and self-control. Many alcoholics can be mean while others become meek as mice. Either way, the patient is not normal.

Symptoms of an overdose of alcohol:

- Slurred speech.
- Passed out.
- Odor of alcohol.
- Red streaks in the whites of the eyes.
- Abnormal breathing.
- Lack of coordination.
- Withdrawn behavior.
- Grief and depression.

Over time, heavy drinking can cause permanent damage to the brain and central nervous system, as well as to the liver, heart, kidneys and stomach. Alcoholism can also produce symptoms similar to those of dementia, forgetfulness, reduced attention and confusion. Heavy drinking of alcohol can also mask pain that might serve as a warning sign of a heart attack.

Older people run the greatest risk of a bad drug interaction since they make up 12 percent of the population, but take 25 percent of all medications. Mixing alcohol with drugs can be very dangerous. Alcohol may appear to act as a stimulant but really is a depressant.

In the older population, problem drinkers tend to be one of two types. The first are chronic abusers — those who have used alcohol heavily for many years. Although the most chronic users die by middle age, some survive into old age. Approximately two-thirds of older alcoholics are in this group.

The second type begins excessive drinking late in life, often in response to factors such as retirement, lowered income, declining health, loneliness or the deaths of friends or loved ones.

Signs of a drinking problem:

- Drinking to calm nerves, forget worries, or reduce depression.
- Losing interest in food.
- Gulping drinks and drinking too fast
- Lying about drinking habits.
- Drinking alone a lot.
- Injuring oneself, or someone else.
- Getting drunk often (more than 3 times a year).
- Needing to drink more to get the affect of the alcohol.
- Acting irritable, resentful or unreasonable during nondrinking periods.
- Experiencing medical, social, or financial problems caused by drinking.

Help for drinking problems can be obtained from a doctor, minister, Alcoholics Anonymous chapter or a local health or social service agency. Older problem drinkers and alcoholics have a good chance for recovery because older people tend to stay with treatment. Detoxification followed by long term treatment may be necessary.

Family members may find it difficult to live with an alcoholic. There are support groups for family and friends of alcoholics where they can learn about the illness and how best to live with an alcoholic. There are also groups for adults who grew up with an alcoholic parent(s). They tend to suffer long term effects from living and being raised in an alcoholic home.

What to do:

Contact Alcoholics Anonymous. Look in the phone book for your local chapter. Or write them at P.O. Box 459, Grand Central Station, New York, NY 10163. You can obtain a free pamphlet on alcoholism and the older patient entitled *Time to Start Living.*

Contact the National Clearinghouse for Alcohol Information. It is a federal information service. You can write for information at P.O. Box 2345, Rockville, MD 20852.

Contact the Council on Alcoholism and Drug Dependence, Inc. Their number is in your local phone book or you can write them at 733 Third Avenue, New York, NY 10017.

Contact American Council for Drug Education. 1-800-488-DRUG (3784). Or write to them at 204 Monroe Street, Rockville, MD 20850. The organization provides information on drug use and publishes a newsletter.

Contact Al-Anon Family Group Headquarters. 1-800-356-9996. If in New York or Canada call (212) 245-3151. Look for the local chapter's telephone number in the White Pages of your phone book. There are more than 30,000 groups. They provide materials on alcoholism specifically aimed at families.

Contact the National Council on Alcoholism. 1-800-622-2255. They provide information on local affiliates and written information on alcoholism.

Alzheimer's Disease

ALZHEIMER'S DISEASE is a degenerative brain disorder. Early stages of Alzheimer's Disease (AD) are characterized by memory loss — such as forgetting recent events, the names of familiar persons, or the ability to perform simple math problems. The disease gradually worsens, with the patient becoming confused, disoriented or frustrated. The patient may have difficulty communicating and making decisions. Personality and behavior changes occur, such as wandering, inappropriate undressing, aggressiveness, asking repetitive questions, yelling for no apparent reason, pilfering items, and visual and auditory hallucinations. In the later stages of AD, the patient may be in a vegetative condition and completely bedridden.

Approximately four million Americans have AD. It primarily affects people over 65 years old. Nearly 50 percent of those over age 85 may have the disorder. Although the risk of having AD increases as one grows older, the disease is not an inevitable process of aging.

Unfortunately, there is no known cure for AD and there are no simple diagnostic tests for AD. The lack of options available to cure or predict AD makes it one of the most difficult disorders to handle as a caregiver. Patients with AD have highly variable life expectancies. Some live for 20 years or more after the symptoms emerge.

The admission by former President Ronald Reagan of his Alzheimer's diagnosis brought a new awareness of the disease to the American public. In Reagan's 1994 letter to the public, he wrote of his illness, that "Unfortunately, as Alzheimer's Disease progresses, the family often bears a heavy burden."

The Caregiver Role

Some doctors question whether patients should even be told that they may have AD. Doctors have reported that while they are generally comfortable with communicating the diagnosis of cancer to their patients, many are unnerved at the prospect of revealing a diagnosis of Alzheimer's disease. However, informing the patient of the affliction in the early stages of the illness allows the patient to organize their personal, spiritual and financial affairs. The patient will need to settle financial and family matters before the later stages of the dementia arise. They also may want to seek another medical opinion. The still uncertain origins of AD has prompted a variety of laboratory studies, and patients informed of their AD diagnosis may wish to participate in scientific studies for a cure.

Several arguments can also be made for why a patient should not be told of the memory disorder. Severely demented patients may be unable to understand their condition and an explanation is futile. Some believe that being told of their possible AD diagnosis may make the disease more likely to occur (the "ostrich" theory).

Agitation is a predominant trait among AD patients. Nearly 90 percent of AD patients exhibit some form of agitation, such as verbal aggressiveness, physical attacks, restlessness and wandering.

Episodes of wandering are one of the most frightening aspects of caregiving. The patient, who is unable to gauge temperature variations, may leave the home unannounced, dressed only in pajamas and walk in the snow barefoot. Some patients may get lost and forget their addresses, even after living at the same location for decades.

Wandering behavior is not just restricted to patients who are able to walk. Patients confined to wheelchairs will also wander, so making the home safe for unsupervised wheelchair and gerichair movement is important. Blocking stairs with gates or locked doors will reduce the possibility of falls. Putting socks over door knobs will make it difficult for an Alzheimer patient to open doors.

The "Alzheimer's Association Safe Return Program" uses an identification system to help locate missing persons. For a $25 registration fee, an individual can be listed in a nationwide database. Clothing labels, a bracelet or necklace, and wallet cards are issued to help identify a missing person. No matter what type of identification is used, be sure that the patient cannot remove it.

For physically and verbally agitated patients, drugs may be prescribed to reduce the incidence of violent behavior.

The patient in the later stages of AD is disoriented and confused, and sometimes fails to recognize family members. Sometimes they cannot even remember how to use household appliances like a can opener and might use a knife instead. They may even become frightened at seeing their own image reflected in a mirror.

Advanced stages of AD may also force dietary changes. Feeding of a demented patient can be an increasingly time-consuming task. Finger foods will need to be served for those incapable of handling eating utensils. Some patients will require spoonfeeding.

Caregiving for an AD patient can be extremely demanding. As the disease progresses and worsens, the individual becomes more demented and requires more supervision. The coping strategies for the caregiver often have direct effects on the patient. Studies have shown that caregiver behavior is significantly associated with patient behavior. For the caregiver, a greater understanding of the processes of the disease and improved skills in taking care of the patient leads to improved morale. The informed caregiver is better able to separate feelings of low morale and burden from intolerance of the patient's behavior. Positive verbal exchanges between the patient and the caregiver instead of negative comments help create a more pleasant environment. Encouraging the AD patient to participate in pleasant activities, such as listening to music, looking through a photo album, and dancing will also help both the caregiver and the patient. Try and establish as much of a routine as possible to help overcome the patient's confusion.

Married patients in the early stages of the disease are still highly aware of the stress and burden the ailment causes the spouse. The afflicted spouse is aware that joint activities may have declined and that the caregiving spouse may want other companionship and feels a "need to escape." Such feelings sometimes lead to false accusations of infidelity, and add to the stress level of an already stressful situation.

One study at a New York nursing home saw improvement in patient behavior result from the creation of a "Wanderer's Lounge." An area was created in the facility where patients prone to incessant wandering were allowed to freely explore and touch objects in the room. A similar type environment can be created in the home.

Tips on establishing and maintaining contact with someone who has Alzheimer's disease:

- Lower your voice and talk in a calm manner.
- Do not give more than one direction at a time.
- Maintain eye contact when talking with the patient.
- Give the patient simple repetitive tasks such as folding napkins, picking up the newspapers.
- Do not put pressure on the patient to be ready at specific times — take your time and let the patient do the same.
- Disguise exits with screens and by painting the door the same color as the wall.
- Play music. Many patients respond to music.
- Wear name tags and repeat your name.
- Provide a bright living area.

Safety Check List

Lock all medicines away (use medicine bottles with child resistant caps). ☐
Dispose of plastic bags that are big enough to fit over the patient's head. ☐
Lock away all power tools. ☐
Remove poisonous plants from the home. ☐
Remove locks from bathroom doors. ☐
Cover or remove mirrors (later stages). ☐
Post poison control number by phone. ☐
Disconnect or lock switch on the garbage disposal. ☐
Remove and/or lock away all alcohol. ☐
Remove and/or lock away matches. ☐
Remove clutter (tape down throw rugs or remove). ☐
Keep the refrigerator and pantry clean of spoiled food. ☐
Store hazardous chemicals in a secure place. ☐
Take knobs off kitchen stove or use knob covers. ☐
Install fire extinguishers, smoke alarms and other electronic alert alarms. ☐
Reduce temperature of the hot water heater to a maximum of 120° degrees F. ☐
Lock away any guns. ☐
Remove fish tanks. ☐
Give a neighbor a key and obtain their phone number. ☐
Install secure locks on all exterior doors (hide a spare key outside the home in case the patient locks you out). ☐

Nobody can live with Alzheimer's Disease alone.

Presented on the following pages are products and services that will make life easier for the caregiver and the patient. Remember you will never be alone. **LeBoeuf's ☎ 1-800-546-5559** will endeavor to assist you in every way possible.

Beginnings of Alzheimer's — 2 to 4 Years

Symptoms:　　Memory begins to affect job performance
　　　　　　Gets lost going to work
　　　　　　Loses zest — becomes lethargic
　　　　　　Can't begin anything
　　　　　　Makes bad decisions
　　　　　　Has trouble paying bills — might pay none or
　　　　　　　　pay some 2 or 3 times
　　　　　　Loses things
　　　　　　Has trouble finding right words

　　Check the list below for safety products and services to purchase prior to the patient moving into your home. We will provide you with suggestions of how to rearrange or remodel your home to make life easier for both the patient and the caregiver. All you need to do is follow the instructions in the section titled "Modifying Your Home and Making It Safer." (pages 15-52)

　　It would also be a good idea for you and/or the patient to inform the neighbors that the patient has Alzheimer's. Most neighbors will be happy to assist in keeping watch over the patient and the home. There is nothing to be ashamed about in asking for help. In fact, if more people did ask for help, their life could be much easier. We all have to learn to help each other.

　　In addition to the products shown, **we** can find and/or supply you with just about any product made. If you have a special need, we and our suppliers will work with you to find a solution. Call **LeBoeuf's** ☎ 1-800-546-5559.

Products That Will be Needed

	Yes	No
Smoke Detectors	☐	☐
Pill Counter or dispenser	☐	☐
Telephone that automatically dials special number	☐	☐
Hot water sensor	☐	☐
Exercise programs (mental and physical)	☐	☐
Bath supplies		
Grab bars	☐	☐
Safety rails	☐	☐
Scale	☐	☐
Shower spray (hand held)	☐	☐
Safety bath mat	☐	☐
Phone answering machine	☐	☐
Install:		
Secure locks on all exterior doors (hide a spare key outside the home in case the patient locks you out.)	☐	☐
Light movement sensors outside the home	☐	☐
Childproof plugs for electric outlets	☐	☐
Safety grip strips on carpet and stairs	☐	☐
Bright or reflective tape on stair edges	☐	☐

Helpful Hint:
Use different colored tape to mark
the first and last steps so patient
will know when they have reached
the top or bottom of stairs.

Over 70 percent of Alzheimer's
patients are cared for in the home.
The cost of home care can run up to
$18,000 per year.

Middle Phase of Alzheimers — 2 to 10 Years

By the time an Alzheimers patient reaches this phase, they are usually provided for in the home of the caregiver.

Symptoms:
- Memory loss and more confusion
- Can't recognize close friends or family
- Keep repeating themselves
- Shorter attention span
- Very restless, especially in late afternoon and at night
- Occasional muscle twitching or jerking
- Problems with reading, writing and math
- Become suspicious, irritable, cry or act silly
- Become sloppy — won't bathe, bad table manners
- Trouble dressing — may undress at any time or in the wrong place

Products That Will be Needed	Yes	No
Bright tape to mark edge of steps	☐	☐
Swimming pool alarm	☐	☐
Light and movement sensors outside the home	☐	☐
Put up a "NO SOLICITATION" sign	☐	☐
Child proof latches on cabinet doors	☐	☐
Night lights, motion sensor light for rooms	☐	☐
Intercom device to warn of a fall or a need for help for bedrooms and bath	☐	☐
Bed rails	☐	☐
Blanket support	☐	☐
Bedding (sheets, pillows and cover, pads)	☐	☐
Wall-to-wall washable carpeting for bath	☐	☐
Foam rubber cover for faucet in tub	☐	☐
Decals for large glass doors or windows	☐	☐
Put mail box outside gate or purchase mail box you can lock	☐	☐
Equip a "wandering" room with lots of objects the patient can touch and handle	☐	☐
Bathtub thermometer	☐	☐
Childproof latch on refrigerator and oven	☐	☐
Install a kill switch on the auto(s)	☐	☐
Bathing supplies		
Soaps	☐	☐
Creams and oils	☐	☐
Bath seats	☐	☐
Hand held shower set	☐	☐
Bath grab rails	☐	☐
Diverter valve for shower	☐	☐
Bathtub safety grabs	☐	☐
Bath/shower safety mat	☐	☐
Bath carpet	☐	☐
Blood pressure monitor	☐	☐
Pill dispenser	☐	☐
Thermometer	☐	☐
Exercise equipment	☐	☐

Talking books, videos, mind games .... ☐ ☐
Lingerie .... ☐ ☐
Bedside chest .... ☐ ☐
Wardrobe .... ☐ ☐
Recliner chair (waterproof) .... ☐ ☐
Cubicle curtains .... ☐ ☐

Alzheimer's Association Safe Return Program

The Alzheimer's Association Safe Return Program was developed to assist police, community agencies and private citizens to identify people with Alzheimer's disease and related disorders, and help return them home. In addition to identification, you also have access to the Alzheimer's Association help-lines, education and support groups for caregivers. There are 35,000 Alzheimer's Association volunteers who serve in all 50 states.

The Safe Return Program provides:

- An identification bracelet or necklace, clothing labels and wallet cards to identify the memory-impaired patient.
- Registration in a national database
- A 24-hour toll-free 800 number to contact when a patient is lost or found
- Access to the National Crime Information Computer, a national network of 17,000 local law enforcement agencies, to help find missing patients.
- A nationwide network of 220 community-based Alzheimer's Association chapters to provide education, training and support to families and caregivers

You should allow six weeks for delivery of the identification products.

The cost for the Alzheimer's Association Safe Return Program is $25.00. You can also register directly by calling 1-800-272-3900 or writing:

Safe Return
P.O. Box A-3956
Chicago, IL 60690

If you wish to write the Alzheimer's Association national headquarters, the address is:

Alzheimer's Association
919 North Michigan Avenue
Chicago, IL 60611

There is also a TTY number: (312) 335-8882

Keep your mailbox locked. AD patients often hide or throw away mail.

Last Phase of Alzheimers — 1- 3 Years

Patients are not able to assist themselves. Nursing or hospice support is needed to assist the caregiver in the home. The number of possible friends and relatives who can provide respite care for a patient in this phase of the disease is reduced because many people cannot handle this type of stress. Young people do not understand the disease and can become frightened of the patient and their behavior. It takes a knowledgeable and mature person to handle many patients in the later stages of Alzheimer's disease. Even then, constant support for the caregiver(s) must be expressed every day.

Symptoms:
- Can't recognize family or talk to themselves looking in a mirror
- Loses weight even with a good appetite
- Unable to communicate with words (groans or grunts; or even screams)
- May put everything in their mouths or touch everything
- Can't control bowels or bladder
- May have seizures
- May have difficulty swallowing
- Skin infections
- Sleep more

Products That Will be Needed	Yes	No
Hospital bed	☐	☐
Overbed table	☐	☐
Wheelchair	☐	☐
Wheelchair accessories (cushions, tables)	☐	☐
Wheelchair ramps	☐	☐
Walker	☐	☐
Helmet	☐	☐
Transfer board	☐	☐
First aid kits	☐	☐
Medication helpers (pill cases, spoons, etc.)	☐	☐
Bath supplies		
Transfer bench for bathtub	☐	☐
Toilet safety frame	☐	☐
Commode	☐	☐
Bath or shower seat	☐	☐
Incontinence supplies		
Disposable underpads	☐	☐
Undergarments	☐	☐
Disposable washcloths	☐	☐
Disposable towels	☐	☐
Rubber/flannel sheet	☐	☐
Bed pad and alarm	☐	☐
Reusable quilted underpads (waterproof)	☐	☐
Disposable gloves	☐	☐
Fecal containment device	☐	☐
Perineal foam cleanser with odor control	☐	☐
Body wash and shampoo	☐	☐
Barrier and moisturizer creams	☐	☐
Protective clothing (disposable)	☐	☐

Collection bags . . . . ☐ ☐
Cleaning supplies . . . . ☐ ☐
Hand degerming soap . . . . ☐ ☐
Bed sore and wound products
Gauze sponges . . . . ☐ ☐
Bandages . . . . ☐ ☐
First aid kit . . . . ☐ ☐
Tape . . . . ☐ ☐
Wound dressing . . . . ☐ ☐
Wound packing . . . . ☐ ☐
Wound dressing kit . . . . ☐ ☐
Skin cleanser . . . . ☐ ☐
Bed sore prevention and care products
Pressure sore pads and mattresses . . . . ☐ ☐
Heel, foot and elbow protectors . . . . ☐ ☐
Wound cleaner . . . . ☐ ☐
Bedding . . . . ☐ ☐
Lifting device . . . . ☐ ☐

What to do

One third of all falls in and around the home occur in the bathroom.

Contact a doctor — Have the patient make and keep the appointment. There is no single or simple test for Alzheimer's Disease. It will take a lot of testing to be sure that the patient has Alzheimer's. It is important to have this diagnosis done as soon as the first signs of Alzheimer's appear. If you have a family doctor, he may recommend you take the patient to see a neurologist. If the diagnosis determines that the patient has Alzheimer's, the following will provide the caregiver with information, support and services to assist in coping with the initial onset of the disease through the final stages.

Contact the Alzheimer's Association — 1-800-272-3900. They will provide the caregiver and the patient with lots and lots of information to assist in understanding the disease. Very responsive and understanding. There are 220 Alzheimer's Association chapters, 1,800 support groups and 35,000 volunteers throughout the United States.

Contact the Alzheimer's Disease Education and Referral Center — (301) 587-4352. The address is P.O. Box 8250, Silver Spring, MD 20907. This is an information clearinghouse run by the National Institute on Aging. They can provide information on such topics as home safety, managing stress, caregiving skills and other useful information.

Contact the Alzheimer's Disease and Related Disorders Association, Inc. (312) 335-8700 or TDD: (312) 335-8882. 919 N. Michigan Ave., Suite 1000, Chicago, IL 60611-1676. Over 3,000 support groups and 200 chapters exist nationwide.

Contact the local social services organizations. There are many agencies that will provide information and listings of resources available in your area. Agencies such as the offices on aging, local health agencies as well as religious-affiliated service groups also provide information, training and support. There are also associations and companies that provide care management services to serve as the link between you and community-based services. They charge for their services; so be sure you understand what it will cost to have them provide assistance.

Contact a lawyer — It is very important to act quickly to protect the future security of the patient. There are lawyers who specialize in elder law. You will need to execute a durable power of attorney, a living will and/or a living trust. Living trusts appear to be the best way to handle an estate because you can avoid probate and not have an estate's assets tied up by the courts. Contact **LeBoeuf's** ☎ 1-800-546-5559 for a listing of lawyers in your area.

Safety — Organize the home to permit the patient to carry on as much of the normal daily routines as possible. Take precautions concerning wandering and especially bathing. Other tips and items that make for a safer home are listed below and in the section titled "Modifying Your Home and Making it Safer."

Communication — Explain to the patient what is happening. Tell only as much as the patient wants to know. Tell family and friends. Explain the symptoms and tell family and friends that you need their support and love. Tell them how and when they can help. Be specific about your needs. Draw up a plan of action that allows everyone to understand the role that they can (and must) play.

LeBoeuf's Services

Call **LeBoeuf's** ☎ 1-800-546-5559 for the following services. Please have ready the patient's name, address, zip code, age, telephone number and physical circumstances (Alzheimer's, heart problem, arthritis, etc.) when you call.

- Consulting Service
    - Wheelchairs (design, ultra-light, sports chairs, etc.)
    - Van Conversions
    - Electronics
        - Hearing
        - Vision
        - Security
        - Communication (TTY, Call Buttons, Telephones, etc.)
        - Television, VCR's, Radio, Stereo
        - Computers and Software

- Home Healthcare Workshops

- Caregivers Speakers Bureau

- Incontinent Supply Service

- Respite Network

- Home Modification Planning Service

- Assistive Travel Agency

- Employment Screening Service

- Referral Service for:
    - Hospitals
    - Nursing homes
    - Hospice
    - Visiting nurse associations
    - Adult day care programs
    - Respite care (nursing homes, support groups,)
    - Social services case workers
    - Household help

LeBoeuf's

PHONE **1-800-546-5559**

FAX **1-800-233-9692**

Hearing Impaired with TDD
CALL **1-800-855-2880**

Arthritis

HALF OF ALL PEOPLE over the age of 65 have arthritis. Of the more than 100 forms of arthritis, osteoarthritis, rheumatoid arthritis and gout are the most common in older people. There are about 37 million adults and an estimated 200,000 children with arthritis. Three out of four are women. While the causes of most arthritis are unknown, and most forms cannot be prevented or cured, there is much that can be done to overcome or cope with the disease.

Sometimes, a common disease known as fibromyalgia — a disease that causes the muscles to become too tight in response to pain — is misdiagnosed as arthritis. Most of the people affected by fibromyalgia are women and there are about 10 million Americans with the disease. It affects the soft tissues around the joints, unlike arthritis which affects the joints themselves.

Osteoarthritis (OA)

Osteoarthritis (OA) is sometimes called degenerative joint disease. Symptoms can range from a mild problem with only occasional stiffness and joint pain to a serious condition with much pain and disability. Osteoarthritis most often affects the hands and large weight-bearing joints of the body such as the feet, knees, hips, neck and back. Early in the disease pain occurs after activity and rest brings relief. Later on, pain can occur with minimal movement or even while at rest.

Several factors may produce osteoarthritis in different joints. OA in the hands or hips may run in families. Being overweight has been linked to OA in the knees. Injuries or overuse may relate to OA in joints such as the knees, hips and elbows.

Rheumatoid Arthritis (RA)

Rheumatoid arthritis (RA) can be one of the more disabling forms of arthritis but varies in severity. Signs of RA include morning stiffness, swelling in three or more joints, swelling of the hands and wrists and swelling of the same joints on both sides of the body. RA can occur at any age and affects women about three times more often than men. If the patient's drug program for controlling RA is not properly managed, the pain from RA can become very intense and joint damage and deformities can be irreversible. An exercise program is also important to maintain the patient's muscle strength and mobility. Scientists believe that RA may result from a breakdown in the immune system. It is also likely that people who get RA have certain inherited traits that cause this process to go awry.

Gout

Gout often occurs in young men. Later in life both men and women are equally affected. Gout affects the toes, ankles, knees, elbows, wrists and hands. An acute attack of gout is very painful. Swelling may cause the skin to pull tightly around the joint and make the area red or purple and very painful to

Medications can cause unwanted
side effects.such as:
   Heartburn
   Nausea
   Stomach pain
   Vomiting
   Diarrhea
   Headaches
   Dizziness
   Blurred vision
   Black Stools
Call the doctor if in doubt about
what is happening with the patient.

touch. Medication can now stop gout attacks, as well as prevent future ones. Drinking alcohol can be a problem and should be limited.

Treatment, Therapy and Medication

Treatment for arthritis may include medications, special exercises, use of heat or cold therapy, diet and/or surgery. Plenty of sleep is also highly recommended. The patient should sleep 8 to 10 hours a night and lie down for about half an hour twice or more a day. Correct body position during rest is to extend joints rather than flexing them. A firm mattress, a straight backed chair, a raised toilet seat and other assistive aids will help in reducing fatigue and allow the patient to minimize discomfort.

Medications help relieve pain and reduce inflammation. The medications used most often are aspirin and nonsteroidal anti-inflammatory drugs, such as ibuprofen. These drugs block the production of chemicals in the body that cause pain and inflammation. Most of the medications used are only available by prescription. It often takes two to three weeks before the full benefits of the medicines are felt.

Corticosteroids also may reduce arthritis inflammation and can be taken by mouth or by injection. While corticosteroids rapidly relieve the pain, swelling and redness caused by arthritis, these drugs have serious side effects including lowered resistance to infection, indigestion, weight gain, loss of muscle mass and strength. You should make sure that the patient is under close doctor's supervision when taking this or any medication.

Medications can cause unwanted side effects in some people. Make sure you keep the doctor informed so that an adjustment in the patient's treatment can be made to keep side effects to a minimum. Things to watch out for include: heartburn, nausea, stomach pain, vomiting, diarrhea and, occasionally, gastrointestinal bleeding. Gastrointestinal bleeding can be especially serious for older people and can be recognized by very black or very dark stools or blood in the stool. Some medicines can also cause headaches, dizziness and blurred vision. Follow the doctor's directions very carefully to prevent and/or minimize side effects.

There are many other medications that are being used to treat arthritis and the doctor will provide the patient with the most current and effective treatment, or combination of treatments. Tell the doctor what other drugs the patient is taking and follow the doctor's instructions exactly. Take the amount specified and ask what to do if you miss a dose. Make sure the patient keeps all doctor appointments. Don't fall for quack remedies. Over a billion dollars is spent each year on useless pills, gadgets and diets hoping to find a cure for arthritis.

Symptoms:
- Swelling in one or more joints.
- Early morning stiffness that lasts for more than an hour.
- Recurring pain or tenderness in any joint.
- Inability to move a joint normally.
- Obvious redness or warmth in a joint.
- Unexplained weight loss, fever, or weakness combined with joint pain.

If any of these symptoms last for more than two weeks, the patient should see a doctor.

What to do:

Contact a doctor — Have the patient make and keep the appointment. There is no single or simple test for arthritis. It will take a lot of testing to be sure that the patient has arthritis. Testing may include blood tests, x-rays, and drawing fluid from an affected joint. It is important to have this diagnosis done as soon as the first signs of arthritis appear. If the diagnosis determines that the patient has arthritis, the following sources will provide the caregiver with information, support and services that will help the patient to cope with the initial onset of the disease.

Contact the Arthritis Foundation — 1-800-283-7800. They will provide the caregiver and the patient with information to assist in understanding the disease. They are very responsive and understanding. Have your zip code number ready when you call and the voice mail system will provide the number of the closest office.

Contact the National Institute of Arthritis and Musculoskeletal and Skin Diseases — Building 31, Room 4C05, Bethesda, MD 20892. This is an information clearinghouse run by the National Institute on Aging. They can provide information on such topics as home safety, managing stress, caregiving skills and other useful information.

Contact local social services organizations — There are many agencies that will provide information and listings of resources available in your area. Agencies such as the offices on aging, local health agencies and religious-affiliated service groups also provide information, training and support. There are also associations and companies that provide care management services to serve as the link between you and community-based services. They charge for their services — so be sure you understand what it will cost to have them provide assistance.

Safety — Organize the home to permit the patient to carry on as much of their normal routines as possible. Take precautions concerning walking (remove loose rugs, etc.) and especially bathing. For additional tips for patient's safety see the section "Modifying Your Home and Making if Safer." There are many products that will help to make things easier for an arthritis patient.

Communication — Tell family and friends how they can help the patient cope with arthritis.

If you have any questions, please call **LeBoeuf's** ☎ 1-800-546-5559

LeBoeuf's Services

Call **LeBoeuf's** ☎ 1-800-546-5559 for the following services. Please have ready the patient's name, address, zip code, age, telephone number and physical circumstances (Alzheimer's, heart problem, arthritis, etc.) when you call.

- Consulting Service
    - Wheelchairs (design, ultra-light, sports chairs, etc.)
    - Van Conversions
    - Electronics
        - Hearing
        - Vision
        - Security
        - Communication (TTY, Call Buttons, Telephones, etc.)
        - Television, VCR's, Radio, Stereo
        - Computers and Software

- Home Healthcare Workshops
- Caregivers Speakers Bureau
- Incontinent Supply Service
- Respite Network
- Home Modification Planning Service
- Assistive Travel Agency
- Employment Screening Service
- Referral Service for:
    - Hospitals
    - Nursing homes
    - Hospice
    - Visiting nurse associations
    - Adult day care programs
    - Respite care (nursing homes, support groups,)
    - Social services case workers
    - Household help

LeBoeuf's

PHONE **1-800-546-5559**

FAX **1-800-233-9692**

Hearing Impaired with TDD
CALL **1-800-855-2880**

Arthritis Aids

THERE ARE A NUMBER OF low-cost steps that a patient can take to help relieve the discomfort and pain caused by arthritis. Here are some products and a few ideas that will assist the patient.

- Use lighter weight aluminum utensils when cooking.
- Use lightweight plastic dishes.
- Use double handled pots to allow the use of both hands when lifting.
- Use slow cookers, toaster ovens and microwaves to lessen the bending required when using the oven.
- A few rustproof nails in a cutting board will hold the food, which allows for the use of both hands when cutting.
- Use an electric can opener.
- Tell the pharmacist not to use child proof caps on medicine bottles.
- Buy a key holder that allows the patient to have leverage when turning the key.

For heat therapy — have the patient take a warm shower, soak in a tub, or apply warm wet cloths where needed. A heating pad wrapped in a towel is also good heat therapy — and heating pads are relatively inexpensive. Some patients will benefit more from cold therapy. Ice bags and cold moist towels are an inexpensive way to obtain relief.

Be sure that the patient takes medication as prescribed. Sometimes many different drugs need to be taken to achieve desired results. Set up a schedule for medication and follow it closely. There are medication helpers (pill crushers, pill cutters, oral medication syringes) available to assist in taking the medication. There are also a number of products designed to help you and the patient keep track of the medication schedule. If the patient's symptoms become worse during drug therapy, let the doctor know at once. Ointments and liniments provide some relief, but these substances are absorbed through the skin and can cause problems if used excessively.

There are many good products and therapies that can help the patient overcome pain and discomfort. If the patient complains about pain, contact your doctor for assistance. Why "tough it out" when there are products and therapies that will help? Again, a little common sense goes a long way toward helping the patient reduce pain and reduce the cost of treatment. A good example of using common sense would be working with an overweight patient to develop a weight reduction diet if there is pain in the knees, ankles or feet.

Always contact your doctor before the patient takes any medication, treatment or uses any device. Be especially careful that the patient does not fall for expensive and quack therapies, devices and treatments. If you cannot contact the doctor, call the Arthritis Foundation at 1-800-283-7800 for help and information. The Arthritis Foundation will set you and the patient straight on what works and what doesn't.

Arthritis Aids

Pride Lift Recliner Chairs. Sealed single-switch hand control. These chairs help the patient get up from the chair without assistance. They are good looking, very comfortable and recline to two or three positions. The chairs have double plate, wide base, steel frames. Arm covers and headrest are included. Oak chair frame. Fire retardant foams and fabrics. Weight capacity 300 pounds. Lifetime warranty on steel frame.

If you already have a good recliner, or similar comfortable chair, LeBoeuf's has an electric lift frame that attaches to the chair to make it a lift chair. Call LeBoeuf's for more information.

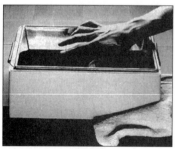

Le 112-5897 / Le 112-6283

Pride Gentle Lift 2-position recliner.

Le 121-9971	Camel color	$879.95
LE 122-1209	Mauve color	$879.95
Le 121-8528	Deep Blue color	$879.95

Pride Luxury 3-position recliner.

Le 112-5897	Aztec color	$949.95
Le 112-6283	Cinnamon color	$949.95

Pride Body Lounger 3-position recliner.

Le 148-0169	Aztec color	$1,059.95
Le 148-0839	Cinnamon color	$1,059.95

Thermamed Paraffin Bath. Safe smooth heat therapy. Stimulates circulation. Faster, longer lasting heat penetration. Preset at 128 to 132 degrees. Three-year warranty. Five-pound pan of wax comes with unit.

Le 220-7892	$189.95

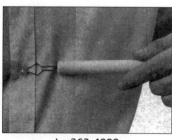

Le 220-7892

Thermamed Paraffin Bath. Wax refill. Five-pound pan. Just lift out old pan, drop in new pan. Lanolin rich paraffin wax formula.

Le 220-8031	$25.95

Thermamed Cloth Wraps. Makes hard-to-reach body areas easily treatable. Cotton/polyester terrycloth 24″ × 6″. Convenient, sanitary and easy to store.

Le 220-8023	$5.95

SunMark Daily Helper Foam Tubing. Ideal for building up handles of forks, pencils, toothbrushes. Easy to hold and clean.

Le 363-4821	$5.95

SunMark Daily Helper Button Aid. Allows user to fasten buttons with only one hand.

Le 363-4888	$7.95

Le 363-4888

SunMark Daily Helper Jar Opener. Loosens any jar lid with a twist of the wrist.

Le 363-4649	$7.95

LILA Lidbuster. For vacuum sealed jars. Simple and easy to use. Lidbuster goes under lid and handles are squeezed until vacuum is broken.

Li 436781	Works on paint cans, Tupperware, etc.	$4.95

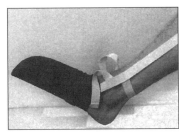

Le 363-4706

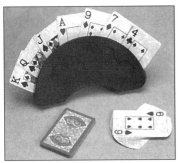

Li 147622

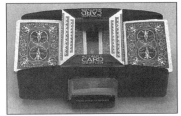

Li 151400

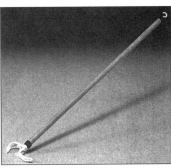

Ca 843500

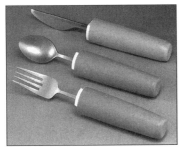

Ca 849000 / Ca 849100 / Ca 849200

LILA Book/Recipe Holder. Handcrafted by a furniture designer who signs each holder. Solid base is made from selected hardwood and the protecting screen is of washable lucite.

Li 828426   9 × 5½ × 6¾ inches   **$19.95**

SunMark Daily Helper Sock Aid. Easy to use. Convenient cords to pull sock over foot and up leg. Can be used sitting or standing.

Le 363-4706   **$14.95**

Carex Extra Long Metal Shoe Horn. 24″ chrome-plated shaft with loop hole on handle for hanging.

Le 139-8999   **$13.95**

LILA Card Player, Card Holder. Solid, light and easy to hold, yet built to stand up. Self adjusting action. Inner liner that spaces cards farther apart and hold the cards even when the hand is turned down. ABS plastic. Great for those patients with arthritis.

Li 147622   Weighs 5 ounces   **$9.95**

LILA Disc Card Holder. Simple device allows those without finger strength or dexterity to hold a hand of cards. Single cards can be added or removed without disturbing other cards.

Li 257418   Weighs only ½ ounce   **$2.95**

LILA Playing Card Holder. Unique tension device holds up to 13 cards. Metal with walnut wood grain finish. Weighted to stay on the table without tipping.

Li 614600   Card holder is 10¾ inches long   **$6.95**

LILA Playing Card Shuffler. Shuffles two decks of cards at the touch of a lever. Two "C" batteries are required and not included.

Li 151400   Unit is 8 × 4¼ × 3½ inches   **$14.95**

Carex Exerciser Ball. Strengthens hand and finger muscles. Long lasting rubberized construction.

Ca 512500   **$4.95**

Carex Dressing Stick. Provides added convenience while dressing. Unique design of ends allows easier access to hard-to-reach places such as shoelaces, socks, zippers, etc.

Ca 843500   **$6.95**

Carex Knife, Fork and Spoon. Large handle provides easy grasp. Dishwasher safe.

Ca 849000	Knife	**$10.95**
Ca 849100	Fork	**$10.95**
Ca 849200	Spoon	**$10.95**

Carex Pen/Pencil Gripper. Triangular gripper fits over writing instruments.

Ca 847000   **$6.95**

LILA Arthwriter. Helps the patient with arthritis to eat, write and brush their teeth. Lightweight plastic ball. Weighs 2 ounces.

Li 089010   3-inch diameter with ¾-inch center hole   **$7.95**

Carex Key Holder. Holds two keys. Handle provides leverage for easy use.

Ca 845000   **$5.95**

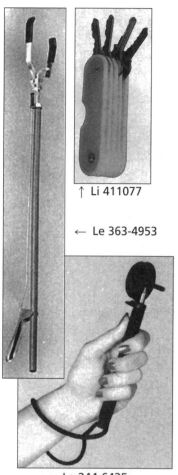

↑ Li 411077

← Le 363-4953

Le 244-6425

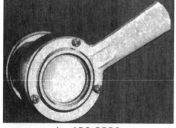

Le 139-3339

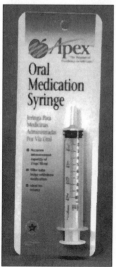

AP 7004L

LILA Giant Key Holder. Holds four keys. Handle provides leverage for easy use.
Li 411077   3¼ inches long $9.95

LILA Push Button Padlock. Keyless high security lock. Push buttons to open lock. Rust resistant.
Li 569400   Chrome plated $6.95

LILA Klik-Lok Padlock. Combination lock works with parallel levers instead of a dial. Can be opened by feeling or hearing the clicks.
Li 411322 $7.95

Sun Mark Daily Helper Reacher. 30-inch reach. Strong metal shaft with sturdy grasping claw and nonslip rubber tips. Easy-to-use mechanism and easy to grasp handle.
Le 363-4953 $11.95

SunMark Daily Helper Deluxe Reacher. 32″ reach. Lightweight with trigger mechanism that requires only light pressure to operate.
Le 115-3329 $16.95

SunMark Daily Helper Scissors with pouch. Easy-to-squeeze handles that reopen automatically after being squeezed. Can be used with either hand.
Le 363-4763 $19.95

LILA E-Z Grip Scissors. Stainless steel cutting blades with molded-on nylon handles. Scissors have round safety blades. 8″ overall length.
Li 275717   With hang-up holder to protect blades $21.95

Carica 2200 TeleStik™ Portable Retriever. Retrieves objects weighing up to 1.5 pounds, with hook or adhesive disk. Folds to 8″ and extends to 34″. Portable.
Le 244-6425 $25.95

Carica 2400 TeleStik™ Portable Retriever. Retrieves objects weighing up to 1.5 pounds. Comes with with hook, hook/loop, adhesive disk or magnet. Folds to 8″, extends to 34″. Portable.
Le 244-7373 $41.95

Carica Ultrastik Adhesive Disk (pad only). Adhesive disk retrieves objects up to 1.5 pounds. Gentle enough to retrieve paper products without tearing. Adhesive rejuvenates with soap and water. Guaranteed for 2,000 pick-ups.
Le 211-0674 $5.95

Carex Metal Door Extension. Provides leverage for easy gripping. Fits over standard door knob.
Le 139-3339 $11.95

LILA Tab Puller. Helps open cans with tabs.
Li 755888 $1.95

Apex Oral Syringe. Helps dispense liquid medication accurately. Easy-to-read black highlighted calibration markings with free filler tube.
AP 70004L $1.55

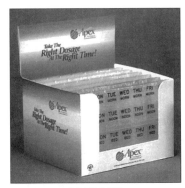

AP 70013L

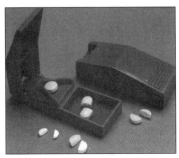

AP 70028L

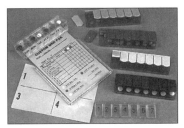

Bo MD 1001 / Bo MD Liner

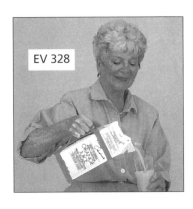

EV 328

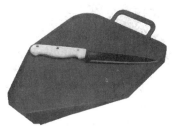

Li 206862

Apex 7-Day Pill Organizer. Seven compartment weekly organizer. Raised highlighted letters and braille markings for the sight impaired.

AP 70010L $1.75

Apex Mediplanner II. Allows for weekly medication planning. Each organizer has 28 pill compartments. Lids are marked morning, noon, bedtime and evening. Features a living hinge that strengthens as it is used.

AP 70013L $7.95

Apex Pill Splitter. Stainless steel bale to divide pills and vitamins of all types. Requires only light pressure of a single finger. Reduces crumbling and uneven dosages.

AP 70028L $5.95

Borin-Halbich The 7 Pack. One color per day with 4 compartments for each day marked morning, noon, evening and bedtime. Extra large compartments.

Bo 6001 $8.95

Borin-Halbich Multi-Dose Pill Box. Revolutionary system for accurate medication dispensing. A pharmacist-prepared legal container with a built-in visible means of entry detection. After trays are filled, a tight, light-resistant and disposable lid is secured to the trays. When the lids are opened, they break off and the residual tab becomes the visible means of entry detection. Starter kit comes with 40 amber bottoms and 200 colored lids (50 each of yellow, red, white and blue). If your pharmacist says that the medication must be dispensed in disposable units, liners are available in lots of 200.

Bo MD 1001 $139.95
Bo MD Liner   200 Liners $8.95

Apex Pill Pulverizer. Easy to use and clean and has a powerful pulverizing point. Handy pill storage in lid.

AP 70029 $5.95

Handi-Holder Deluxe for half-gallon paper milk and juice cartons. For pouring or carrying.

EV 328 $1.95

Handi-Holder for 1 quart paper milk and juice cartons. For pouring or carrying.

EV 324 $1.55

Handi-Holder for 1 gallon cartons.

EV 923 $2.25

Handi-Holder for oblong glass bottles.

EV 1259 $1.95

LILA Cutting Board with Food Chute. Easy to hold and has enough cutting space for most daily cutting needs. Guides food to bowl or container. Sturdy, lightweight and dishwasher safe.

Li 206862 $5.95

LILA Extra Long Kitchen Tweezers. 10-inch long tweezers are made of stainless steel. Great for getting olives out of those tall jars.

Li 307846   For serving hors d'oeuvres, turning food, etc. $5.95

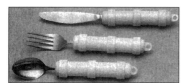

Le 197-6332 / Le 197-6414 /
Le 197-6877

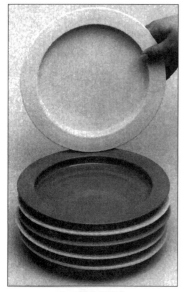

Le 197-5572

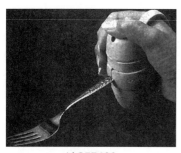

Li 357400

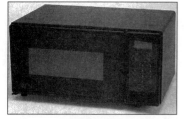

Li 481500

LILA Boxtopper. Easy way to open boxes. Molded plastic blade quickly slices through any box.

| Li 126544 | Also opens food bags and frozen juice cartons | $4.95 |

Southwest Technologies Elasto-Gel Therapy Mitten (hot or cold). Excellent treatment for arthritic hands. For cold therapy, mitten may be cooled in a freezer for 45 minutes. For heat therapy mitten can be heated in a microwave or crock pot. Heating times: 30-45 seconds each side in microwave or 15 minutes in a crock pot set on high.
Note: Extreme care must be taken when applying the mitten. Even though the surface may feel warm, after being applied, the heat becomes quite intense and can cause burns if the mitten is too hot.

| So TM7001 | | $43.95 |

Southwest Technologies Elasto-Gel Hand Exercisers for hot and cold therapy. For cold therapy cool in freezer for 30 minutes. For heat therapy heat for 30-45 seconds in microwave or 10-15 minutes on high in a crock pot.

| So HE 5001 | Small Hand Exerciser (1½″ × 4½″) | $12.95 |
| So HE 5005 | Large Hand Exerciser (3″ × 4½″) | $16.95 |

Maddak Built-up Handle Cutlery. Stainless steel utensils with secure lock-in handles. Space in handles for adding weights. Three grip rings to support fingers comfortably. Dishwasher safe handles are ⅞″ diameter and 4½″ long.

Le 197-6232	Teaspoon	$7.95
Le 197-6414	Knife	$8.95
Le 197-6877	Fork	$8.95

Soup spoons can be special ordered

Maddak Inner Lip Plate. Aids in self feeding. Inner lip holds food on plate. Prevents spills and makes eating more enjoyable. 9½″ diameter. Off-white color.

| Le 197-5572 | | $5.95 |

LILA Grip Mate. Designed as an aid for those patients who have arthritis or a hand disability. Soft plastic with Velcro® closure strap provides secure fit for any hand size. The unit opens for insertion of any utensil, such as a toothbrush, comb, knife, fork, spoon, etc. Two latches keep a tight grip and release is quick and easy.

| Li 357400 | Weighs 7 ounces | $17.95 |

LILA Black and Decker Toaster Oven-Broiler. Best for cooking fast snacks and even full meals. Will not heat up whole kitchen. Removable tray for easy clean-up.

| Li 793550 | Can be marked with braille tape | $68.95 |

LILA General Electric Microwave Oven. Cooks fast, clean and easy. Transparent brailled templates are available for the vision impaired from General Electric upon request.

| Li 481500 | 0.4 cubic feet oven for smaller kitchens | $185.95 |

LILA Touch Light Lamp Control. Turn lamp on or off with a touch. Touch any metal part of the lamp to switch it on or off. Turns any lamp into a three-way lamp. No tools needed for installation. Takes any incandescent 25- to 150-watt bulb.

| Li 798640 | UL Listed | $10.95 |

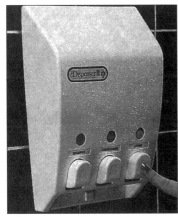

Li 258714

LILA Dispenser™. Perfect way to eliminate all the bottles in the shower and bath. Three 16-ounce chambers can be filled with soap, shampoo and conditioner. Ideal for those patients who have arthritis.

Li 258714   Mounts on wall using tape or screws, which are included $31.95

LILA Easy Hold Fingernail and Toenail Clippers. Unique thumb and finger grips are slip-proof and easy to squeeze. Toenail clipper has convex cutting edge to help prevent ingrown toenails. Built-in compartment collects nail clippings.

Li 275794   Sold as a set $8.95

LeBoeuf's Services

Call **LeBoeuf's** ☎ 1-800-546-5559 for the following services. Please have ready the patient's name, address, zip code, age, telephone number and physical circumstances (Alzheimer's, heart problem, arthritis, etc.) when you call.

- Consulting Service
    - Wheelchairs (design, ultra-light, sports chairs, etc.)
    - Van Conversions
    - Electronics
        - Hearing
        - Vision
        - Security
        - Communication (TTY, Call Buttons, Telephones, etc.)
        - Television, VCR's, Radio, Stereo
        - Computers and Software

- Home Healthcare Workshops

- Caregivers Speakers Bureau

- Incontinent Supply Service

- Respite Network

- Home Modification Planning Service

- Assistive Travel Agency

- Employment Screening Service

- Referral Service for:
    - Hospitals
    - Nursing homes
    - Hospice
    - Visiting nurse associations
    - Adult day care programs
    - Respite care (nursing homes, support groups,)
    - Social services case workers
    - Household help

LeBoeuf's

PHONE **1-800-546-5559**

FAX **1-800-233-9692**

Hearing Impaired with TDD
CALL **1-800-855-2880**

Pain Control

THERE ARE OVER 23 MILLION SURGICAL OPERATIONS performed in the United States every year. Most of them involve some type of pain management. Unfortunately, standard pain relief techniques fail to relieve pain in about half of postoperative patients. Recognition of inadequate pain management has prompted recent corrective efforts on the part of doctors, nurses and others who are involved in pain management. It is estimated that about 80 percent of the elderly have at least one chronic condition that involves pain. The three most common ailments in the elderly associated with acute pain are:

- Cancer
- Arthritis
- Vascular disease

Pain is caused by injury or disease of special sensory nerve endings called nociceptors. When the nerve endings are stimulated, they send a message to the brain. People vary greatly in their pain thresholds. A patient's response to pain is tempered by past experience. Insomnia, apprehension, fear and depression that often accompany a serious illness can greatly lower pain tolerance. Pain has an impact on the patient's physical, psychological and social makeup as well as the patient's family and loved ones.

Because patients vary greatly in their responses to pain, rigid prescriptions for the management of pain are not appropriate. Pain must be assessed and reassessed throughout the patient's stay at the hospital and this process of assessment must continue when the patient goes home or enters a nursing home. The patient determines what is or is not pain and their needs must be respected. It is no longer appropriate to not have relief from pain. It is a mistake to consider pain as a normal part of aging — it isn't.

Unrelieved pain has negative physical and psychological consequences. Aggressive pain prevention, during and after surgery, can yield both short and long-term benefits. Techniques are now available that can bring pain reduction to acceptable levels. The development of a plan for pain management and reduction is realistic and is now a common medical practice. Pain in the postoperative period should be assessed every two hours during the first 24 hours after the operation. Prevention of pain is better than treatment because pain is dynamic. Without pain control, sensory input from injured tissue reaches the spinal cord neurons and causes later responses to pain to be amplified. Once pain becomes established, it is difficult to control.

The patient should know the importance of factually reporting pain and avoid unconcern and exaggeration. Pain control will provide greater comfort while the patient heals. The patient will get well faster, walk sooner and may even leave the hospital sooner. The patient should not worry about getting "hooked" on drugs. This is a very rare occurrence unless the patient already has a problem with drug abuse.

Set up with the doctors and nurses a schedule for pain medicines. It is no longer appropriate to have pain prescribed on an "as needed" schedule.

Patient controlled analgesia (PCA) may be available at the patient's hospital. With PCA, patients control when they get pain medicine. When they begin to feel pain, they press a button to inject the pain medication through the IV in their vein.

There are a number of steps that can be taken to help keep pain under control and reduce anxiety:

- Find out from the doctor or nurse what, where and how much pain there will be after surgery.
- Have the doctor and nurse prepare a pain control plan from before the operation through complete recovery at home. The plan should include instructions for timing and use of pain control drugs. There should also be a description of when and how to perform non-drug pain control methods.
- Talk with the doctor and nurse and let them know what pain control methods worked in the past.
- Tell the doctors and nurses about any allergies to medicines.
- Tell the doctors and nurses what medicines are currently being taken.
- Ask about side effects from the pain medicine.
- Set up a schedule for pain medicines with the doctors and nurses. It is no longer appropriate to have pain medicine prescribed on an "as needed" schedule.
- Ask about "patient controlled analgesia" (PCA). It allows the patient to control when to get pain medicine.
- Take action against pain when it first starts. This is the key to successful pain control.
- Tell the doctor or nurse about any pain that will not go away.

Symptoms of Pain:

- Increased heart rate.
- Perspiration.
- Increased arterial blood pressure.
- Dilated pupils.
- Crying, screaming, grimacing, clenched fists.
- Immobility.

Breathing for Relaxation

The following breathing exercises will help relieve tension and reduce pain:

- Breathe in slowly and deeply.
- Let breath out slowly and relax.
- Breathe in slowly and regularly at a comfortable rate. Try abdominal breathing. If the patient does not know how to do abdominal breathing, ask the nurse or doctor to demonstrate it.
- Focus on breathing and breathe in rhythm.
- Do the breathing exercise for up to 20 minutes.

PAIN CONTROL PLAN

(Make copies of this form and work with the doctor to complete)

Patient's Name: _____

Date Surgery is Scheduled: _____

Doctor (s): _____ Telephone _____

_____ Telephone _____

Before surgery the following medication will be taken:

_____ How to use _____

_____ How to use _____

After surgery the following medication will be given:

Medication: _____ Every _____ hours for _____ days
How Given: ☐ Pill ☐ Shot ☐ Liquid ☐ In a vein ☐ Through a tube ☐ In the back

Medication: _____ Every _____ hours for _____ days
How Given: ☐ Pill ☐ Shot ☐ Liquid ☐ In a vein ☐ Through a tube ☐ In the back

Medication: _____ Every _____ hours for _____ days
How Given: ☐ Pill ☐ Shot ☐ Liquid ☐ In a vein ☐ Through a tube ☐ In the back

Medication: _____ Every _____ hours for _____ days
How Given: ☐ Pill ☐ Shot ☐ Liquid ☐ In a vein ☐ Through a tube ☐ In the back

Medication: _____ Every _____ hours for _____ days
How Given: ☐ Pill ☐ Shot ☐ Liquid ☐ In a vein ☐ Through a tube ☐ In the back

Patient Controlled Analgesia (PCA): ☐ Yes ☐ No   Name: _____

Patient will also use the following non-drug pain control methods:

Breathing exercises:	☐ Yes	☐ No
Jaw relaxation:	☐ Yes	☐ No
Nerve stimulation (TENS):	☐ Yes	☐ No
Massage:	☐ Yes	☐ No
Hot therapy :	☐ Yes	☐ No
Cold therapy:	☐ Yes	☐ No

Note: According to the U.S. Department of Health and Human Services, there are no risks related to the use of physical techniques for managing pain.

Patient should learn how to: (get out of a chair, cough, etc.)

_____

_____

_____

_____

_____

What to do:

See the doctor — Set up a pain control plan and develop a schedule prior to any surgery. The doctors and nurses want to make the patient's surgery as pain free as they can. The patient needs to understand they play a key role in defining what levels of medication will be required to minimize pain.

Contact Center for Research Dissemination and Liaison, AHCPR Publications Clearinghouse, P.O. Box 8547, Silver Spring, MD 20907. They have copies of booklets that will provide information on topics such as pain in the lower back, pain in children, pain in the elderly non-cognitive patient and many others.

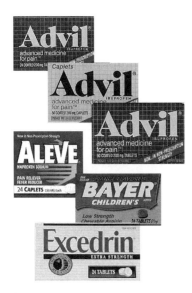

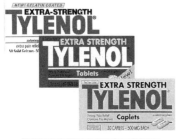

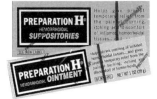

Analgesics

Mc 173-3567	Advil Tabs.	24s	$4.35
Mc 173-3583	Advil Tabs.	50s	$7.45
Mc 173-3609	Advil Tabs.	100s	$12.55
Mc 196-5169	Advil Caplets	24s	$4.35
Mc 196-5920	Advil Caplets	50s	$7.45
Mc 135-3358	Aleve Caplets	24s	$4.35
Mc 135-2509	Aleve Caplets	50s	$7.25
Mc 135-3580	Aleve Tablets	24s	$4.35
Mc 164-9839	Bayer Childrens' Chew Tabs	36s	$2.85
Mc 114-9103	Bonine Tabs	8s	$3.25
Mc 145-6219	Ecotrin Reg-Strength Tabs.	100s	$8.75
Mc 118-3441	Excedrin Tabs	24s	$4.15
Mc 321-7601	Tylenol X-Strength Gelcaps	24s	$4.35
Mc 321-7668	Tylenol X-Strength Gelcaps	50s	$7.35
Mc 321-7742	Tylenol X-Strength Gelcaps	100s	$11.45
Mc 270-1837	Tylenol X-Strength Caplets	24s	$4.05
Mc 270-1845	Tylenol X-Strength Caplets	50s	$6.75
Mc 270-1852	Tylenol X-Strength Caplets	100s	$10.55
Mc 140-8913	Tylenol X-Strength Tabs.	30s	$4.75
Mc 140-8939	Tylenol X-Strength Tabs.	60s	$7.75
Mc 140-8954	Tylenol X-Strength Tabs.	100s	$8.75
Mc 134-3664	Tylenol Infants Drops Fruit	5oz	$6.75
Mc 134-3672	Tylenol Childs Suspension Liquid Cherry	4oz	$6.95
Mc 162-7678	Preparation H Ointment.	1oz	$6.15
Mc 162-7694	Preparation H Suppositories	12s	$7.75

Caution! Be sure that you check with the patient's doctor and/or pharmacist before purchasing any of the analgesics, antacids and laxatives. You must be certain that they will not interfere with the patient's medication and/or they can be taken along with the patient's current medication. As with any medication, follow the instructions on the package and do not exceed recommended dosage.

Caution! According to the American Medical Association, children should not be given aspirin for viral infections or fever of unknown origin. Always check with the doctor before giving any medication to your patient.

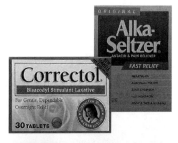

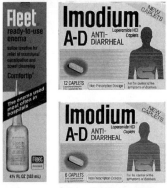

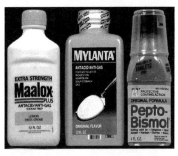

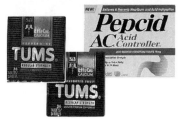

Antacids/Laxatives

Mc 136-1252	Alka-Seltzer Blue+Aspirin	36s	$5.85
Mc 140-3336	Correctol Tab	30s	$5.25
Mc 127-0230	Dulcolax Tab 5mg	25s	$5.65
Mc 126-3300	Fleet Enema Disposable	4.5 oz	$1.25
Mc 197-8493	Imodium A-D Caplets	6s	$3.55
Mc 197-8329	Imodium A-D Caplets	12s	$5.95
Mc 146-2639	Imodium A-D Anti-Diarrheal	2 oz	$5.45
Mc 350-1012	Imodium A-D Caplets	18s	$7.65
Mc 2263283	Maalox Plus X/Str Lemon	12 oz	$7.65
Mc 197-2199	Maalox Plus X/Str Mint	12 oz	$7.65
Mc 147-1069	Mylanta Rs Liquid	12 oz	$5.75
Mc 135-4026	Mylanta Ds Liquid	12 oz	$7.95
Mc 176-5759	Pepcid Ac Tab	6 Ct	$3.95
Mc 176-6724	Pepcid Ac Tab	12 Ct	$7.15
Mc 176-9769	Pepcid Ac Tab	18 Ct	$8.95
Mc 137-7472	Pepto-Bismol Liquid Reg	8 oz	$3.95
Mc 137-7464	Pepto-Bismol Liquid Reg	4 oz	$2.95
Mc 137-7498	Pepto-Bismol Tab Reg	30s	$3.95
Mc 271-8773	Rolaids Tab Reg	3pk	$1.95
Mc 223-8475	Tagamet Hb Tab 100mg	16s	$4.35
Mc 223-8954	Tagamet Hb Tab 100mg	32s	$7.55
Mc 243-0650	Tums Peppermint	3pk	$2.35
Mc 243-0684	Tums Assorted	3pk	$2.35
Mc 131-2875	Tums Tab Assorted	75s	$3.45
Mc 132-8400	Tums Tab Peppermint	150s	$5.65

Caution! Be sure that you check with the patient's doctor and/or pharmacist before purchasing any of the analgesics, antacids and laxatives. You must be certain that they will not interfere with the patient's medication and/or they can be taken along with the patient's current medication. As with any medication, follow the instructions on the package and do not exceed recommended dosage.

Pain Management

TRANSCUTANEOUS ELECTRIC NERVE STIMULATION (TENS) is a noninvasive pain control technique that helps a patient manage acute and chronic pain. Most users of TENS have chronic pain such as lower back pain, pain from an incision, headaches, or pain from hip, knee and thigh surgery. The use of a TENS unit helps reduce the need for pain controlling drugs.

TENS units consist of a portable battery-operated generator, electrodes which are attached to the skin, and wires that carry the current from the generator to the electrodes. A doctor or nurse should teach the patient how to operate the unit. If the patient has a pacemaker, other heart problems or is suffering from confusion, it is unlikely that the doctor will prescribe the procedure.

TENS units will require some trial and error to find the best settings for getting the most effective pain relief. The electrodes are usually placed on both sides of an incision, along peripheral nerve areas, at an acupressure point or along the spinal column. More intensity is not necessarily better with a TENS unit. Sometimes, a lower setting will prove to be better for the most effective pain relief. The patient should not use the TENS unit for more than 45 minutes at a time. Prolonged use may result in decreased effectiveness and possible skin irritation.

Always make sure the unit is off prior to attaching the electrodes and follow the manufacturer's instructions carefully. If the patient places the electrodes too close together, they may receive a shock and possibly a burn. Do not submerge the unit in water. Once the desired relief from pain is reached, write the settings on some tape and tape the settings to the unit or — if the unit has dials — tape the dials in place.

Pain Control Products

Stimtech PT-1 TENS Unit. Three different modes allow for different types of stimulation from one unit. Two 9-volt batteries, two 36-inch lead wires, one package of 16 Stimflex/M electrodes.

Mc 135-2715   Carrying case included $615.95

Stimtech SDM TENS Unit. Four distinct stimulation modes. Two 9-volt batteries, two 36-inch lead wires, and 1 package of 16 Stimflex/M electrodes.

Mc 141-5637   Carrying case included $645.95

Stimtech Stimflex/M TENS Electrodes. Dry gel, self adhesive. Disposable, last 3 to 4 days. 2 inches by 2 inches. Pin connection 1 inches by 1 inches.

Mc 240-7872   16 per package $21.95

Stimtech Stimgel, II. Conductive gel for use with electrodes.

Mc 220-5037   3 oz. tube $3.95

Stimtech Twin Lead Wires

Mc 220-3586   36 inches long   Black $24.95

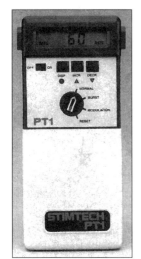

Mc 135-2715

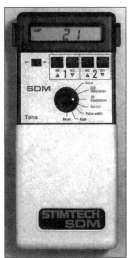

Mc 141-5637

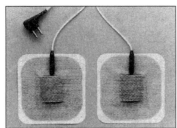

Mc 240-7872

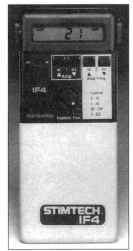

Mc 161-5327

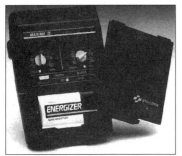

Mc 219-6079

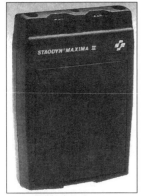

Mc 326-4421

Stimtech Interferential Therapy Unit. Deep muscle stimulation. Four-electrode interferential therapy. Adjustable treatment timer with automatic shut-off. Compliance meter. Nicad power pack, charger, two 36-inch lead wires, one package of 4 RS electrodes (reusable). May also be powered by two 9-volt batteries.

Mc 161-5327   Carrying case included $1395.95

Stimtech Stimflex/RS Electrodes. Reusable. Pin connection.

Mc 139-4527   1⅝″ × 1¾″,   4 per package $18.95

Staodyn Maxima III TENS Unit. True strength modulation, normal, burst, and modulation operating modes. Modulation cycle adjusts from .5 to 12 seconds per cycle. Push-button mode selection with memory; LED indicators for operating modes. Soft turn-on allows current to ramp-up gently. 40-inch wire leads, 4 Staoderm R electrodes, 9-volt battery.

Mc 219-6079   Carrying case included $665.95

Staodyn Maxima II TENS Unit. Adjustable rate and width; modulation and burst modes. Dual output jacks. Built-in testing allows lead and electrode check. 30-inch leads, 4 Staoderm R electrodes, 9-volt battery.

Mc 326-4421   Carrying case included $645.95

Staodyn Staoderm, Reusable Electrode. Used properly, may be reused 10 to 20 times. Pin connection.

Mc 149-8690   1⁹⁄₁₆″ × 1¾″   Pouch of 8 $24.95

Staodyn Disposable Electrodes. Flexible tan-tone fabric backing. Can be used from 1 to 4 days.

Mc 149-8245   Snap connection   Pouch of 16 $16.95
Mc 149-9292   Pin connection   Pouch of 16 $16.95

Pills & Shots

Taking more medication than the doctor or pharmacist has directed will not help the patient feel better sooner or get well faster.

Hint: It is a very good idea to choose a pharmacist and stick with the one chosen. The pharmacist will maintain a record of all the patient's prescriptions and can warn you and/or the patient of the dangers of combining medications.

OTC drugs don't cure conditions, they treat symptoms.

THE NATIONAL ASSOCIATION OF RETAIL DRUGGISTS estimates that 25 percent of hospital admissions for people over 60 are the result of drug errors. A 1993 study by a team of Harvard University researchers in two of the United States' most prestigious hospitals found that nearly one out of three patients in the two hospitals had an adverse reaction to medication because of an error by the doctor or by hospital personnel. Twelve percent of the errors were considered life threatening. It is very important that you and the patient discuss in detail with the doctor what treatment the patient will receive, what medications will be administered, when and how much. This holds true whether in a hospital or at home. While this may seem intrusive of the doctor's domain, if satisfactory responses are not provided to the patient or the caregiver, change doctors. You may save the patient's life.

People over age 60 have over 600 million prescriptions filled every year. People over 65 make up 11 percent of the population, but take 25 percent of all prescription drugs sold in the United States. It is also thought that 25 percent of nursing home admissions are the result of the patient's inability to take drugs properly. The U.S. Department of Health and Human Services found in a recent study that drug induced falls cause 32,000 fatalities each year among older people. Taking more medication than the doctor or pharmacist has directed will not help make the patient feel better sooner or get well faster. In fact, it can lead to serious side effects.

It is not only prescription drugs that can cause problems. Over-the-counter (OTC) medicines contain strong agents and, when large quantities are taken, they can equal a dose that would normally be available only by prescription. OTC drugs don't cure conditions, they treat symptoms. The Food and Drug Administration requires extensive labeling information on OTC labels to help patients take the drugs safely and effectively.

Drugs that interact with other drugs (drug-drug interaction) may cause an adverse reaction. If the patient is taking the following types of drugs, make sure that you have told the doctor or pharmacist about all the other medications that are currently being taken or have been taken recently:

antibiotics	blood thinners
anticonvulsants	decongestants
antidepressants	high blood pressure medications
antidiabetic drugs	sedatives

The basic rules for taking medicine — whether prescription or over-the-counter — include the following:

- Take the exact amount prescribed by the doctor.
- Follow dosage schedule as closely as possible.
- Ask your doctor about the use of over-the-counter drugs.
- Never take drugs prescribed for someone else.
- Tell the doctor about past problems with any drug.

From a United States General Accounting Office study dated July 1995, a panel of experts considered the following 20 drugs inappropriate for the elderly:

Diazepam

Clordiazepoxide

Flurazepam

Meprobamate

Pentobarbital

Secobarbital

Amitriptyline

Indomethacin

Phenylbutazone

Chlorpropamide

Propoxphene

Pentazocine

Isoxsuprine

Cyclandelate

Dipyridamole

Cyclobenzaprine

Methocarbamol

Carisoprodol

Orphenadrine

Trimethobenzamide

Note: While these drugs are generally considered inappropriate for elderly patients, consult with the patient's doctor before making any changes in medication.

If your pharmacist will work with you and your patient, you have found valuable support.

- Keep a daily record of drugs taken. This is especially important if the patient is taking more than one drug at a time. The record should show the name of the drug, the doctor's name, amount to be taken and when it should be taken.
- Keep drugs out of the reach of children.
- Make sure that you and the patient understand the directions on the label.
- Throw out old medicines. They lose their effectiveness over time.
- When the patient starts taking a new drug, ask the doctor what side effects may occur.
- Understand how to store the drug.
- Call the doctor if any unusual reactions occur.

Pharmacists are now required to offer customers information on a drug's side effects, dosage, and how the drug interacts with food and other medication. Do not hesitate to ask your patient's pharmacist about the medication. Compare information that the pharmacist provides to what the doctor has said. If there is a difference, be sure that you tell the doctor and the pharmacist about the difference. Insist that both the pharmacist and the doctor agree that the prescription is right and that the dosage is correct.

In addition, many pharmacies offer services such as "brown bag days" (take all the drugs the patient is taking to the pharmacist in a brown paper bag) to review all the medications the patient has to insure that they are up to date and that there are no harmful combinations. If the patient is seeing more than one doctor, it is important to make a list of all their prescriptions as well as all the over-the-counter drugs the patient is taking and review them with the pharmacist. Take *LeBoeuf's Handbook* with you to update the medical information in the "Personal Information" section. The pharmacist will spend time counseling the patient about the dangers of not using medication as prescribed.

The American Pharmaceutical Association recommends that you and the patient ask the doctor and/or pharmacist the following questions before taking any prescription or over-the-counter medication:

- What is the name of the medication and what is it supposed to do?
- When and how often should the patient take it? Should the patient take the medication with water, juice, another liquid or food? Can the medicine be taken on an empty stomach?
- How long should the patient take the medicine?
- Based upon the patient's allergy history, will the medication contain anything that could cause a reaction? (Take *Handbook* with you and let the doctor and/or pharmacist see the list of other medications the patient is taking. Always make sure you include all over-the-counter drugs that the patient is taking)
- How many times can a prescription be refilled? When should you get it refilled?
- Should the patient avoid alcohol or any other drugs, food or activities such as driving, exposure to sun, etc.
- What side effects, if any, could the patient experience? What should you do if adverse side effects occur?

- What should the patient do if a medication dose has been missed?
- Is there a generic version of the drug?
- How should you store the medication?

Some substances, including vitamins, laxatives, cold remedies, antacids and alcohol can also lead to serious problems if used too often or in combination with other drugs. Foods and drinks that you should be wary of when giving medications to the patient:

- Dairy products.
- Alcohol.
- Caffeine (soft drinks, tea, coffee).
- Salt.
- Fruit juices.

Symptoms of reaction to a drug or drugs:

- Rashes.
- Indigestion.
- Dizziness.
- Loss of appetite.
- Blacking out or fainting.
- Agitation or anxiety.
- Fatigue.
- Depression.
- Weakness.
- Decreased sexual drive.
- Confusion or memory loss.

To safely store medications, keep them on a high shelf in the kitchen, bedroom or in a closet. Bathrooms are usually too warm and humid to store medications. Do not place the patient's medication in direct light or on a TV or radio (both get very warm). If there is no expiration date on the medication, check with the pharmacist to see if it is still okay to use. If you or the patient need to discard any medication, flush pills and liquid medicines down the toilet. Ointments and creams should be removed from their containers and also flushed down the toilet before throwing out the tubes or containers. If a medication is not labeled, destroy it. Never store medications in another medication container. Use a pill box and label it.

Flu (Influenza) and Pneumonia Shots

Pneumonia and influenza are the sixth most common causes of death in the United States.

Pneumonia and influenza are the sixth most common causes of death in the United States. Between 15 and 50 percent of all adult pneumonia is caused by pneumococcal bacteria, and these infections are the leading cause of pneumonia requiring hospitalization.

Despite antibiotic therapy, pneumonia remains a leading cause of death. 268,000 cases of pneumonia are reported each year in the United States among the 36 million people who are 65 or older. On average, 32,800 elderly die each year from pneumonia.

There are two main kinds of pneumonia — viral pneumonia and bacterial pneumonia. Bacterial pneumonia is the most serious. At least 20 percent of persons who get bacterial pneumonia will die from it. In 1994, there

The best time to get a flu shot is in October or November.

Flu shots are free under Medicare.

Check with the doctor before obtaining a flu shot if the patient is allergic to eggs. The flu vaccine is made in egg products and can cause serious reactions in patients who have such allergies.

Contrary to myth, it has never been possible to get the flu from a flu shot in the United States because the vaccines are only made from killed viruses which cannot cause infection.

were approximately 17,000 cases of bacterial pneumonia and there were 7,300 deaths (about 43 percent). According to the most recent available data (from the 1993 National Health Interview Survey) 73 percent of older Americans had never received the pneumococcal vaccination, despite its coverage under Medicare, and 49 percent of the elderly had not been vaccinated against influenza during the 1992-1993 flu season.

While the number of older people obtaining flu shots has increased each year, about 40 percent still do not get flu shots, even though many have visited a doctor. Believe it or not, even persons visiting a doctor five or more times a year were unlikely to have received a flu shot.

Everyone age 65 or older should consult with the doctor about the pneumococcal vaccine. This one-time vaccine protects against 87 percent of the kinds of bacteria that cause pneumococcal disease. The vaccine protects against other pneumococcal diseases as well and is covered by Medicare.

Three shots that older people should have:

- **Pneumococcal shot** — Given once to protect against pneumococcal bacteria that cause infections, including those affecting the lungs (pneumonia), the covering of the brain (meningitis) or the blood (bacteremia).
- **Flu shot** — Taken every year because of the new and different strains of the flu virus that develop every year.
- **Tetanus and diphtheria** — A booster shot is needed every ten years. Usually they are given together.

Mild side effects, such as swelling and pain where the shot was given, occur in about half the people who are given pneumonia vaccine. However, fever, muscle pain and more serious local reactions have been reported in less than one percent of those receiving shots. Although most individuals have no side effects from flu shots, some patients may have soreness where the shot was given or body aches for a day or two. Contrary to myth, it has never been possible to get the flu from a flu shot in the United States, because the vaccines are only made from killed viruses which cannot cause infection.

Studies of flu shots for older people indicate that they reduce hospitalization by about 70 percent and death by 85 percent among the noninstitutionalized elderly.

What to do:

Contact the doctor. When visiting with the doctor, make sure that the doctor is aware of all the medicines the patient is taking, even if they are over-the-counter drugs such as aspirin. Have the doctor give the patient the annual flu shot and make sure that the patient has received the pneumococcal shot. Check with the doctor to see if the patient is due for tetanus and diphtheria shots.

Contact the NIDA Helpline 1-800-662-HELP (4357). It provides information on drug abuse. It is a service of the National Institute on Drug Abuse.

Contact the National Parent's Resource Institute for Drug Education. 1-800-241-7946. It provides materials on drug-related issues. They can refer you to related organizations for additional information.

Orthopedic Products

Easing Back & Neck Pain

Over 80 million people suffer from neck and back pain in the United States. A proper sitting position can help decrease the chances of your patient being among the 7 million increase in people who suffer from back pain each year. When sitting, keep feet flat on the floor, knees level with the hips and support the lower back. Avoid slumping in the chair. Sit with the neck and back as straight as possible.

In order to have correct posture in bed, a firm mattress is a must. If you do not have a firm mattress, use a piece of plywood to add support to a soft mattress. Patients should not use high pillows or sleep on their backs or stomach. These positions strain the neck and shoulders. Patient should lie on their sides with knees bent and a pillow between the knees to flatten the back. A flat pillow for supporting the neck is okay.

For back pain from a sudden wrenching back injury in a localized area of the back, immediately apply cold packs for 10 to 20 minutes, several times a day during the first 48 hours. If the pain does not subside, call the doctor. To treat a wide-spread backache that sets in hours after injury, or for chronic discomfort, apply moist heat.

Some do's and don't for improving the patient's posture and avoiding back problems:

Do
- Keep neck and back as straight as possible when sitting, standing or lying in bed.
- Cross legs to rest back during long periods of sitting.
- Use a footrest during long periods of standing.
- Bend from the hips and knees, not from the waist.
- Obtain permission from your doctor before doing any exercises.
- Wear shoes with low to moderate heels.
- Face any object to be lifted.
- Hold heavy objects close to the body.

Don't
- Carry anything heavier than can be managed with ease.
- Lift a heavy object above the waist.
- Move heavy furniture.
- Strain to open windows or doors.

Common Joint Injuries

For common joint injuries to knees, ankles, wrists, elbows and shoulders, rest and elevate injured area. Apply cold pack for 30 minutes. If swelling or pain is more than slight after the application of the cold pack, see the doctor. Apply ice for 30 minutes on, and 15 minutes off for the next few hours. Bear weight cautiously. Heat may be applied, but only after 24 hours.

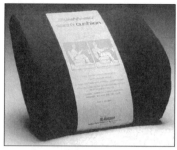

Le 221-5663

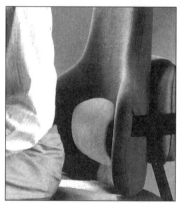

Le 115-0119

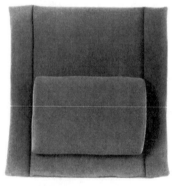

Le 119-3309 / Le 197-7024

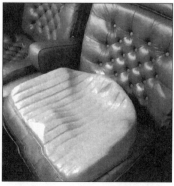

Le 218- 6492

Back and Cervical Aids

SunMark Sacro Cushion. Form fitted to relieve back discomfort and fatigue. Perfect for use in the home or automobile

Le 221-5663	Brown	$19.95
Le 211-6952	Blue	$19.95
Le 211-7075	Maroon	$19.95

Wahl, Home & Auto Back Massager. Dual motors provide unique oscillating massage. Includes adapter to plug into car cigarette lighter (not battery operated). Soft cushion with plush cover.

Le 329-5862 $49.95

Futuro Lumbar Support Cushion. Adds comfort to chairs, wheelchairs and car seats. Molded of polyurethane foam. Machine washable. Dark blue.

Le 341-9199 $13^1/2'' \times 13^1/2''$ $36.95

Futuro Back Buddy® Lumbar Support. Facilitates proper sitting posture. Winged ridged frame and adjustable lumbar cushion maximizes support and comfort.

Le 115-0119 $128.95

Homedics SP-1 Spine Ease Deluxe Massage Cushion. Massage action for soothing tired muscles. Fits back contour. Battery operated for use in home auto or office. Uses 2 "D" batteries, not included.

Le 247-7529 $29.95

Accu-Back Orthopedic Cushion. Contour Design. Lightweight and portable. Fits all types of seats — car or home. Made of stain resistant fabric. Flame retardant.

| Le 178-8389 | Grey | $24.95 |
| Le 329-2711 | Black | $24.95 |

Accu-Back Rest with Adjustable Lumbar Pillow. Easily adjusted to individual comfort zone. Flexible side panels and adjustable strap.

| Le 119-3309 | Beige | $36.95 |
| Le 197-7024 | Black | $36.95 |

RoLoKe Buttoms Up Pelvic Spinal Posture Seat. Designed to relieve back, neck and buttocks pain and sitting fatigue by supporting spine from pelvis. Multi-contoured surface distributes body weight and stabilizes pelvis. For use in autos, at home, in wheelchairs.

Le 218- 6492	Petite 16" , Blue	$62.95
Le 218-6617	Small 18", Blue	$62.95
Le 218-6708	Medium 20", Blue	$62.95
Le 218-6807	Large 22", Blue	$62.95

RoLoKe Back Me Up Adjustable Support. Pump-up control adjusts support for upper, middle or lower back. For use in home or car. Blue gray color. Adjustable strap.

Le 192-8738 $32.95

SunMark Breathe Easy Foam Pillow. Adjusts to six positions for individualized comfort. Convoluted foam surface. 14" wide × 21" long and 3¼" high.

Le 270-1639 $29.95

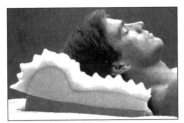

Le 363-6586 / Le 321-3501

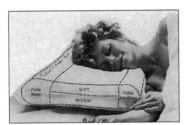

Le 132-2254 / Le 132-0076

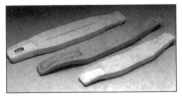

Le 220-5367

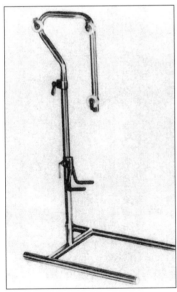

Le 220-0152

RoLoKe Wal-Pil-O Neck Pillow. Patented design of firm narrow/firm wide borders plus soft and medium firm centers provides four combinations of neck and head support. Helps relieve tension, headaches, stiff necks, muscle spasms, jaw pain and lower back pain. 25″ × 15″ × 4″ high. Fits a standard pillow case. Flame retardant.

Le 363-6586		$39.95
Le 321-3501	Travel Pillow 12¼″ × 15½″ × 4¼″ high	$42.95

Bio Clinic Pro Pillow. Anatomically shaped for comfort. Surface is convoluted to mold to body shape. Two sizes—regular for home use and Mini-Traveler.

Le 132-2254	Regular, 19½″ × 26″	$42.95
Le 132-0076	Mini-Traveler, 14″ × 14″	$38.95

Futuro Cervical Pillow. Dual support provides two different support levels. 8″ support for lying on back. 5″ firm support for lying on one's side. Washable cotton/polyester cover. White.

Le 370-2982	4½″ diameter × 18″ long	$24.95

Caution:

All cervical collars, traction equipment, and braces with aluminum (metal) stays are prescription items. Be sure that you check with the patient's doctor prior to ordering these items. It is always wise to check with the doctor prior to purchasing or using any orthopedic product. Be especially careful with those patients who have diabetes or circulatory problems.

SunMark Deluxe Soft Foam Cervical Collar. One size fits all. Comfortable polyurethane foam with soft stockinette covering. Long Velcro tabs for easy adjustment.

Le 220-5250	$10.95

SunMark Hard Adjustable Height Cervical Collar. Rigid plastic construction. Reinforced and contoured chin rest. Soft, washable chin pad. One size fits all. Front adjusts from 3″ to 5″. Long Velcro tabs for adjustment. Soft padding top and bottom.

Le 220-5367	$29.95

Invacare Overbed Traction Floor Stand with Offset Head. Can be used at head or foot of any bed for cervical or pelvic traction. Vinyl-coated panel hooks adjust height from 34″ to 51″. Chrome plated welded steel.

Le 221-1605	$105.95

SunMark Pelvic Traction Kit. Includes pelvis traction belt of canvas with flannel lining, Y-shaped pull straps, hook and buckle adjustment and closure. 7″ deep front and back. Kit also has steel spreader bar, bed traction bracket that allows height adjustment and features strong steel pulley support, section of rope and 20 lb. water weight bag. For use with regular beds or hospital beds.

Le 220-0152	Complete Kit	$106.95
Le 228-1574	Rope Only	$1.95
Le 220-0335	Water Weight Bag Only	$5.95
Le 220-0210	Pelvic Traction Belt Only	$46.95

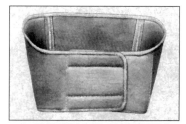

Le 242-2814 / Le 242-3606 /
Le 242-5353

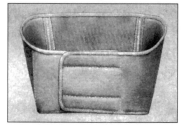

Le 243-2045 / Le 240-3764 /
Le 240-5603

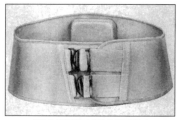

244-2309 / 244-3166 /
244-3166

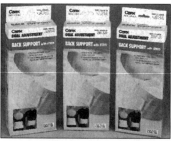

Le 116-7311 / Le 117-6866
Le 117-5314

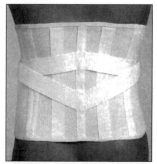

Le 242-3051 / Le 242-3127
Le 242-3184 / Le 242-3267

Excel Supporter Belt. Wide band and detachable pouch. Hand washable. Measure around waist.

Le 248-2388	Small—31" to 34"	$24.95
Le 248-3444	Medium—35" to 38"	$24.95
Le 248-5787	Large—39" to 42"	$24.95

Excel Rib Belt. Women's. Adjustable. Hand washable. Measure around chest and over lower ribs.

Le 242-2814	Small—23" to 26"	$18.95
Le 242-3606	Medium—28" to 32"	$18.95
Le 242-5353	Large—34" to 38"	$18.95

Excel Rib Belt. Men's. Adjustable. Hand washable. Measure around chest and over lower ribs.

Le 243-2045	Small—26" to 32"	$19.95
Le 243-3068	Medium—34" to 40"	$19.95
Le 243-5014	Large—42" to 48"	$19.95

Excel Hernia Belt. Adjustable, cotton. Hand washable. Measure around widest area of hips.

Le 240-2709	Small—30" to 35"	$22.95
Le 240-3764	Medium—35" to 41"	$22.95
Le 240-5603	Large—41" to 46"	$22.95

Excel Sacro Brace. Adjustable. Canvas. Hand washable. Measure around widest area of hips, 3" below waist.

Le 244-2309	Small—30" to 34"	$22.95
Le 244-3166	Medium—34" to 40"	$22.95
Le 244-5039	Large—40" to 46"	$22.95

Carex Back Brace. Provides support to abdomen and lumbosacral areas. Elastic dual adjustment panels. Aluminum stays provide additional support.

Le 116-7311	Small—26" to 38"	$41.95
Le 117-6866	Medium—36" to 50"	$41.95
Le 117-5314	Large—44" to 62"	$41.95

Jerome Criss-Cross Brace–9-inch. All elastic crisscross for lower lumbar support. Flexible uprights. Criss-cross Velcro closure, front and back. Semi-rigid A-PM-L control. Measure hips.

Le 215-7022	Small	30" to 33"	$25.95
Le 215-7212	Medium	33" to 37"	$25.95
Le 215-7519	Large	37" to 41"	$25.95
Le 247-6273	Universal	30" to 44"	$25.95

Jerome Flexible Cinch Belt–10-inch. All elastic diamond crisscross for added abdominal and lower lumbar support. Velcro closure. Semi-rigid A-P M-L control. High-tempered aluminum stays. Measure hips.

Le 242-3051	Small	30" to 33"	$28.95
Le 242-3127	Medium	33" to 37"	$28.95
Le 242-3184	Large	37" to 41"	$28.95
Le 242-3267	X-Large	41" to 44"	$28.95

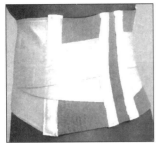

Le 242-3432 / Le 242-3499
Le 242-3556

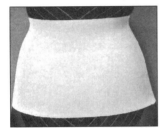

Le 215-3856 / Le 215-3948

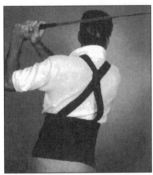

Le 166-4929 / Le 166-5215
Le 166-5363 / Le 166-5678

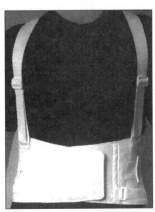

Le 133-7757 / Le 133-7831
Le 133-7922 / Le 133-8367

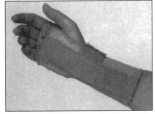

Le 227-2383 / Le 227-3191
Le 227-5055

Jerome Compression Brace with Neoprene. Dual elastic panels adjust compression as needed. Neoprene lumbosacral pad provides added warmth. Semi-rigid A-P M-L control. Measure hips.

Le 242-3432	Small	26″ to 38″	$25.95
Le 242-3499	Medium	36″ to 50″	$25.95
Le 242-3556	Large	44″ to 62″	$25.95

Jerome 9-inch Abdominal Supports. Provides circular compression to patient's abdomen. Recommended as postoperative dressing binder. 3-Panel elastic. Measure hips.

Le 215-3856	Small/Medium	30″ to 45″	$12.95
Le 215-3948	Medium/Large	45″ to 62″	$12.95

Accu-Back Action Belt™. Designed to reduce possibility of low back strain and injury at work, at play and at home. Designed for both men and women. Ventilated, lightweight and durable. Adjustable side bands for snug custom fit. Stays provide bilateral support. Measure waist.

Le 166-4929	Small—24″ to 30″	Black	$28.95
Le 166-5215	Medium—30″ to 36″	Black	$28.95
Le 166-5363	Large—36″ to 42″	Black	$28.95
Le 166-5678	X-Large—42″ to 48″	Black	$28.95

Jerome Utility Healthcare Belt. Support to abdomen and lumbosacral area during lifting and carrying heavy patients. 9-inch elastic rear panel; full front Velcro closure. Adjustable, removable suspenders; adjustable utility straps and lateral elastic double-pulls. Measure hips.

Le 133-7757	Small—26″ to 40″	White	$28.95
Le 133-7831	Medium—36″ to 49″	White	$28.95
Le 133-7922	Large—44″ to 59″	White	$28.95
Le 133-8367	X-Large—55″ to 68″	White	$28.95

Orthopedic Products

Excel Wrist Brace, Splint, Adjustable. Sewn with live rubber cord yarn, seamless. Hand washable. One size fits all.

Le 227-2383	Small—5½″ to 7½″	$!6.95
Le 227-3191	Medium—6½″ to 8½″	$16.95
Le 227-5055	Large—7½″ to 9½″	$16.95

Excel Wrist Brace. Comes with Velcro tab. Once size fits all.

Le 228-8496	Hand Washable	$9.95

Excel Wrist Brace. Slip-on type. Hand washable. Measure around wrist.

Le 226-2756	Small—5½″ to 6½″	$4.95
Le 226-3689	Medium—6¾″ to 7¼″	$4.95
Le 226-5080	Large—7½″ to 8″	$4.95
Le 226-6187	Extra Large—8¼″ to 9″	$4.95

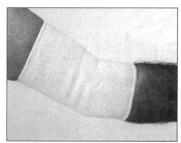

Le 222-2032 / Le 222-3402 /
Le 222-5423

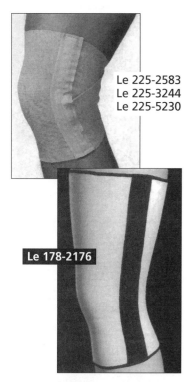

Le 225-2583
Le 225-3244
Le 225-5230

Le 178-2176

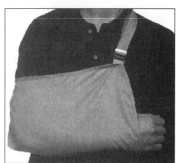

Le 186-0592

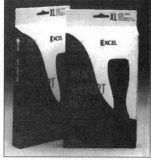

Le 328-5202

Excel Elbow Brace. White. Sewn with live rubber cord yarn. Seamless and hand washable. Measure around arm just below elbow when bent.

Le 222-2032	Small—8½" to 10"	$6.95
Le 222-3402	Medium—10" to 11½"	$6.95
Le 222-5423	Large—11½" to 13"	$6.95

Excel Tennis Elbow Brace. Hand washable.

| Le 138-9915 | One size fits all | $13.95 |

Excel Knee Brace, X-Cross. Two-way stretch. Sewn with live rubber cord yarn. Hand washable. Measure around knee at widest point.

Le 225-2583	Small—10" to 12¾"	$12.95
Le 225-3155	Medium—13" to 15¾"	$12.95
Le 225-5230	Large—16" to 18¾"	$12.95

Jerome Exerlite® Economy Knee Support. Recommended for mild inflammatory conditions. Provides graduated, circular compression—helps reduce swelling. Seamless 4-way stretch elastic knit sleeve with soft, comfortable interior. Allows freedom of movement and will not gap behind the knee or roll down. Measure circumference of knee at patella (kneecap).

Le 178-2176	X-Small—11¼" to 12½"	$21.95
Le 178-1426	Small—12½" to 13¾"	$21.95
Le 178-0766	Medium—13¾" to 15"	$21.95
Le 178-0311	Large—15" to 16¼"	$21.95
Le 178-0113	X-Large—16¼" to 17½"	$21.95
Le 177-9768	XX-Large—17½" to 18¾"	$21.95

Excel Squid Ankle Brace. Sewn with live rubber cord yarn. Hand washable. Measure around ankle at smallest point.

Le 137-2168	Small—6½" to 7¾"	$19.95
Le 137-4347	Medium—7¾" to 9"	$19.95
Le 138-0484	Large—9" to 10¼"	$19.95
Le 138-6929	Extra Large—10¼" to 11½"	$19.95

Excel Arm Sling. One size. Gray. Hand washable.

| Le 186-0592 | Adult | $9.95 |

Excel Men's Support Hose. Knee length. Medium weight with graduated compression. Greater compression at ankle than knee to improve circulation. Small fits shoe sizes 9-10, Medium fits shoes sizes 10-11, Large fits shoes sizes 11-12 and X-Large fits shoe sizes 12-13. Per pair.

Le 328-5202	Small	Black	$6.95
Le 328-5269	Small	Blue	$6.95
Le 328-5327	Small	Brown	$6.95
Le 328-5384	Medium	Black	$6.95
Le 328-5442	Medium	Blue	$6.95
Le 328-5509	Medium	Brown	$6.95
Le 328-4767	Large	Black	$6.95
Le 328-4825	Large	Blue	$6.95
Le 328-4882	Large	Brown	$6.95
Le 328-4957	X-Large	Black	$6.95
Le 328-5079	X-Large	Blue	$6.95
Le 328-5145	X-Large	Brown	$6.95

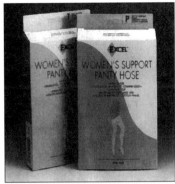

Le 348-0530

Excel Women's Support Pantyhose. Ultra sheer 84% nylon, 16% Lycra spandex. Graduated, moderate compression. Control top, cotton panel. See chart below to determine proper size. Not recommended for women with a thigh over 25 inches.

Le 348-0530	Small	Taupe	$8.95
Le 348-0597	Medium	Taupe	$8.95
Le 348-0654	Large	Taupe	$8.95
Le 348-0712	X-Large	Taupe	$8.95
Le 348-0290	Small	Beige	$8.95
Le 348-0357	Medium	Beige	$8.95
Le 348-0415	Large	Beige	$8.95
Le 348-0472	X-Large	Beige	$8.95

Size Chart for Excel Women's Support Pantyhose

Height	WEIGHT (IN POUNDS)															
	90	95	100	105	110	115	120	125	130	135	140	145	150	155	160	165
4'11"	S	S	S	S	S	S	S	S	S	M						
5'0"	S	S	S	S	S	S	S	S	M	M	M	M				
5'1"	S	S	S	S	S	S	S	M	M	M	M	M	M	M	L	L
5'2"	S	S	S	S	S	S	M	M	M	M	M	M	L	L	L	L
5'3"	S	S	S	S	S	M	M	M	M	M	M	L	L	L	L	L
5'4"		S	S	M	M	M	M	M	M	L	L	L	L	L	L	
5'5"		S	M	M	M	M	M	L	L	L	L	L	L	L	XL	
5'6"			M	M	M	M	L	L	L	L	L	L	L	XL	XL	
5'7"			M	M	M	L	L	L	L	L	L	XL	XL	XL		
5'8"				L	L	L	L	L	L	XL	XL	XL	XL			
5'9"					L	L	L	L	XL	XL	XL	XL	XL			
5'10"					L	L	L	L	XL	XL	XL	XL	XL			
5'11"					L	L	XL	XL	XL	XL	XL	XL				

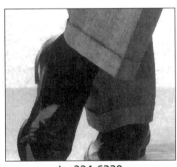

Le 324-6329

Jobst Pumpers, Men's Dress Support Socks. Over the calf length. Nylon and orlon blend. Graduated compression; greater counterpressure at ankle than knee to improve circulation. Bubble-toe and heel pocket for good fit. "Stay-up" top. Small fits shoe sizes 7-8, Medium fits shoe sizes 8½ to 10, Large fits shoe sizes 10½ to 12½ and X-Large fits shoe sizes 13 and over. Per pair.

Le 324-6329	Small	Black	$12.95
Le 324-6832	Medium	Black	$12.95
Le 324-7673	Large	Black	$12.95
Le 324-9547	X-Large	Black	$12.95

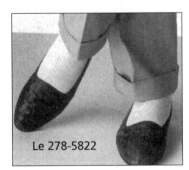

Le 278-5822

Jobst Pumpers Women's Casual Support Socks. Knee length. Nylon and orlon blend. Graduated compression; greater compression at ankle than calf to stimulate circulation. Bubble toe and heel pocket for good fit. "Stay-up" top. Small fits shoe sizes 5-6½ , Medium fits shoe sizes 7-8½ , Large fits shoe sizes 9-11. Per pair.

Le 278-5822	Small	White	$12.95
Le 278-6044	Medium	White	$12.95
Le 278-6200	Large	White	$12.95
Le 278-6325	Small	Cream	$12.95
Le 278-6440	Medium	Cream	$12.95
Le 278-6622	Large	Cream	$12.95
Le 278-6788	Small	Blue	$12.95
Le 278-3058	Medium	Blue	$12.95
Le 278-3330	Large	Blue	$12.95
Le 278-3520	Small	Charcoal	$12.95
Le 278-3637	Medium	Charcoal	$12.95
Le 278-3785	Large	Charcoal	$12.95

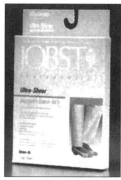

Le 228-8660

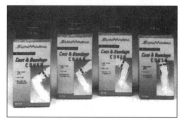

Le 365-9257 / Le 365-9315 /
Le 365-9372 / Le 365-9430

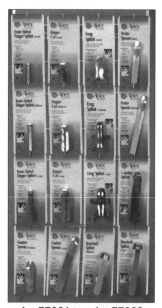

Ap 77001 . . . Ap 77009

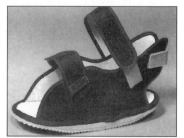

Le 349-6353 / Le 349-6437
Le 349-6544 / Le 349-6650

Jobst Ultra-Sheer Support Knee-Hi. Ultra-sheer 84% nylon, 16% Spandex. Graduated compression; firmer at ankles to help relieve leg fatigue. Sandal-foot styling; wide, non-constricting top. Small fits shoe sizes 4-5, Medium fits shoe sizes 5½ to 7½, large fits shoe sizes 8-10½.

Le 228-8660	Small	Suntan	$8.95
Le 229-2159	Medium	Suntan	$8.95
Le 229-3504	Large	Suntan	$8.95

SunMark Cast and Bandage Covers. Made from highest quality polyurethane plastic and other materials. Keeps casts and bandage completely dry. Convenient Velcro band seals top of cover. Durable and large enough for fiberglass casts.

Le 365-9257	Lower leg, 27"	$13.95
Le 365-9315	Full leg, 40"	$14.95
Le 365-9372	Lower arm, 24"	$10.95
Le 365-9430	Full arm, 32"	$11.95

Apex Finger Splints. Aluminum and foam. Protects and promotes healing.

Ap 77001	Small,4- Sided	$2.95
Ap 77002	Medium, 4-Sided	$2.95
Ap 77003	Large, 4-Sided	$2.95
Ap 77004	Small, Finger cot	$2.95
Ap 77005	Medium, Finger cot	$2.95
Ap 77006	Large, Finger cot	$2.95
Ap 77010	Medium, Gutter/Spoon	$2.95
Ap 77011	Large, Gutter/Spoon	$2.95
Ap 77008	Medium, Frog type	$4.95

Jerome Cast Shoe. Protects cast from damage and weather. Soft rubber, rocker-bottom soles for durability and secure footing. Straps adjust for easy application and proper fit. Heavy duty navy duck upper.

Le 349-6353	Small—Women's 4 to 6, Men's 5 to 7 shoe size	$15.95
Le 349-6437	Medium—Women's 6 to 8, Men's 7 to 9 shoe size	$15.95
Le 349-6544	Large—Women's 8 to 10, Men's 9 to 11 shoe size	$15.95
Le 349-6650	X-Large—Men's 11 to 13	$15.95

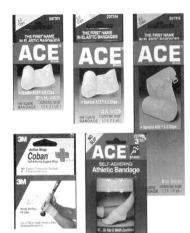
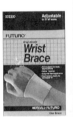
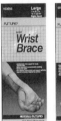
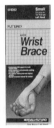
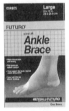
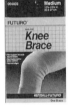
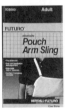
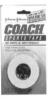

Elastic Products

Le 116-3070	Ace Elastic Bandage 2.5" 207311	$5.45
Le 116-3088	Ace Elastic Bandage 3" 207314	$5.85
Le 116-3104	Ace Elastic Bandage 4" 207313	$7.25
Le 116-3112	Ace Elastic Bandage 6" 207315	$12.35
Le 278-1318	Ace Athletic Bandage 2" Width	$5.25
Le 278-1326	Ace Athletic Bandage 3" 207461	$6.65
Le 112-7117	Ace Athletic Bandage 4" 207462	$7.95
Le 212-3081	Ace Cold Compress Wrap 207511	$1.95
Le 173-6438	Ace Reusable Cold Compress	$5.65
Le 274-1106	Coban Action Wrap 2" × 5 yd. Cr-2	$4.85
Le 130-7040	Futuro 3392 Wrist Brace Right Sml	$20.85
Le 130-7032	Futuro 3382 Wrist Brace Left Sml	$20.85
Le 130-7065	Futuro 3393 Wrist Brace Right Med	$20.85
Le 130-7057	Futuro 3383 Wrist Brace Left Med	$20.95
Le 130-7081	Futuro 3395 Wrist Brace Right Lrg	$20.85
Le 130-7073	Futuro 3385 Wrist Brace Left Lrg	$20.85
Le 130-6000	Futuro 4303 Wrist Brace Med	$5.85
Le 270-4013	Futuro 2300 Wrist Brace Adjustable	$5.75
Le 130-6075	Futuro Ankle Brace Large	$8.75
Le 130-6067	Futuro Ankle Brace Med	$8.75
Le 130-6034	Futuro Knee Brace Med	$8.75
Le 130-6042	Futuro Knee Brace Lrg	$8.95
Le 161-4510	Futuro 3080 Arm Sling Pouch Adult	$13.95
Le 216-4713	J&J Coach Sport Tape 1½" × 10'	$4.05
Le 129-2549	3M 2646 Cold Comfort Cold Pack	$6.45
Le 116-0365	Cold Comfort Inst Pack 2640	$2.45

Hot & Cold Therapy

CARE MUST BE TAKEN when using heat as part of any therapy for back pain. Maximum benefits are derived from heat therapy in the first 20 to 30 minute range. After that amount of time, the patient may be at risk of burns because the blood vessels will have constricted and are unable to dissipate the heat via blood circulation.

The normal temperature of a hot water bottle used for adults is 125°F. If your patient is feeble, a temperature between 105°F and 115°F would be better. The hot water bottle should be wrapped in a towel or a hot water bottle cover. Make sure that all the air is out of the bottle or it will not mold itself to the patient's body.

During cold therapy, blood vessels will reach maximum constriction when the skin reaches a temperature of 60°F. Below 60°F, blood vessels will become larger to protect the tissue from freezing. That's why the face and ears turn red in cold weather. Make sure you ask the doctor how long, where and when cold therapy is to be applied.

Your doctor, therapist and/or nurse will assist you with any therapy whether it is hot or cold. It pays to use a little common sense and err on the side of caution when using hot and cold therapy on the patient. If pain persists, call the doctor.

Hot and Cold First Aid.

Using cold therapy:

- *Suspected Bone Fracture:* Apply cold pack; stabilize injury; see doctor immediately.
- *Joint Injury:* Elevate injured area; apply ice pack.
- *Moderate Burns:* Apply cold pack for 5 minutes at a time; do not break blisters or apply creams/sprays.
- *Hives:* Apply cold pack for itching.
- *Back Pain:* Apply cold pack for 10 to 20 minutes several times a day.

Using hot therapy:

- *Arthritis, Neck Pain, Aching Muscles:* Apply heat packs frequently.
- *Chronic Back Pain:* Apply moist heat frequently.

Using cold or hot therapy:

- *Headaches:* Place hot or cold packs around head or neck. Hot baths also help.

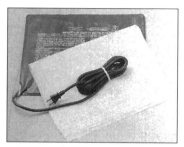

Le 114-2850 / Le 198-2842

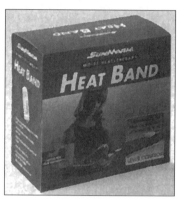

Le 215-9622

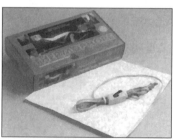

Le 221-4930 / Le 221-5374 /
Le 221-4948

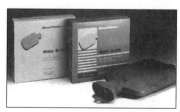

Le 114-2926 / Le 114-2975

Hot and Cold Therapy Products

SunMark Heating Pads. Three heat settings, lighted controls, washable covers and Braille touch switch.

Le 114-2850	Deluxe with push-button switch	$24.95
Le 198-2842	Hospital low temperature with 5 disposable covers. 100% wetproof, safety sealed vinyl.	$28.95

SunMark Moist/Dry Heating Pads. Can be used for both dry and moist heat. Sponge for applying moist heat. Three heat settings, lighted controls. Wet-proof pad construction. Braille touch switch.

Le 114-2868	Deluxe with washable cover	$28.95
Le 220-3537	King-Size Deluxe 12" × 24"	$31.95

SunMark Moist Heat Band. Flexible, wraparound heating pad for soothing moist or dry heat application. Sponge provides penetrating moist heat. Three heat settings with indicator light. Removable washable cover with snaps. Braille touch lever. Wet-proof pad construction.

Le 215-9622	6" × 19½"	$29.95

Dunlap Moist Heat Therapy Wrap. Microwaveable Therabeads. No gels, plastic, electricity or boiling water. No special cover needed. Adjustable and reusable.

Le 248-0192	6½" × 22"	$29.95

Dunlap Moist Heat Pack. Heat in microwave. Contains Therabeads — no gels or plastic. Reusable.

Le 353-9202	9" × 12"	$25.95

Dunlap Moist Heat Therapy Wrap. Microwaveable Therabeads. Up to 30 minutes of moist heat. Reusable.

Le 247-9715	6" × 40"	$29.95

SunMark Moist Heat Sinus Mask. Three heat settings. Relieves chronic sinusitis symptoms. Lighted controls, Braille touch push-button switch and wet-proof pad construction.

Le 220-3123	Economical and easy to use	$29.95

Dunlap Moist Heat Sinus Compress. Heats in microwave — moist heat in minutes. Contains Therabeads — no gels or plastics. Soft and flexible; reusable.

Le 247-9608	10" × 7½"	$14.95

Battle Creek Thermo-phore Moist Heat Pack. Absorbs moisture from the air instantly — no sponge to moisten. Pressure sensitive on/off switch. Temporary relief for arthritis, sore muscles, and sinus discomfort.

Le 221-4930	14" × 27"	$69.95
Le 221-5374	4" × 17"	$49.95
Le 221-4948	14" × 14"	$59.95

SunMark Water Bottle. Textured surface for added strength and style.

Le 114-2926	2 quart with 5 year guarantee	$8.95
Le 114-2975	2 quart with lifetime guarantee. Ribbed surface on one side	$13.95

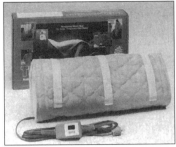

Le 220-6480

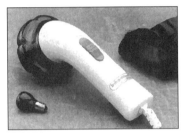

Le 247-8691

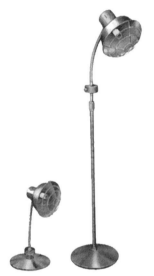

Br 51101 / Br 51102

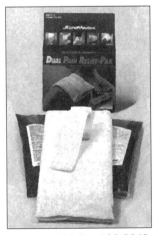

Le 114-2850 / Le 198-2842

Baxter Kwik-Heat™ Instant Hot Pack. Attains controlled temperature of 110°F seconds after bag is squeezed. Disposable.

Le 271-3691 $3.95

Battle Creek Thermophore Moist Heat Muff. Designed to temporarily relieve pain and stiffness in hands, elbows and ankles. Adjustable strap for comfortable fit.

Le 220-6480 $47.95

Health Team Infrared Heating Unit. Therapeutic infrared heat. Relieves pain due to arthritis, bursitis and overexertion. Eases pain by dilating blood vessels. Heat penetrates 10mm of skin tissue. Handy flashlight size.

Le 127-2541   Comes with carrying case $29.95

Homedics Infra-Wave Heat Therapy. Penetrating infrared heat for aching muscles. Similar to units used by therapists. Lightweight, contoured shape. Includes 1 replacement bulb.

Le 247-8691   Comes with carrying case $39.95

Brandt Infra-Red Lamps. All lamps are equipped with a 12″ flexible arm for positioning. Three conductor cord set and protective wire guard.

Br 51101	300 watt table model	$154.95
Br 51102	300 watt pedestal base. Height adjustment 35″ to 58″	$205.95
Br 53103	300 watt Mobile. Variable control or timer. Height 35″ to 58″	$324.95
Br 053	300 watt replacement unit	$37.95

Brandt Sun/Heat Lamp. You can produce a beautiful tan with the lamp's 800 watt u.v. generator or use the 600 watt heating elements to relieve arthritis, bursitis, back pain, muscular cramps, decubitis ulcers (bed sores) or muscular soreness. Black matte chassis is mounted on a 3-way adjustable floor stand. Adjusts for height, tilt and folds for compact storage. 10-minute timer switch. 7¼″ × 8″ reflector.

Br 62023   Adjusts from 52″ to 63½″ $364.95

SunMark Ice Bag. Made from strongest rubber available — supple and durable.

Le 241-6618	1 Pint capacity, 6″	$8.95
Le 114-3023	1 Quart capacity, 9″	$9.95
Le 114-3031	3 Quart capacity, 11″	$11.95

Baxter Kwik-Kold, Instant Ice Packs. Attains controlled temperature of 34°F seconds after bag is squeezed. Disposable.

Le 220-1671   6¼″ × 9″ $6.95

SunMark Dual Pain Relief Pak. Includes separate reusable hot and cold gel packs. Store blue cold pack in freezer and heat red hot pack in microwave oven or boiling water. Heat guide indicates heat level of hot pack.

Le 168-2822   Cover has elastic strap and Velcro tape $18.95

SunMark Cold Therapy. Reusable gel packs store in freezer. Flexible when frozen. Velcro and tie bands for convenience. Nontoxic.

Le 168-1956	Removable cover with elastic strap and Velcro closure	$9.95
Le 168-4125	Elastic wrap combines cold and compression therapies	$11.95

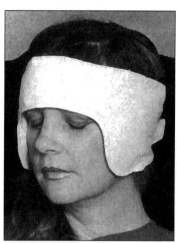

Le 354-7866

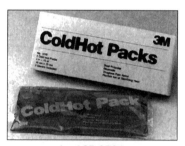

Le 165-9721

Sub I.P. Headache Ice-Band. Designed to position gel pack across forehead and temples — Velcro strap. Helps in treatment of migraine in advanced stages.

Le 354-7866   Two sided band, cool velour side and cold vinyl side $18.95

Sub I.P. Headache Ice-Pillo. Helps relieve tension and migraine headaches. Reusable gel pack slips inside contoured pillow.

Le 328-4247 $34.95

Le 363-2197   Massage vibrating unit for relaxing massage $45.95

3M ColdHot Pack. Reusable dual purpose cold and hot pack. Remains flexible between -20°F and 212°F. Nontoxic. Can be safely stored in freezer, refrigerator or hot water bath. Microwaveable.

Le 165-9721   4½" × 10½" $14.95

Cancer

CANCER IS THE SECOND LEADING CAUSE OF DEATH in the United States (heart disease is number one). In 1995, it is estimated that 1,250,000 new cancer cases were diagnosed and about 547,000 people died from cancer. By the year 2000 it is estimated that cancer will be the leading cause of death in the United States. Over 80 types of cancer are known to exist and, if detected early, many can be treated successfully. About one in three people will eventually have cancer. Currently, an estimated eight million people with a history of cancer live in the United States. Advancing age has the most significant impact on the incidence and mortality of cancer.

Cancer may develop in any tissue of any organ at any age. The research that the United States has put into cancer has resulted in a substantial increase in survival rates. In 1960, only 25 percent of patients survived five or more years. Now, survival rates are approaching 50 percent. Five years without further symptoms after treatment is the accepted term for "cured."

Cancer is a disease in which cells grow and multiply uncontrollably. If the patient has a tumor, the tumor will increase in size as the cells multiply. Tumors that spread throughout the body are called metastatic tumors and commonly spread to the lungs, liver, bones and brain.

Successful treatment of cancer depends on early detection. Early detection decreases cancer mortality, leads to less radical therapy and reduces financial costs. The American Cancer Society recommends a cancer check-up by a doctor every three years for people who are 20-39 years of age and annually for those over 40. The check-up should always include health counseling and exams for cancer of the breast, uterus, cervix, colon, rectum, prostate, mouth, skin, testes, thyroid and lymph nodes.

Tests include fecal occult blood test (blood that is not visible) for colon or rectal cancer, rectal exam for prostate and rectal cancers, sigmoidoscopy "procto" for colon and rectum cancers, pelvic exam and Pap test for cancers of the female reproductive organs, breast exam and mammography for breast cancer. If cancer is suspected, a biopsy may be performed. In this procedure, a piece of the tumor is removed surgically (the new needle biopsy method for breast biopsies called Fischer Imaging system eliminates the need for an incision) and examined under a microscope to determine if it is cancerous (malignant) or noncancerous (benign).

Women should perform breast self-examinations once a month. Just after the period, check breasts all over — including the armpit. Look at the breasts in the mirror for any changes in size or shape. The most common site of a breast tumor is the upper and outer part of the breast. In most cases, the lump is not painful. The doctor can teach the right way to check. If the patient finds a lump, see the doctor. Don't take a chance.

If lumps in the breast are found, women should also have a mammogram — the most reliable method for detecting breast cancer. There are different opinions on how often to have a mammogram. Check with your doctor for advice. If the patient's mother, sister or other close relative has developed breast cancer, the chances of the patient developing the disease increases. When breast cancer is detected in its early stages, 90 percent of

Mammography is the X-ray procedure for detecting breast cancer at an early stage. It simple, safe and causes minimal discomfort.

Breast cancer is the most common cancer in women. One woman in 14 develops breast cancer. Over 80% of all breast cancers occur in women over the age of 50.

Call LeBoeuf's and we will send a pamphlet showing the methods used for a breast self-examination. The patient's doctor can also demonstrate the correct way to perform a breast self-examination.

Breast cancer warning signs to watch for:

A lump or thickening in or near the breast or in the underarm area.

A change in breast shape.

Swelling, redness or heat in the breast.

A discharge from the nipple.

A retraction of the nipple.

A change in the color or feel (texture) of the skin of the breast or nipple area.

the women can be treated successfully. In many cases, less extensive surgery can be used to treat the tumor and the breast can often be saved.

Men can perform testicular self-examination to increase the chances of finding a tumor early. Men should perform this test once a month after taking a hot (warm) shower or bath. Examine each testicle gently with both hands. The index and middle fingers should be placed underneath the testicle while the thumbs are placed on top. Roll the testicle gently between the thumbs and fingers. One testicle may be larger than the other and this is normal. There is a cord-like structure on the top and back of the testicle that stores and transports sperm. Do not confuse the cord-like structure with an abnormal lump. Feel for an abnormal lump — about the size of a pea — on the front or side of the testicle. These lumps are usually painless. If a lump is found, call the doctor for an appointment right away. Testicular cancer is highly curable if detected and treated early. Testicular cancer almost always occurs in only one testicle and the other testicle is all that is needed for full sexual function.

Symptoms:

- **Lungs** — cough that won't go away, coughing up blood, shortness of breath, chest hurting all the time
- **Breast** — lump or thickness in the breast, change in breast shape, discharge from the nipple
- **Colon and rectum** — changes in bowel habits, bleeding from rectum, blood in the stool
- **Uterus, ovary, and cervix** — bleeding, unusual discharge from the vagina, swelling of the stomach, pain during intercourse
- **Skin** — a sore that doesn't heal, change in the size or color of a wart or mole, sudden appearance of a mole
- **Prostate** — painful or burning urination, blood in urine, can't urinate or difficulty in starting to urinate
- **Testicular** — painless swelling or a feeling of heaviness in the testicles, lump the size of a pea or if you have been told that your testicles never descended
- **Throat** — difficulty in swallowing

The three major kinds of treatment for cancer are surgery, radiation therapy and chemotherapy (anti-cancer drugs).

No one knows exactly what causes cancer, but it is not contagious. Cancer is a serious illness and, while it often can be cured, treatment can be intense and prolonged. The three major kinds of treatment for cancer are surgery, radiation therapy and chemotherapy (anti-cancer drugs).

The control of pain is a vital factor in caregiving for the cancer patient.

Surgery is performed to remove all or part of a tumor. Surgery is the oldest effective form of cancer therapy. Mastectomy, laryngectomy and colectomy are three of the most common types of cancer surgery.

Chemotherapy is treatment with special drugs that destroy cancer cells. The drugs may be taken by mouth or through a needle inserted into a vein. Drugs enter the blood stream and are carried to cancer cells anywhere in the body. Treatment is usually given many times over several months. Chemotherapy is designed to work on cancer cells, but noncancerous cells can be harmed as well and side effects such as nausea, vomiting, loss of appetite, sores on gums, tongue and cheeks and hair loss. Also, chemotherapy can affect the bone marrow that produces blood cells.

Radiation therapy is the application of high energy x-rays or rays from radioactive substances to the tumor. The radiation prevents cancer cells from dividing and they die. Radiation therapy does not hurt and takes only a few minutes, but like chemotherapy there are side effects. The skin may be burned and/or hair loss may occur in the area receiving radiation. If treatment is in the stomach area, nausea, vomiting and/or diarrhea may result. If treatment is in the head area, the patient may develop sores in the mouth or headaches. In some cases, the radiation source is surgically implanted in the tumor. The patient is not radioactive during or after treatment and none of the treatment will harm other people. However, when the patient has an radioactive implant in place, you will not be allowed to get too close until it is removed. The patient generally, but not always, will be in the hospital while the implant is in place.

Control of pain is a vital factor in caregiving for the cancer patient. The U. S. Agency for Health Care Policy and Research claims that 90 percent of cancer patients can have pain effectively controlled. Treatment of pain is complex, but pain can be controlled and should not be considered a part of the disease or part of the inevitable process of growing old (see section on "Pain Control").

Risk of cancer can be reduced by:

- Maintaining a desirable body weight.
- Eating a varied diet.
- Including a variety of vegetables and fruits in the daily diet.
- Eating more high-fiber foods such as pasta, whole grain cereals, breads, vegetables, and fruit
- Cutting down on total fat intake.
- Limiting consumption of alcoholic beverages.
- Limiting consumption of salt-cured, smoked and nitrate-preserved foods.
- Not smoking.
- Limiting exposure to sunlight — use sunblock
- Not using smokeless tobacco such as snuff or chewing tobacco – may lead to cancer of the mouth, larynx, throat and esophagus.
- Consulting with doctor on risks of estrogen treatment.

The Caregiver Role

The caregiver who is treating a cancer patient may be needed for a wide range of assistance. The caregiver should monitor the patient to insure that medications are taken exactly as prescribed. Let the doctor or nurse know if there any side effects and make sure that all chemotherapy pills and other medications are out of the reach of children.

Danger Signs

Notify the doctor and/or nurse as soon as possible if you observe any of the following symptoms:

- Weight changes of five pounds or more in a week and a nauseated feeling for more than a day.
- Dehydration caused by vomiting, diarrhea or fever and lasting for more than 24 hours.
- Swallowing problems causing the patient to gag, cough or choke, if there are red shiny ulcers in the mouth or on the tongue.
- Hiccoughs (hiccups) that last for more than a day.
- Mouth sores caused by a cut or sore in the mouth, white patches appearing on the tongue or on the inside of the mouth and/or if redness or shininess in the mouth lasts for more than 48 hours.
- Bleeding in the mouth happens for the first time and continues for more than half an hour. The patient may also vomit blood.
- Dry mouth persisting for more than three days and the patient has trouble breathing.
- Nausea and vomiting more than three times an hour for more than three or more hours, some of the vomited material has been inhaled, if blood or a material that looks like coffee grounds appears in the vomit and if the patient cannot take medications.
- Diarrhea that causes 6-8 or more loose bowel movements per day for two days in a row, if you notice blood in or around anal area or in the stool, if abdominal cramps last for two or more days, if the abdomen suddenly becomes blown-up.
- Constipation and no bowel movement for more than three days and persistent cramps or vomiting.
- Blood in the urine and/or stool on toilet tissue two or more times, you notice blood streaks in the stool and if you notice bright red blood from the rectum.
- Fever that lasts for one or more days and temperature is 100.5 degrees orally or 101.5 degrees rectally or higher.
- Shortness of breath and chest pain causing the nostrils to flare during breathing, there is a wheezing, the skin is pale or blue and the skin is cold and clammy and if there is a thick yellow/green or bloody sputum.

Risk factors associated with suicide for cancer patients include:

- *Depression*
- *Prior psychiatric diagnosis of depression*
- *Poorly controlled pain*
- *Family history of suicide*
- *Delirium*
- *Substance abuse*
- *Advanced disease*
- *Disfiguring disease*
- *Disfiguring surgery*
- *Poor social support*
- *Increased age*

- Skin rash or color changes that cause the skin to turn yellow, severe itching and bruises that do not go away within a week, new bruises continuing to appear for three days.
- Skin that becomes very rough or painful.
- Excessive sweating, shaking chills and a fever that is 101.5°F or higher for more than 24 hours.
- Falls that cause bleeding or unconsciousness, breathing has stopped and you are concerned about possible injury from a fall.
- Swelling that spreads up legs or arms, that if you press your finger into the swollen area and the fingertip mark stays.
- Leg cramps that last more than 6-8 hours, the legs become red, swollen or hot and cramping is not relieved by heat or massage.
- Uncontrolled movement of the muscles or a seizure requires the attention of the doctor as soon as possible.

There are numerous other symptoms that will require the attention of a doctor and/or nurse. Common sense, and instructions from the doctor, should provide the caregiver with enough information to make appropriate decisions. If in doubt about the condition of the patient always call the doctor.

The caregiver needs to monitor the patient's pain level and symptoms closely. Changes in types of medication and dosages may produce adverse side effects.

The patient's method of taking medication sometimes needs to be changed. Difficulty swallowing may require giving some oral medications by rectal or transdermal means. There are also some drugs that can be given through the nasal passages.

Patients who are not able to swallow a whole tablet should never be given *crushed* controlled-release drugs. Crushing the tablet immediately releases the drug and can produce undesirable side effects. Before you crush *any* tablet or capsule, ask your pharmacist or doctor if the medication is a controlled-release drug.

The taking of some medications will require that the caregiver watch the patient to make sure that the pill(s) are swallowed. The patient may fear that taking the prescribed drug will result in addiction, nausea or some other adverse event. The caregiver may also need to search the room for signs of hoarding or hidden pills. Caregivers should also be alert for prescription forgery. The patient may also be seeing more than one physician in hopes of securing additional medication.

Some patients will deliberately exceed their dosage intake. Security locks, timed pill dispensers and programmable pill dispensers will help prevent abusing the prescription.

Both the National Cancer Institute and the American Cancer Society will furnish a list of reputable doctors.

Contact the National Cancer Institute — 1-800-422-6237. It is located at 31 Center Drive, Bethesda, MD 20892.

Contact the Susan G. Komen Breast Cancer Foundation — 1-800-462-9273. It is located at 5005 LBJ Freeway, Suite 370, Dallas, TX 75244

What to do:

Contact your doctor — Regular check-ups are the most important way to reduce the risk of cancer. Early detection increases survival rates significantly. Check-ups should always include exams for cancer of the breast, uterus, cervix, colon, rectum, prostate, mouth, skin, testes, thyroid, and lymph nodes.

Contact the American Cancer Society — 1-800-ACS-2345 (1-800-227-2345). Or you can write to: 1599 Clifton Road, N.E. Atlanta, GA 30329. Their local number is (404) 320-3333. The Society has over 3,400 local units, over 2 million volunteers and information and programs for patients and care-givers that are invaluable.

Contact the American Cancer Institute — 1-800-4-CANCER (1-800-422-6237). Or you can write to: 9000 Rockville Pike, Building 31, Room 10A24, Bethesda, MD 20892. The Cancer Information Service will provide answers to your questions and free booklets about cancer.

Contact the American Institute for Cancer Research — 1-800-843-8114, (202) 328-7744. Or write to them at: 1759 R Street, N.W., Washington, DC 20069. The institute provides public education and publications about diet nutrition and cancer.

Contact local social services organizations — There are many agencies that will provide information and listings of resources available in your area. Agencies such as the offices on aging, local health agencies as well as religious-affiliated service groups also provide information, training and support. There are also associations and companies that provide care management services to serve as the link between you and community-based services. They charge for their services — so be sure you understand what it will cost to have them provide assistance.

Contact a lawyer — It is very important to act quickly to protect the future security of the patient. There are lawyers who specialize in elder law. You will need to execute a durable power of attorney, a living will and/or a living trust. If the estate is of any size, living trusts appear to be the best way to handle the estate because you can avoid probate and not have the estate's assets tied up by the courts. Contact **LeBoeuf's** ☎ **1-800-546-5559** for a listing of lawyers in your area.

Safety — Organize the home to permit the patient to carry on as many of their normal routines as possible. Other tips and items that make for a safer home are listed in the "Home Modification and Safety Products" section.

Communication — Explain to the patient what is happening. Tell only as much as the patient wants to know. Tell family and friends. Explain the diagnosis and tell family and friends that the patient needs their support and love. Tell them how and when they can help. Explain to family and friends that feelings of guilt, anxiety, anger and a feeling of uselessness are all normal for the cancer patient, their families and friends. Try to have all parties be compassionate and understanding as possible. Be honest with each other. Be specific about your needs. Draw up a plan of action that allows all parties to understand the role that they can (and must) play.

Prostate Problems

Prostate problems are not uncommon in men 50 years of age and older. More than 300,000 surgeries on the prostate are performed annually in the United States. Most of these surgeries are the transurethral resection of the prostate (TURP).

The prostate is a small organ about the size of a walnut. It lies below the bladder (which holds the urine) and surrounds the urethra (the tube that carries urine from the bladder). The prostate makes a fluid that becomes part of semen. Semen is the white fluid that contains sperm. If the prostate becomes enlarged, it squeezes the urinary tube (urethra) and causes problems with urination.

Noncancerous prostate problems include:

- **Acute Prostatitis** — A bacterial infection of the prostate. It can occur in men at any age. Symptoms include fever, chills and pain in the lower back and between the legs. Treatment consists of antibiotics and instructions to drink more liquids.
- **Benign Prostatic Hypertrophy (BPH)** — An enlargement of the prostate gland. This condition is more common in older men. More than 50 percent of men in their 60s and as many as 90 percent of men in their 70s and 80s have this condition. Symptoms include difficulty in urinating, dribbling after urination and the urge to urinate often. In rare cases, the patient is unable to urinate. Treatment may include doing nothing but monitoring the problem and having regular checkups to insure that the condition does not get worse, balloon dilation, drugs to relax the muscles near the prostate to relieve symptoms and/or surgery. Surgery is the treatment most likely to relieve the symptoms but has the most complications. Men should carefully weigh the risks and benefits of each option.
- **Chronic Prostatitis** — A prostate infection that comes and goes. Symptoms are similar to those of acute prostatitis, but without the fever. Treatment is difficult and antibiotics work in those cases where bacteria are present. In some cases, it helps to massage the prostate to release fluids. Warm baths also are a big help. Sometimes the problem clears up by itself.

Prostate Cancer

Prostate cancer is one of the most common forms of cancer among American men. About 80 percent of all cases occur in men over 65. In 1995, it is estimated that over 200,000 new cases of prostate cancer were diagnosed. For unknown reasons, prostate cancer is more common and more virulent at an earlier age among African-American men than white men. In the early stages, the disease usually is a slow-growing malignancy and is not life threatening. However, without treatment, the cancer can spread to other parts of the body and cause death. About 40,000 men die every year from prostate cancer that has spread.

Treatment for prostate cancer can include surgery, radiation therapy or hormone therapy. The choice of treatment depends on many factors, such as the patient's general health and whether or not the cancer has spread beyond the prostate.

Radical prostatectomy surgery removes the entire prostate and surrounding tissues. New surgical techniques can preserve the nerves to the penis so that men can still have erections after prostate removal. Incontinence is common for a time after surgery and, in most cases, the patient will regain urinary control after several weeks. Those who continue to have a problem will have to wear a device that collects the urine. As with all surgeries, it is recommended that a second opinion be obtained. It is possible to find surgeons who have performed hundreds of prostate operations. Impotence may occur.

Balloon dilation is less effective than surgery, but has fewer complications. At present, balloon dilation is a reasonable treatment for patients with smaller prostates. Recent studies indicate that improvement of symptoms is temporary and symptoms will recur within two years.

Transurethal resection (TURP) is another kind of surgery which cuts the cancer from the prostate but does not take out the entire prostate. The doctor inserts a special instrument into the urethra through the penis to remove part of the prostate. No skin needs to be cut. This procedure can be performed in ambulatory settings or during a one-day hospitalization. This procedure is the most effective of all, with improvement of symptoms in 75 to 96 percent of cases.

Radiation therapy uses high-energy rays to kill cancer cells and shrink tumors. It is used when cancer cells are found in more than one area. Impotence may occur in men treated with radiation therapy although statistically in far fewer cases than medical prostatectomy.

Hormone therapy uses various hormones to stop cancer cells from growing. It is used for prostate cancer that has spread to other parts of the body. A common side-effect of hormone treatment is enlargement of breast tissue.

There is no self-examination protocol to detect prostate cancer. The American Urological Association and the American Cancer Society recommend annual screening for prostate cancer for men over 50. For African-American men, and for men who have a family history of prostate cancer, annual exams should begin at age 40.

The diagnosis evaluation will include digital rectal examination and/or inserting a gloved, lubricated finger into the rectum to check the prostate, urinalysis to rule out urinary tract infection and hematuria, a general medical history focusing on the urinary tract, measurement of serum creatinine and assessment of renal function, blood test and always testing for prostate-specific antigen (PSA). Testing for PSA increases the detection rate for prostate cancer over the digital rectal examination and tends to detect cancer at an earlier stage. However, the PSA test does not discriminate well between patients with symptomatic BPH and those with prostate cancer.

Symptoms:

- Progressive urinary frequency and urgency.
- Difficulty in urinating.
- Dribbling of urine.
- Sensation of incomplete emptying.

- Complete urinary retention (will require catheterization).
- Almost continuous overflow incontinence.
- Blood in the urine.
- Painful ejaculation.
- Continuing pain in the lower back, hips or upper thighs.
- Painful or burning urination.

What to do:

See a doctor — The doctor can determine if you have BPH or if another disease is the cause of the problem through testing. There are numerous tests that can be performed and they are neither costly nor painful.

Contact the American Cancer Society — 1-800-227-2345. They can provide you with information on the over 3,400 local Units and over 2 million volunteers. The American Cancer Society has 57 chartered Divisions and a professional staff of over 4,800.

Contact the National Cancer Institute — 1-800-4-CANCER (1-800-422-6237). The National Cancer Institute operates the Cancer Information Service that can answer questions and provide free booklets about cancer.

Ostomy Products

Ileostomy is an operation that is normally performed for people who have Crohn's disease or an ulcerative colitis. The lower part of the small intestine is brought through an incision in the stomach wall and formed into an artificial outlet (stoma) for the discharge of feces into a pouch attached to the skin. Fecal drainage is constant and cannot be regulated. The drainage contains enzymes which are very damaging to the skin, so you and the patient should make sure that there is no skin breakdown. An ileostomy is usually permanent. Recovery from the operation will normally take about six weeks.

An ostomy is a surgical opening in the stomach wall for the elimination of feces or urine. A colostomy is a surgical opening into the colon (large bowel). The location of the ostomy determines the character of the fecal drainage.

A healthy stoma will appear red. Pale or dark-colored stomas indicate poor blood circulation to the area and you should contact the doctor. The skin must be kept clean and dried thoroughly before attaching the pouch (appliance). Most ostomy appliances have three things in common: a pouch that can be emptied or a disposable pouch, a faceplate and an adhesive wafer. A burning sensation may indicate that the skin beneath the faceplate is breaking down. Pouches should be emptied when they are about one-third to one-half full. Make sure that you have received instructions from the doctor or nurse about how to change the appliance.

After an ileostomy, most patients feel much better. The patient should be able to return to normal activities and life-style. The doctor will recommend that the patient drink increased amounts of water and make sure that the patient is getting enough salt (the colon's main function is the absorption of water and salt).

Diet Tips for Ostomy Patients:

- Ileostomy blockage may be caused by high fiber foods, seeds, corn, celery, popcorn, nuts, coleslaw, Chinese vegetables, coconut macaroons, grapefruit, raisins, dried fruit, fried apples, apple skins and orange rinds.

- Loose bowels may be caused by larger more liquid meals eaten at temperature extremes, highly spiced foods, raw fruits and beer.

- Gas may be caused by cabbage, onions, beans, cucumbers, radishes and beer.

- Odor causing foods include cheese, eggs, fish, beans, onions, cabbage, asparagus and some vitamins and medications.

- Reduction of odors can be obtained by drinking cranberry juice, buttermilk or yogurt.

Ostomy products (appliances) should be selected with the following criteria:

- Odor resistance
- Close-fitting faceplate opening
- Faceplate should stay tight for at least 3 to 5 days
- Affordable and readily available
- Invisible under clothing and rustle-free.

We have a complete line of ostomy products from Convatec, Hollister, Smith & Nephew United, Bard and Coloplast. Many of the ostomy products are described on the following pages. For other products, call **LeBoeuf's** ☎ **1-800-546-5559** to obtain pricing or additional information.

DRUGS THAT DISCOLOR FECES

Drug	Feces Color Produced
Antacids, aluminum hydroxide types	Whitish or speckling
Antibiotics, oral	Greenish gray
Anticoagulants	Pink to red to black*
Bismuth-containing preparations	Black
Charcoal	Black
Chlorophyll	Green
Ferrous salts	Black
Heparin	Pink to red to black*
Indomethacin (Indocin®)	Green
Phenazopyridine (Pyridium®)	Orange-red
Phenylbutazone (Butazolidin®)	Pink to red to black*
Pyrvinium pamoate (Povan®)	Red
Salicylates, especially aspirin	Pink to red to black*
Senna	Yellow

*These colors may indicate intestinal bleeding.

What to do:

Contact the United Ostomy Association, Inc. 1-800-826-0826. You can write it at 36 Executive Park, Suite 120, Irvine, CA 92714. It helps ostomy patients return to normal living.

Ostomy Management from Convatec®

Sur-Fit Two-Piece System—Body-Side Skin Barriers

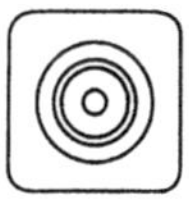

Stomahesive® Wafer, Sur-Fit Flange.

Le 116-4318

4″ × 4″ WAFER		BOX OF 5
Le 116-4318	1¼″ flange	$22.95
Le 248-4780	1½″ flange	$22.95
Le 248-4798	1¾″ flange	$22.95
Le 248-4806	2¼″ flange	$22.95
Le 277-8215	2¼″ flange	$22.95
6″ × 6″ WAFER		**BOX OF 5**
Le 215-6727	4″ flange	$34.95

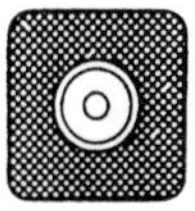

Sur-Fit Flexible.®

Le 241-3482

4″ × 4″ TAN COLLAR		BOX OF 5
Le 241-3482	1¼″ flange	$23.95
Le 241-3524	1½″ flange	$23.95
Le 241-3532	1¾″ flange	$23.95
5″ × 5″ TAN COLLAR		**BOX OF 5**
Le 241-3540	2¼″ flange	$24.95
Le 227-9321	2¾″ flange	$24.95
4″ × 4″ WHITE COLLAR		**BOX OF 5**
Le 186-3463	1¼″ flange	$23.95
Le 186-4198	1½″ flange	$23.95
Le 362-5514	1¾″ flange	$23.95
5″ × 5″ WHITE COLLAR		**BOX OF 5**
Le 186-4297	2¼″ flange	$24.95
Le 181-0050	2¾″ flange	$24.95

Sur-Fit Flexible with Pre-Cut Opening.

4″ × 4″ TAN COLLAR	To fit 1¾″ pouch flange size	BOX OF 5
Le 213-0789	½″ opening	$23.95
Le 213-1019	⅝″ opening	$23.95
Le 213-1100	¾″ opening	$23.95
Le 213-1282	⅞″ opening	$23.95
Le 213-1605	1″ opening	$23.95
Le 213-2017	1⅛″ opening	$23.95
Le 213-2256	1¼″ opening	$23.95
Le 213-2462	1⅜″ opening	$23.95
5″ × 5″ TAN COLLAR	To fit 2¾″ pouch flange size	**BOX OF 5**
Le 213-0334	1½″ opening	$24.95
Le 213-0508	1⅝″ opening	$24.95
Le 21 3-0649	1¾″ opening	$24.95

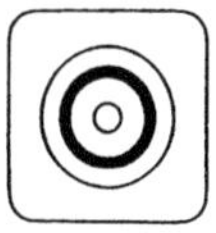

Durahesive Wafer,® Low-profile Flange.

Le 220-8577

4″ × 4″ WAFER		BOX OF 5
Le 220-8577	1¼″ flange	$33.95
Le 220-8676	1½″ flange	$33.95
Le 220-8767	1¾″ flange	$33.95
Le 220-8866	2¼″ flange	$33.95

Durahesive Wafer with Convex-It.

4″ × 4″ WAFER	To fit 1¾″ pouch flange size	BOX OF 5
Le 353-2793	½″ opening	$46.95
Le 353-2868	⅝″ opening	$46.95
Le 353-2967	¾″ opening	$46.95
Le 353-3031	⅞″ opening	$46.95
Le 353-3148	1″ opening	$46.95
Le 353-3221	1⅛″ opening	$46.95
Le 353-3338	1¼″ opening	$46.95
Le 353-1019	1⅜″ opening	$46.95

4″ × 4″ WAFER	To fit 2¼″ pouch flange size	BOX OF 5
Le 353-1084	1½″ opening	$47.95
Le 353-1183	1⅝″ opening	$47.95
Le 353-1258	1¾″ opening	$47.95
Le 353-1324	2″ opening	$47.95

Sur-Fit Pouches for Colostomy and Ileostomy Patients

Sur-Fit Drainable Pouches.

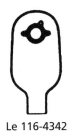

Le 116-4342

12″ OPAQUE	One tail closure per box	BOX OF 10
Le 116-4342	1¼″ flange	$24.95
Le 126-1981	1½″ flange	$24.95
Le 248-8864	1¾″ flange	$24.95
Le 248-8872	2¼″ flange	$24.95
Le 277-8231	2¾″ flange	$24.95
10″ OPAQUE		BOX OF 10
Le 116-4565	1¼″flange	$24.95
Le 248-8898	1½″ flange	$24.95
Le 116-4375	1¾″ flange	$24.95
Le 248-8922	2¼″ flange	$24.95
Le 215-3088	2¾″ flange	$24.95
12″ TRANSPARENT		BOX OF 10
Le 217-7210	1¼″ flange	$24.95
Le 179-7000	1½″ flange	$24.95
Le 121-4500	1¾″ flange	$24.95
Le 217-3961	2¼″ flange	$24.95
Le 215-4169	2¾″ flange	$24.95
14″ TRANSPARENT		BOX OF 10
Le 217-4175	4″ flange	$30.95

Sur-Fit Closed-End Pouch.

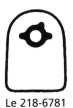

Le 218-6781

OPAQUE		BOX OF 30
Le 218-6781	1½″ flange	$42.95
Le 218-9777	1¾″ flange	$42.95
Le 227-9404	2¼″ flange	$42.95
Le 227-9594	2¾″ flange	$42.95

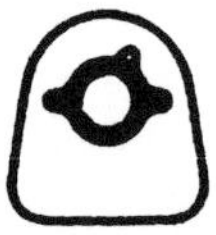

Sur-Fit Mini-Pouch.

Le 228-0139

SUITABLE FOR PEDIATRIC USE		BOX OF 20
Le 228-0139	1¼″ flange	$26.95
Le 228-0196	1½″ flange	$26.95
Le 228-0261	1¾″ flange	$26.95
Le 227-0402	2¼″ flange	$26.95

Active Life® One-Piece System

One-Piece Drainable Pouches with Stomahesive Skin Barrier.

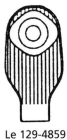

Le 129-4859

10″ OPAQUE		BOX OF 10
Le 129-4859	¾″ opening	$37.95
Le 129-1913	1″ opening	$37.95
Le 128-6459	1¼″ opening	$37.95
Le 128-4173	1½″ opening	$37.95
Le 128-1385	1¾″opening	$37.95
Le 127-7797	2″ opening	$37.95
Le 127-6575	2½″ opening	$37.95
12″ OPAQUE		BOX OF 10
Le 127-3291	¾″ opening	$37.95
Le 116-3609	1″ opening	$37.95
Le 116-3617	1¼″ opening	$37.95
Le 116-3674	1½″ opening	$37.95
Le 116-3807	1¾″ opening	$37.95
Le 116-3823	2″ opening	$37.95
Le 127-2632	2½″ opening	$37.95

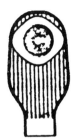

Le 225-5040

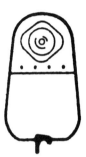

Le 175-6311

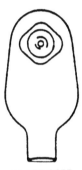

Le 175-8655

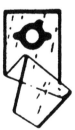

Le 116-3856

Le 277-3448

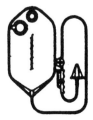

Le 116-4342

12" TRANSPARENT		**BOX OF 10**
Le 127-1469	3/4" opening	$37.95
Le 216-3046	1" opening	$37.95
Le 216-3756	1 1/4" opening	$37.95
Le 216-3855	1 1/2" opening	$37.95
Le 216-4184	1 3/4" opening	$37.95
Le 216-4366	2" opening	$37.95
Le 216-4788	2 1/2" opening	$37.95

One-Piece Drainable Custom Pouch with Stomahesive Skin Barrier.

12" TRANSPARENT		**BOX OF 10**
Le 225-5040	Can be enlarged to accommodate stoma sizes from 3/4" to 2 1/2"	$39.95

Active Life Convex Pouches

One-Piece Urostomy Pouch with Durahesive Skin Barrier.

STANDARD POUCH—TRANSPARENT		**BOX OF 5**
Le 175-6311	1/2" opening	$48.95
Le 175-6717	5/8" opening	$48.95
Le 175-6758	3/4" opening	$48.95
Le 175-6964	7/8" opening	$48.95
Le 175-7178	1" opening	$48.95
Le 175-7384	1 1/8" opening	$48.95
Le 175-7608	1 1/4" opening	$48.95
Le 175-7954	1 3/8" opening	$48.95
Le 175-8291	1 1/2" opening	$48.95

One-Piece Drainable Pouch with Durahesive Skin Barrier.

12" TRANSPARENT		**BOX OF 5**
Le 175-8655	3/4" opening	$55.95
Le 175-8770	7/8" opening	$55.95
Le 175-8929	1" opening	$55.95
Le 175-9315	1 1/8" opening	$55.95
Le 175-9547	1 1/4" opening	$55.95
Le 175-9687	1 3/8" opening	$55.95
Le 175-0404	1 1/2" opening	$56.95
Le 175-0768	1 3/4" opening	$56.95
Le 175-2004	2" opening	$56.95

Visi-Flow® Irrigation System

Sur-Fit Irrigation Sleeve.

		BOX OF 5
Le 116-3856	1 1/2" flange	$27.95
Le 116-3971	1 3/4" flange	$27.95
Le 116-4011	2 1/4" flange	$27.95
Le 116-4029	2 3/4" flange	$27.95

Sur-Fit Disposable Flange Cap.

		BOX OF 5
Le 277-3448	1 1/2" flange	$43.95
Le 277-3562	1 3/4" flange	$43.95
Le 277-3695	2 1/4" flange	$43.95

Visi-Flow Irrigator with Stoma Cone.

		BOX OF 10
Le116-4342	1 1/4" flange	$24.95

Sur-Fit Urostomy Pouches. Two Accuseal adapters per box.

SUR-FIT STANDARD POUCH—TRANSPARENT		**BOX OF 10**
Le 216-4861	1 1/4" flange	$35.95
Le 217-4225	1 1/2" flange	$35.95
Le 217-4233	1 3/4" flange	$35.95
Le 216-4994	2 1/4" flange	$35.95
Le 198-6470	2 3/4" flange	$35.95

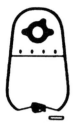

Le 216-5652

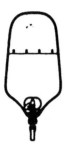

Le 241-3342

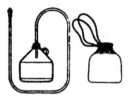

Le 116-9929

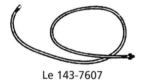

Le 143-7607

Visi-Flow® Irrigation System

Sur-Fit Urostomy Pouches.

SUR-FIT SMALL POUCH—TRANSPARENT		BOX OF 10
Le 216-5652	1¹⁄₄″ flange	$35.95
Le 217-7079	1¹⁄₂″ flange	$35.95
Le 216-7583	1³⁄₄″ flange	$35.95
Le 217-0025	2¹⁄₄″ flange	$35.95

Sur-Fit Urostomy Pouches with Accuseal® Tap. Two Accuseal adapters per box.

STANDARD POUCH—TRANSPARENT		BOX OF 10
Le 241-3342	1¹⁄₄″ flange	$38.95
Le 241-3359	1¹⁄₂″ flange	$38.95
Le 241-3391	1³⁄₄″ flange	$38.95
Le 227-9719	2¹⁄₄″ flange	$38.95
Le 227-9818	2³⁄₄″ flange	$38.95
Le 218-7086	4″ flange	$43.95
STANDARD POUCH—OPAQUE		BOX OF 10
Le 241-3409	1¹⁄₄″ flange	$38.95
Le 241-3417	1¹⁄₂″ flange	$38.95
Le 241-3466	1³⁄₄″ flange	$38.95
Le 217-1890	2¹⁄₄″ flange	$38.95
Le 217-0553	2³⁄₄″ flange	$38.95
SMALL POUCH—OPAQUE		BOX OF 10
Le 271-0101	1¹⁄₄″ flange	$38.95
Le 217-5941	1¹⁄₂″ flange	$38.95
Le 272-1976	1³⁄₄″ flange	$38.95
Le 272-2452	2¹⁄₄″ flange	$38.95

Sur-Fit Night Drainage Container Set. Includes container, universal adapter, cover.

	BOX OF 1
Le 116-9929	$32.95

Sur-Fit Night Drainage Container Tubing.

	BOX OF 1
Le 143-7607	$8.95

TO ORDER CALL TOLL FREE

LeBoeuf's

PHONE 1-800-546-5559
FAX 1-800-233-9692

Hearing Impaired with TDD
CALL **1-800-855-2880**

Ostomy Management from Hollister®

Hollister Ostomy Pouch Sizing

Type of Pouch	Sizing Instructions	Example
First Choice™ Pre-Sized	Pouch size and stoma size are equal	A 2″ pouch size accommodates a 2″ stoma
Pouches Without Skin Barriers	Pouch size and stoma size are equal	A 2″ pouch size accommodates a 2″ stoma
Pouches With Skin Barriers	Pouch size should be a ¼″ larger than stoma size	A 1¾″ pouch size accommodates a 1½″ stoma
Guardian™ Two-Piece System	Pouch size and skin barrier size should equal stoma size	A 1½″ pouch size and 1½″ skin barrier accommodate up to a 1½″ stoma
Hollister® Two-Piece System	Pouch size and skin barrier size should be ¾″ larger than stoma size	A 2¼″ pouch size and 2¼″ skin barrier accommodate up to a 1½″ stoma

Premium Drainable Pouches

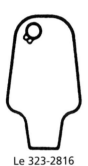

Le 323-2816

Premium Drainable Pouches with Replaceable Filter. Karaya™ 5 Seal Ring, Microporous II Adhesive, and Transparent Quiet Film.

INCLUDES 20 FILTERS AND 2 PLUGS		BOX OF 10
Le 323-2816	1″ opening	$43.95
Le 320-1597	1¼″ opening	$43.95
Le 320-1746	1½″ opening	$43.95
Le 320-1951	1¾″ opening	$43.95
Le 320-2256	2″ opening	$43.95
Le 323-3277	2½″ opening	$43.95

SAME AS ABOVE, BUT WITHOUT REPLACEABLE FILTER		BOX OF 10
Le 340-5776	1″ opening	$32.95
Le 320-2611	1¼″ opening	$32.95
Le 320-2934	1½″ opening	$32.95
Le 320-3262	1¾″ opening	$32.95
Le 320-3593	21/2″ opening	$32.95
Le 323-5834	3″ opening	$32.95

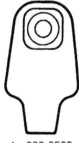

Le 323-3509

Premium Drainable Pouches with Synthetic Seal Ring. Microporous II Adhesive, and Transparent Quiet Film.

		BOX OF 10
Le 323-3509	1″ opening	$34.95
Le 321-9482	1¼″ opening	$34.95
Le 321-7239	1½″ opening	$34.95
Le 321-7312	1¾″ opening	$34.95
Le 321-7411	2″ opening	$34.95
Le 323-3780	2½″ opening	$34.95

First Choice™ Drainable Pouches

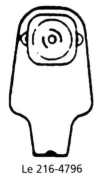

Le 216-4796

First Choice Drainable Pouches with Convex Synthetic Skin Barrier. CushionFit Backing, Microporous II Adhesive, Transparent Odor Barrier Quiet Film and Belt Tabs.

		Box of 5
Le 216-4796	¾″ opening	$30.95
Le 216-5157	⅞″ opening	$30.95
Le 216-5280	1″ opening	$30.95
Le 216-5454	1⅛″ opening	$30.95
Le 216-5553	1¼″ opening	$30.95
Le 216-5645	1⅜″ opening	$30.95
Le 216-5777	1½″ opening	$30.95
Le 216-5918	1⅝″ opening	$30.95
Le 216-6049	1¾″ opening	$30.95
Le 216-9811	2″ opening	$30.95

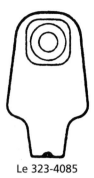

Le 323-4085

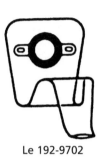

Le 192-9702

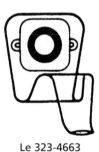

Le 323-4663

TO ORDER CALL TOLL FREE

LeBoeuf's

PHONE 1-800-546-5559
FAX 1-800-233-9692

Hearing Impaired with TDD
CALL **1-800-855-2880**

First Choice™ Drainable Pouches

First Choice Drainable Pouches with Synthetic Skin Barrier.
CushionFit™ Backing, Microporous II Adhesive and Quiet Film.

TRANSPARENT		BOX OF 10
Le 323-4085	¾″ opening	$36.95
Le 321-7569	1″ opening	$36.95
Le 321-7627	1¼″ opening	$36.95
Le 321-7692	1½″ opening	$36.95
Le 321-7767	1¾″ opening	$36.95
Le 323-4176	2″ opening	$36.95
OPAQUE		**BOX OF 10**
Le 184-0842	¾″ opening	$36.95
Le 182-3327	1″ opening	$36.95
Le 182-4721	1¼″ opening	$36.95
Le 1S2-5827	1½″ opening	$36.95
Le 182-6924	1¾″ opening	$36.95
Le 182-7401	2″ opening	$36.95
Le 182-7773	2½″ opening	$36.95

Karaya Seal Drainable Pouches with Karaya 5 Seal and Microporous Adhesive.

12″ TRANSPARENT		BOX OF 30
Le 192-9702	1″ opening	$75.95
Le 320-4229	1¼″ opening	$75.95
Le 320-4740	1½″ opening	$75.95
Le 320-4849	1¾″ opening	$75.95
Le 320-4955	2″ opening	$75.95
Le 320-5234	2½″ opening	$75.95
Le 320-5891	3″ opening	$75.95
9″ TRANSPARENT		**BOX OF 30**
Le 193-0080	1″ opening	$72.95
Le 320-5762	1¼″ opening	$72.95
Le 320-5929	1½″ opening	$72.95
Le 320-6083	1¾″ opening	$72.95
Le 320-6182	2″ opening	$72.95
16″ TRANSPARENT		**BOX OF 30**
Le 117-6569	1″ opening	$76.95
Le 320-6307	1¼″ opening	$76.95
Le 320-6448	1½″ opening	$76.95
Le 320-6661	1¾″ opening	$76.95
Le 320-0177	2″ opening	$76.95
Le 320-0326	2½″ opening	$76.95
Le 193-0585	3″ opening	$76.95

Karaya Seal Drainable Pouch with Karaya 5 Seal Ring and Adhesive.

12″ TRANSPARENT		BOX OF 30
Le 323-4663	1″ opening	$83.95
Le 321-7825	1¼″ opening	$83.95
Le 321-7882	1½″ opening	$83.95
Le 321-7957	1¾″ opening	$83.95
Le 321-8013	2″ opening	$83.95
Le 321-8070	2½″ opening	$83.95
Le 323-4754	3″ opening	$83.95
16″ TRANSPARENT		**BOX OF 30**
Le 323-4846	1″ opening	$85.95
Le 321-8161	1¼″ opening	$85.95
Le 321-8229	1½″ opening	$85.95
Le 321-8302	1¾″ opening	$85.95
Le 321-8393	2″ opening	$85.95
Le 321-8468	2½″ opening	$85.95
Le 323-4960	3″ opening	$85.95

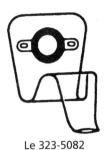

Le 323-5082

Karaya Seal Drainable Pouch with Karaya 5 Seal Ring.

12″ TRANSPARENT		BOX OF 30
Le 323-5082	1″ opening	$70.95
Le 321-8526	1¼″ opening	$70.95
Le 321-8591	1½″ opening	$70.95
Le 321-8666	1¾″ opening	$70.95
Le 321-8757	2″ opening	$70.95
Le 321-8823	2½″ opening	$70.95
Le 321-5231	3″ opening	$70.95

16″ TRANSPARENT		BOX OF 30
Le 323-5348	1″ opening	$72.95
Le 321-8914	1¼″ opening	$72.95
Le 321-9128	1½″ opening	$72.95
Le 321-9201	1¾″ opening	$72.95
Le 321-9292	2″ opening	$72.95
Le 321-9409	2½″ opening	$72.95
Le 340-5966	3″ opening	$72.95

Closed Pouches

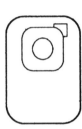

Le 110-3704

Filter Closed Stoma Pouch with Adhesive and Deodorizing Filter.

TRANSPARENT		BOX OF 30
Le 110-3704	1″ opening	$44.95
Le 193-4439	1¼″ opening	$44.95
Le 320-3973	1½″ opening	$44.95
Le 320-4690	1¾″ opening	$44.95
Le 320-4815	2″ opening	$44.95
Le 212-8981	2½″ opening	$44.95
Le 323-5538	3″ opening	$44.95

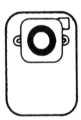

Le 244-8520

Premium Closed Pouch with Karaya 5 Seal Ring, Microporous Adhesive, Deodorizing Filter and Quiet Film.

TRANSPARENT		BOX OF 15
Le 244-8520	1″ opening	$35.95
Le 320-3510	1¼″ opening	$37.95
Le 320-3759	1½″ opening	$37.95
Le 320-3957	1¾″ opening	$37.95
Le 320-4658	2″ opening	$37.95
Le 320-4807	2½″ opening	$37.95
Le 323-4309	3″ opening	$37.95

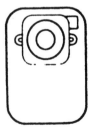

Le 340-6634

Holligard™ Seal Closed Pouch with Karaya 5 Seal Ring, Microporous II Adhesive, Deodorizing Filter, and Quiet Film.

TRANSPARENT		BOX OF 30
Le 340-6634	1″ opening	$70.95
Le 340-6691	1¼″ opening	$70.95
Le 320-6265	1½″ opening	$70.95
Le 320-6380	1¾″ opening	$70.95
Le 320-6620	2″ opening	$70.95
Le 340-6758	2½″ opening	$70.95
Le 340-6816	3″ opening	$70.95

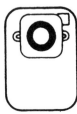

Le 323-5132

Karaya Seal Closed Pouch with Karaya 5 Seal Ring, Microporous Adhesive, and Deodorizing Filter.

TRANSPARENT		BOX OF 30
Le 323-5132	1″ opening	$64.95
Le 320-6703	1¼″ opening	$64.95
Le 320-0243	1½″ opening	$64.95
Le 320-0482	1¾″ opening	$64.95
Le 320-0540	2″ opening	$64.95
Le 320-0813	2½″ opening	$64.95
Le 110-3514	3″ opening	$64.95

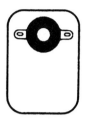

Le 340-6873

Le 320-5124

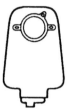

Le 323-5124

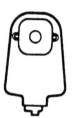

Le 321-8534

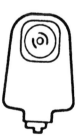

Le 323-5595

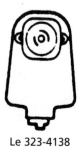

Le 323-4138

Closed Pouches

Karaya Seal Closed Pouch with Karaya 5 Seal Ring.

TRANSPARENT		BOX OF 30
Le 340-6873	1″ opening	$57.95
Le 320-1183	1¼″ opening	$57.95
Le 320-1530	1½″ opening	$57.95
Le 320-1712	1¾″ opening	$57.95
Le 320-1936	2″ opening	$57.95
Le 320-2181	2½″ opening	$57.95
Le 340-6980	3″ opening	$57.95

The Hollister Two-Piece Ostomy System

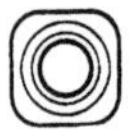

Skin Barrier with Floating Flange and Microporous Adhesive.

		BOX OF 5
Le 320-3916	1½″ opening	$22.95
Le 320-4591	1¾″ opening	$22.95
Le 320-4773	2¼″ opening	$22.95
Le 321-7809	2¾″ opening	$22.95
Le 340-6154	4″ opening	$22.95

Premium Urostomy Pouch with Flange.

		BOX OF 10
Le 323-5124	11/2″ flange	$36.95
Le 320-6372	1¾″ flange	$36.95
Le 320-6596	21/4″ flange	$36.95
Le 340-6279	23/4″ flange	$36.95

Urostomy Drainable Pouches

Lo-Profile™ with Microporous II Adhesive, Belt Tabs, and Drain Tube.

TRANSPARENT		BOX OF 10
Le 321-8534	¾″ opening	$40.95
Le 320-6695	1″ opening	$40.95
Le 320-0235	1¼″ opening	$40.95
Le 320-0474	1½″ opening	$40.95
Le 320-0789	1¾″ opening	$40.95
Le 320-7932	2″ opening	$40.95

First Choice™ Urostomy Pouch with Convex Synthetic Skin Barrier and CushionFit Backing, Microporous II Adhesive, and 2 Drain Tube Adapters.

TRANSPARENT		BOX OF 5
Le 323-5595	½″ opening	$38.95
Le 321-9227	⅝″ opening	$38.95
Le 321-9318	¾″ opening	$38.95
Le 321-9417	⅞″ opening	$38.95
Le 321-9532	1″ opening	$38.95
Le 323-5694	1⅛″ opening	$38.95

First Choice Urostomy Pouch with Convex Synthetic Skin Barrier and CushionFit Backing, Microporous II Adhesive, Belt Tabs, and 2 Drain Tube Adapters.

TRANSPARENT		BOX OF 5
Le 247-4138	½″ opening	$37.95
Le 247-4229	⅝″ opening	$37.95
Le 247-4286	¾″ opening	$37.95
Le 247-4351	⅞″ opening	$37.95
Le 247-4476	1″ opening	$37.95
Le 247-4542	1⅛″ opening	$37.95
Le 247-4609	1¼″ opening	$37.95
Le 247-4666	1⅜″ opening	$37.95
Le 247-4823	1½″ opening	$37.95
Le 247-4922	1¾″ opening	$37.95

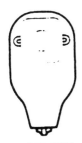

Le 323-5777

Urostomy Pouch with Standard Adhesive, Belt Tabs, and 1 Standard Drain Tube.

9″ TRANSPARENT		BOX OF 20
Le 323-5777	3/4″ opening	$58.95
Le 191-3367	1″ opening	$58.95
Le 191-3441	1¼″ opening	$58.95
Le 191-3532	1½″ opening	$58.95
Le 191-3623	1¾″opening	$58.95
Le 323-5876	2″ opening	$58.95

16″ TRANSPARENT		BOX OF 20
Le 340-6337	1″ opening	$59.95
Le 340-6394	1¼″ opening	$59.95
Le 340-6451	1½″ opening	$59.95
Le 340-6519	1¾″ opening	$59.95
Le 340-6576	2″ opening	$59.95

12″ TRANSPARENT		BOX OF 20
Le 323-6205	3/4″ opening	$59.95
Le 323-6338	1″ opening	$59.95
Le 193-7069	1¼″ opening	$59.95
Le 323-6452	1½″ opening	$59.95
Le 323-2667	1¾″ opening	$59.95

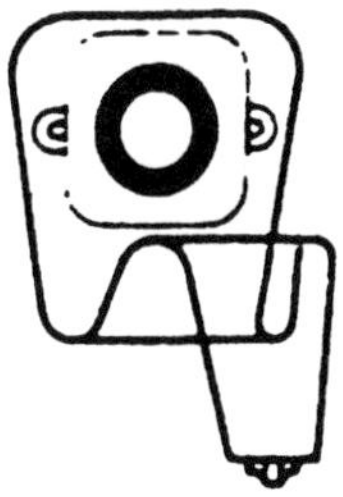

Urostomy Pouch with Karaya 5 Seal Ring, Standard Adhesive, Belt Tabs, and 1 Standard Drain Tube.

16″ TRANSPARENT		BOX OF 20
Le 323-3400	1″ opening	$86.95
Le 191-3680	1¼″ opening	$86.95
Le 191-3797	1½″ opening	$86.95
Le 191-3920	1¾″ opening	$86.95

12″ TRANSPARENT		BOX OF 20
Le 323-3863	3/4″ opening	$84.95
Le 191-3995	1″ opening	$84.95
Le 191-4050	1¼″ opening	$84.95
Le 191-4126	1½″ opening	$84.95
Le 191-4191	1¾″opening	$84.95
Le 323-4119	2″ opening	$84.95

Le 323-3400

Stoma Caps

Stoma Cap with Microporous Adhesive and Deodorizing Filter.

TRANSPARENT		BOX OF 30
Le 320-4914	2″ opening	$51.95
Le 320-5143	3″ opening	$51.95

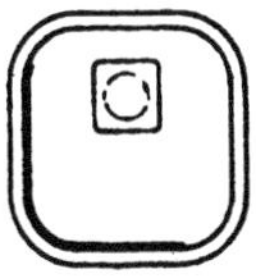

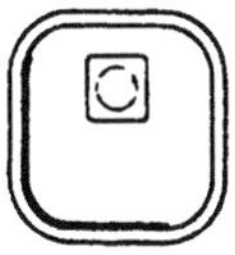

Le 320-4914

Stoma Cap with Standard Adhesive and Deodorizing Filter.

TRANSPARENT		BOX OF 30
Le 320-5457	2″ opening	$51.95
Le 320-5861	3″ opening	$51.95

Ostomy Accessories

Ostomy Belt.

Le 321-8542	Small 17″ to 26″	$7.95
Le 321-8625	Medium 26″ to 43″	$7.95
Le 321-8690	Large 29″ to 49″	$7.95

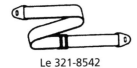

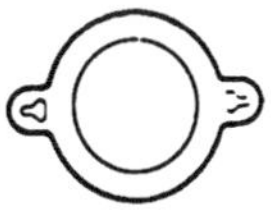

Le 321-8542

Belt Adapter.

		BOX OF 30
Le 321-8773	1″	$1.45
Le 321-8856	1½″	$1.45
Le 321-8948	2″	$1.45
Le 321-9144	2½″	$1.45
Le 321 -9235	23/4″	$1.45

Le 321-8773

Skin Gel.

		BOX OF 20
Le 321-7916	1 oz each	$3.95

Ostomy Accessories

Skin Gel Wipes. 50 sheets each
Le 321-7973 $9.95

Karaya Paste. 4.5 oz each
Le 321-7494 $10.95

Karaya Powder. 2.5 oz puff bottle
Le 321-7643 $10.95

Universal Removal Wipes.
Le 321-8120 $11.95

Medical Adhesive Remover. 6 oz spray can
Le 321-8328 $15.95

Deodorizer / Germicide. 12 oz spray can
Le 340-5487 $9.95

Pouch Clamp. For drainable pouches   **BOX OF 20**
Le 191-3888 $2.95

Ostomy Management from Smith & Nephew United®

Colostomy Pouches

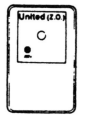

Le 329-1358

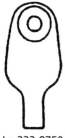

Le 323-8750

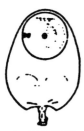

Le 141-6817

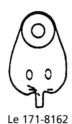

Le 171-8162

Z.O. Colostomy Pouches.

CLOSED-END POUCH—8" CLEAR		PACKAGE OF 10
Le 329-1358	3/4" opening	$11.95
Le 329-1895	1" opening	$11.95
Le 141-7526	1 1/4" opening	$11.95
CLOSED-END POUCH		**PACKAGE OF 10**
Le 328-4312	10" clear, 1 1/4" opening	$21.95
Le 329-1598	5" beige, 3/4" opening	$20.95

Feather-Lite® **Odorproof Ileostomy Drainable Pouch with Center Spout.** Can be used with any standard size face plate.

SMALL POUCH		BOX OF 5
Le 328-8750	5 3/8" × 11 1/4", 14 oz	$40.95
MEDIUM POUCH		**BOX OF 5**
Le 328-8925	5 3/8" × 12 1/4", 19 oz	$40.95
LARGE POUCH		**BOX OF 5**
Le 328-9212	6 1/4" × 12", 24 oz	$40.95

Bongort Trim 'n' Fit Urinary Diversion Pouches. Anti-reflux valve, Stent guides, Starter Hole.   **PACKAGE OF 5**

MEDIUM POUCH		
Le 141-6817	6" × 8", 19 fl oz	$39.95
LARGE POUCH		
Le 171-7693	6" × 8", 32 fl oz	$39.95

Feather-Lite Urinary Diversion Pouches.   **PACKAGE OF 6**

Le 171-8162	5 3/8" × 10 3/4", 12 fl oz	$56.95

Feather-Lite Dri-Flo Urinary Diversion Pouches.   **BOX OF 5**

Le 171-6968	Clear, 6 3/4" × 10 1/8", 13 fl oz	$58.95

Ostomy Management from Bard®

Closed End One-Piece Adhesive Pouches.

Extra Closed-End Pouches. Extra gauge and soft pliable form, Rustle free and odorproof, Rounded corners for comfort, No belt necessary.

5″ × 8″ POUCH #1		**BOX OF 10**
Le 137-2010	15/16″ opening	$18.95
5¹/₂″ × 8″ POUCH #2	**BOX OF 10**	
Le 120-1656	1³/₁₆″ opening	$20.95
6¹/₂″ × 10″ POUCH #3	**BOX OF 10**	
Le 120-1730	1³/₁₆″ opening	$21.95

Regular Closed-End Pouches. Reliable adhesive, Lightweight film.

5″ × 8″ POUCH #1		**BOX OF 10**
Le 120-1813	15/16″ opening	$18.95
5¹/₂″ × 8″ POUCH #2	**BOX OF 10**	
Le 120-1896	1³/₁₆″ opening	$15.95
6¹/₂″ × 10″ POUCH #3	**BOX OF 10**	
Le 243-0809	1³/₁₆″ opening	$17.95

Ostomy Management from Coloplast®

One-Piece Ostomy Products

Drainable Pouches. Custom cut, with Secure Life.

13″—POST-OP, TRANSPARENT		**BOX OF 10**
Le 121-9955	3¹/₈″ × 3¹/₈″ cutting size	$39.95
11″—OPAQUE		**BOX OF 10**
Le 121-9385	¹/₂″ × 2¹/₂″ opening	$36.95

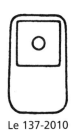

Le 137-2010

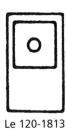

Le 120-1813

TO ORDER CALL TOLL FREE

LeBoeuf's

PHONE **1-800-546-5559**
FAX **1-800-233-9692**

Hearing Impaired with TDD
CALL **1-800-855-2880**

Urologicals

THE DIAMETER OF A CATHETER is measured in a unit called French (FR). When prescribing a 14 FR catheter, the physician is requesting a specific tube diameter size. The smaller the number, the smaller the diameter. Catheters used for intermittent catheterization range from 5 to 20 FR, with 12 and 14 FR being the most common for adults.

For many patients with urinary incontinence, it is possible to manage the problem by using catheterization and/or for males, an external catheter (drainage condom). There are two common types of catheterization: intermittent and indwelling.

The doctor or nurse will teach the patient how to perform their own intermittent catheterization. Normally patients will drain their bladders every 3 to 6 hours. Care must be exercised to prevent infections to the urinary tract (UTI). There are products on the market that make self-catheterization easy and less susceptible to risk of infection.

For the patient who requires an indwelling catheter, the Foley catheter seems to be the one recommended by a majority of doctors. There a few simple guidelines to avoid possible problems with the patient's Foley catheter.

Maintain closed drainage system

- Never remove the catheter unless instructed to do so by the nurse or doctor.
- Both patient and caregiver must wash hands with soap and water before handling the catheter. Wash the area around the catheter with soap and water daily.
- After the patient has had a bowel movement, wash the area immediately to reduce the risk of infection.
- Do not disconnect the catheter from the tubing. If for some reason disconnection does happen, clean both ends with alcohol and reconnect immediately. Call the nurse and/or doctor.
- Anchor tubing securely.
- Anchor catheter securely to the thigh with a Velcro leg strap.
- Make sure that the strap is not too tight.
- Do not clamp the catheter or the tubing.
- Leave some slack on the catheter between the leg strap and the point where the catheter enters the patient to prevent the catheter from tugging uncomfortably or pulling out.

Maintain steady urine flow

- Unless the doctor has prescribed otherwise, the patient should drink eight to ten 8-ounce glasses of water a day.
- Keep drainage bag below the level of the lower abdomen at all times.
- Make sure there are no kinks or loops in the tubing.
- Empty drainage bag every four to eight hours — or if it becomes filled before then.
- When emptying the bag, do not let the drain tube touch the container into which the urine is draining.
- Do not touch the drain tube.

Call the nurse and/or doctor if there is:

- Strong odor or cloudy urine.
- Blood in urine.
- Chills, fever above 99.4 degrees.
- Lower back pain.
- Abnormal leakage around catheter (occasional leakage is not unusual).
- Swelling of catheter insertion site, especially in men.
- Disorientation or change in mental status.

Sometimes, the doctor will order a bladder irrigation to wash out the bladder. Usually an irrigation is carried out to remove pus or blood clots that may be blocking the catheter.

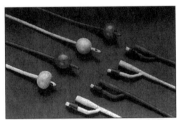

Le 323-3962, . . ., Le 323-3384

Urological Equipment

Bard Bardia Urethral Catheter Trays. Trays are sterile and contain waterproof underpad, drape, gloves, 5 gram lubricant, 3 BZK swab sticks, graduated container tray and specimen container and label. A 15 French catheter is included.

Le 160-7878	$6.95

Bard Bardia Foley Catheter Insertion Trays. Trays are sterile and contain waterproof underpad, gloves, 5 gram lubricant, pre-filled inflation syringe with sterile water, 3 antibacterial swab sticks and graduated peel top tray.

Le 164-7833	10 cc syringe	$7.95
Le 166-2121	30 cc syringe	$8.95

Bard Davol, Intermittent Female Catheter. Sterile with graduated specimen tube with cap, 8 French, 5½ inches long. Includes gloves and prep swabs.

Le 146-6622	$7.95

Bardia Foley Catheters Silicone Elastomer Coated Latex. 100% tested for performance. Sterile. 12 per box.

Le 323-3962	12 French	5cc	$6.95
Le 323-4028	14 French	5cc	$6.95
Le 323-2212	16 French	5cc	$6.95
Le 323-2378	18 French	5cc	$6.95
Le 323-2436	20 French	5cc	$6.95
Le 323-2493	22 French	5cc	$6.95
Le 323-2550	24 French	5cc	$6.95
Le 323-2626	26 French	5cc	$6.95
Le 323-2683	28 French	5cc	$6.95
Le 323-2741	30 French	5cc	$6.95
Le 323-2808	12 French	30cc	$8.95
Le 323-2865	14 French	30cc	$8.95
Le 323-2949	16 French	30cc	$8.95
Le 323-3004	18 French	30cc	$8.95
Le 323-3061	20 French	30cc	$8.95
Le 323-3137	22 French	30cc	$8.95
Le 323-3194	24 French	30cc	$8.95
Le 323-3251	26 French	30cc	$8.95
Le 323-3319	28 French	30cc	$8.95
Le 323-3384	30 French	30cc	$8.95

Bardia Foley Catheter all Silicone, Ribbed Balloon. 100% tested for performance. Sterile. 12 per box.

Le 276-6806	14 French	5cc	$13.95
Le 276-6863	16 French	5cc	$13.95
Le 276-6996	18 French	5cc	$13.95
Le 276-7275	20 French	5cc	$13.95
Le 276-7382	22 French	5cc	$13.95
Le 276-7473	24 French	5cc	$13.95
Le 168-3408	16 French	30cc	$14.95
Le 276-7556	18 French	30cc	$14.95
Le 276-7655	20 French	30cc	$14.95
Le 276-7820	22 French	30cc	$14.95
Le 276-7929	24 French	30cc	$14.95

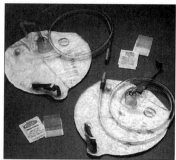

Le 274-0181, Le 127-7706

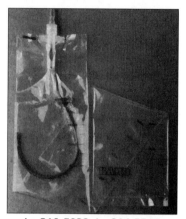

Le 210-5039, Le 214-5514

Bard Bardia, Urinary Drainage Bags. Sterile fluid path. 2000cc drainage bag. Sample port. Anti-reflux/drip chamber.

Le 274-0181	Living hinge hanger	Each	$8.95
Le 127-7706	Adjustable hook and loop hanger	Each	$7.95

Bard Wide Leg Bag Strap. Designed for use with all Bard leg bags. 1¾″ wide straps to keep bag from slipping. Fabric straps help minimize skin irritation. Washable.

Le 378-9856	Small — 9 to 13 inches long	$10.95
Le 378-9922	Medium — 13 to 20 inches long	$10.95
Le 378-9989	Large — 20 to 27 inches long	$10.95

Bard Touchless, Plus Unisex Intermittent Catheter System. Designed for patients with limited dexterity. 1100cc chamber, gloves, swabs and underpad. Reduces trauma, discomfort and risk of infection. Sterile.

Le 210-5039	14 French red rubber catheter	$8.95
Le 214-5514	14 French vinyl catheter	$8.95

External Catheters

The time the patient can wear a condom catheter will vary, but you can expect him to wear one for at least 24 hours. Sometimes, the patient can wear one for up to 72 hours. Ask the doctor and/or the nurse for guidance. Many leg bags that hold the urine come with latex straps. As the bag fills, these straps may pull the hair on the legs and can restrict blood circulation. Soft mesh elastic straps may be safer and more comfortable for the patient.

For the patient to obtain the best results from an external catheter:

- Make sure the condom catheter is the correct size and fit.

  Small is the width of the thumb

  Medium is the width of two fingers

  Large is the width of three fingers

- Clip the hair on the patient's penis and any hair that may get caught as the condom catheter is rolled to the base of the penis.

- Make sure the skin is clean and dry before the catheter is put on.

- Apply a polymer skin sealant. Allow the sealant to dry until it is slick and smooth.

- Make sure the tip of the penis is positioned in the cone of the catheter but the head does not rub against the inside of the condom.

- Make sure the catheter is changed when it is loose.

- Make sure the patient inspects the skin each time the catheter is changed.

- Make sure the patient empties the leg bag regularly.

- Watch for kinks in the tubing.

- Make sure the patient keeps the tubing and bag clean and odor free.

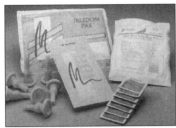

Le 126-4878, Le 126-4852,
Le 126-4845

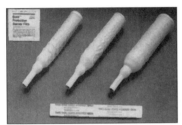

Le 323-3764, Le 125-0737,
Le 136-2953

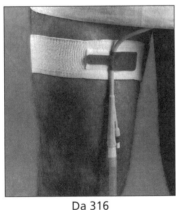

Da 316

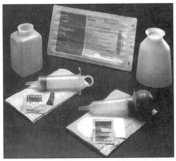

Le 167-0306, Le 168-1725

Mentor Freedom Pak™ Seven. 7 day kit. Contains 7 male external catheters, 7 Shield Skin wipes, leg bag kit with 19 oz. disposable bag and 18-inch latex-free extension tubing and universal connector. Comes with instruction book.

Le 126-4878	Small	Each kit	$19.95
Le 126-4852	Medium	Each kit	$19.95
Le 126-4845	Large	Each kit	$19.95

Bard Disposable Male External Catheters. 100% latex sheath. Pre-rolled for easy application. Bulb tip for kink prevention. Double-sided adhesive strip. Barrier film included. Individually packed.

Le 323-3764	Small/Geriatric	$1.95
Le 125-0737	Medium	$1.95
Le 136-2953	Standard	$1.95

Bard Extension/Connective Sterile Tubing with Adapter. Connects Dispoz-A-Bag to Bard male external or Bard Foley catheter.

Le 127-7912	$4.95

Bard Dispoz-A-Bag, Leg Bags. Disposable and odorproof. Anti-reflux valve reduces back flow risk. 100% inspected for quality. Has rubber cap. Made of heavy duty PVC film.

Le 164-8211	9 oz. capacity	$6.95
Le 273-0414	19 oz capacity	$6.95
Le 164-8237	32 oz. capacity	$6.95

Bard Dispoz-A-Bag with Flip-Flo™ Drain. Opens and closes with a simple flip. No rubber caps to misplace or drop. Wide diameter for fast drainage. Box of 4.

Le 165-9358	19 oz. capacity	$27.95
Le 134-8341	32 oz. capacity	$27.95

Bard Leg Bag Holder. Designed for use with Bard Dispoz-A-Bag leg bags. Discreet — conceals and protects leg bag. Leg bag straps not required. Polyester and spandex for a soft and comfortable fit. Minimizes possibility of skin irritation. Washable. 16 inches long.

Le 379-1043	Small 8 to 14 inches wide	Each	$13.95
Le 379-1118	Medium 14 to 20 inches wide	Each	$14.95
Le 379-1183	Large 16 to 26 inches wide	Each	$15.95

Dale Medical Foley Catheter Holder. Velcro, locking device anchors the Foley catheter in place. Made of stretch material that has a hypo-allergenic backing for added skin comfort. Washable. If the patient has diabetes or a circulatory problem, check with the doctor before using.

Da 316	One size fits all	$6.95

Bard Bardia Irrigation Trays. Trays are sterile and contain an underpad, 500cc solution container, irrigation syringe, 1200cc graduated tray and a drainage tube tip protector.

Le 167-0306	With bulb syringe	$4.95
Le 168-1725	With piston syringe	$4.95

Baxter General Specimen Container. 4 oz. sterile with screw cap.

Le 162-7934	Box of 20	$38.95

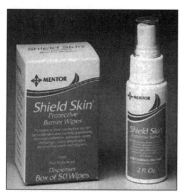

Le 322-3716, Le 149-5746

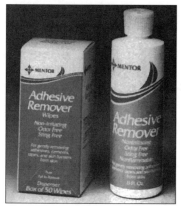

Le 345-7918, Le 345-7843

Mentor Shield Skin Wipes and Spray. Helps protect skin from irritation caused by adhesives. Moisture resistant, non-staining, easy to apply.

Le 322-3716	Box of 50 wipes	$7.95
Le 149-5746	2-ounce spray bottle	$5.95

Mentor Adhesive Remover. Gently emulsifies and removes adhesives. Non-toxic and non-irritating to skin. Will not sting broken skin areas.

Le 345-7843	8-ounce bottle	$7.95
Le 345-7918	Box of 50 wipes	$10.95

Mentor Ultra-Fresh™ Room Deodorizer. Hospital strength odor eliminator. Leaves powder-fresh scent. Non-aerosol pump spray. Nonflammable and nontoxic.

Le 194-4032	2-ounce bottle	$5.95
Le 194-4131	8-ounce bottle	$11.95

We also carry a full line of Baxter, Mentor and Hollister urological products. Call ☎ 1-800-546-5559 for product listing and pricing.

TO ORDER CALL TOLL FREE

LeBoeuf's

PHONE **1-800-546-5559**
FAX **1-800-233-9692**

Hearing Impaired with TDD
CALL **1-800-855-2880**

Dental Health

Taking care of the teeth and mouth is very important for good health, good hygiene and patient comfort. About 40 percent of the older population wear dentures. Over 90 percent of people who wear dentures do not think it is necessary to visit a dentist and only about a third of people 65 years old or older visit a dentist at least once a year. Oral and dental problems are a leading cause of discomfort in older Americans.

Nutrition is extremely important to the well being of the patient. Problems with teeth and gums can cause malnutrition because the patient is not eating the right foods or cannot eat properly.

Tooth Decay

Tooth decay is not just a children's problem. Tooth decay is caused by bacteria that normally live in the mouth. The bacteria cling to the teeth and form a colorless film called dental plaque. These bacteria live on sugars and produce acids that dissolve the teeth, thereby causing cavities. Each time sugar is eaten, it triggers an acid attack on the teeth that lasts for 20 minutes.

Tooth decay can be prevented by regular brushing with a fluoride-containing toothpaste, rinsing with fluoride mouthwashes, flossing, application or use of fluoride gels as prescribed by the dentist and regular visits to the dentist. Fluoride is the most effective agent available to prevent tooth decay.

You can check for plaque on the teeth by chewing red "disclosing tablets" found in drug stores. The red color left on the teeth will show you where you still have plaque and where you have to brush and/or floss again.

Gum Disease (Periodontal Disease)

Gum disease is the most common cause of tooth loss after age 35. Infections of the gum and bone that hold the teeth in place are also caused by dental plaque. The bacteria cause the gums to become inflamed and to bleed easily. If not treated, the disease causes receding gums and loss of supporting bone. If you lose enough bone support, your teeth will fall out.

Gum disease caused by plaque can usually be reversed by daily brushing, flossing and frequent (twice a year) visits to the dentist for cleaning. More serious gum and bone problems need to be treated by a gum disease specialist or a dentist who has received special training in treating gum disease. Brushing and flossing alone will not control the disease.

Dry Mouth (Xerostomia)

Dry mouth is common in many adults and it makes it hard to eat, swallow, taste and speak. Dry mouth happens when salivary glands fail to work and is commonly caused by medical treatments such as chemotherapy, nerve damage to the head and neck area or as a side effect of medications. There are over 400 commonly used medications that contribute to dry mouth. Until recently, dry mouth was thought to be a normal part of aging. This is not true — healthy older adults produce as much saliva as younger adults.

Approximately 32 million Americans wear full or partial dentures.

Patients who have had a heart attack within the past three months should inform the dentist prior to any work being done on the teeth, especially if a tooth is to be pulled.

A tooth is made up of four main tissues:
Enamel — hardest part of the tooth
Dentin — inner body of both the crown and root of the tooth
Pulp — soft and sensitive tissue which fills the inner tooth
Cementum — thin layer of hard tissue which covers the root and meets the enamel at the neck of the the tooth

Enamel is the hardest tissue in the body.

Gingivitis is the earliest form of periodontal disease. It begins as an inflammation of the gums

Hint:
Those patients with dry mouth can obtain relief by sucking on ice chips during the day.

There are a number of artificial saliva products available for the patient. Check with the patient's dentist. If the product recommended is not a prescription item, we can obtain it for you.

The adult body contains about 3 pounds of calcium. If the body does not get enough calcium from food, it takes the mineral from the bones.

While not correcting the underlying cause of dry mouth, the following should be done to preserve your teeth and make you more comfortable. Brush your teeth twice a day. Use dental floss daily. Use a toothpaste that contains fluoride. Avoid sticky, sugary foods. See the dentist at least twice a year. Drink frequently — especially when eating — but avoid caffeine and sugary drinks. Chew sugarless gum and eat sugarless mints or hard sugarless candies. Use a humidifier — especially at night.

Cancer therapies — especially radiation to the head and neck and/or chemotherapy — can cause tooth decay, dry mouth, sores and cracked and bleeding lips. You should contact your dentist prior to any cancer therapy to the head and/or neck. The dentist will show you how to care for your teeth before, during and after the cancer treatment to prevent problems. Even if you wear dentures, you need to contact your dentist so that a treatment plan can be put in place.

Fever Blisters

Fever blisters are sometimes called cold sores and occur in epidemic proportions. There are about 100 million cases of fever blisters yearly in the United States. Up to 80 percent of all adults and children have experienced fever blisters, which are caused by a highly contagious virus called Herpes simplex (kissing is one way of spreading the virus). The onset of fever blisters starts with a tingling or burning in the lip area. The fluid-filled fever blisters can form on the inside and outside of the mouth, lips and throat and can be accompanied by fever, swollen neck glands or sore throat. There is no cure for fever blisters, but recurrent episodes are usually less severe. Fever blisters generally heal within two weeks and do not leave scars.

Treatment of fever blisters consists mainly of relieving the pain and discomfort. There are a number of numbing ointments that can be applied to the blisters, antibiotics that control secondary infections and ointments that soften the crusts of the sores.

Canker Sores

Canker sores affect about 20 percent of the population. Beginning as small oval or round reddish swellings on the tongue, lips or cheek, canker sores can range in size from an eight of an inch to an inch and a quarter. Fever is rare and usually only one or two canker sores will occur at one time. These sores will normally heal within two weeks.

There does not appear to be a virus or a bacteria that causes canker sores. Some suggest that they are caused by an allergic reaction to certain foods. Canker sores are not contagious.

Treatment of canker sores consists of numbing preparations such as xylocaine that is applied on the sores or mouthwashes containing tetracycline. Anti-inflammatory steroid mouthwashes containing tetracycline may reduce the unpleasant symptoms and speed healing. Before using any tetracycline treatments, patients should contact their doctor or dentist as the tetracycline can permanently stain teeth. There are also anti-inflammatory steroid mouthwashes or gels for patients with several sores. Again, close supervision by a doctor or dentist is a must.

Patient Toothbrushing Tips

You will need a towel, bowl of water (cup), mouthwash, toothbrush, toothpaste, towel and chapstick. If possible, have the patient sit up. If the patient

Symptoms of oral health problems:

- *Loss of appetite*
- *Pain in the mouth*
- *Lack of interest in wearing dentures*
- *Swelling of gums*
- *Bad breath and/or a bad taste in the mouth*
- *Trouble chewing*

Tooth decay, gum disease, cancer therapies, fever blisters, canker sores and dry mouth are the major reasons for oral and mouth problems.

To keep a healthy bright smile, regular dental care is essential.

Note:

If the patient is on oxygen, do not use petroleum based lip balms.

Dentures are made to fit precisely and the use of adhesives can mask infections and cause bone loss in the jaw. If the dentures feel loose or cause discomfort, see the dentist immediately.

is not able to sit up, have him lie on his side or turn his head to the side (you do not want him to choke on the toothpaste and water). If the patient can brush his own teeth, by all means, let him do it.

- Place the head of the toothbrush at a 45 degree angle to the gums and move the brush back and forth with short, gentle strokes.
- Use a soft nylon toothbrush. Replace once a month.
- Use fluoride toothpaste. Do not use hydrogen peroxide or baking soda containing toothpastes in those persons shown to be sensitive to them, especially if debilitated.
- Rinse toothbrush in cold water, shake off excess water and store where air can circulate with the bristle part upright.
- Brush after every meal if at all possible. If you only brush once a day, brush at night.
- Brush the tongue to freshen breath (forward stroke).
- Floss between teeth (use a piece of floss about 18″ long). There are commercial floss holders that make flossing somewhat easier.
- Electric toothbrushes can be used by those who are not able to use a regular toothbrush. The toothbrush should be rechargeable with an on-off switch, a pressure-sensitive head and lightweight.
- Oral irrigation can be used but it is not a substitute for brushing. Oral irrigation is especially useful for those patients who are undergoing treatment for gum problems or to refresh the mouth.
- Use chapstick or vaseline on the lips to help prevent them from drying out or cracking.

Generally, doctors will have patients remove their dentures prior to throat surgery, general anesthesia or shock therapy. However, some anesthesiologists believe that leaving the dentures in place helps the patient to breath easier. They also believe that the face mask used to administer anesthesia will fit better and leaving the dentures in prevents patients with natural teeth from damaging the gums.

For those patients who are missing teeth, a bridge or partial denture can be made. Bridges are usually smaller than a partial denture and permanently fixed to other teeth. Partial dentures are usually removable and are supported in the mouth by the gums and clips that fit over other teeth.

Denture Cleaning

Dentures should be cleaned at least once a day.

- Use warm, not hot, water.
- Clean in sink half filled with water to avoid breaking the denture if dropped.
- Brush all areas (inside and outside) using a denture cleaner or toothpaste.
- Rinse with cool water.

Caring for Dentures

The patient should see the dentist regularly for an oral examination. The dentist will check for signs of oral cancer and examine the gum ridges, tongue and jaw joints. Signs that the dentures need attention:

- *Looseness caused by tissue changes.*
- *Bad odor caused by absorption of fluid and bacteria.*
- *Color change due to age or a reaction to mouth fluids.*
- *Stains and calculus deposits resulting from mouth fluids.*

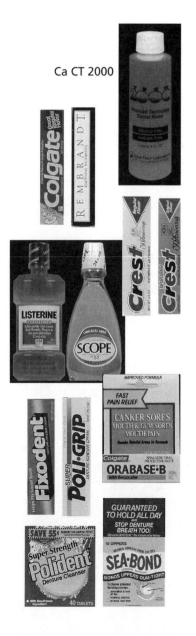

Ca CT 2000

- Soaking in a commercial solution is a supplement to brushing, not a substitute.
- If stains or yellow deposits remain, take the dentures to the dentist for ultrasonic cleaning.
- Massage the gums with a soft brush.
- Store the dentures in clean water.
- Do not wear dentures while asleep at night. The gums need a chance to breathe.

What to do:

Contact the American Society for Geriatric Dentistry. Write them at Suite 1616, 211 East Chicago Avenue, Chicago, IL 60611. The society will provide you with information on ways to maintain and improve the dental health of older people. They also can provide a listing of dentists who have a special interest in treating older people.

Contact the American Dental Association. Call the number in the local phone book. It will be able to provide information on which dentists are able to work on patients in wheelchairs; dentists who provide home visits and information of the various specialties of each dentist.

Oral Care Products

Care-Tech TECH 2000, Oral Rinse. Advanced formula neutralizes odor while providing humectancy for aging gum tissues. Antibacterial oral rinse which counteracts "dry mouth syndrome."

Ca CT 2000	4-ounce bottle		$1.95
Le 143-5460	Anbesol Gel	.25 oz	$5.85
Le 242-5692	Anbesol Liquid	.31 oz	$5.85
Le 121-5375	Colgate	7 oz	$3.55
Le 121-5367	Colgate	4.6 oz	$2.65
Le 141-4754	Crest	4.6 oz	$2.65
Le 141-4762	Crest	6.4 oz	$3.55
Le 126-7392	Crest Tartar	4.6 oz	$2.65
Le 126-7525	Crest Tartar	6.4 oz	$3.45
Le 161-6879	Efferdent Tabs	40 Ct	$3.95
Le 121-3800	Fixodent Adhesive Cream	2.5 oz	$5.65
Le 121-3818	Fixodent Adhesive Cream	1.5 oz	$3.85
Le 160-7589	Fixodent Denture Cream Frsh	1.4 oz	$3.85
Le 173-7923	Listerine	8.5 oz	$3.65
Le 173-7618	Listerine	16.9 oz	$5.15
Le 173-7402	Listerine	33.8 oz	$7.95
Le 142-9307	Orabase-B/Benzocaine	5 gm	$3.95
Le 172-9151	Polident Tabs	40 Ct	$3.95
Le 148-1522	Rembrandt Whitening T/P	3 oz	$9.65
Le 165-2676	Sea Bond Denture Adh Uppers	15 Ct	$3.65
Le 165-2759	Sea Bond Denture Adh Lowers	15 Ct	$3.65
Le 141-5231	Scope	12 oz	$3.95
Le 141-5256	Scope	24 oz	$4.95
Le 168-2954	Stim-U-Dent	100 Ct	$2.15
Le 149-9607	Super Poligrip	2.4 oz	$5.75
Le 161-2068	Benzodent Denture Ointment	0.25 oz	$2.95

Diabetes

D IABETES MELLITUS is a disorder in which the pancreas produces insufficient or no insulin. Insulin is the hormone responsible for the absorption of glucose into cells for their energy needs and into the liver and fat cells for storage. Glucose is the sugar in the blood. When insulin levels are low, the level of glucose in the blood becomes abnormally high, causing excessive urination and constant thirst and hunger. The glucose can build to dangerous levels and can cause serious damage to body organs. Long term complications such as stroke, blindness, heart disease, kidney failure, gangrene and nerve damage can result from uncontrolled blood glucose levels. Diabetes is nothing to fool around with. If you suspect that the patient has any one or more of the symptoms described, arrange a doctor's appointment as soon as possible. There are almost 14 million people with diabetes — more than 95 percent have non-insulin-dependent Type II.

Diabetes tends to run in families but factors other than heredity are responsible as well. For example, becoming overweight can trigger diabetes in susceptible older people. About half of the estimated 14 million people with diabetes mellitus are undiagnosed and not receiving medical treatment.

There are two main types of diabetes. Type I, or insulin-dependent diabetes, is the most severe form of the disease. Although this type of diabetes can appear at any age, it generally starts during childhood or adolescence. The disease most commonly appears in people between the ages of 10 and 16. Type I develops rapidly. Lifelong treatment with insulin is required, along with exercise and a controlled diet. Without regular injections of insulin, the patient will lapse into a coma and die. Insulin will start acting in about 30 minutes after injection. However, there is ongoing research to come up with an insulin that starts acting in five minutes. There is also research on a laser device that will sense the amount of blood sugar in blood vessels of the fingertips.

Diabetes affects the circulation when blood sugar levels are too high and glucose coats the red blood cells, making them more rigid. Tiny blood vessels are damaged when the more rigid red blood cells pass through them. While the body will regenerate the blood vessels, regenerated blood vessels are more fragile than original ones. Blood circulation to areas served by the small blood vessels, such as the feet and eyes, is affected.

Noninsulin-dependent diabetes, or Type II, is the most common form of diabetes among older people. Also known as "adult-onset" diabetes, this form accounts for over 95 percent of all cases. Most people with this type of diabetes do not need insulin injections. They can usually keep their blood glucose levels near normal by controlling their weight, exercising and following a sensible diet.

Diabetes cannot be cured, but it can be controlled by proper diet, exercise and insulin injections or oral medications. The patient who is taking oral medication and/or insulin should self-monitor blood glucose levels before beginning exercise and again 30 minutes after exercising. Diabetic patients should not exercise for at least 90 minutes after a meal. They should also

Food eaten turns into glucose (a kind of sugar) in the stomach and goes into the blood stream. Insulin helps the glucose get into the bodies cells. Insulin and glucose work together so the cells can make energy from food.

Diabetic patients should not go without food for more than five hours.

avoid exercising during periods of poor blood glucose control and carry a snack high in sugar in the event that blood sugar is too low to exercise.

A recent 10-year government study indicated that keeping blood glucose levels as close to normal is the best way to prevent or delay complications from diabetes. Those Type I Diabetes patients who intensely managed their blood glucose levels had fewer rates of complications than those patients who took the conventional approach aimed at avoiding extremely high or low blood glucose levels. With the new testing devices on the market, it is much easier to test for blood glucose levels more often.

It is essential for people with diabetes to inspect their feet every day and note any redness or patches of heat. In addition, any sores, blisters, breaks in the skin, infections or buildup of calluses on the feet should be reported to the doctor immediately. According to the American Diabetes Association, about one in five people with diabetes end up in the hospital with foot problems. If the patient complains of cold feet, tell them to wear socks. Do not use heating pads, hot water or electric blankets to warm their feet. The patient may not feel the heat and there is a possibility that they may burn their skin. People with diabetes are less able to resist infection and should protect their skin against injury, keep it clean, use skin softeners to treat dryness and take care of minor cuts and bruises. The patient should soak the feet before cutting toe nails. If the toenails are too thick, have a doctor or nurse cut them. Patients with diabetes should not go barefoot, even at home. Teeth and gums must also receive special attention — the dentist should be told if the patient has diabetes.

With modern treatment and sensible self-monitoring, most diabetics can look forward to a normal life. It is very important to keep an accurate daily record of the patient's blood glucose levels, what the patient has eaten, amount of insulin or oral hypoglycemic medication taken, amount of exercise and whether or not the patient has had an illness or stress. This information will enable you and the patient to better manage the disease and help the patient feel better.

People who have diabetes must know the warning signs of problems and what to do if problems occur.

High Blood Sugar is caused by:
- Not enough insulin.
- Too much food.
- Infection, fever and illness.
- Emotional stress.

Symptoms (symptoms noticed within hours to several days):
- Fatigue — feeling "run down".
- Increased thirst.
- Frequent urination.
- Large amounts of sugar in the blood.
- Weakness, pains in the stomach and patient aches all over.
- Labored and heavy breathing.
- Loss of appetite, nausea and vomiting.

What to do:
- Call the doctor immediately.
- Take fluids without sugar if the patient is able to swallow.
- Test blood sugar frequently.
- Test urine for ketones.

Low Blood Sugar is caused by:
- Too much insulin.
- Not enough food.
- Unusual amount of exercise.
- Delayed meal.

Symptoms (symptoms noticed within minutes to hours):
- Cold sweats, faintness and dizziness.
- Headache.
- Pounding of heart, trembling and nervousness.
- Blurred vision.
- Hungry.
- Inability to waken.
- Grouchiness.
- Personality change.

What to do
- Call the doctor — take liquids, tablets or food containing sugar (e.g. orange juice, regular soda).
- Check blood sugar level.
- Do not give insulin.
- Do not give anything by mouth if the patient is unconscious.

Other symptoms of diabetes include:
- Pain or numbness in legs or feet.
- Numerous skin infections.
- Slow healing cuts or scratches.
- More than 20 pounds overweight.
- Pale skin color.
- Chest pain.
- Vaginal itching.
- Unexplained weight loss.

Insulin has to be injected because it's protein and would be digested by the stomach.

Insulin and Insulin Therapy

A ten year study of 1,400 patients with Type I diabetes who had intensive therapy by The Diabetes Control and Complications Trial found that keeping blood sugar as close to normal as possible reduced damage to the eyes by 76 percent, to the kidneys by 35 to 56 percent and to the nerves by 60 percent. Overall, the people in the intensive treatment group had fewer and less severe complications than the people in the conventional treatment group. Complications from diabetes cause blindness to 15,000 to 39,000 people each year.

Intensive insulin therapy in older people has not been well studied and should only be used with great care and under the supervision of the patient's doctor. Older people with hardening of the arteries risk permanent injury from low blood sugar. These people are at risk of suffering heart attacks or strokes during episodes of low blood sugar.

Intensive insulin therapy may not be worthwhile in a person over 70. Complications take years to develop. If an older person has no sign of complications, tight control may sometimes not be worth the effort. But if the patient is mentally fit and comes from a family with a history of living to a ripe old age, intensive therapy may be a good idea. Check with the doctor to see if intensive therapy is right for your patient.

Those patients with Type II diabetes are at risk for all of the complications as those with Type I diabetes. Most people with Type II are overweight and not getting enough exercise. By sticking to a diet, losing weight and starting and maintaining a regular exercise program, the patient can often make their blood cells more sensitive to insulin. The patient should check their blood sugar regularly. If the patient is managing their diabetes by exercise and diet alone, they may only need to test once a day, once a week or less. Keep records of test results. These records can help the doctor make adjustments to improve the patient's control of diabetes. Since diabetes can be very dangerous, constant vigilance is required by both the caregiver and the patient to head off as many complications as possible.

Blood sugar levels before eating stay between 70 and 115 in people who don't have diabetes. After eating, blood sugar levels will be between 80 and 140.

One of the most important goals of diabetes care is to keep sugar levels near the normal range. This can be accomplished by balancing the effects of food, exercise and diabetes medicine. According to Novo Nordisk Pharmaceuticals, Inc., acceptable blood sugar levels range (for those patients with diabetes) before eating is between 80 and 140. After eating the range (for those with diabetes) that is acceptable is between 80 and 200.

Eating, stress and illness make glucose levels go up. Insulin and exercise make glucose levels go down.

Blood Sugar Level Tests

People cannot tell what their blood sugar level is by the way they feel. Testing is the only way to be sure. The patient's blood sugar level can be found by testing a small drop of blood. This is usually done by placing a drop of blood on a small specially treated plastic strip. Sugar causes the strip to change color. By comparing changes in the strip's color to a color chart, the level of blood sugar can be estimated. More exact results can be obtained by using a special meter that detects changes in the strip's color. All the blood testing methods are accurate if the patient follows directions exactly. Testing is important for those who are taking insulin and for those who have severe low blood sugar reactions.

Blood sugar should be checked before meals and at bedtime. Records of the tests should be kept so the patient can determine what changes need to be made in meals, exercise and medication to improve blood sugar levels.

What to do:

Contact the doctor — The doctor will test the urine for glucose level and/or will obtain blood samples after an overnight fast to determine glucose levels. They will determine whether or not insulin needs to be taken by injection and will provide advice on diet for the patient. The doctor will also teach the patient how and when to measure blood glucose levels and/or urine ketones, how to keep records and how to treat low blood glucose reactions. The patient should see the doctor at least four times a year.

Contact the American Diabetes Association — 1-800-232-3472. The Association will provide you with many free or low-cost publications. Their address is 1660 Duke Street, Alexandria, VA 22314.

Contact the National Diabetes Information Clearing House — 1-301-654-3327. Or write to them at 1 Information Way, Bethesda, MD 20892-3565. The Information Clearing House is a part of the National Institute of Diabetes and Digestive and Kidney Disease.

Contact the National Institute of Diabetes and Digestive and Kidney Diseases — 1-301-499-3583. You can write them at Building 31, Room 9A04, Bethesda, MD 10892 for information on how to deal with diabetes.

Contact LeBoeuf's — ☎ 1-800-546-5559 for free pamphlets courtesy of Becton-Dickinson on blood glucose monitoring, drawing insulin from its vial and injecting insulin, fast-food guide (how to eat smart) and mixing insulin.

Diabetes Testing & Other Diagnostic Devices

BLOOD PRESSURE IS MEASURED with an instrument called a sphygmo-manometer. A cuff (rubber bag that can be inflated with air and called a bladder) is wrapped around one arm above the elbow and inflated to cut off circulation temporarily. As air is slowly released, a stethoscope is placed over the artery at the bend in the arm.

The top number of a blood pressure reading is called systolic pressure and is measured when the first sound of rushing blood is heard. The bottom number, called diastolic pressure, is measured when the sound stops. Have the doctor or nurse show you how to use this equipment. It is very simple to operate but you must be sure that everything is done correctly to get an accurate reading. There are electronic blood pressure monitors that make taking blood pressure very simple and eliminate the need to listen through a stethoscope.

Early warning signs of hypertension can be diagnosed by a systolic reading of 120 and above and/or a diastolic reading of 90 and above. Blood pressure readings can go up and would be normal in response to stress and exercise. However, hypertension is a high blood pressure reading taken while at rest. Because blood pressure increases with age, a somewhat higher blood pressure is normal for older patients. The patient's doctor can tell you what would be normal for your patient.

Tips to obtain the most accurate blood pressure readings:

- Avoid taking blood pressure within 30 minutes of eating, smoking or exercising.
- Make sure the cuff is the right size and wrap the cuff (bladder) evenly and smoothly around the arm.
- Position the stethoscope appropriately in the ears and make sure the stethoscope is not rubbing against clothing or an object such as a table.
- Have the patient relax for at least two minutes before taking blood pressure.
- Rest patient's arm on table even with their heart.

Signs and symptoms of hypertension:

- Headache
- Ringing in the ears
- Flushing of face, nosebleeds

Complications that can result from untreated hypertension can include, heart failure, stroke, kidney damage and damage to the retina.

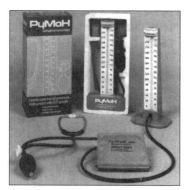

Py 6793 / Py 6792

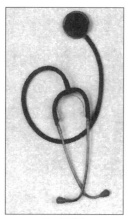

Py 5906

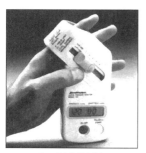

Le 119-2111

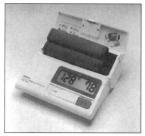

Le 139-4147

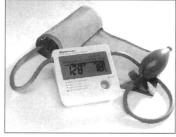

Le 220-4238

Diagnostic Equipment

PyMaH Corporation Home Care Sphygmomanometers. Virtually unbreakable mercury instrument. Just like the doctor uses. Complete inflation system includes cuff, old-style bladder, stethoscope, bulb and valve. D-ring cuff is designed to permit individuals to take their own blood pressure.

Py 6793	Adult	$81.95
Py 6792	Large adult	$87.95

PyMaH Corporation Travel Sphygmomanometers. Aneroid sphygmomanometer with carrying case, D-ring cuff and stethoscope. Designed to permit patient to take their own blood pressure.

Py 2893	Adult	$67.95
Py 2892	Large adult	$74.95

PyMaH Corporation Stethoscopes. Single head, flat diaphragm.

Py 5906	Nurse type	$11.95

SunMark Finger Cuff Blood Pressure Kit and Pulse Monitor. Reads blood pressure accurately from left index finger 2 inches to 3 inches in circumference. Adjustable oscillometric cuff for finger; photo-electric cell reads blood pressure. Automatic inflation and deflation. Simple warning on large LCD display. Automatic shut-off. Portable. Needs 2 AA batteries.

Le 119-2111	1 year limited warranty	$105.95

Omron Fuzzy Logic Blood Pressure Monitor. Uses fuzzy logic to determine the ideal cuff inflation level according to the patient's systolic blood pressure and arm size. Virtually eliminates patient arm discomfort and misreadings due to incorrect inflation. D-ring cuff automatically deflates when measurement is complete. Systolic, diastolic and pulse measurements are alternately displayed on an extra large LCD panel. Error indicators and automatic power-off. Needs 4 AA batteries. Cuff will fit arm circumference of 9 inches to 13 inches.

Le 271-3618	Adult	$133.95

SunMark Sensor Cuff™ Electronic/Digital Blood Pressure Kit. Deluxe D-ring, contoured oscillometric (no microphone) cuff provides uniform fit. Large, easy to read digital display. Manual cuff inflation; automatic deflation. Audio indicators. Portable, lightweight and compact. Soft vinyl carrying case. 4 AA batteries included.

Le 220-4238	Fits 9- to 13-inch arm circumference	$59.95

SunMark Wrist Cuff Blood Pressure Kit and Pulse Monitor. Pre-formed wrist cuff inflates faster than arm cuff. Cuff fits wrist 5¼ inches to 7¾ inches in circumference. User can preset proper cuff inflation level. Extra large LED display. Error indicators and automatic shut-off. 4 AA batteries included.

Le 124-5455	Built-in storage compartment	$136.95

3M Littman Lightweight Stethoscope. Lightweight and easy to carry. Aluminum combination chestpiece. Durable long-life PVC, single lumen tubing for better sound transmission. Affordable

Le 165-8194	$51.95

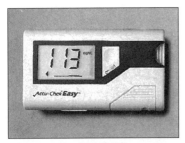

Le 188-2505

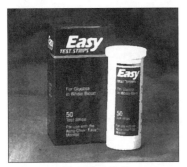

Le 188-2406

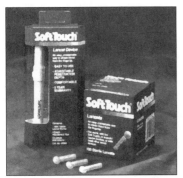

Le 364-6759 / Le 364-6817

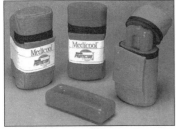

Ap 01950

Boehringer Mannheim Accu-Chek, Easy™ Diabetes Care Kit. No wiping. Results in as little as 15 seconds. 350-value memory, plus time and date. Two week average high and low blood glucose. Kit contains Accu-Chek Easy Test strips, Soft Touch lancet device, 10 lancets, Easy Glucose Control Solution, user's manual and pocket testing guide.

Le 188-2505	Comes with carrying case	$121.95
Le 188-2406	Easy Test Strips, Box of 50	$53.95

Boehringer Mannheim Accu-Chek Advantage™ Diabetes Care Kit. Simple to use; no timing, wiping, blotting or cleaning. Accurate results in as little as 40 seconds. Less blood needed. Multiple value memory. Kit contains Accu-Chek Advantage Monitor, 10 Advantage test strips, Soft Touch lancet device, 10 lancets, batteries. Advantage Glucose Control Solution and quick reference English and Spanish. Self-test diary.

Le 119-1428	Carrying case	$84.95
Le 119-1857	Advantage Test Strips, Box of 50	$53.95

Boehringer Mannheim Soft Touch™ Lancet Device. Quiet, comfortable, and easy to use. Adjustable. Includes 100 lancets.

Le 364-6759	5 Year warranty	$17.95
Le 364-6817	Soft Touch lancets, Box of 100	$13.95

Becton Dickinson Alcohol Swabs. High alcohol concentration. Thick, soft convenient. Individually foil-wrapped.

Le 116-5133	Box of 100	$2.95

Becton Dickinson Glucose Tablets. For fast relief from low blood sugar. Dissolve quickly. Convenient, stay-fresh package. 19 calories—no fat.

Le 218-9587	Orange flavor	$1.95

Becton Dickinson Automatic Injector. Holds filled syringe and quickly inserts needle into skin at the touch of a button. Easy to use.

Le 181-9739	$35.95

Becton Dickinson Safe-Clip™. Insulin syringe needle clipper.

Le 115-3915	$5.95

Apex Medicool Insulin Protection System. Keeps insulin cool for eight or more hours. Stores up to two vials of insulin. Pockets for syringes, swabs, or test strips. Hand or belt strap for easy carrying. Can be used to keep insulin from freezing during cold weather. Comes with two freezeable coolers; one for immediate use and one to be ready when needed.

Ap 01950	$28.95

LILA Large Print Diabetes Register. Allows a low vision diabetic to keep a simple accurate record or date and time of measurements, blood glucose readings, insulin or pill dosage administered, meal times, etc. Each register has enough pages for one month's record keeping.

Li 234675	Blue Cover	$2.95
Li 234680	Yellow Cover	$2.95

Diabetic Travel Case.

Le 322-4474	$22.95

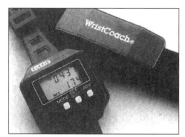
Le 247-3684

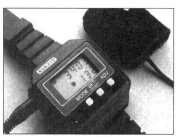
Le 140-1892

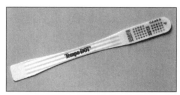
Py 5122

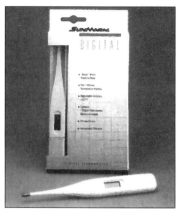
Le 220-8049

Generally, if your patient's total cholesterol level is less than 200, their cholesterol level is okay; between 200-239, moderate risk; over 240 high risk of developing heart disease. You should have the patient's doctor administer a blood cholesterol test when they go in for a check-up.

Elexis Salt Chek. LED scale indicates sodium level in moist foods and beverage. Low voltage indicator. Includes batteries and Guide to Lower Sodium.

Le 140-1298		$19.95

Biomerica DZ Detect. Home test for detecting hidden blood in the stool. One-step, two minute test. No handling of stool — test pad is just dropped in toilet bowl. No diet restrictions.

Le 365-9562	Reliable and accurate	$7.95

Elexis FM-118 Wristwatch Heart Rate Monitor. Wireless chestband heart-rate monitor. Watch/stopwatch for runners and cyclists. Features include maximum heart rate, time in target zone, high/low limit alarms. Audio and visual pulse indicators. Monitors heart rate and displays EKG reading.

Le 247-3684	$119.95

Elexis FM-111 Pulse-Coach Heart Rate Monitor. Unit mounts on stationary exercise equipment. Ear lobe sensor monitors heart rate using infrared technology. High/low limit alarms. Includes batteries and mounting adapter. Target range indicator and elapsed time.

Le 247-3478	$59.95

Elexis FM-135 Pulsewatch. Designed for walking or stationary exercise equipment. Fingertip heart rate monitor with audio pulse indicator. Functions as watch, stopwatch and lap timer. Batteries included. High/low limit alarms.

Le 140-1892	$59.95

PyMaH Tempa-Dot, Single Use Clinical Thermometers. Individually wrapped. Sterile. Oral and axillary use.

Py 5122	Box of 100	$17.95

SunMark Glass Thermometers. Certified accurate. Tri-top safety grip. Large easy to read numbers. Tempered glass.

Le 218-7011	Rectal	$2.95
Le 218-6989	Oral	$2.95
Le 218-7029	Baby rectal	$2.95

SunMark Electronic Digital Thermometers. Fast accurate reading in about 1 minute. Large easy to read digital display. Automatic shut-off. Safe for children-no mercury. Retains previous reading in memory.

Le 220-8049	Beeps when peak temperature is reached	$8.95

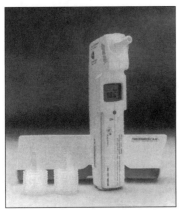

Le 122-0318 / Le 227-7382

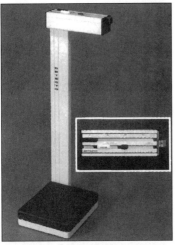

Le 366-2368

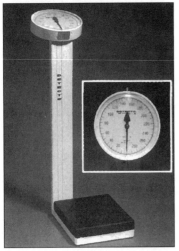

Le 168-9249

Thermoscan HM-2 Instant Thermometer. Accurately reads temperature in ear in 1 second. Displays temperature in oral or rectal equivalent. Can be used on sleeping patient. Large digital display. Auto shut-off.

Le 122-0318	Includes 21 lens filters and storage case	$95.95
Le 227-7382	Lens filters for above, Pack of 40	$7.95

SunMark Electronic Digital Scale. Digital accuracy with bright easy-to-read LED display. Automatic zeroing. Modern styling. Durable construction. Accurate to 300 pounds. White.

Le 220-2414	10¹/₈″ × 10³/₄ ″ × 2¹/₁₆″	$30.95

SunMark Platform Scale. Oversize steel platform. Easy to read dial. Accurate to 325 pounds.

Le 352-8585	Lifetime warranty	$48.95

Detecto 057 Waist-High Doctor Scale – Beam Type. Waist-high viewing eliminates stooping and squinting. Platform size 11″ × 13″. Height is 38″. Professional quality scale that should last for many years.

Le 366-2368	340 pound capacity	$205.95

Detecto 080 Waist-High Doctor Scale – Dial Type. Large, easy-to-read dial with 7½-inch reading line. Easy zero adjustment.

Le 168-9249	340 pound capacity	$219.95

Fever

ANY BODY TEMPERATURE above 98.6°F when measured in the mouth, or 99.8° F in the rectum, is known as a fever. A fever usually indicates that the body is fighting an infection. Fever can be accompanied by symptoms such as shaking chills, back pain, severe headaches, drenching sweats, thirst, confusion or delirium, flushed face, hot skin and faster than normal breathing.

Consult a doctor if a fever lasts longer than three days in a child under 6 months of age, or in an elderly person, and one or more of the following symptoms appear:

Check with the doctor prior to giving children aspirin.

- Shaking chills, back or flank (fleshy side of a person between the ribs/upper part of the thigh) pain — which may indicate bacteria in the blood stream.
- Severe headache with vomiting — which could signal infections around the brain.
- Abdominal pain — which could indicate appendicitis, gall bladder infection, inflammatory bowel disease or a severe ulcer.
- Fatigue and rash — which could indicate scarlet fever, Rocky Mountain spotted fever or Lyme disease.
- Medication triggers a fever.
- Sore throat — which may indicate strep throat.
- Persistent fever that returns four or more times in a three week period.
- History of febrile seizures (twitching or jerking of the limbs with a loss of consciousness after a rapid rise in temperature).
- Frequent burning or blood urination — which may indicate infection of the urinary tract, bladder, kidneys, or prostrate gland.

Treatment may include temperature-lowering drugs such as aspirin or Tylenol, which will also help to relieve the aches and pains associated with a fever. Treatment also consists of treating the underlying cause, such as giving antibiotics for a bacterial infection. Febrile seizures can often be prevented by cooling the entire body as soon as a fever starts by taking a lukewarm bath or sponging with lukewarm water.

To take a patient's temperature:

- Wear disposable rubber gloves if in contact with patient's body secretions or substances.
- Shake down the mercury in the thermometer until the reading is below 35°C or 95°F by holding the thermometer at the farthest end from the bulb between the thumb and forefinger and snapping your wrist.

Most suppliers will indicate if the thermometer is oral or rectal. A round bulb indicates that it can be used as a rectal thermometer. Some thermometers are color coded; blue for rectal, and silver for oral and armpit. If electronic, follow the instructions with the unit. Electronic units may have separate probes for oral, rectal or armpit. Warm up the unit by switching it on. Listen for a sound indicating that the maximum measurement has been reached. If the probe has a disposable cover, discard when done.

Oral Temperature

Determine when the patient last took hot or cold food or fluids, or smoked. Allow at least five minutes after eating, drinking or smoking to get an accurate reading. Place the thermometer under the patient's tongue at the base. Tell the patient to close their lips — not their teeth — around the thermometer. Thermometers can be broken if gripped too firmly with the teeth. Leave the thermometer in place for 2 to 3 minutes. If an electronic oral thermometer is used, keep it in place 10 to 20 seconds, or until it finishes registering. Avoid taking oral temperatures of patients who are under 6 years of age, are irrational, unconscious or who have had recent oral surgery.

Rectal Temperature

Place the patient in a lateral position. Lubricate the thermometer by placing lubricant on a tissue, then on the thermometer. Put on a disposable glove. Raise the patient's buttock to expose the anus. Tell the patient to take a deep breath and insert the thermometer from .5 inch to 1.5 inches, depending on the age and size of the patient (.5 inches for an infant and 1.5 inches for an adult). Having the patient take a deep breath will often relax the external sphincter muscles, making it easier to insert the thermometer. Hold in place for 2 minutes (for newborn up to a month old, hold in place for 5 minutes). Hold children firmly while thermometer is in the rectum or it may become displaced inside or outside the anus.

Armpit Temperature

If the armpit is moist, pat it dry with a towel. Be sure you do not rub, since rubbing can cause the temperature of the armpit to rise. Place the thermometer in the armpit and move the patient's arm across the chest to keep the thermometer in place. Leave the thermometer in place 9 minutes for adults and 5 minutes for infants and children.

To read the thermometer, hold it at eye level and rotate it until the mercury is clearly visible. The end away from the bulb is the patient's temperature. After the reading, wash the thermometer in tepid soapy water, making sure that any organic material is completely removed. Rinse the thermometer in cold water, dry and store it. To disinfect before storage, use 70 percent isopropyl alcohol. If electronic, return to battery case for recharging.

Other types of thermometers include:

- *Temperature-sensitive tape, which is used to obtain a general indication of body surface temperature. Usually applied on the forehead or the abdomen. Readings are not as accurate, but are useful for infants whose temperature needs to be monitored.*

- *Infrared thermometers that sense body heat. The infrared thermometer is inserted into the outer portion of the ear canal. The probe tip seals the ear opening and in one or two seconds the temperature reading is complete.*

- *Chemical sensitive disposable thermometers are used in the same manner as a mercury oral thermometer. The temperature is determined by reading the dots.*

Flu

See also section on "Pills and Shots" — pages 217 and 218.

Fʟᴜ ᴏʀ ɪɴꜰʟᴜᴇɴᴢᴀ is a viral infection of the nose, throat and lungs. Flu is caused by viruses that enter the system and multiply rapidly. The viruses can be passed by droplets from coughs or sneezes that enter the body through the nose or mouth. Normally a mild disease in healthy children, young adults and middle-age people, flu can be life-threatening in older people and people of any age who have chronic illnesses such as heart disease, emphysema, asthma, bronchitis, kidney disease or diabetes.

Flu reduces the body's ability to fight off other infections, especially pneumonia. It is very important for older people to take flu prevention measures by getting a shot. Because flu viruses change every year, *people over 50 need to get a flu shot annually.* If the patient is allergic to eggs, flu shots may cause a serious reaction. The doctor should ask you or the patient if the patient is allergic to eggs prior to giving a flu shot.

It is easy to confuse a common cold with the flu. Normally a cold doesn't cause a fever and flu does. Cold symptoms are usually milder and do not last as long as the flu. Flu symptoms include: feeling weak, a cough, a headache, a sudden rise in temperature, aching muscles, chills and red, watery eyes.

While flu is rarely fatal, older people and people with chronic diseases have the greatest risk of developing pneumonia from a case of the flu. Pneumonia, an inflammation of the lungs, is one of the five leading causes of death among people who are 65 years of age or older.

Pneumonia

The usual treatment of flu, and to reduce the aches and pains, is to take aspirin, drink plenty of fluids and stay in bed until the fever has been gone for one or two days. For children, aspirin is not recommended due to the incidence of Reye's syndrome. Call the doctor if the fever lasts, as a more serious infection may be present. An antiviral drug, amantadine, also is recommended to prevent and treat many types of flu — particularly in high-risk people. Steam inhalation may relieve respiratory symptoms and prevent drying of discharges.

Pneumonia symptoms are similar to those of flu, but are much more severe. Shaking chills are very common. Coughing becomes more frequent and may produce a colored or bloody discharge. The fever will continue and remain high. Pain in the lungs will occur as they become more inflamed. One of the most dangerous complications of pneumonia is the body's loss of fluids. The doctor will prescribe extra fluids to prevent shock, a serious condition caused by inadequate blood supply.

Pneumonia can also be caused by bacteria. Bacterial pneumonia is usually treated with antibiotics, such as penicillin. Antibiotic drugs that kill bacteria are very effective if given when you first get pneumonia.

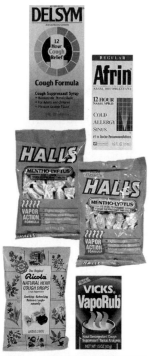

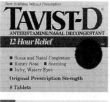
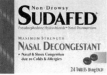

Cough\Cold Products

Le 143-7391	Afrin Nasal Spray Reg	15 ml	$6.15
Le 115-6504	Benadryl Kap 25mg	24s	$5.45
Le 115-6397	Benadryl Elix (Otc)	4 oz	$5.85
Le 228-2341	Benadryl Tab 25mg	24s	$5.45
Le 114-3213	Blistex Ointment 2288	0.21oz	$1.85
Le 248-6512	Carmex Tube B/P	0.35 oz	$.95
Le 228-9270	Carmex Jar	1/4 oz	$.95
Le 194-0766	Chap Stick Lip Reg B/P	0.15 oz	$1.15
Le 115-1745	Delsym Liquid	3 oz	$7.55
Le 136-8380	Fisherman/F Loz Orig X/S 19	Bag	$1.45
Le 116-0498	Halls Mentho-Lypt	Bag/30	$1.75
Le 149-4939	Halls Cherry	Bag/30	$1.75
Le 149-4962	Halls Honey Lemon	Bag/30	$1.75
Le 216-4317	Halls Mentho-Lypt Stick	Each	$.75
Le 186-4891	Halls Cherry Stick	Each	$.75
Le 131-1455	Halls Ice Blue	Bag/30	$1.75
Le 216-5769	Ocean Nasal Mist	45 ml	$2.95
Le 320-2363	Ricola Drop Herbal	3 oz	$1.85
Le 134-8127	Robitussin-CF Syrup	4 oz	$4.95
Le 142-6469	Robitussin-DM Syrup	4 oz	$4.95
Le 274-8283	Robitussin-DM Syrup	8 oz	$8.65
Le 119-1105	Sudafed Tab 30mg	24s	$5.75
Le 146- 8263	Tavist-D Tab 12hr Cold/Relief	8s	$4.85
Le 147-3891	Tavist-D Tab 12hr Cold/Relief	16s	$8.75
Le 161-1854	Vicks Vaporub Ointment	1.5 oz	$3.35

TO ORDER CALL TOLL FREE

LeBoeuf's

PHONE **1-800-546-5559**
FAX **1-800-233-9692**

Hearing Impaired with TDD
CALL **1-800-855-2880**

Foot Problems

S EVENTY-FIVE PERCENT OF ALL AMERICANS have problems with their feet at some point in their lives. Foot problems can be caused by a number of factors:

- Heredity.
- Unaddressed health problems such as diabetes, arthritis and circulatory problems.
- Improper foot wear, ill-fitting socks and poor hygiene.
- Exposure to cold and water.
- Smoking.
- Long periods of sitting.

See also section on "Diabetes," pages 267 through 271.

The average person takes between 8,000 to 10,000 steps per day. This is the equivalent of walking around the world four times over a lifetime. Because foot problems tend to accumulate over a lifetime, older persons are much more likely to have problems than younger persons. And women have four times as many problems with their feet as men, primarily due to wearing high-heeled shoes. Doctors say that there are over 300 different foot ailments. However, most foot problems can be prevented and treated by practicing healthy behavior and seeking help from a doctor when trouble first develops.

Athlete's foot is a fungal infection that occurs because the feet are usually enclosed in a dark, damp and warm environment. If not treated promptly, an infection may become chronic and difficult to cure. To prevent this problem you must keep the feet dry and clean, especially between the toes. If your patient has athlete's feet symptoms, it is also a good idea to dust the feet daily with a fungicidal powder. Exposure to the air is also a good idea.

Itching and burning feet are normally caused by dry skin. To reduce this problem, use mild soap sparingly and a body lotion on legs and feet every day. The best moisturizers contain petroleum jelly or lanolin. If you add oils to the bath water, use extra caution as the oils will make the bathtub very slippery.

The foot contains 26 bones and 33 joints joined together by over 100 ligaments. There are 19 foot muscles.

Corns and calluses are caused by friction and pressure of the bony areas of the feet rubbing against the shoes. Corns usually develop on the toes and calluses on the soles of the feet. A doctor can determine the cause of this condition and suggest treatment. It is important that a doctor be consulted because many over-the-counter medicines contain acids that destroy the tissue, but do not treat the cause. This is especially true if the patient has diabetes or poor circulation.

Bunions are deformities at the big toe joints that are swollen and tender. Bunions may be hereditary or can be aggravated by poor fitting shoes. Treatment includes wearing shoes that are wide at the instep, protective pads, application or injection of drugs, and whirlpool baths. Surgery may also be an option if the pain persists.

Warts are skin growths caused by viruses. Sometimes these warts are called plantar warts and usually invade the skin through abrasions. To help prevent getting warts, avoid walking barefoot in public places where the virus may be lurking. Warts can be painful and may spread if untreated. A doctor can apply medications, burn or freeze the wart off or remove it surgically.

Hammertoe is caused by shortening of the tendons that control toe movement. The toe knuckle is usually enlarged, drawing the toe back. Over time, the joint enlarges and stiffens as it rubs against the shoes. Balance may be affected. Hammertoe is treated by wearing shoes and socks with plenty of toe room. In some advanced cases, surgery may be recommended.

Spurs are calcium growths that develop on the bones of the feet. They are caused by muscle strain in the feet and are irritated by standing for long periods of time, wearing badly fitted shoes, or being overweight. If the spurs are painful, treatment includes using proper foot support, heel pads, heel cups or other recommendations by the doctor.

Ingrown toenails occur when toenails pierce the skin. Normally they result from improper nail trimming, but can also occur from injury or fungus infection. If your patient has toenails that are too thick to be cut with normal toe trimming tools, you may have to take the patient to a podiatrist.

Symptoms of problems with the feet include:

- Redness
- Blisters
- Peeling and itching
- Pain in the joints
- Warts
- Pain in the heel
- Sores

What to do:

Contact the doctor — The doctor may recommend that a podiatrist be contacted to discuss the pros and cons of the patient's particular problem. Podiatrists are specialists in the diagnosis and treatment of diseases and problems with the foot. Much of the treatment for foot problems can be given in the doctor's office.

Contact the American Podiatric Medical Association — 1-800-366-8273 (Footcare). Or you can write them at 9312 Old Georgetown Road, Bethesda, MD 20814.

Foot Care Products

Le 141-8037	Blue Star Ointment . . . . 2 oz	$5.85
Le 229-6143	Compound W Wart Gel 25oz	$8.35
Le 170-5417	Dr Scholl Air-Pillo Insole W7-8 30300	$2.55
Le 170-5474	Dr Scholl Air-Pillo Insole M8-9 30200	$2.55
Le 170-5490	Dr Scholl Air-Pillo Insole M10-11 30220	$2.55
Le 144-6798	Dr Scholl Callous Cushion 10390	$2.65
Le 182-5272	Dr Scholl Callous Remover 10042	$3.25
Le 144-8307	Dr Scholl Corn+Callous Rem Liq . . . . 1/3 oz	$4.95
Le 144-6806	Dr Scholl Corn Cushion 10140	$2.65
Le 144-6814	Dr Scholl Corn Cushion Sml 10150	$2.65
Le 274-5586	Dr Scholl Corn Cushion Soft 10200	$2.65
Le 186-3653	Dr Scholl Corn Remover 10002	$3.25
Le 186-3661	Dr Scholl Corn Remover Sml 10013	$3.25
Le 182-5819	Dr Scholl Corn Remover Soft 10521	$3.25
Le 144-7960	Dr Scholl Moleskin 4¹⁄₈ × 3³⁄₈ 1480.	$3.15
Le 144-8026	Dr Scholl Molefoam 4¹⁄₈ × 3³⁄₈ 14900.	$2.85
Le 144-6962	Dr Scholl Foot Pwd 7oz	$5.35
Le 350-2606	Duofilm Wart Remv Liq 05oz	$11.65
Le 189-2801	Lotrimin AF Cream. .24gm	$13.95
Le 345-2273	Lotrimin AF Cream. .12gm	$9.85
Le 143-9397	Tinactin Cream . . . . 15 gm	$8.55

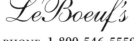
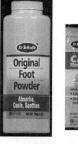
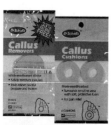
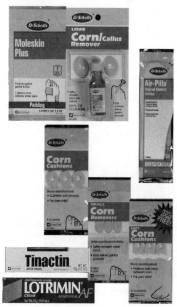

Hearing Loss

NEARLY ONE IN FOUR PEOPLE between the ages of 65 and 74 have a hearing impairment. Between the ages of 75 and 84 the ratio increases to one in three. Of those over age 85 one out of every two people are affected. Over 10 million people in the United States are hearing impaired. Total deafness is rare and is usually congenital (present from birth), occurring in about one out of every 1,000 babies.

All deafness is either the faulty transportation of sound from the outer to the inner ear (conductive) or because of damage to the structures within the inner ear or to the acoustic nerve (sensorineural) which connects the inner ear to the brain.

The most common cause of conductive deafness in adults is earwax. In children, the most common cause of deafness is an infection in the middle ear resulting in a collection of fluid. As many as one quarter of children starting school have some degree of hearing loss as the result of middle-ear infections. Sometimes, but rarely, damage to the eardrum or the middle ear can happen due to sudden changes in pressure in an aircraft or under water.

Sensorineural deafness can be caused by prolonged exposure to loud noise, Meniere's disease, drugs such as streptomycin or by viral infections. Damage to the inner ear can also happen naturally with old age. Damage to the acoustic nerve can be the result of a benign tumor (acoustic neuroma) on the nerve. Meniere's disease is an inner ear disorder where the patient has recurrent vertigo, deafness and tinnitus caused by an increase in the amount of fluid in the canals of the inner ear. Usually, only one ear is affected (80-85 percent of the time). The cause is Meniere's disease is unknown in most cases and is usually not found in patients under 50.

Hearing loss can lead to social isolation, depression, reduced mobility and worsening of an existing psychiatric condition. Denial is a common reaction. It is very important for the caregiver and the patient to recognize and deal with hearing loss.

Audiologists measure hearing loss and can provide information regarding treatment for hearing impairment. Normally, audiologists will dispense hearing aids and other hearing assistive devices (Medicare will not pay for hearing aids). Most states license hearing aid dispensers and it is a good idea to check with the local Better Business Bureau, the local or state consumer protection agency and your doctor. There are a large number of hearing assistive devices and services to help the patient cope with most levels of hearing loss.

Symptoms:
- Tunes out from conversations when more than one person is talking.
- Lets someone else do the talking.
- Long conversations make patient tired and irritable.
- Family and friends avoid conversation with patient.
- Frequently misunderstands people and has to ask them to repeat what they have said.

Each ear has three parts:
- *Outer ear*
- *Middle ear*
- *Inner ear*

For the eardrum to function properly, the air pressure must be equal on each side. Pressure is equalized by the eustachian tube.

- Ringing or hissing background noise.
- Certain sounds are overly loud or annoying.
- TV programs, concerts, movies or social gatherings are less enjoyable.
- Words are difficult to understand.
- Speech sounds slurred or mumbled, especially when there is background noise.

A hearing aid consists of a tiny microphone, an amplifier and a speaker.

Tips for your patient on coping with a hearing loss:

- Don't hesitate to ask people to repeat what they have said.
- Try to reduce background noise (TV, radio, etc.).
- Tell people you have a hearing problem.
- Tell people how best to talk to you.
- Anticipate difficult situations and plan how to minimize them.
- Pay attention to the person who is speaking.
- Don't bluff. Admit if you don't understand in order to avoid trouble.
- Look at the person who is speaking.

Tips for your patient on talking to someone who has a hearing loss:

- Speak at your normal rate.
- Do not overarticulate or shout.
- Speak to the person at a distance of 3 to 6 feet.
- Position yourself so that your lip movement and facial expressions can be clearly seen.
- Don't hide your mouth, chew gum or smoke while talking.
- Never speak directly into the person's ear.
- Take your time and don't get frustrated.
- Treat the hearing impaired person with respect.

What to do:

Contact a doctor — Have the doctor perform a hearing exam or ask the doctor where the patient can get a hearing exam by a trained audiologist. The audiologist can test the degree of hearing loss, and the ability to understand speech in different settings. The doctor may also perform a caloric test if the patient is experiencing vertigo (dizziness).

Contact American Academy of Otolaryngology — (703) 836-4444. Or write to them at Head and Neck Surgery, Inc., One Prince Street, Alexandria, VA 22314

Contact National Information Center on Deafness — (Voice) 202-651-5051, (TTY) 202-651-5052. Or write to them at Gallaudet University 800 Florida Avenue, NE, Washington, DC 20002

Contact Self Help for Hard of Hearing People, Inc. — (301) 657-2248. Or write to them at 7800 Wisconsin Avenue, Bethesda, MD 20892. They stay on top of what's new in hearing assistive equipment.

There are many other associations that will provide information on hearing loss. You can call **LeBoeuf's** ☎ **1-800-546-5559** for additional information and associations in your area. We do does not sell hearing aids.

Hearing Assistive Devices

Assistive listening devices can be very helpful to the patient and the caregiver. There are a number of products that will allow the hard-of-hearing patients to listen to a TV or stereo at normal listening levels or will allow them to hear well enough so they do not have to fear the embarrassment of not hearing when meeting people at social functions. There are also a number of products that will help provide for the patient's safety and convenience in the home or when traveling, if the patient has severe or total hearing loss.

The most important thing to remember is that patients will most likely be in denial about having a hearing problem. They will resist trying products that will help them hear better and, in many cases, withdraw from social contacts. You need to encourage your patient to use and wear the device. If you make fun of them or the device, make a big issue out of using the equipment or if it is not comfortable or easy to use, you will have paid for a hearing assistive device that will sit on a shelf and not be used. To encourage a patient to use the assistive equipment, it may be that two devices will have to be purchased, one for the caregiver and one for the patient. This has proven to weaken a patient's resistance to the use of a device. Once they become used to the benefits that hearing assistive equipment provides, the patient will want to continue using them. In many cases the caregiver can use the assistive listening device in other settings such as listening to TV in bed while the spouse is sleeping, or listening to the stereo while the rest of the family is watching TV.

There are a number of ways that sound can be connected to the ear. The most common methods include: direct wire to the source such as a TV or radio with headphones or an ear bud (small earphone that fits in the ear instead of over the ear), move speakers closer to the patient's ear, send the sound via infrared light, send the sound via FM radio waves, and induction loop. The purpose of all these assistive devices is to improve the sound to noise ratio. In other words, increase the sound that is wanted and reduce the sound that is unwanted.

Induction Loop Systems

Conventional induction assistive listening systems consist of a loop of wire which creates a magnetic field that is placed around the listening area such as a room or an auditorium, a special amplifier and a microphone for the primary speaker. Speech signals are amplified and circulated through the loop wire. The resulting energy is picked up and amplified by the "telecoil" found in many hearing aids or by portable induction receivers. Intelligibility is increased because background noise is dramatically reduced and because the patient is using a personal hearing aid (must have telecoil) which has been carefully adjusted to give the best sound quality. The patient can move freely about the room without wires.

FM Systems

FM for people with hearing disabilities operates on 40 FM channels in the 72 to 76 MHz range designated by the Federal Communications Commission (FCC). FM is a narrow band radio wave signal. Typically, FM can be broadcast 150 to 300 feet and is ideal for outdoor use. FM is wireless and no connecting cable is required. Many FM systems are used in public schools and other public places such as churches. You need to be careful that both the amplifier and receivers are on the same frequency. Only the factory or a factory service store can change the frequency on single frequency units. It is possible to buy FM systems that have more than one frequency that can be changed by the users. This type is probably the best because you can switch to another frequency if there is interference.

Infrared Systems

Infrared is invisible and harmless light. It is immune to outside interference. Infrared systems consist of three parts: the transmitter, the emitter and the receiver. Sometimes, the transmitter and emitter are in the same unit. The transmitter converts the audio signal into a signal that the emitter converts into infrared light. The receiver decodes the infrared light into the original sound. Infrared is used in many movie theaters in the United States and you can take your receiver with you when you go to movies that have infrared capability. Theaters use the 95 kHz frequency. Usually, infrared cannot be used in bright daylight and the receiver has to be in line with the emitter. Infrared can be used in multiple screen theaters because the light does not go through the walls.

LeBoeuf's is an authorized dealer for Williams Sound, Ultratec, Ameriphone, Chorus, Sennheiser, Oval Window and many others. We will work with you on any hearing assistive problem to obtain the best possible solution and/or equipment for you and your patient. We also have a number of associate sound technology companies throughout the United States and Canada that can install custom equipment in the home or automobile.

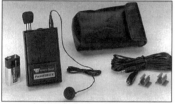

Wi PKT SYS B1

Williams Sound Pocketalker™ Personal Amplifier. Compact amplifier that can be used for TV listening, riding in a car, in small groups or for one-on-one conversations.

Wi PKT SYS B1	Basic system consisting of amplifier, microphone, mini earphone, belt clip case, 12-foot TV listening cord, 9V battery and carrying case.	$159.95
Wi TEL 100	Telelink adapter allows the Pocketalker to be used as a telephone amplifier.	$44.95

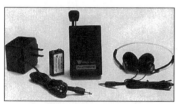

Wi PKT PCS B1

Williams Sound Pocketalker™ Consultation System. Designed for one-on-one consultation situations. Perfect for the patient who needs to hear and understand what the doctor and/or nurse in instructing them to do.

Wi PKT PCS B1	Pocketalker amplifier, microphone, headphones, belt clip case, rechargeable 9V battery and charger.	$169.95

Williams Sound Hearing Helper, Personal FM System. Wireless listening system for TV listening, riding in the car, meetings. 150 feet of range and easy to operate. Can be used with or without a hearing aid. Transmitter, receiver, microphone, earphone, rechargeable 6V batteries and charger included.

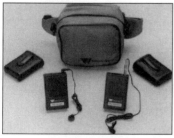

Wi PFM 100E

Wi PFM 100E	Belt clip cases and storage case	$589.95

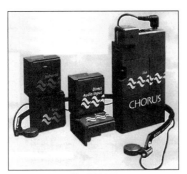

Ch CSRUP

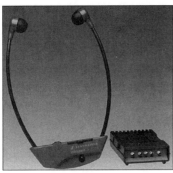

Se Set 100

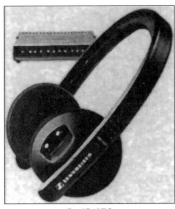

Se IS 450

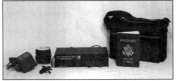

Ov Mic II/II, Ov Rec

Williams Sound Conference Microphone. Table-top microphone that conceals an FM transmitter (not included). For use in small groups or meetings.

Wi MIC 061	Available in natural walnut	$219.95

Williams Sound Speechmaker Voice Amplifier. An amplifier system for those persons who have lost their vocal power or need to rest their voice. Set consists of headset microphone, amplifier with volume control, rechargeable battery with charger and speaker.

Wi PKT SYS G	Belt clip case included	$329.95

Chorus™ Universal Listening System. An "all-in-one" assistive listening device that comes with modules for about any audio transmitting system for the hearing impaired. Includes infrared, FM and induction loop transmissions. Includes microphone, headphones, 2 AAA alkaline batteries, lanyard and instruction manual. The AAA batteries have a life of 90 hours or more.

Ch CSRUP	Complete system includes FM, infrared, telecoil, direct audio input and radio	$419.95

Chorus™ Transmitters

Ch CSTFM	FM Transmitter with microphone, 6V rechargeable battery	$459.95
Ch CSTIR	Infrared transmitter, 95 kHz	$149.95
Ch CSTML	Audio loop transmitter with 90 feet of wire	$295.95

Sennheiser Audiolink™ Infrared System. Lightweight and portable infrared system designed for hearing impaired patients so they can hear TV or stereo with enhanced sound. Includes transmitter and featherweight headset that can be used for hours at a time without discomfort. Rechargeable battery good for about 7 hours. Transmitter also acts as battery charger. Best on the market for TV listening. For continuous listening, we recommend that you buy an extra battery.

Se Set 100	Frequency 95 kHz	$199.95
Se BA 90	Extra battery for Set 100	$9.95

Sennheiser IS 450 Stereo Infrared System. Includes HDI 450 headphone with adjustable volume control and rechargeable Nicad battery. T200 transmitter also serves as battery charger. Perfect headphone for those who desire high performance audio without cords. For continuous listening, we recommend that you buy an extra battery.

Se IS 450	Stereo infrared system with both 95 and 250 kHz	$259.95
Se BA 90	Battery	$9.95

Sennheiser R1100-A Receiver. Additional receiver with battery, charger not included.

Se R1100-A	Receiver	$119.95

Oval Window Audio Microloop II/II FM. Easily transported and contains 90 feet of loop wire with wireless microphone. Ideal for larger rooms and TV viewing. Can be used in an automobile with the optional auto kit. If your patient has a "T" coil in their hearing aid, or has an induction receiver, this will be all you need to communicate with the patient. If the patient has neither, you will need to purchase a receiver.

Ov Mic II/II	Basic system	$549.95
Ov Rec	Receiver with earphone, battery and charger	$115.95

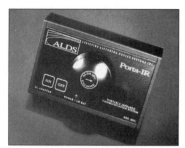

Al PIR S300/OM

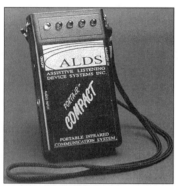

Al COM L 100

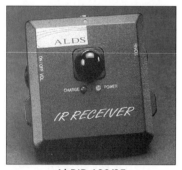

Al RIR 100/95

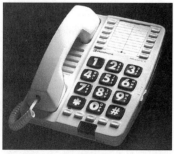

Am 76572

Williams Sound Power Loop Receiver. Battery powered pocket receiver that can be used with any audio induction loop system (Not an FM receiver).

Wi PWL LR1	Includes mini earphone and 9V battery	$76.95

ALDS PORTA-IR Infrared Communication System. Can be used with or without a hearing aid. Very useful when patient is in a group. Speakers talk normally and their sound is picked up and transmitted by infrared light to the patient with receiver. Great for family gatherings and at the dinner table. Range is up to 20 feet. Operates on either 95 or 250 kHz.

Al PIR S300/OM	Omnidirectional emits 360 degree signal	$749.95

ALDS PORTA-IR Compact. Converts sound to invisible infrared light to be picked up by the receiver. About the size of an eyeglass case and can be carried in the patient's pocket. Comes with 9V rechargeable batteries that last up to two hours, or you can use the AC adapter that is supplied. Has audio input feature to connect the Compact to earphone jack or audio output. Great for listening to TV and stereo.

Al COM S100	Each	$199.95

ALDS PORTA-IR Lavaliere One-to-One Infrared Transmitter. Worn around the neck of the speaker. Provides improved hearing with less background noise to listeners wearing any infrared receiver. Great for use in restaurants or doctor's offices. Can be either 95 or 250 kHz. Standard 9V rechargeable batteries provide power for up to two hours. Charger is included.

Al COM L 100	Each	$199.95

ALDS IR Receiver. State of the art infrared technology combined with excellent amplification. Lightweight and unobtrusive with adjustable neck strap. Has tone control and a unique daylight filtering lens. Can be used with or without a hearing aid. Operates 35 hours on rechargeable batteries. Can be ordered either in 95 or 250 kHz. Need to order either earbuds or headset to go with receiver.

Al RIR 100/95 or 100/250	Receiver	$130.95
Al AT-538S	Earbuds	$18.95
Al WM-HED001	Headset	$18.95

Ameriphone XL-25 Amplified Telephone. Makes voices coming through louder and clearer than ever before. Adjustable 75 decibel tone ringer with hearing aid compatible handset. Anti-feedback filter, 12 memory buttons for one-touch buttons. Extra large buttons, last number redial, bright incoming call flasher and electronic hold with auto release.

Am 76571	Telephone line powered	$99.95

Ameriphone XL-30 Amplified Telephone. Gives clearer and more natural sounding voices. Adjustable 85 decibel tone ringer. Hearing aid compatible handset. Anti-feedback filter, frequency screening tones, super bright incoming ring flasher, last number redial, electronic hold with auto release. Amplifier can be set to amplify outgoing voice. Extra large buttons. AC adapter with battery back-up (battery not included).

Am 76572	Tone amplification selector	$119.95

Ameriphone Amplification Handset Model AR-22. Amplifies the volume of incoming calls up to 20 decibels, hearing aid compatible and powered by the telephone. Built in volume control. For use with traditional (non-electric) telephones with a modular handset cord (plug-in type).

Am 01901	Ivory color	$29.95

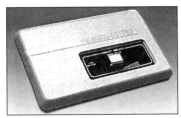

Am 01929

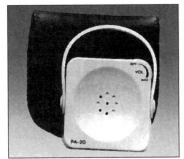

Am 01961

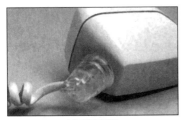

Li 603537

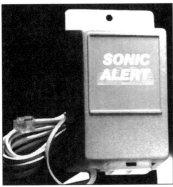

So TR 75

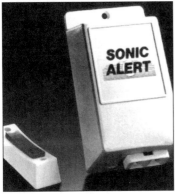

So TD 500M

Ameriphone In-Line Telephone Amplifier Model HA-25. Auxiliary amplifier connects between the handset and the telephone base. It increases the volume of the incoming voice by 20 decibels. Comes with sliding volume control and can be used with all telephones that have a modular handset cord (plug-in type). Battery powered and 9V battery is included.

| Am 01929 | Low battery indicator | $34.95 |

LILA Telephone Answering Machine. Easy to operate. Has call screening function so you can know who is calling. Has only four buttons which are large and easy to use.

| Li 764287 | Compact size 4½ × 6½ inches | $57.95 |

Ameriphone Portable Telephone Amplifier Model PA-20. Lightweight amplifier can be easily strapped onto a telephone handset. It increases the volume of the incoming voice by 20 decibels. It is hearing aid compatible and is ideal for use with telephones that are not modular (hard wired) handsets.

| Am 01961 | AAA battery and carrying case included | $24.95 |

LILA Phone Coil Twisstop. Stops phone cords from twisting.

| Li 603537 | Easy to install | $5.95 |

Sonic Alert Telephone Ring Signalers Model TR 75. When the telephone rings, the signaler flashes any lamp plugged into it. Comes with a switch to allow lamp to be used for room lighting. Can transmit signal to remote receivers in other rooms.

| So TR 75 | Great for TDD locations | $49.95 |

Sonic Alert Doorbell/Telephone Ring Signalers. Allows the patient to be alerted by the flashing of a remote receiver whenever the phone rings or the doorbell is pushed. Different flashing codes for the telephone and doorbell. You will need to order at least one remote receiver.

So TD 500M	For homes with existing doorbells	$89.95
So TD 500	For homes without existing doorbell (Doorbell button and wire included)	$79.95
So SA 201	Remote receiver flashes lights	$45.95
So RH 100	Remote receiver sounds horn (78-85 decibel)	$45.95

Ameriphone Super Phone-Ringer Model SR-100. Loudest telephone ringer on the market. Generates up to 95 decibels of ringing sound. Adjustable volume settings and frequency tone controls. Just plug it into any phone jack. Powered by the telephone line.

| Am 75173 | Easy installation | $36.95 |

Ameriphone Call Alert Model CA-100. Lets the patient know the phone is ringing by flashing a connected lamp. See the telephone ring. Works whether the lamp is on or off. Ideal for those patients using text telephone terminals. Never miss a call again.

| Am 08009 | Switch for turning lamp on or off | $36.95 |

TTY/TDD

Telecommunication companies offer a free service that allows people who are hard or hearing or deaf to talk with people who use a standard telephone. The patient needs to call the relay service and a person called a Communications Assistant (CA) will answer. The CA calls the person the patient wishes to talk to and relays voice or text (TTY/TDD) messages between parties.

In a voice carry over call, the person with the hearing loss speaks directly to the other party. The CA relays the response from the other person via a text message that shows up on the voice carry over phone screen. The patient then reads and responds.

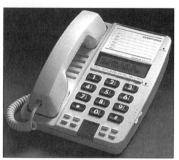

Am 76570

Ameriphone Dialogue VCO Read and Talk Telephone. Enables the very hard of hearing or deaf patient to communicate. Comes with a powerful hearing aid compatible amplifier and automatic tone enhancement. Incoming voices can be amplified up to 30 decibels for loud and clear conversation. Automatically switches between voice and text messages.

Am 76570	Bright ring flasher, lighted 2-line 20 character screen	$189.95

Ameriphone Dialogue III-P With Built in Printer. Text telephone (TTY/TDD) that offers automatic answering system, phone directory, electronic voice, emergency call announcer which sends out emergency signals when 911 is dialed. User friendly 51 key keyboard. Large 20 character fluorescent display. Heavy duty rechargeable batteries allow hours of portable TTY/TDD use. Date and time stamping of all calls. Printer comes with standard or large letter sizes for easy reading. Bright call signaler.

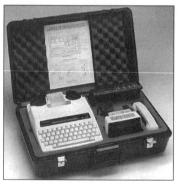

Am 79063

Am 79063	Built-in handles for easy portability.	$489.95
Am 79019	Dust cover/carrying case	$24.95
Am 79080	Dialogue III-P training video	$24.95
Am 79066	Printer paper pack (3 rolls)	$4.95
Am 79067	Printer paper pack (12 rolls)	$16.95

Ameriphone Guest Room Kit Number 6. An all-in-one kit that allows your hearing-impaired patient to have all the communication tools at home or while traveling. Kit includes TTY/TDD telephone, bed shaker and flashing lamp when door is knocked or phone is ringing, visual smoke detector, TV closed caption decoder (for TVs without built-in decoder), telephone amplification handset.

Am	Comes with carrying case	$795.95

Other kits range in price from $499.95 to $789.95. Call for brochure.

Am

Care must be exercised in the purchase of any hearing assistive device. The equipment is expensive, but it can make a huge difference in your patient's attitude, safety and your peace of mind. If at all possible, talk with other people who have hearing problems and find out what has worked for them. Ask if it would be possible to see a demonstration or try the equipment. If you find a device that works for your patient and it is not in our catalog, call us. We will help you locate the device.

Ear Care Products

Le 1295054	Debrox Earwax Control	.5 oz	$6.35
Le 1329390	Ear Plug Soft	2s	$1.75
Le 2224392	Murine Ear Drops w/Syringe	.5 oz	$7.65

Heart Disease

During the average person's lifetime, their heart will beat more than 2.5 billion times.

OVER 66 MILLION AMERICANS have one or more forms of a heart and/or blood vessel disease. Heart disease, along with arthritis and mental retardation, is one of three the biggest reasons for long-term home health care. In 1988, 32 percent of all hospital stays were because of diseases of the circulatory system. With the control of high blood pressure (hypertension), a major risk factor in heart disease, there has been a marked decline in death rates for heart disease. Even so, heart disease remains the largest single cause of death.

Coronary artery disease (CAD) is the most common reason for heart failure in the United States and continues to be the leading cause of death. Nearly 1.25 million new cases of heart failure are diagnosed in the United States each year and about 500,000 people will die from it. About half the heart attacks will occur suddenly with little or no warning. There are about 350,000 bypass surgeries done annually and nearly as many angioplasties

There are three types of heart pain:

- **Ischemic** — the most common form of heart disease. Caused by a reduced blood supply from the narrowing or obstruction in the coronary arteries.
- **Pericardial** — inflammation of the membrane that encloses the heart. Causes include fungal infections, viral infections, cancer from lungs, injury from an accident.
- **Atypical Pain Syndrome** — includes pain from rupture of vessels, obstruction of the pulmonary artery or one of its branches, and the collapse of the valve in the left side of the heart. It can be caused by rheumatic fever, birth defect, heart disease or enlargement of the heart.

Symptoms of heart disease:

- Pain in the chest (crushing heavy feeling).
- Painful breathing.
- Weakness.
- Palpitations due to abnormal heart rhythm.
- Swelling of ankles and legs.
- Indigestion.

A person with cardiac arrest will not have a pulse, not be breathing and collapses suddenly. If the person is breathing, a cardiac arrest has not occurred. The only way to be sure is to measure the electrical activity of the heart with an (EKG machine). Between 20–30 percent of patients who have had a cardiac arrest will recover enough to leave the hospital. The balance of the patients will have damage to the brain and the heart so extensive that they will not recover.

There are a number of ways to treat the heart attack patient:

- **Pacemaker** — a device usually implanted under the skin of the collarbone. It normally operates for years without any problems. The pacemaker sends an electrical signal to the heart to stimulate the heart to beat properly.

- **Angioplasty** — the doctor will thread a catheter through the artery until it reaches the blockage. A tiny balloon will be inflated to squeeze the plaque into the lining of the artery. About 30 percent of the patients will experience re-clogging of the artery and need to have the procedure done again.

- **Coronary Atherectomy** — a small rotating blade inside a catheter is used to clean the arteries by shaving off the plaque in the artery.

- **Bypass surgery** — a surgery that can take 5 hours or more. Surgeons take parts of the veins from the legs or mammary arteries in the chest to replace the damaged arteries and graft them to the affected aorta and arteries. It is very important that you and/or the patient check the hospital to find out how many bypass surgeries are done weekly and what the success rate is. Mortality rates can range from 1 percent to as high as 15 percent. It pays to check.

- **Heart transplant** — heart transplants were first achieved in 1959 and early results were not successful. However, by 1984, 85 percent of heart transplant patients were surviving a year or more. Patients need to consult with their doctor for the criteria to receive a heart transplant.

The risk factors for developing heart disease are numerous. These factors include obesity, tobacco usage, age, alcohol consumption, poor nutrition, exercise regime, high blood pressure, diabetes mellitus, hereditary influences, environmental conditions, alcohol and drug abuse.

Educating the Patient and the Caregiver

Education of the patient and the caregiver are important for the recovery of the heart failure patient. When the patient is discharged from the hospital, detailed written (and oral) instructions for post-treatment care should be given. The caregiver will most likely be instructed by the doctor or nurse on how to measure the patient's blood pressure, take the patient's pulse rate, how to manage the patient's diet, maintain the skin to prevent infection from arterial ulcers, and administer medications such as nitroglycerin.

Noncompliance with doctor recommendations is a major reason for recurring problems to the heart failure patient and for hospital readmission. The patient must understand the severity of the illness when suffering from heart failure. The unwillingness of the patient to follow instructions regarding exercise, smoking cessation, medication dosages or dietary changes is an invitation for an unscheduled visit back to the hospital emergency room.

The caregiver needs to understand the preferences of the patient. A patient may decline to undergo surgery despite medical advice to the contrary. The patient's expectations may be far different from the caregiver's prognosis.

Plans that acknowledge the patient's expectations should be in place in case the patient stops breathing. If the patient does not want to be resuscitated, an "advance directive" will help guide the doctor, attending staff and emergency personnel for the extent of their efforts to revive the patient. The "advance directive" is sometimes called a "living will" or a "do not resuscitate" ("DNR") order (see the section titled "Legal Guidelines" for more detailed instructions on a living will). If the patient wants to be resuscitated, the family should be instructed in the latest cardiopulmonary resuscitation (CPR) techniques (the local chapter of your Red Cross or YMCA/YWCA frequently offers training classes).

Patients of course, can change their mind. They are free to change their DNR request any time. While it is hard to predict the exact behavior of family members when they are faced with an unconscious loved one, dialing 911 may not be the patient's desire. An already frightening scene can be made worse when emergency personnel begin heroic efforts to revive a patient who didn't want to be revived. Wristbands are available to help identify those who have made advance directives. Patients who have made their DNR wishes known should instruct the caregiver and family members of the persons to contact in the event of sudden death.

Dietary changes are likely after a diagnosis of heart failure. The doctor may make recommendations for changes in salt intake, alcohol and fluid consumption, vitamin supplements, and the eating of fatty foods. Limits on salt (sodium) intake are often prescribed, with a recommended limit of 3 grams a day. Nutritionist are able to design a reduced salt diet that is both healthy and flavorful. Caregivers need to be aware of the nutritional components of foods preferred by the patient to monitor salt intake. A totally salt-free diet is never recommended.

Some patients will receive instructions from their doctor to reduce fluid consumption in order to decrease the amount of water stored in the body. Sometimes diuretic drugs are prescribed to help reduce the amount of water in the body. Diuretics, in turn, increase urination. Increased urination may pose a unique sequence of events, particularly for those who are incontinent or find it difficult to move fast enough to get to the bathroom in time to relieve themselves.

One of the adverse side effects of the use of diuretics are blood imbalances, particularly low potassium. Eating fruits and vegetables will aid in replenishing the lost potassium.

Heart failure patients who continue to drink alcohol after their discharge need to be watchful of their consumption levels. A limit of one bottle of beer, a glass of wine or one drink of hard liquor per day may be acceptable.

Heart failure patients can be expected to receive doctor's orders to stop smoking or stop chewing tobacco. For homes with oxygen equipment in use, lighted tobacco products are a hazard.

The weight of the patient should be monitored closely. The patient should be weighed daily — preferably in the morning, after urinating and before eating breakfast. A written record of the daily weighing should be kept and brought to the patient's next doctor's visit. Patients who have gained more than 3 to 5 pounds since their last clinical evaluation should contact their doctor.

Should the patient have bed rest or exercise regularly? Again, education of the patient and the caregiver is crucial on this topic. Some heart ailments will require very limited physical exertion, while others will call for a dedicated and active exercise schedule.

Temperature extremes are also important to keep in mind. Moving from a warm house outside into the frigid cold for the day's walk sometimes causes a shortness of breath even for a healthy person. It's not unusual to hear of someone who suffered a heart attack after leaving a cozy house to shovel a snow-packed driveway. Wearing a scarf or mask over the mouth will help warm the air before it enters the lungs.

Patients should receive specific instructions from the doctor about when it is permissible to resume driving.

It is common for heart failure patients to experience sexual difficulties. Resumption of sexual behavior by heart failure patients may be inhibited for fear of overexertion. The patient should be reassured by the doctor about when sexual activity can resume.

When the patient returns to the doctor for a follow-up examination, the caregiver or other family members should also attend. The doctor may have questions that the patient doesn't answer truthfully or adequately, and the caregiver can supplement the patient's responses.

The caregiver and/or patient can be expected to answer questions about the most strenuous activities that the patient can perform without showing symptoms of over exertion. Topics will most likely cover:

- Walking
- Climbing stairs
- Activities of daily living such as bathing and dressing
- Sleeping patterns
- Morale
- Sexual function
- Concentration
- Alertness
- Work habits
- Diet
- Medicine side effects

What to do:

Contact a doctor — Have the patient make and keep the appointment. The doctor will perform a number of non-invasive tests to find out what, if any damage the heart has sustained. Tests may include an electrocardiogram (EKG), a stress test, an Echocardiogram and sometimes a thallium stress test. Unfortunately, cardiac catheterization — the most informative test — is invasive and usually requires a stay at the hospital.

Contact the American Heart Association — Call 1-800-242-8721 or write to them at 7272 Greenville Avenue, Dallas, TX 75231-4596. They will provide the caregiver and the patient with lots of useful information to assist in understanding the disease. Very responsive and understanding.

Contact the The Coronary Club, Inc. — Call (216) 444-3690 or write to them at 9500 Euclid Avenue, #E37, Cleveland, OH 44195. Offers support groups for heart patients and their families.

Contact the International Society on Hypertension in Blacks, Inc. — Call (404) 875-6263 or write to them at 69 Butler Street, S.E., Atlanta, GA 30303

Contact the National Heart, Lung and Blood Institute Information Center
Call (301) 251-1222 or write to them at P.O. Box 30105, Bethesda, MD 20824.

Contact the National Institute on Aging Information Center — Call 1-800-222-2225 or 1-800-222-4225 or write to them at P.O. Box 8057, Gaithersburg, MD 20898-8057. (TTY) Resource of health and aging issues, including nutrition, exercise and smoking.

Contact The Mended Hearts, Inc. — Call (214) 373-6300 or write to them at 7320 Greenville Ave., Dallas, TX 75231-4596. Founded in 1981, Mended Hearts is a non-profit volunteer organization providing a support network for heart patients. Over 200 chapters are located in the U.S.

Contact the local social services organizations — There are many agencies that will provide information and listings of resources available in your area. Agencies such as the offices on aging, local health agencies as well as religious-affiliated service groups also provide information, training and support. There are also associations and companies that provide care management services to serve as the link between you and community-based services. They charge for their services, so be sure you understand what it will cost to have them provide assistance.

Contact a lawyer — It is very important to act quickly to protect the future security of the patient. There are lawyers that specialize in elder law. You will need to execute a durable power of attorney, a living will and/or a living trust. Living trusts appear to be the best way to handle the estate because you can avoid probate and not have the estate's assets tied up by the courts. Contact us at ☎ 1-800-546-5559 for a listing of lawyers in your area.

Safety — Organize the home to permit the patient to carry on as many normal routines as possible. Other tips and items that make for a safer home can be found in the section titled "Modifying Your Home and Making it Safer."

Communication — Explain to the patient what is happening. Tell family and friends. Explain the symptoms and tell family and friends that you need their support and love. Tell them how and when they can help. Be specific about your needs. Draw up a plan of action that allows everyone to understand the role that they can (and must) play.

LeBoeuf's Services

Call **LeBoeuf's** ☎ 1-800-546-5559 for the phone numbers and addresses of the following service providers in your area. Please have the patient's name, address, zip code, age, telephone number and physical circumstances (Alzheimer's, heart problem, arthritis, etc.) when you call.

- LeBoeuf's Consulting Service

    Wheelchairs (design, ultra-light, sports chairs, etc.)

    Van Conversions

    Electronics
    - Hearing
    - Vision
    - Security
    - Communication (TTY, Call Buttons, Telephones, etc.)
    - Television, VCR's, Radio, Stereo
    - Computers and Softwear

- LeBoeuf's Incontinent Supply Service
- LeBoeuf's Respite Network
- LeBoeuf's Home Modification Planning Service
- LeBoeuf's Assistive Travel Agency
- LeBoeuf's Employment Screening Service
- Hospitals in your area, or in area patient is traveling to
- Nursing homes
- Hospice
- Visiting nurse associations
- Adult day care programs
- Respite care (nursing homes, support groups,)
- Social services case workers
- Household help

Heat Stroke, Heat Exhaustion & Hypothermia

Heat stroke, heat exhaustion and a below normal body temperature called hypothermia all can be very serious and even fatal if not detected and treated promptly. Those with heart and circulatory problems, stroke or diabetes are especially vulnerable.

Heat Stroke

Heat stroke is usually caused by overexposure to extreme heat — severe fever (rare), working in a very hot environment, or unaccustomed exposure to the sun in a hot, humid climate — and a breakdown of the body's heat-regulating mechanisms. Heat stroke is a condition that requires immediate attention and treatment.

Symptoms include:

- Fainting.
- Dizziness.
- Headache.
- Nausea.
- Loss of consciousness.
- Body temperature of 104°F or higher (rectal); may reach 107°F.
- Rapid pulse.
- Flushed skin.
- Profuse sweating.

Immediate emergency help should be sought. Wrap the patient without clothes in a cold, wet sheet. Keep the sheet wet all the time. You can also continually sponge the patient with cold water. Cooling can be increased by fanning the patient. If the patient has lost consciousness, place in the recovery position while being cooled. Treatment should continue until the patient's rectal temperature reaches 101°F or the victim feels cool to the touch. If the patient is conscious, give salt tablets or a weak salt solution to sip. To make the weak salt solution, dissolve 1/4 of a teaspoon of salt in a glass (about a pint) of water. If heat stroke is treated early, the patient will usually recover fully.

Heat Exhaustion

Heat exhaustion results from a loss of body water and salt. The main reasons are insufficient water intake, insufficient salt intake and not sweating. If untreated, it can lead to heat stroke.

Symptoms include:

- Fatigue.
- Fainting.
- Dizziness.

- Nausea
- Giddiness
- Heat cramps in legs, arms, back or abdomen
  (only when salt loss is heavy)
- Pale and clammy skin

If conscious, the patient should lie down in a cool place with their head 12 inches lower than their feet. Have the patient take salt tablets or sip water with 1/4 teaspoon of salt dissolved in it. If unconscious, place the patient in the recovery position. With rest and the replacement of water and salt, the patient will usually recover fully. You should contact the doctor immediately.

Hypothermia

Hypothermia (body temperature below 95°F) can occur when a patient is exposed to mild to severe cold without protection. If the patient's body temperature drops below 93.2°F, the heart may stop beating. More susceptible to hypothermia are the chronically ill, the poor who cannot afford heating fuel and those who do not dress warmly. There are some people who, for unknown reasons, cannot feel cold or shiver and do not produce body heat when they need it. Most cases of hypothermia occur in poorly heated homes of elderly people.

The only way to detect hypothermia is to use a low-reading thermometer or a regular thermometer that has been shaken down below 95°F. If the patient's temperature is below 95°F, emergency help should be sought immediately.

Symptoms include:

- Slurred speech.
- Pale, puffy faced, waxy skin.
- Decreased urine output.
- Sluggishness.
- Confusion.
- Drowsiness.
- Cold armpits.
- Faint and irregular heart beats.
- Severe shivering at the onset of symptoms.

If hypothermia is suspected, call for emergency help. Give the patient warm drinks and cover the head. Do not let the patient walk. Do not warm the skin by rubbing. Do not give the patient any alcohol. Warm the patient by moving to a warm place and, if the patient is young, giving a hot bath. **Do not give the elderly a hot bath.** It can cause a rush of blood to the surface of the body, thereby reducing the amount of blood to the heart and brain, which could cause death. If elderly, raise the temperature in the room to at least 78°F, cover with blankets and warm the patient at a rate of 1 degree an hour.

Steps to lessen the risk of hypothermia include keeping the temperature of the home or apartment at a minimum of 65°F. Make sure that the patient dresses warmly and eats properly. Elderly people should eat hot food and drink warm drinks several times a day. Always wear a warm hat during cold weather — more than 20 percent of body heat loss is through the head.

Hip Replacement

HIP REPLACEMENTS are most often performed in older people because of falls and osteoarthritis or rheumatoid arthritis that has spread to the hip. The head and neck of the femur (thigh bone) are replaced with a metal ball. The damaged socket is lined with a metal backed plastic socket. The operation normally takes about two hours and hospitalization is for three to five days. Full recovery takes about four months. Younger patients will not usually have this operation because their greater activity puts more strain on the joint and an artificial joint won't hold up.

This operation has been very successful and has allowed many patients to lead normal lives again. Continuing development in the operation is on-going to make the artificial joint last longer.

Before leaving the hospital make sure that you and the patient know:
- How to dress.
- How to turn in bed.
- How to get in and out of bed, shower, car and bathtub.
- Safety precautions to prevent dislocation.
- What medication and the dosage to take.

The patient should take it easy for a week or two after the operation and:
- Sit in chairs with arms the patient can use for support when getting up.
- Keep the leg that has been operated on facing forward whether walking, sitting or lying down.
- Exercise as the doctor and/or therapist has prescribed.
- Lie down and raise the legs if they swell after walking.
- Place a pillow between the legs when lying on the side.
- Wear support stockings except when in bed at night.
- Learn how to use the crutches and walker (usually for about 6-10 weeks).
- Learn how to use a cane (usually for about 4 weeks).

When climbing stairs, the patient should have someone standing behind to assist. The patient should begin by putting the good foot onto the step. Then, while pushing up with the crutches, straighten the good leg. Next, bring the repaired leg up to the step followed by the crutches. Repeat this sequence. Going down the stairs, the patient's helper should stand in front. Place the crutches on the step in front of the patient. Then move the repaired leg. Shift body weight to crutches and bend the knee of the good leg. Remember — good leg first up and bad leg first down. The doctor and/or the therapist will demonstrate for the patient.

The patient should not:
- Sit on low couches or chairs.
- Bend way over when picking something up.
- Twist when reaching for objects.
- Turn toes in.
- Cross the legs or turn the knee or hip inward or outward.
- Take a tub bath.
- Scrub the hip incision.
- Lift heavy items.
- Drive a car until doctor gives permission.
- Have sexual intercourse until doctor says it is okay (about 6 weeks).

If a tooth needs to be pulled, or there will be other oral surgery performed, make sure that you tell the dentist about the surgery (doctor will probably prescribe antibiotics a couple of days before and after)

Call the doctor if:
- Redness or swelling develops around the incision.
- There is drainage from the incision.
- A fever or chill develops.
- There is severe hip pain.
- A sudden pain and a clicking or popping sound in the hip.
- One leg becomes shorter and the foot turns outward.
- There is a complete loss of leg motion.

Ambulatory Aids

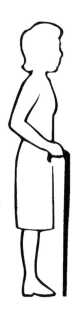

Canes

If the patient is experiencing periods of dizziness, weakness, pain and/or poor coordination, a walker or cane can be purchased to assist in walking. The cane should be held on the stronger side of the body (opposite the weaker leg) and moved forward at the same time the weaker leg moves forward. If you are walking with the patient, walk on the side with the weaker leg. If the patient loses balance and starts to fall, it will usually be to the weaker side.

Selecting a cane:

- Height of handle should be at the top of the hip joint.
- Weight of the cane should be such that the patient has no trouble lifting it.
- Grip should be comfortable and secure (does not turn in the hand).
- Select either a single-tip base or 4-legged base (quad cane).
- In some cases, the patient may prefer to use two canes instead of a walker.

How to fit a cane

- Make sure the patient has on shoes normally worn.
- The top of the cane should be even with the top of the hip joint.
- The cane fits properly when, while standing straight with the cane tip six inches forward and six inches to the side, the elbow is bent at approximately a 30 degree angle.

Wooden Canes. All of our canes are crafted from northern hardwoods, come with a rubber safety tip, weather resistant finish and are 36″ long. To cut a cane to size, take off the rubber tip, measure the height (allow ¼″ for the thickness of the rubber tip) and use a saw to cut it to size. Use a miter box to get a straight cut. If you do not have a saw or a miter box, call your local hardware store and ask if they will cut the cane to size for you. Most will be willing to assist you at no charge.

SunMark Standard Wooden Canes. Available in ⅞″ or 1″ diameter with heavy-duty rubber tips.

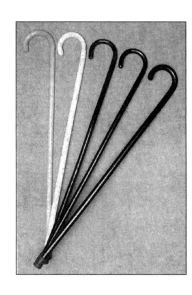

Le 277-9809	Walnut finish 7/8″ diameter	$9.95
Le 114-2728	Natural finish 7/8″ diameter	9.95
Le 116-1827	Black finish 7/8″ diameter	9.95
Le 114-2736	Natural finish 1″ diameter	9.95
Le 116-1884	Black finish 1″ diameter	9.95
Le 144-8836	Walnut finish 1″ diameter extra long 42″	14.95

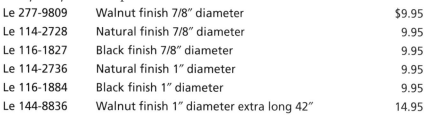

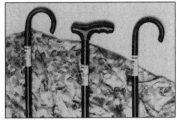

Le 277-9825   Le 116-1793
          Le 116-1850

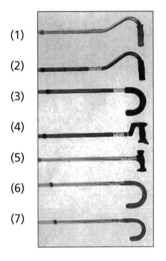

(1)

(2)

(3)

(4)

(5)

(6)

(7)

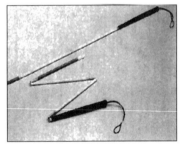

Le 174-7021

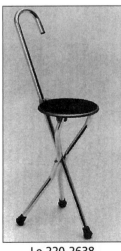

Le 220-2638

SunMark Ladies Wooden Canes. Canes are 13/16″ diameter with heavy duty rubber tips.

Le 277-9825	Standard handle, Rosewood finish	$10.95
Le 116-1850	"T" handle, Walnut finish	10.95
Le 116-1793	Standard handle, Ebony finish	10.95

SunMark Adjustable Aluminum Canes (300 pound weight limit). ⅞″ diameter sturdy anodized aluminum, adjustable from 29″ to 38″ with locking nut. Tips are steel reinforced and come with heavy duty rubber tips. Each cane is adjustable in 1″ increments.

Le 242-8423	Orthopedic handle, aluminum finish	(1)	$19.95
Le 183-0546	Hypalon handgrip, bronze-tone finish	(2)	22.95
Le 221-6844	Hypalon handgrip, bronze-tone finish	(3)	24.95
Le 138-6283	Orthopedic handle offset, bronze-tone finish	(4)	25.95
Le 220-1762	Devon handle, aluminum finish	(5)	19.95
Le 114-2751	Standard handle, aluminum finish	(6)	13.95
Le 220-3164	Ladies standard handle, aluminum finish	(7)	13.95

SunMark Folding Cane (250 pound weight limit). Orthopedic handle for secure grip. Bronze finish. Folds to less than 12″ and unfolds automatically. Adjusts from 33″ to 36″.

| Le 197-6893 | Folding cane w/ orthopedic handle | $26.95 |

SunMark Folding Cane. Pistol Grip Handle. Black finish aluminum with walnut handle and clear vinyl carrying case. 36″ long. A very handsome cane for the man about town.

| Le 116-1629 | Folding cane w/ pistol grip handle | $23.95 |

SunMark Folding Cane for the Blind. Putter grip, wrist strap and nylon tip. White reflective tape and red bottom, heavy duty but lightweight aluminum. For use as a guide cane, not a support cane.

| Le 174-7021 | Folding guide cane for the blind | $38.95 |

SunMark Seat Cane. Folds out into a sturdy and stable seat. Aluminum finish and folds to 36″. Seat is 8½″ diameter and 18″ high, holds 200 pounds.

| Le 220-2638 | Folding seat cane | $36.95 |

Momentum Medical Supercane™. Second lower handle helps the patient stand up easily from chair or bed. Adjustable, lightweight and easy to use.

Le 172-6918	Large	Black	$54.95
Le 172-5985	Medium	Black	$54.95
Le 172-6397	Small	Black	$54.95

Cane Replacement Tips and Accessories. It is a good idea to order replacement tips when ordering a cane. Tip life will vary. You never want the patient to use a cane that does not have the rubber tip on and in good shape.

Le 188-3834	Package of two fits 13/16″ or 3/4″ shaft	$2.19
Le 144-8943	Package of two fits 3/4″ aluminum shaft	$2.95
Le 188-3842	Package of two fits 7/8″ shaft	$2.19
Le 360-3495	Package of two fits 1″ shaft	$2.29
Le 144-8729	Ice grips for canes. Flips up for indoor use.	$10.95
Le 197-5846	Cane holder holds cane against table or desk. Fits shafts from 5/8″ to 1″ in diameter.	$4.95
Le 168-3960	Cane wrist strap for all wooden canes	$5.95

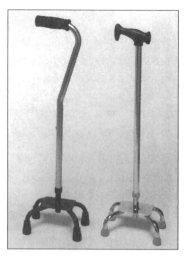

Le 220-3198 / Le 379-5416

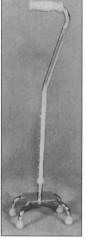

Le 379-5531

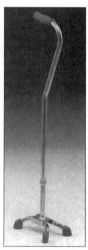

Le 220-6613

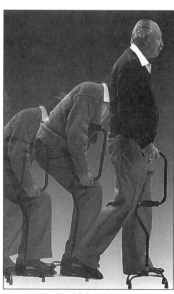

Le 220-6704

| Le 187-5418 | Quad cane tips. Fit 5/8" shaft. Package of 4 suction type tips, black. | $3.95 |
| Le 220-3032 | Quad cane tips. Fit 3/4" shaft. Package of 4 nonsuction type tips, gray. | $3.95 |

SunMark Quad Canes. Quad canes provide more stability. The patient can make an adjustment to use the cane with either the right or left hand without tools. Height adjustable with spring button. All carry a lifetime warranty on workmanship and materials.

SunMark Quad Cane. Adjustable from 29″ to 38″. ⅞″ diameter, chrome plated steel base, gray rubber tips and gray rubber handgrips.

Le 379-5473	Orthopedic handle, large base.	$32.95
Le 220-3198	Orthopedic handle, small base. Bronze color shaft with black base.	$49.95
Le 379-5416	Devon handle, small base. Aluminum finish. Height adjustable from 29" to 38"	$41.95

SunMark Orthopedic Handle Quad Cane. Low profile. Anodized aluminum tubing ⅞″ in diameter. Adjustable from 29″ to 38″. Chrome-plated steel base. Gray rubber handgrips and reinforced gray rubber tips.

| Le 379-5531 | Small base quad cane | $32.95 |

Lumex Quad Canes (250 pound weight limit). Uni-Line design places the patient's weight directly over base for maximum stability. Positive push-button height adjustment with locking nut. Height adjusts from 29½″ to 38½″. ⅝″ tubing at the tips. Small base.

| Le 220-6613 | Small base quad cane | $54.95 |

Ortho-Ease Hand Grip. Angle of grip adjusts to hand and wrist angle. Rounded edge plate on base prevents scraping and bruising of ankles. Base size 7½″ × 12″.

| Le 220-5664 | | $49.95 |

Ortho-Ease Hand Grip. Angle of grip adjusts to hand and wrist angle. Rounded edge plate on base prevents scraping and bruising of ankles. Base size 6″ × 8″

| Le 220-4253 | | $49.95 |

ActiveAid Quad Cane. Attractive chrome finish. Full 7″ height adjustment (31″ to 38″) with a built-in tool for easy adjustment. Base size 5½″ × 8″ weighs 2 pounds and 9″ × 13″ base size weighs 2½ pounds. Wood handles

| Ac Quad 101 | Small base | $48.95 |
| Ac Quad 102 | Large base | $48.95 |

Momentum Medical Superquad™. Strong, four-legged steel base designed for people who need extra stability while getting up and walking. Features built-in lower hand grip.

Le 220-6704	Large	Black, Standard base	$79.95
Le 222-5944	Medium	Black, Standard base	$79.95
Le 221-7644	Small	Black, Standard base	$79.95

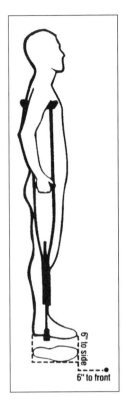

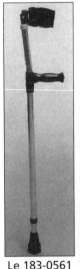

Le 183-0561

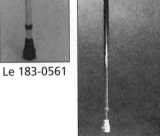

Tu 2624/1

How to fit crutches

Align the crutch tips approximately 6″ to the front and 6″ to the outside of the feet. Crutches fit correctly when the top of the crutches rest on the chest cavity 2″ below the armpit and the elbow is bent at approximately 15 to 30 degrees. The weight of the patient's body should be borne by the arms and not the armpits. Continued pressure on the armpit can cause crutch palsy — a weakness of the forearm, wrist and hand. Be especially careful when using crutches when it is wet outside. Dry the tips as soon as you get inside.

How to use crutches

There are a number of different manners of walking for a patient using crutches. The method of walking depends on the patient's ability to take steps, the patient's ability to bear weight on one or both legs and the patient's ability to hold their body erect. The doctor or therapist will decide what is best for the patient. If you are in doubt, be sure that you ask the doctor or therapist. Be sure that you and the patient are taught by the doctor and/or therapist how to go up and down stairs. Remember, the affected leg is always supported by the crutches.

Crutches

SunMark Crutches (300 lb. recommended weight limit). Laminated wooden crutches. Come with underarm pads, solid handgrips and tips. Preformed bows make adjustments quick and easy. High-gloss, weather resistant finish.
Le 276-1567 $32.95

Aluminum Crutches. Include underarm pads, solid handgrips and extra large tips. Adjust from 46″ to 60″ for patient height 5′4″ to 6′6″. Plastic tops are light yet strong and handgrips are contoured around bows to prevent rotation.
Le 220-3107 $42.95

Aluminum Crutches with Push-Button Adjustment. Adjust for patient heights from 5′2″ to 5′10″. Fitting scale printed on crutch allows for quick and easy adjustment. Includes pads, tips and grips.
Le 221-1563 $45.95

Adult Forearm Crutch. 1″ anodized aluminum. Swivel-jointed cuff section of vinyl coated steel. Handgrip is heavy steel welded and epoxy coated with deluxe vinyl contour grip. Extra large crutch tips with molded metal inserts for added strength. Leg and cuff adjust independently with spring-loaded buttons. Adjusts from 30½″ to 38½″ for patient's 5′2″ to 6′2″. Lifetime warranty on workmanship and materials.
Le 183-0561 $66.95

Tubular Fabricators Tall Adult Platform-Forearm Crutches. Hook and loop fastening system. Push button adjustment. Easy change pad with adjustable grip angle.
Tu 2624/1   Height adjusts from 42 to 51 inches $95.95

Crutch Replacement Tips and Accessories

SunMark Crutch Accessory Kit. Outfits one pair of standard crutches with pads, grips and tips.

Le 220-0863 $12.95

Care Products Sheepskin Covers for Crutches. Synthetic sheepskin covers for axillary pad and handgrip. Fastens securely with Velcro, 2-ply cushioning. Patented protection against soreness, rashes, blisters, pain and chafing. Machine washable and dryer safe.

Le 189-2199 $20.95

SunMark Crutch Tips. 100% natural rubber, extra tread for longer wear, safety and skidproof traction. Extra large base absorbs shocks. Fits 3/4″ and 7/8″ diameter crutches.

Le 188-3859	Pack of 2	$3.95
Le 188-3867	SunMark crutch tips super size. For long term use Base diameter of tip 2″. Fits 3/4″ and 7/8″ crutches Pack of 2	$4.95

Selecting walkers

Walkers are used by patients of all ages. Patients with recent amputations, hip surgery, hip replacements, arthritis, etc. use walkers to reduce strain on hips and knees. Walkers are usually divided into four groups:

- RIGID — Lift up and put down. Patient will need partial strength in both hands and wrists to lift and place the walker.
- FOLDING — lift up and put down, but fold for storage or in an auto or closet.
- TWO-WHEELED — Wheels are in the front. The back legs without wheels act as a brake. Most walkers have either 3-inch or 5-inch wheels. The back legs act as brakes when you put weight on them.
- FOUR-WHEELED — Only those with hand brakes are listed in our catalog. While more unstable than walkers without wheels, wheeled walkers make it possible for a patient with little upper body strength to move about.

The doctor or the physical therapist must assist the patient in choosing the right walker. You should also consider where the walker will be used before you buy. If the area in which the patient will be traveling is unpaved, or there are a number of stairs, a wheeled walker would be impractical. A little common sense will save you and the patient a lot of aggravation and money as well as improving the patient's safety. For those patients who are living in a two story home, it would be a good idea to buy two walkers – one for downstairs and one for upstairs. Walkers and steps just don't mix.

When shopping for a walker, the patient should consider the following:

- Height — The walker height should be adjustable so elbows are 20-30 degrees from vertical.
- Width — The patient must be able to stand within the frame.

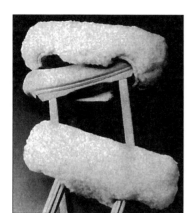

Le 189-2199

Hint: If the button on an adjustable cane, walker or crutch disappears, it has not fallen out. It probably has twisted and/or moved up or down in the shaft. If you are out of town and this happens, ask the hotel if they can have the maintenance staff move the button back into place. It will take them just a minute or two to fix. You can normally get the button back in place yourself using a coat hanger (a good stiff one), a pair of pliers and a flashlight.

TO ORDER CALL TOLL FREE

LeBoeuf's

PHONE **1-800-546-5559**

FAX **1-800-233-9692**

Hearing Impaired with TDD
CALL **1-800-855-2880**

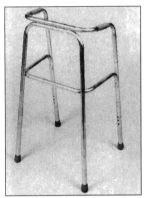

Le 119-5882

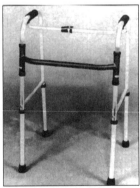

Le 220-3701

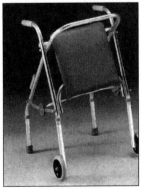

Le 323-9845

- Depth — The patient must be able to stand within the frame.
- Weight — The patient must be able to lift the walker without undue strain.
- Handgrips — Must be comfortable and positioned to support the patient's weight.
- Wheels — The use of 5-inch or larger wheels makes navigating over difficult terrain easier.

Using a walker

If one leg is weaker than the other, move the walker and the weak leg ahead together about 6 inches, then move the stronger leg ahead while the patient's weight is borne by the weaker leg and both arms. The doctor and/or the physical therapist along with a good dose of common sense will dictate what type of walker is appropriate for the patient. It is important to work with the doctor and/or the therapist to insure that the patient will benefit from the walker and the patient will know how to use the walker safely.

There are a number of accessories that can be attached to the walker:

Baskets	Cane or crutch clips
Bags	Oxygen tank holders (on wheeled models only)
Trays	Forearm support
Seats	

SunMark Walkers (250 recommended weight limit). Rigid walker constructed of 1″ aluminum. Reinforced stress points, cushioned handgrips. Height adjustment 32″ to 36″. Width between hand grips 16½″ depth 19½″. Overall width 22½″.
Le 119-5882 $44.95

SunMark Folding Walker. Easy to store. Bronze finish accented in black. Durable black sponge grips. Height adjustment 32″ to 37″. Cross braces for optimum stability. Easy folding action.
Le 220-3701 $89.95

SunMark Folding Walker. With height adjustment from 32″ to 37″. Cross brace fits over toilet. Width between handgrips 17¾″. Chrome plated steel front cross brace. Gray cushioned handgrips. Lifetime warranty. Special open/close design for easy folding.
Le 379-5655 $69.95

Carex Folding Walker with Seat. Vinyl seat folds down for use when needed. 5″ front wheels allow for easier movement of walker without lifting. Skid resistant rubber tips on back act as brakes. Height adjustment 31″ to 36″. Seat height 19½″, width between handgrips 17″.
Le 323-9845 $134.95

SunMark Extra Wide Folding Walker. Width between handgrips is 19½″. 1″ aluminum tubing with cross brace that fits over toilet. Special open/close design for easy folding. Height adjusts from 32″ to 37″.
Le 348-0787 $112.95

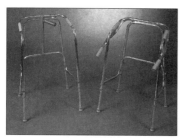

Tu 2112/1

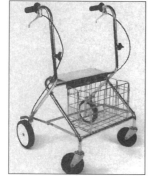

Le 111-0550 ↓   Le 111-0899 ↑

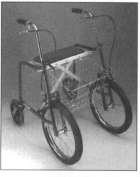

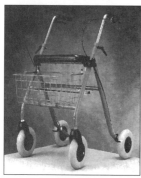

Le 162-0293

SunMark Walkerette Folding Aluminum Walker. Especially useful as a support for the user who has trouble rising from a sitting position. Angled legs for full tip contact with floor. Height adjustment 32″ to 36″. 14″ depth

Le 220-0756		**$55.95**
Le 179-5822	5″ Mag wheels for the folding walker with extensions (Le 220-3701)	**$28.95**
Le 197-3254	Glide brakes for folding walker (Le 220-3701)	**$34.95**

Tubular Fabricators Universal Stroke Walker. Walker is designed to use with one hand. The balanced center grip can be positioned for either right or left hand use. Over the toilet design. Height adjustable in 1-inch increments.

Tu 2112/1	Capacity of 250 pounds	**$94.95**

Wheeled Walkers

American E-Z Wheeled Walker. With adjustable handlebars 30″ to 36″. Front wheels swivel for easy maneuverability. Folds easily. 24″ wide and weighs only 17 pounds. Locking handbrakes.

Le 111-0899   **$399.95**

American Comb-O-Cycle with 8″ rear swivel wheels and 16″ airless front tires for the roughest terrain. Handlebars adjust from 29″ to 42″. Locking handbrakes and backrest. Folds to 8″ wide and stands alone.

Le 111-0550   **$529.95**

American Out-N-About Walker with adjustable handlebars. 8″ wheels, front wheels swivel. Padded seat. Can accommodate bracket for holding an oxygen cylinder. Locking handbrakes and backrest. Can be folded to 6″ wide and stand alone.

Le 111-0444   **$499.95**

Accessories for American Walkers:

Le 111-0253	Small wire basket for E-Z walker, Out-N-About and Comb-O-Cycle. 8½″ × 13″ × 9″ deep.	**$30.95**
AM 0031	Large wire basket for Comb-O-Cycle only 8½″ × 13″ × 16″ deep	**$59.95**
AM 0037	Cane holder for Comb-O-Cycle and Out-N-About only	**$34.95**
AM 0041	Food and beverage tray for Comb-O-Cycle and Out-N-About only	**$59.95**
AM 0051	Plaid pouch for E-Z Walker, Comb-O-Cycle and Out-N-About	**$34.95**
AM 0065	Oxygen cylinder holder for Out-N-About only	**$53.95**

Guardian Easy Care™ Walker has dual folding mechanism that allows sides to fold independently. Reinforced front cross brace. Folds to less than 4″ depth. For patients 5′4″ to 6′2″. 300 pound recommended weight limit.

Le 363-8194   **$116.95**

Jadestone Wheeled Walker with seat and basket, 2″ wide soft tires, orthopedic grip. Handles adjust from 30″ to 38¼″, push button wheel stops for more stability when seated. Folds for storage.

Le 162-0293   **$308.95**

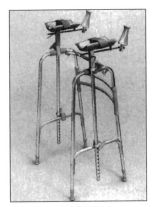

Le 220-8544

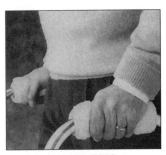

Le 189-2322

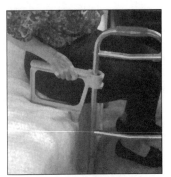

Le 116-8426

Walker Accessories

Le 220-8544	Lumex forearm walker attachments with universal pair clamp that will fit on all walkers. Forearm rests can be adjusted and angled. Velcro strap for security and comfort. Sold in pairs only.	$169.95
Le 355-3435	Carex walker basket fits most walkers. Velcro straps for easy attachment.	$19.95
Le 189-2322	Care Products synthetic sheepskin covers with 2-ply cushioning reduce irritation. Machine washable and dryer safe.	$15.95
Le 348-9762	Guardian pouch attaches easily with Velcro tabs. Zippered pouch with three side pockets. Machine washable 19½" long, 7" deep and 12" high.	$46.95
Le 116-8426	Crestline Easy Up Handle for all walkers. Provides support while getting out of bed, chairs, autos and couches.	$29.95
Le 220-0731	Walker tips for 1⅛" tubing. Packs of 4. Rubber tips with steel washer.	$4.95
Le 221-3130	Walker tips for 1" tubing. Packs of 4. Rubber tips with steel washer.	$4.95

Wheelchairs and Scooters

Wheelchairs were first used in the United States during the Civil War. In 1907, the first patent application for a wheelchair was made – a folding wheelchair with a steel frame. Since then the number and combination of options available on wheelchairs has become virtually unlimited.

Wheelchairs enable the patient to have freedom of movement and many people in wheelchairs can get around as quickly as someone who can walk. The appropriate selection of a wheelchair should be made by you, the patient, the doctor and/or the physical or occupational therapist. You and the patient should investigate different types of wheelchairs and available options. Your investigation of the wheelchairs, along with the patient's preferences, plus the knowledge and experience of the doctor and the therapist will insure that the wheelchair will meet the needs of the patient.

Pick out options that the patient believes are needed and discuss these options with the doctor and/or the therapist prior to having the prescription written. Under Medicare, only a doctor can make the determination of the patient's medical need for a wheelchair and its options. Check with **LeBoeuf's** ☎ **1-800-546-5559** for the latest requirement under Medicare. Even if the doctor has prescribed a lightweight wheelchair, Medicare may disallow it and the patient will either have to accept a standard wheelchair or pay for the difference in price. If the patient is turned down by Medicare for the wheelchair that you, the patient and the doctor believe to be the best for the patient, you and the patient can file additional documentation which justifies the medical necessity of the wheelchair.

If the patient is non-ambulatory, but has some upper body strength, always buy or rent wheelchairs with removable and/or swing-away arms to facilitate patient transfers in and out of the wheelchair. In many cases, the patient can perform transfers to the toilet, bed, bathtub, shower, chair, etc. without your assistance. This is true only if proper thought has gone into the wheelchair purchase and there are appropriate grab bars, hoists, and other assistive devices available for the patient to use.

Most wheelchairs are from 27 inches to 29 inches in width and about 3 feet 6 inches in length. Turning space needed is from 4 feet 11 inches to 5 feet 2 inches. Most folding wheelchairs will collapse to about 11 inches in width and 3 feet 6 inches in length.

Typical chair armrest levels are 2 feet 5 inches, thigh level is 2 feet 3 inches and the chair seat level is 18 inches to 20 inches with pad. Pads are a necessary part of the wheelchair if the patient is using the chair for sitting for long periods and not just transferring from bed to auto, from bed to shower, etc. To prevent pressure sores (bed sores), you will need to have the physical therapists and/or the doctor prescribe the type of seat cushion that would be suitable for your patient.

Manual wheelchairs range in price from about $600 to as much as $4,000 for a special design. Most of the lightweight sporty wheelchairs range in price from $1,800 to $2,800.

Wheelchairs come in dozens of sizes, types, shapes and varieties and there are well over 2,500 different manufacturers and distributors. Basically, there are two types of wheelchairs:

- Manual wheelchairs — For those who have enough upper body strength to propel themselves.
- Power wheelchairs — A wheelchair or a three or four wheeled scooter with a seat and powered by batteries.

When working with the doctor or therapist to fit the wheelchair to the patient, you need to know why they have chosen:

- Frame — Can the wheelchair be folded? What options are available such as stainless steel, chrome, aluminum, magnesium, steel, titanium? The frame determines the strength and most of the weight of the wheelchair.
- Upholstery — Is it rugged enough for daily use? What is the material? How do you take care of the upholstery (e.g. nylon, velour, polyester, parapack cloth, vinyl and leather)?
- Seating System — If part of the chair, will it prevent pressure sores? What should the posture of the patient be? Is the frame compatible with the seating system being considered? Is the back rest of sufficient height? There are many pads used with wheelchairs that will prevent pressure sores and make a very comfortable seat.
- Brakes — Will the patient be able to set the brake? There are many types of brakes and you must be sure that the patient can operate the brake without undue effort.
- Wheels and Tires — Most wheelchairs have four wheels. Two large wheels in the back and two small wheels in the front. The rear wheels are normally about 24 inches in diameter and the front wheels 8 inches in diameter. Wheels can be pneumatic or solid rubber, oversize width for off the road use (beach), steel-reinforced radials and semi-pneumatic.
- Footrests — Can be fixed, detachable, swing-away, elevating or a combination. Some may have a leg rest attachment that supports the leg below the knee.
- Armrest — Can be full length, desk-length, detachable, height adjustable, flip-up or a combination of these features. Some of the sports model wheelchairs are designed without armrests.

The wheelchair is usually fitted to the patient by a physical or occupational therapist and/or a doctor. Be sure that if a cushion is going to be used, the measurements are done with the cushion in place and the patient is wearing the type of clothing normally worn. Wheelchairs are usually fitted using the following measurements:

- Seat width 2 or more inches wider than the hips or thighs.
- Seat depth 2 to 3 inches deeper than the back of the buttocks to behind the knee.
- Seat height 2 inches or more from knee to bottom of heel.

Normally the typical reach of a patient in a wheelchair is 5 feet 8 inches high and 4 feet 8 inches forward reach. Eye level is typically 4 feet and the foot height on the foot rest is 9 inches from the floor.

- Back height low as possible. Four fingers should fit between the top of the seat back to under the armpits.
- Arm height 1 to 2 inches from under seat to under elbow. The arm should rest comfortably and form a triangle between the back, armrest and arm.

It is very important that the patient be properly fitted to avoid pressure sores and to make the user as comfortable as possible.

Manual Wheelchairs

Manual wheelchairs are usually broken down into five groups. Lightweight/ Sports, Standard, Child/Adolescent, Specialty and Institutional. The wheelchairs will range from a low of 12 pounds to a high of 45 pounds. Many can be folded and placed in the trunk of a car or out of the way for storage.

- Lightweight wheelchairs were originally developed for use in sports such as basketball, tennis, road racing, etc. Because of their lighter weight, many wheelchair users realized that they could get around with much less effort and they have become very popular. But, because of their lighter frames, very heavy people may be unable to use them. There are variety of colors and models. There are even three-wheeled models for tennis and basketball. Most of these chairs weigh from 14 to 25 pounds.
- Standard wheelchairs prior to the 1980s were very heavy and hard to maneuver. Most standard wheelchairs have removable arm rests, swing-away footrests and push handles to allow the caregiver to push the chair.
- Child/Adolescent wheelchairs are designed to meet a child's needs as they grow. Many are now designed to be colorful and have some style to them. The doctor or the therapist will determine how much support the chair must provide, how it will be propelled and what special features are needed.
- Specialty wheelchairs are built to meet the specific needs of the patient. They may be designed to allow for one-handed operation, be powered by the feet, to allow the patient to change from a sitting to a standing position, and many other special designs to allow the patient as much help as and flexibility as possible.
- Institutional wheelchairs are the least expensive and are designed for the movement of patients in a hospital or nursing home. The chairs are not fitted for the patient, are not normally supplied with a pad to prevent pressure sores (bed sores) and are only for temporary use. These types of chairs are what you usually get when you rent a wheelchair.

Powered Wheelchairs

Powered wheelchairs are usually divided into two types:

- A powered wheelchair that looks like a regular wheelchair and weighs from 85 pounds to more than 300 pounds. Some can be folded for storage and transport after the batteries are removed. Drive systems are gear driven, direct drive or belt driven. Most are powered by two 12-volt batteries — normally group 22 or 24 batteries. If you are considering any airline travel, most airlines require gel cell batteries. Gel cell batteries are also less of a maintenance problem and are the best battery choice in most, if not all, cases. Depending on the weight and terrain, a battery powered chair will go from 7 to 40 miles between charges. Pricing ranges from $3,500 to $12,000 or more. Rarely are any priced under $3,500, unless you can find a used one.

- Scooter type. Scooters are usually less expensive than powered wheelchairs. Prices are in the $1,500 to $3,500 range. Scooters generally require upper body strength and arm function. Patients should also be able to support themselves in an upright position. Be sure to consider what type of lift or ramp will accommodate both a wheelchair and a scooter. Basically, the scooter is a golf cart with special features. Most scooters have a narrower wheelbase and width than a wheelchair and, therefore, are somewhat more maneuverable.

There are many options available for wheelchairs. These options include bags, pouches, ash trays, transfer boards, trays, seat belts, crutch or cane holder, clothing guards, I.V. holders, oxygen holders, cushions and many others.

Options that are available for wheelchairs and/or scooters include bags, pouches, transfer boards, trays, seat belts, oxygen holder, IV holder, crutch or cane holder, clothing guards and cushions. There are many cushions on the market that will prevent pressure sores when sitting in a wheelchair. If the patient will be spending a good part of the day in a wheelchair, choosing the best cushion you can afford is a wise investment. Your doctor or therapist will work with the patient to prescribe the best cushion.

Things to consider when buying a power wheelchair or scooter include:

- What is the warranty period, if any, and who will perform warranty work?

- Are repair parts available and how long for delivery?

- Does the seller have a toll-free customer service number?

- What is the maximum weight capacity of the unit? (Maximum weight should be the highest weight a wheelchair or scooter can safely carry without risk of structural failure.)

- Does the power unit have the speed and power to transport the patient over the terrain they will encounter daily? (Ask for a list of buyers and call them to see if the power unit performs as advertised.)

- Does the power unit have adequate range? (Rough terrain will significantly reduce the range of any power unit.)

- How will the power unit be transported? (Make sure any lift matches the power unit.)

- Are the controls easy to use, easy to read, accessible and simple? Make sure the controls are on the side that is most comfortable for the patient and the unit has a battery condition indicator that is easy to read.
- How easy is it to set the parking brake?
- How comfortable is the seat?
- Lifts for wheelchairs and scooters should be purchased based upon two primary criteria:
  - A. Physical ability level of the patient and caregiver.
  - B. Type of vehicle patient will be transported in. (auto, van, pick-up, etc.)

Wheelchair and Scooter Lifts

Lift manufacturers will provide you and the patient with guidelines to insure that the right lift is purchased. Items that should be taken into consideration when deciding what type of lift will be the easiest to operate and will fit the vehicle include:

- Type of vehicle (van, auto, etc.)
- Dimensions of the trunk.
- Dimensions of the van door.
- If the vehicle can support a specific type of hitch.
- Where are the tail lights of the vehicle? (Some will be blocked by a wheelchair or scooter carried outside the vehicle.)
- How long can the patient or caregiver stand and how far can the patient walk?
- Can the caregiver or patient maneuver the unit and push the unit into place?

Call ☎ 1-800-546-5559 and we can provide you with a listing of manufacturer trained lift installation and sales dealers in your area.

Deciding to Purchase or Rent

For those patients who do not require a specially-designed wheelchair, it is wise to rent a chair before buying one to make sure it fits the patient's needs. There are so many different types of wheelchairs that it is impossible to provide all the models in one book. If the patient's disability is temporary, buying a wheelchair may not be the wisest investment. Usually, you can rent a decent wheelchair for about $70 a month. Wheelchairs are like automobiles — you can order anything you want — if you have the money to pay for it.

Because there are so many different types of wheelchairs, it will be worth your while to work with a physical/occupational therapist or a specialist in designing wheelchairs to make sure that your patient is getting a wheelchair that meets requirements and is within your budget. Many wheelchair and scooter manufacturers will not sell their products direct and you must buy from a trained and qualified supplier who can instruct the patient on how to use and care for the wheelchair or scooter. We agree with that policy and will assist you and the patient to find a supplier in your area. If your patient has special needs, we can recommend a wheelchair consultant who can work with you and the patient to design a chair that fits the patient's requirements.

You have to be careful when buying a wheelchair that all the necessary parts come with the unit and that it meets all the requirements you, the patient and the doctor have determined are needed. Some chairs are sold without footplates (footrests). Some are sold without elevating leg rests with calf pads. Some are sold without removable arms. Some are sold without padded arms. Some are made of aluminum and some are made of carbon steel. Some fold and others don't. Some come in 18-inch width seats and some come in 16-inch width seats. Some come with 17½-inch seat heights and some come with 19¾-inch seat heights. The variables can go on forever. Take your time and be sure that the wheelchair is the best it can be for your patient.

You will spend anywhere from $600 to many thousands of dollars for a quality wheelchair. It will pay you to shop carefully and make sure that the wheelchair you are buying has all the features needed by the patient included in the final price. Do not let yourself be rushed into buying a wheelchair. If possible, rent the one that you and the patient believe to be the right wheelchair for a month or so to be sure you have the right one.

Wheelchair safety tips:

- Have the nurse or therapist show you how to transfer the patient to and from the bed, from the bath and toilet, into and out of the car, etc. They will show you how to position the wheelchair and yourself to minimize the risk of hurting yourself or the patient. You will find that you can do things you never thought possible when you know how to correctly move the patient.

- Plan ahead every time you move the patient.

- If the patient has an IV, plan on how you can move the patient without disconnecting the IV.

- Make sure you have the transfer board, transfer belt, and other equipment ready.

- Use a utility belt to help prevent injury to your back.

- When using the patient transfer belt, always keep your thumb pointing down to prevent a wrist injury to yourself.

- Take your time and let the patient know what you are planning to do each step of the way. Do not let the patient grab your neck during transfers.

- If there is help in the home, use the assistance. Two people helping to move the patient is almost always better than one. Try and always use the transfer belt, if possible, and make sure it is snug and securely fastened.

- Always lock the brakes on both wheels of the wheelchair when transferring the patient.

- Raise the footplates before transferring the patient to or from the wheelchair.

- Make sure the patient is sitting well back in the seat and make sure that the feet are on the foot plates before moving the wheelchair.

- Use a seat belt if the patient is confused or ill.
- Back the wheelchair into or out of an elevator (large wheels first)
- You should have your body between the wheelchair and the bottom of a ramp.
- Do not leave your patient unattended if they cannot maneuver the wheelchair.

Caring for the wheelchair

- Use a car polish or chrome polish on metal parts.
- Use vinyl cleaner or a mild soap and water on vinyl parts.
- Check axle nuts on the large wheels weekly for tightness.
- Check the spokes on the wheels weekly for tightness.
- Lubricate squeaking parts with WD-40, or light machine oil.

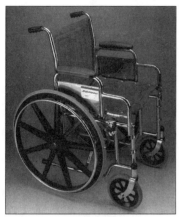

Le 133-9879

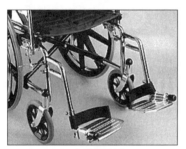

Le 340-0785

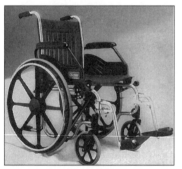

Le 213-7685

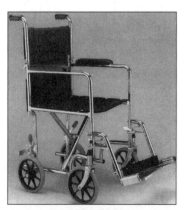

Le 321-3246

Wheelchairs and Scooters

SunMark Standard 1000 Wheelchair. Nickel chrome-plated carbon steel frame. Durable, lightweight 24-inch composite mag style wheels with sealed bearings. Virtually maintenance-free 8-inch composite mag style caster. Toggle wheel locks. Screw-attached clothing guards. Attractive, double embossed tan vinyl upholstery with bacteria resistant liner. Steel seat guides. Padded upholstered armrests.

Le 133-9879	Removable arms, 16″ chair	$459.95
Le 133-0224	Removable arms, 18″ chair	$459.95
Le 189-3031	Removable arms, 20″ chair, 300 pound capacity	$839.95
Le 220-8627	Removable arms, 22″ chair, 300 pound capacity	$859.95
Le 169-4892	Leg rests for 16 and 18″ chair, padded, elevating	$185.95
Le 199-7816	Leg rests for 20 and 22″ chair, padded, elevating	$239.95
Le 340-0710	Footrests for 16 and 18″ chair, swing-away, aluminum	$69.95
Le 199-8244	Footrests for 20 and 22″ chair, swing-away, aluminum	$105.95

Guardian GS-2000 and GL-2000 (lightweight) Wheelchair. One-piece stainless steel sideframe with no-weld joints. Easy to release flip-back arms. Quad-release swing-away footrests. Unique wheel lock lever tip is cushioned and easy to engage. 24-inch composite molded wheels with sealed bearings. Scratch/dent resistant vinyl upholstery. GS model weighs 39 pounds GL model weighs less than 36 pounds. Also available in 14- and 16-inch chair widths. Order either 17½- or 19¾-inch seat heights.

Le 213-7685	18″ chair, swing-away footrests, burgundy upholstery	$714.95
Le 213-3411	18″ chair, swing-away footrests, blue upholstery	$714.95
Le 213-0128	18″ chair, elevating leg rests, burgundy upholstery	$828.95
Le 212-7918	18″ chair, elevating leg rests, blue upholstery	$828.95
Le 210-8264	18″ chair, swing-away footrests, black upholstery (GL)	$850.95
Le 210-8132	18″ chair, elevating leg rests, black upholstery (GL)	$1008.95

Everest & Jennings Premier 2 Companion Chair. Easy to lift and handle. 40 percent lighter than standard wheelchairs; weighs only 24 pounds without footrests. Hinged back folds down. Four 8-inch wheels. Folds to 8 inch width to store easily in car trunk. Rear wheel toggle locks. Padded arm rests. Comfortable padded black nylon upholstery. For the patient who is unable to maneuver a wheelchair.

Le 321-3246	Great travel chair, seat height of 18⅞″	$665.95

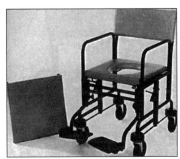

Ac 462-20

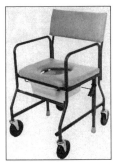

Ac 450

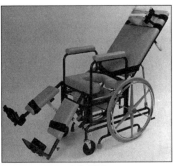

AC 494

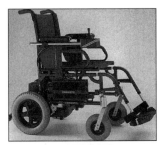

Le 177-9669

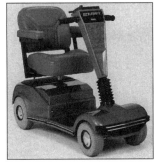

Le 246-2208

Everest & Jennings EZLite Lightweight Wheelchair. Steel frame, integrated crossbraces and reinforced inner rails for durability. Front slide post for easy folding and stability. Flip-back detachable, wraparound desk arm with easy release pin locks. 24 inch black molded wheels with solid rubber snap-on tires. Triple chrome plated tubing. Swing-away footrests.

Le 116-2338	19¾″ seat height	$905.95
Le 116-2460	17¾″ seat height, 22″ wheels	$981.95

ActiveAid Shower/Commode Chairs. 20-inch rear wheels and 5-inch casters with stainless steel bearings. Cushioned removable back. Adjustable, removable swing under footrests. 16½ inch wide seat. Double plunger brake system.

Ac 462-20	19½″ seat height	$945.95

ActiveAid Shower/Commode Chair. Best value. Four uses in one — bedside commode, over toilet commode, shower chair and "get about" chair. Safe, secure steel construction with sturdy plunger brakes. Removable arms, padded seat and back. Corrosion resistant finish, sealed 5-inch casters and sealed upholstery. 17½–inch seat width between arms.

Ac 450	20″ seat height	$456.95
Ac 450I	20″ seat height with footrests	$514.95

ActiveAid Traum-Aid® Shower/Commode Trauma Wheelchairs. Reclining back with eleven independent angle positions starting at 15 degrees from vertical to 25 degrees from horizontal. Elevating leg and foot rests. Head positioning wedge. 4-way padded seat. 24-inch mag wheel with safety sealed bearings. 5-inch caster wheels. Dual-plunger floor brakes. Narrow 24-inch profile.

Ac 494	Seat height of 23″	$1785.95

Quickie Designs P110 Power Wheelchair. Programmable, electronic controller for custom joystick sensitivity. Direct drive motor provide speeds up to 5 mph. Folding frame. Weighs 81 pounds without battery. Range of 20 miles. Adjustable arm and footrests. Requires U1 or 22NF batteries (not included).

Le 177-9669	Seat height of 20″	$3595.95

Invacare Power Drive Wheelchair. Compact and portable. Closed loop system helps maintain speed and direction. Adjustable height back. Comfortable black nylon upholstery. Flip-up arms. Dynamic braking; automatic motor locks similar to parking brake. Batteries not included.

Le 147-8254	Battery charger included	$3495.95

Pride Shuttle Power Scooter. Three wheel design. Modular design fits into most car trunks. 46 inches long and 24 inches wide. Easy to use controls. Top speed of 5½ mph with a 20 mile range per charge. Full wraparound body prevents catching on household objects. 300 pound capacity. Built-in battery charger. Climbs 15 degree grade. Requires two batteries (not included).

Le 141-3756	Easy to transport; no tools required		$2495.95
Le 248-4079	Battery	Each	$109.95

Pride SC-440 Celebrity Scooter. Four wheel scooter. 47 inches long and 24 inches wide. 31 inch turning radius. Top speed 5¼ mph; 25 mile range per charge. Automatic shut-off; built in battery charger. Anti-tip wheels. Gray seat and red body. Climbs a 15 degree grade. Electronic speed control and disc brakes. Requires two batteries (not included).

Le 246-2208	Easy to disassemble for transport		$2995.95
Le 248-4079	Battery	Each	$109.95

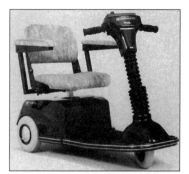

Le 273-2378

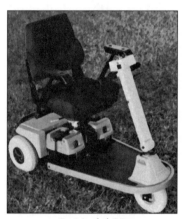

Br Model 55

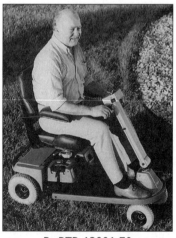

Br BTR-12001-70

Pride Sundancer Scooter. Three wheel scooter, 41 inches long and 24 inches wide. 31 inch turning radius. Top speed 4.5 mph. Built-in battery charger. Easy to disassemble for transport. Anti-tip wheels. Electronic speed control. Batteries not included.

Le 273-2378	Red	$2595.95
Le 272-9499	Teal	$2595.95
Le 248-4079	Battery	$109.95

LeBoeuf's also carries a full line of scooters by Bruno. The Bruno Regal Scooter line is made up of seven models. Each Regal scooter is equipped with:

- E-Z Tilt™ tiller
- Contoured foam seating
- Slant platform
- Powerful 1.32 HP motor and RWD drivetrain
- Custom seating is available

The Regal's durable construction is ideal for outdoor use, while its compact size and short turning radius offer excellent indoor maneuverability. Tiller and platform lengths as well as various seating options can be precisely selected to provide the Regal rider with unparalleled leg room and superior thigh, lateral and lumbar support.

Bruno Regal Standard Model 55. Standard Fish-On® seat with adjustable flip-up armrests. 44 inches overall length. 8½-inch tires.

Br Model 55		$2440.95
Br BTR-12001-55 Battery	Each	$105.95

Bruno Regal Four™ Model 70. Standard Fish-On seat with adjustable, flip-up armrests. 48 inches overall length. Two 8½-inch pneumatic front tires and two 10-inch pneumatic rear tires. Reflective hub-caps.

Br Model 70		$2775.95
Br BTR-12001-70 Battery	Each	$105.95

Bruno Cane Holder. For Fish-On seat.

Br Z-021-030	$25.95

Bruno Oxygen Cylinder Holder. Fits "D" and "E" size cylinders. Rear mount. Specify type of seat.

Br Special	$100.95

Bruno Trailer. 2.0 Cubic foot capacity. 13½ inches deep by 20 inches wide by 13¼ inches high.

Br Z-026-100	$165.95

Other Bruno scooter models are available for small adult and youth-pediatric. There are many other accessories available for the Bruno scooters. Call **LeBoeuf's** ☎ 1-800-546-5559 for brochure.

Battery Chargers for Power Wheelchairs and Scooters

If the battery charger is to be left connected for long periods of times, you should select a battery charger that eliminates the possibility of overcharge. The usage of the wheelchair or scooter determines the amp rating required to have the wheelchair or scooter fully charged and ready to go. Heavy use requires higher amp output, or a constant current type of charge for quick recovery time.

Tips for patients who are using power wheelchairs and scooters

- Charge early and often to avoid severely over-discharged batteries.
- Do not run the batteries till they are dead.
- Over-discharged batteries may take twice as long to charge — don't panic. The charger will eventually charge the battery enough to resume normal charging.
- Batteries must match. Use same type brand, connection, capacity and age.
- Do not connect a twelve volt device to either battery — get a 24 volt phone.
- Be careful with lead-acid batteries. They contain sulfuric acid. If an accident occurs, flush the skin and eyes with lots of water and seek medical attention.
- Care should be used when lifting heavy batteries.
- Store batteries in the coolest place possible. Heat kills lead-acid batteries.
- Make sure batteries are fully charged before placing in storage.
- Choose batteries that match the patient's needs.
- Make sure that the charger is not too big or too small for the application.

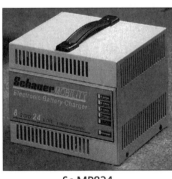

Sc MP824

Schauer Mobility Adaptive Connections System (ACS) Battery Charger. This battery charger works anywhere in the world. Comes with user replaceable connection cords. The AC connection works on 120VAC or 240VAC, with AC cords available for any country. Reverse polarity and short circuit proof. Fully automatic, cannot overcharge, undercharge or damage the battery. Will start charging a fully discharged battery. LED readout for charging status.

Sc MP824	8 AMP, 24 Volt	$410.95
Sc MP524	5 AMP, 24 Volt	$360.95
Sc MP1012	10 AMP, 12 Volt	$350.95

Schauer Mobility Light Weight Battery Charger. Designed for those who need a lightweight (3 pounds) portable battery charger that can furnish recharge times equivalent to most 10 amp chargers. Provides complete cut-off when battery reaches control set points. Temperature compensated to give the correct charge for varying conditions. Lighted on/off switch. LED charging indicator. UL Listed.

Sc LE724	8³/₄″ long × 7″ deep × 3″ high	$210.95

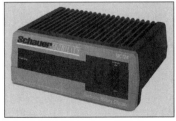

Sc LE724

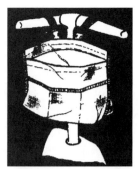
Ro 5025

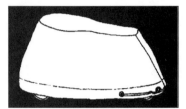
Ro 5015

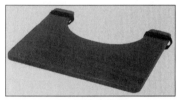
Le 220-0459

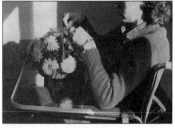
Co 11P

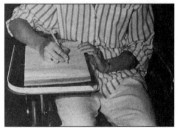
Co 11H

Scooter and Wheelchair Accessories

Roo Express Scooter Bags and Backpack. Made of rugged 600 Denier polyester with vinyl backing. Quick spring action opening. Maintains shape when loaded. All come in black or royal blue. Please specify color when ordering

Ro 5025	Tiller bag with 3 Interior mesh pockets	$16.95
Ro 5026	Armrest bag with 3 interior mesh pockets	$20.95
Ro 5027	Side entry backpack, access from the left or right	$55.95

Roo Express Scooter Covers. Water resistant laminated nylon. Comes in 3 colors: black, gray or navy.

Ro 5015	Small	$95.95
Ro 5016	Medium	$98.95
Ro 5017	Large	$103.95
Ro 5018	Multi-fit cover	$88.95

SunMark Wheelchair Tray. Velcro® fasteners permit installation on any wheelchair. Easy to clean Formica top.

Le 220-0459	$56.95

Maddak Clip-on Ashtray. Plastic clamp attaches easily to most wheelchairs or walkers. Large projections prevent cigarettes from falling out.

Le 197-6059	$12.95

SunMark Wheelchair Safety Belt. Airline-style buckle for easy adjustment and comfort. Attaches easily.

Le 220-2661	10 foot length	$22.95

Consumer Care Products Wheelchair Tray/Desk. Gives complete use of a full size (25¾ inch width and 23¾ inch depth) clear poly-carbonate plastic tray with stomach cutout. Lift tray for instant access to the compartmentalized storage underneath. The entire unit easily slides on and off the wheelchair via telescoping support arms suitable for most wheelchairs.

Co 11P	All hardware included	$295.95

Consumer Care Products Tablet-Arm Tray for Manual Wheelchairs. Designed for those who need a rugged yet portable writing surface without the bulkiness of ordinary full-size trays. Great for those patients who transfer in and out of the chair often. Clear poly-carbonate plastic with ⅝-inch high rim. Lightweight and easy to install. Flips up and away or snaps off. POLY-LOCK, brand tape fastener.

Co 11H	Weighs 3½ pounds	$105.95

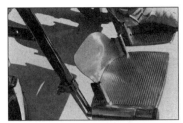

Co 10AV/10:1

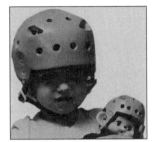

Co 10AV/10:1

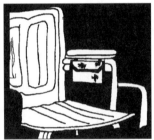

Ro 5028

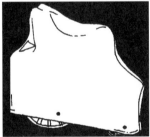

Ro 5014

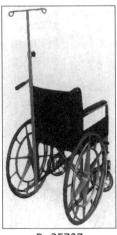

Br 35707

Consumer Care Products Vinyl Heel Loops. 2 inches or 4 inches high and 8 inches long. Soft resilient plastic heel loops are used to provide safe foot positioning and control on foot rests. Per pair.

Co 10AV/10:1	2″ high with mounting hardware	$17.95
Co 10BV/10:1	4″ high with mounting hardware	$21.95

Consumer Care Products Helmet and Chin Guard. Recognized by professionals as the best available. Molded from ½-inch thick shock absorbent vinyl covered foam. Chin guard is molded out of the same soft ½-inch thick plasticized foam. Very light; helmet and chin guard weigh 8 ounces. Handwashable. Special ventilation hole design. Child and youth sizes also available. Can be purchased without chin guard.

Co 15C and 15.2	White Adult size with large chin guard	$54.95

ActiveAid Safety/Transfer Belt. Strong cotton 2-inch wide web belt with cadmium plated safety buckle. A must for transfers.

Ac 71	54″ length	$12.95
Ac 72	60″ length	$12.95
Ac 73	72″ length	$12.95

SunMark Organizer. Convenient carry-all. Can be used on patient's walker or wheelchair.

Le 220-2364	$23.95

Roo Express Wheelchair Pouches and Bags. Simple way of securing valuables, beverages, and other items. Lined for added durability. Flap style allows for easy access to contents. All come in black or royal blue. Please specify color when ordering.

Ro 5028	Security pouch	$9.95
Ro 5029	Beverage bag	$12.95
Ro 5030	Sling bag, 3 interior mesh pockets	$19.95
Ro 5031	Side entry backpack	$44.95
Ro 5032	Top entry backpack, spring action opening	$35.95
Ro 5033	Seatpack fits under wheelchair seat	$43.95

Roo Express Outdoor Wheelchair Cover. Water resistant laminated nylon. Resists fading, mildew and UV damage. Bungy tie-down system. Works well with lifts. Comes in black, gray or navy.

Ro 5014	Specify color when ordering	$82.95

Roo Express Moving Pad. Protects equipment during transport. Covers patient lifts, wheelchairs, bed frames, etc. Comes in gray only.

Ro 5021	Quilted cotton	$31.95

Brandt Wheelchair Infusion Holder and Oxygen Holder. Two ram's horn style hooks. Hooks are 10 inches apart. Adjusts from 40 inches to 77 inches in height. Easy height adjustment by means of a smooth friction clutch. The oxygen holder is added to the infusion holder.

Br 35707	Infusion stand	$79.95
Br 097	Oxygen tank holder	$30.95

Mada Oxygen Holder. Will fit any 18-inch wheelchair. Not for 20-inch and 22-inch manual wheelchairs or power wheelchairs.

Le 379-6562	$47.95

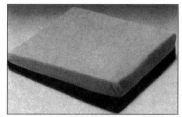

Le 117-3491

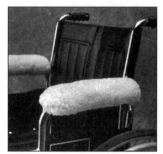

Le 148-2991

Lumex Akros DFD® Seating Cushion. Permanently sealed construction with fluid gel, plastic foam, and sheathing. Gel-cell and foam construction virtually eliminates "bottoming out." Designed to reduce pressure and allow blood to flow freely. Self-leveling and self-adjusting. Dual cover for comfort and protection.

Le 326-2003	18″ × 16″ × 2″, Blue	$110.95
Le 224-3699	18″ × 16″ × 2″, Black	$110.95

Lumex Akros, Economy Gel Cushion. Durable and waterproof. Two color Staph-Chek, cover (blue and black) allows caregiver to track time patient has spent in each position. Convenient carrying handle.

Le 117-3491	18″ × 16″ × 2″	$80.95

Care Products Care Covers. 2-ply cushioning of synthetic sheepskin. Washable and dryer safe. Velcro strap closure. One pair.

Le 148-2991	For 8″ to 9″ length armrest	$27.95
Le 148-2843	For 10″ to 11″ length armrest	$27.95
Le 148-2082	For 13″ to 14″ length armrest	$27.95
Le 148-2454	For 14″ to 15″ length armrest	$27.95

Homecare EZ-Access Wheelchair and Scooter Ramps. Constructed of extruded anodized aluminum with nonskid driving surface. Special snap button catches lock securely.

Le 147-7231	Extends to 5 feet. Locks securely with snap buttons Inside width 4,″ weighs 14 pounds. Holds 350 pounds.	$219.95
Le 147-7439	Van ramp Extends to 7′. Inside width 6½″ Weighs 28 pounds. Holds 600 pounds. Extra safety bolt attachment.	$320.95
Le 249-4946	Roll-up ramp. 3′ long, 30″ wide. Holds 600 pounds.	$245.95
Le 273-1800	Roll-up ramp. 5′ long, 30″ wide. Holds 600 pounds.	$339.95
Le 147-7520	Telescopic 8′ scooter ramp. Extends from 39″ to 8′. Holds 750 pounds.	$499.95

In addition to the ramps shown, we have threshold ramps for scooters and wheelchairs. These ramps provide a 34 inch wide non-skid driving surface for maximum safety and support. Please call for pricing.

Ramp Length Chart

	RAMP LENGTH			
RISE	36"	48"	60"	96"
3"	5°	3.5°	3°	2°
4"	6°	5°	4°	2.5°
5"	8°	6°	5°	3°
6"	9.5°	7°	6°	3.5°
7"	11°	8°	7°	4°
8"	13°	9.5°	7.5°	5°
9"	14°	11°	8.5°	5.5°
10"		12°	9.5°	6°
12"		14°	11°	7°
14"		16°	13°	8.5°
16"			15°	9.5°
18"			17°	11°
20"				12°
21"				13°
28"				17°

To establish the proper length ramp:

- Consult manufacturer's specifications to determine the incline your wheelchair or scooter is designed to climb
- Measure the distance from the top step to the ground (rise)
- Refer to the chart to find the ramp length

Example: If your wheelchair or scooter can climb a 6° incline, and the rise is 5″, then the required ramp length is 48″.

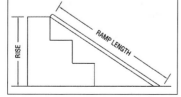

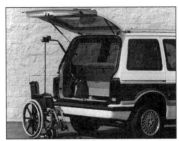

Br AWL-100

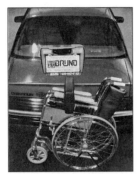

Br AWL-1600

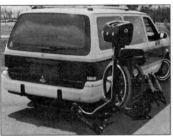

Br AWL-1610

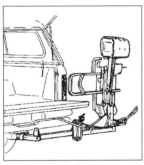

Br ASL-207 T

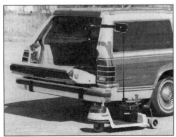

Br VSL-600

Vehicle Lifts for Wheelchairs and Scooters.

Call **LeBoeuf's** ☎ 1-800-546-5559 and we will provide you with the name of a factory trained lift installer in your area. There are so many variables involved in making the best decision for what type of lift would be best for you and the patient, that you must work with factory trained installers to be sure that you have purchased the right lift. Generally, the lift dealer will need to determine the level of physical ability of both the caregiver and the patient as well the type of vehicle(s) the patient will be transported in.

If the patient will be transported in more than one vehicle, be sure that you tell the dealer. Some of the lifts can be switched from one vehicle to another by installing an additional mounting package.

Bruno AWL-100 Wheelchair-Lifter. Raises and stores wheelchairs horizontally for manual swing into the auto trunk or into a hatchback. Maximum capacity is 55 pounds.

Br AWL-100		$795.95
Br AWL-125	Heavy duty with 85 pound capacity	$925.95

Bruno AWL-150 Wheelchair-Lifter. Raises folding wheelchairs vertically for manual swing into the rear opening of full size vans or mini-vans and Suburban® type vehicles with cargo doors or hatch openings. Maximum capacity 55 pounds.

Br AWL-150		$935.95
Br AWL-175	Heavy duty with 85 pound capacity	$1060.95

Bruno AWL-1600 Back-Saver™. Fully automatic rear exterior lift that raises and locks folding wheelchairs under 70 pounds with 22-inch or larger wheels. Installs on Class I hitch.

Br AWL-1600	$865.95

Bruno AWL-1610 Back-Saver Swing-Away. For vehicles with hatch openings or tailgates. Lift can swing away with wheelchair in place. Class III hitch with 2-inch receiver required.

Br AWL-1610	$1200.95

Bruno ASL-207 T Motor Home Out-Sider II. Rear exterior lift that raises and locks down a completely assembled scooter. A fully automatic hold-down bar secures the scooter during transport. The user need only to move the operating lever to the up or down position.

Br ASL-207 T	$1990.95

Bruno VSL-600 Curb Sider®. The 180 degree power rotation of the Curb-Sider makes it ideal for lifting and storing fully assembled scooters or power or manual wheelchairs weighing up to 200 pounds in the rear of full size vans or mini-vans, trucks and Suburbans. It is also an excellent choice for storing partially assembled scooters in vehicles with tailgates, including station wagons and sport utility vehicles.

Br VSL-600	$1915.95

There are many more styles of lifts for autos, pick-ups, vans, motor homes, and station wagons. All the Bruno lifts qualify for rebate programs offered by various auto manufacturers for new vehicles. For more information and free brochures, call **LeBoeuf's** ☎ 1-800-546-5559.

Kidneys

WHEN A PERSON'S KIDNEYS are healthy and functioning normally, they automatically filter waste products and excess fluids from the blood. They help the patient's body keep a normal balance between fluids and chemicals. The kidneys continually control the amount of salt and water in the body, which in turn helps to set the level of blood pressure. They also produce vitamins and hormones which stimulate red blood cell production and promote calcium balance which keeps all of the bones strong.

The kidneys are located above the waist on either side of the spinal column. The kidney on the right is below the liver and the kidney on the left is below the spleen. They are each about 4-5 inches long and each one weighs about six ounces. Each kidney contains about 1 million small round structures, and each of these contains a loop of blood capillaries (glomeruli) that act as filters and starts the process of urine production. Normal urine production is between 60 to 120 ml an hour (about 2 to 4 ounces). These glomeruli are the kidney's primary filtering unit. The glomeruli pass the filtered blood through long and very small tubes (tubules) into the central part of the kidney (medulla). The combination of the glomeruli and the tubules make up the nephrons. Problems occur when the number of functioning nephrons is reduced. However, the number of functioning nephrons gradually reduce as people age and there is nothing that can be done to reverse the process.

What happens when the kidneys fail? First, they are unable to remove the two main wastes that build up in the body; Urea (BUN) and Creatinine. When their levels in the blood become too high, the condition is called uremia. The symptoms of uremia, or uremic poisoning, can include feeling nauseous, a loss of appetite, loss of memory or ability to reason clearly, and an over-all feeling of being sick. When the kidneys do not function, salt and water build up and the individual goes into fluid overload, which in turn leads to shortness of breath, swelling in the hands and feet and high blood pressure. High blood pressure is caused when the blood vessels in the body become narrow, forcing the heart to pump harder to push blood through the body. This hypertension leads to certain chemicals in the body, such as potassium, calcium, and phosphorus, getting out of balance. When potassium is allowed to build up in the body, it can cause the heart to stop beating. If phosphorus and calcium are out of balance, it can lead to bone disease.

There are two kinds of kidney failure: acute and chronic. Acute kidney failure means the kidneys have temporally stopped working because of serious infections, severe diarrhea or vomiting, drug poisoning, surgery, injury or blockage. This type of failure can often be reversed. Chronic kidney failure is a permanent condition and once it occurs, the kidneys will not regain their function. Chronic kidney disease will eventually lead to scarring of the kidney and "End Stage Renal Disease" (ESRD). A person with ESRD will have to depend on medical treatment to replace the lost kidney function.

Some of the main causes of kidney problems include:

- High blood pressure (one of the major causes).

- Diabetes – of the one million Americans with type I insulin dependent diabetes, up to 40 percent will develop kidney damage. Unfortunately, it is not possible to predict whose kidney will be damaged. The damage happens slowly and at first there are no symptoms. The doctor will measure the level of protein in the patient's urine to determine if there is kidney damage.

- Damage from Medication.

- Bladder infections.

- Sickle cell anemia.

When the kidneys stop working, dialysis or a kidney transplant must be performed to make up for the loss of healthy kidneys.

Kidney disease causes are grouped into three categories:

- **Hereditary** – Polycystic which is the most common and, along with simple kidney cysts, is found in almost half of all people over 50. Polycystic kidneys are caused by cysts that gradually increase in size until most of the normal kidney tissue is destroyed. There is no known workable treatment or cure at this time and the patient's only options are kidney dialysis or a kidney transplant. Other hereditary kidney problems include Alport's syndrome, hereditary nephritis and cystinuria.

- **Congenital** – Horseshoe kidneys (two kidneys joined at the base) are fairly common. Some people are also born with only one kidney or have both kidneys on one side of their body.

- **Acquired kidney disease** – Inflammation of the kidneys caused by infection (pyelonephritis) is the most common and is usually caused by an obstruction of the urinary tract that leads to stagnation and subsequent infection coming from the bladder. Problems with infections from improper use of catheters is a big cause of this problem. Cancer, kidney stones, hypertension, diabetes and heart problems can all lead to kidneys not functioning as they should. When kidneys fail to operate properly the result is a build-up of waste products in the body and the inability to control the salt and water balance from lower blood flow.

When kidneys stop working (end state renal failure or 10 percent of less than normal kidney function), dialysis or a kidney transplant must be performed to make up for the loss of healthy kidneys. There are two types of dialysis; peritoneal and kidney machine (artificial kidney).

Peritoneal dialysis gets its name from the peritoneum which is a thin membrane that stretches around the internal organs in the body and acts as a filter that allows wastes to be removed from the blood. During peritoneal dialysis, a catheter is surgically placed in the abdomen and a solution containing water, glucose and normal serum electrolytes is passed through it into the abdominal cavity, which is the space next to the peritoneum. Using the principles of diffusion and osmosis, the sugar in the solution acts like a magnet and draws water and wastes through the semipermeable peritoneum membrane and into the solution. The fluid may stay in the peritoneal cavity from 10 minutes to 4 hours. This is called "dwell time." The contaminated dialysate is then removed and new dialysate is injected. Most patients can perform this exchange themselves. The patient will cycle from 8 to 12 bags of dialysate each treatment through a mechanical fluid regulator and a warmer. The patient may need to do this three to six times a day but is free to perform normal activities between treatments. The doctor and/or nurse will teach you and the patient how to perform this procedure and provide you with a check list of things to do as well as what to do if things are not going right. The supplies and equipment can be easily delivered to the patient's home, or hotel if traveling.

Using an artificial kidney machine to clean the blood is called hemodialysis. During hemodialysis, the patient's blood is passed through tubing into a machine which contains the artificial kidney. After wastes and extra fluids are taken out of the patient's blood, the blood flows back through the tubing and into the body. The machine takes over the kidney function until they start working normally again or, if no kidney transplant is performed, may continue on for the life of the patient. This process can be accomplished at any one of the over 2,400 dialysis centers around the United States or numerous clinics world-wide. Presently, 5 percent of kidney patients carry out their hemodialysis on machines in their own homes. This number is growing as technology improves and the machines get smaller and simpler to operate.

Hemodialysis patients usually have to be hooked up to a kidney machine three or more times a week for three to five or more hours each time. The first three months of dialysis can be extremely traumatic while the patient gets over the shock of being "hooked-up" to the machine and bound to a schedule — to say nothing of recuperating from the surgery required to create a fistula or graft in the arm or leg so that the person's artery and vein can be connected to the artificial kidney. Once the patient is acclimated to the machinery, terminology, the medicines, the routine and the new life style changes (watching out for sodium, phosphorus, potassium and fluid intake), a very normal and happy life can be lead. It is important that you and the patient have someone who has gone through machine dialysis assist you and the patient and help you to understand what is going on.

Today's kidney dialysis patients are truly blessed because they have a fantastic group of individuals prepared and willing to ensure that they receive the most complete treatment possible. Persons on dialysis are backed up by a "Renal Support Team" whose goal is to help them manage their own care while continuing to have full and happy lives. The "Team" consists of the patient, a family member if desired, a nephrologist, a hemodialysis or peritoneal dialysis nurse, a dialysis technician, a dietician and a renal social worker. The registered nurse or licensed practical nurse develops a plan for meeting the medical and learning needs of the patient starting dialysis. Some technicians are trained in the technical aspects of dialysis and are able to care for the patient. Dietitians determine nutritional needs. Renal social workers provide the social, psychological and environmental support to help patients and family adjust. They provide information about treatment availability, insurance, Medicare, Social Security, transportation needs, and help counsel individuals and families in illness-related problems. Patients are encouraged to take advantage of all of the services that the Renal Team offers.

Patients on dialysis soon realize that they have the most important role — staying physically and mentally healthy. The patient has the responsibility for keeping appointments, for taking medication, for eating well and getting enough exercise, and for making good use of time, especially while on the machine (reading, listening to talking books, etc.). Only the individual dialysis patient can decide how to handle this treatment in a positive or negative manner. For those who choose to appreciate the technology and have a positive attitude, life can be as normal and productive as they want it to be.

It is estimated that over 20 million people in the United States suffer from kidney or urinary tract related diseases. The National Kidney Foundation is set up to help these individuals. To find out the local affiliate near you, call 1-800-622-9010. This non-profit voluntary health organization offers many direct patient services, including: medication bank programs, patient emergency funds, patient/family seminars, people-to-people support programs, medical alert jewelry programs, free information services and pre-dialysis education seminars.

Those who have been diagnosed as having chronic renal disease may want to ask their doctors about kidney transplants. Kidney transplants are the use of a donated kidney from a close blood relative, an unrelated living donor, or a person who has donated a kidney after death. To prevent rejection of the implanted kidney, the tissue type and blood type of the donor and the patient must be a close match. Usually the left kidney is removed from a living donor because it is easier to remove safely. The donor kidney is usually placed in the patient's pelvis. The donor's health is not affected by the loss of one kidney and the donor's remaining kidney will grow to take over full function. If the patient has received a kidney from a young child or even an infant, the kidney will grow to be full sized.

Rejection is the main problem of a transplant operation. The body instinctively wants to "fight off" the foreign organ. Thanks to outstanding immunosuppressive medications, improved surgical techniques, preservation of donated kidneys and research advances, the success rate for kidney transplants is very good. If rejection of the kidney occurs, the patient returns to artificial dialysis and can try for another kidney transplant later. Since the anti-rejection drugs have to be taken continually and can cause side-effects, medical supervision will be a lifelong commitment. During the first several months after a kidney transplant, follow-up visits are frequent but they become less so as time goes by. A kidney transplant quickly brings with it a new lease on life.

Symptoms of *chronic renal disease:*

- Decreased need to urinate.
- Confusion.
- Puffiness around the eyes, swelling of the hands and feet, especially in children.
- Poor appetite.
- Nausea.
- Weakness.
- Difficulty concentrating.
- High blood pressure.

Kidney Stones

More than one million people are diagnosed as having kidney stones every year. Kidney stones affect mostly young and middle-aged adults. Kidney stones are more common in men than in women – 4 out of 5 patients are men. Kidney stones tend to recur and successful treatment depends on finding out what causes the stones. 90 percent of kidney stones will pass by themselves within 48 hours of changes in diet and fluid intake. Kidney stones should always be removed when infection, obstruction or kidney damage are present. Sometimes the kidney is so damaged that the doctor will remove the entire kidney. One kidney is enough to keep the body healthy.

The reasons for developing kidney stones are not always clear. Normal urine contains chemicals that prevent crystals from forming. Evidence shows that the following are factors contributing to kidney stone formation:

- Drinking too little fluid.
- Chronic urinary tract infections.
- Misuse of medications.
- Blockage of the urinary tract.
- Limited activity for several weeks or more.
- Genetic and metabolic diseases.
- Certain foods in people with absorptive hypercalciuria (too much calcium is being absorbed).

X-rays and sound waves are used to identify the size and location of the kidney stones. Blood and urine tests are used to find out what is causing the kidney stones and to help the doctor determine the best treatment. Several methods are used to remove kidney stones: surgery, telescopic instrument inserted into bladder or ureter to pull out stones or break them into small pieces with sound waves and laser beams; or extracorporeal shock wave lithotripsy in which the stones are broken down into small fragments by high energy shock waves while in a water bath or on top of a water filled cushion. This last procedure is still being studied for long-term effects. There are also some medications that help prevent kidney stones.

Symptoms of kidney stones:

- Severe pain in the lower abdomen that may move to the groin.
- Nausea and vomiting.
- Burning and frequent urge to urinate.
- Fever, chills and weakness.
- Cloudy or foul smelling urine.
- Blood in urine.
- Blocked flow of urine.
- Severe back pain in the kidney area.

Incontinence

ACCORDING TO THE NATIONAL INSTITUTE OF NURSING RESEARCH, the economic costs of urinary incontinence are estimated at $10.3 billion annually. $4.8 billion of the total is for elderly patients. According to Kimberly-Clark, a leading manufacturer of incontinent products (Depends), the number of patients who are incontinent is currently about 15 million people. The number of people with very light incontinence is estimated to be 7.5 million; light incontinence 5.0 million; moderate 1.5 million and heavy 1.0 million. By the year 2000, it is expected that the number of people using incontinent products will double. Incontinent simply means a person is unable to stop a natural discharge such as urination.

There are two types of incontinence: Urinary and Fecal. Urinary incontinence is broken down into four kinds:

- **Urge** — The involuntary loss of urine associated with an abrupt and strong desire to void (urgency). Once urination starts, it continues until the bladder is empty.

- **Stress** — The involuntary loss of urine associated with coughing, laughing, running, etc., when pressure is placed on the bladder. It is very common in women, especially after childbirth when the urethral sphincter muscles are stretched.

- **Overflow** — The involuntary loss of urine associated with over-distention of the bladder. Can be frequent or constant dribbling. The patient is unable to empty the bladder normally, often as a result of an obstruction such as an enlarged prostate gland. Removal of the obstruction will restore continence.

- **Functional or Total** — A complete loss of bladder control. Urine loss due to environmental factors or barriers such as a hole between the bladder and vagina.

Bladder control involves the urinary system, the pelvic muscles, the spinal cord and the brain. All must be in working order for the process of continence to take place. There are three general categories of treatment.

- Behavioral techniques are low-risk techniques such as bladder training, timed voiding, prompted voiding and pelvic muscle exercises.

- Pharmacological treatment of incontinence by the use of drugs.

- Surgery to remove obstructions such as bladder stones.

Incontinence often affects the elderly because the efficiency of the sphincter muscles surrounding the urethra declines with age. Women are affected more often than men.

Often, exercises (Kegel exercises) to strengthen the pelvic floor muscles are all that is required to regain bladder control if incontinence is caught early. Kegel exercises are also for men. Check with the doctor or nurse to be sure that the exercise is done properly or the exercise will not be effective.

As many as 73 percent of women may suffer from incontinence at some time during their life. As many as 1 in 10 persons age 65 or older suffer from incontinence. According to Help for Incontinent People (HIP), as many as 30 percent of older Americans are troubled by bladder control problems. Often, exercises (Kegel exercises) to strengthen the pelvic floor muscles are all that is required to regain bladder control if incontinence is caught early. Kegel exercises are also for men. Check with the doctor or nurse to be sure that the exercise is done properly or the exercise will not be effective. Incontinence is not inevitable or shameful, but is treatable or at least manageable. The patient does not have to live wet.

People with incontinence often withdraw from social life and attempt to hide the problem from their family, friends and even their doctor. Prompt medical attention to determine the cause is very important to the management of the problem.

A number of medications can be used to treat incontinence. However, these drugs may cause side effects such as dry mouth, eye problems and buildup of urine. Therefore, they must be used carefully under a doctor's supervision.

If normal bladder function cannot be restored, special incontinence undergarments can alleviate discomfort and absorb the urine or contain fecal matter. When buying incontinence products, be sure that they are properly fitted to contain the urine and stool. The patient should also purchase incontinence undergarments that control odor. However, dependency on absorbent pads can be a deterrent to overcoming incontinence because it gives the patient a sense of security that the condition will no longer become a problem socially. If the patient is wearing absorbent products, it is very important to use special care to keep the skin from becoming irritated. Frequent changes of undergarments are needed to prevent rashes and urinary tract infections (UTI).

Men can wear a sheath over the penis — the sheath leads into a tube connected to a portable urine bag. These condom type catheters should not be used on patients with chronic obstruction. Some people can pass a catheter into the bladder four or five times a day to empty it. If these measures are not successful, and the condition is severe, a urinary diversion operation may be necessary to bypass the bladder.

Intermittent self-catheterization is a safe and effective therapy, either long or short term, for those who have overflow incontinence. This type of treatment is preferable to the Foley catheter because of the lower risk of infection and bladder stone formation. The catheter is inserted through the urethra into the bladder every 3 to 6 hours for bladder drainage.

Foley catheterization is an indwelling catheter held in place by a small water-filled balloon that holds the catheter in place inside the bladder. The patient's urine will automatically drain out of the their bladder into a bag which is attached to the catheter. The patient may experience a stinging sensation or spasms in the first few days. This is not unusual and should not be cause for alarm. However, if the discomfort continues for more than three days, call the doctor and/or nurse.

In accordance with AHCPR guidelines for the management of incontinence, an indwelling catheter should be inserted for:

- Urinary retention which cannot otherwise be treated and for which no alternative therapy is possible.
- Monitoring for fluid balance in an acutely ill person where incontinence interferes.
- Patients who are seriously ill, or severely impaired persons for whom bed and clothing changes are painful or disruptive.
- Situations where the severity of incontinence and the complexity of patient care have contributed to skin irritation or pressure ulcers (grade 3 or 4). An indwelling catheter may be indicated for short-term therapy until the skin condition improves.
- In home care, the lack of a caregiver who is able to perform intermittent catheterization or diaper changes may contribute to the use of Foley indwelling catheters.

Fecal incontinence usually involves compromise or impairment of the multiple mechanisms that control bowel movement. Feces lodged in the rectum (constipation) irritate and inflame its lining, resulting in fecal fluid and small pieces of feces to be passed involuntarily. Temporary loss of continence may occur at any age from severe diarrhea. Other causes, though less common, are injury to the anal muscles (childbirth or surgery), paralysis of the legs and lower trunk, mental handicap and dementia.

Constipation can be prevented by a high-fiber diet (eating more vegetables, fruits and whole grains). Water and other liquids add bulk to stools, making bowel movement easier. Older people worry too much about having a bowel movement every day. There is no right number of daily or weekly bowel movements. "Regularity" may mean bowel movements twice a day for some people or twice a week for others. Glycerin suppositories taken daily (or laxative suppositories taken occasionally) may be used if the constipation has persisted for several days. Incontinence due to dementia or nerve injury can be avoided by regularly using enemas or suppositories to empty the rectum.

Patient incontinence cleaning protocol:

- Assist your patient to a comfortable lying position and explain what you are going to do. Place a towel or disposable pad next to patient to prevent soiling bed clothes. Do not overexpose the patient. Appropriate covering will avoid a chill and lessen patient embarrassment.
- Spray cleaner liberally on the area to liquefy feces and urine.
- Clean patient from *front to back*. Repeating if necessary.
- Pat area dry with towel.
- Apply a protective ointment to the area to ensure protection for the skin.
- Report any reddened areas to the doctor or nurse.
- Repeat this procedure after each incontinent episode.

Odors can be controlled. Listed below are some tips on how to prevent and control odors:

- Wash bed linens and patient's clothing immediately (100% polyester may have to be thrown away).
- Store soiled items in an airtight container until taken to the laundry. A plastic bag with a zip-lock seal will work.
- Try adding baking soda *or* white vinegar to wash water to eliminate odors (use only one at a time, not both together). If using vinegar, rinse well to avoid smelling like a salad.
- Buy disposable products with an odor reducing material in the pad or garment. Not just a perfume but a material that prevents odor from forming.
- Urine collection devices such as a condom catheter, leg bag should be cleaned regularly with a commercial cleaner or a solution of one part white vinegar and four parts water.
- Use air fresheners that neutralize odors, not just cover them up with perfume.
- Light a candle in the bathroom after a bowel movement.
- Potpourri and incense will keep the house smelling fresh.
- Drink cranberry juice to help to reduce urine odor.
- Deodorizing tablets such as Derifil® or Nullo® may work. It may take a few days, but it's worth the try.
- Talk to the doctor about giving the patient vitamin C to combat urine odor.

What to do:

See a doctor — Make and keep the appointment. Many patients are embarrassed to talk with anyone about their incontinence problem. Incontinence can be controlled and the doctor will treat it like the common and treatable medical condition it is. The doctor will work with the patient to find the best solution for bladder and bowel control. Research is continuing at an increasing rate and a cure for the majority of people with incontinence is possible.

Contact Help For Incontinent People (HIP) — 1-800-Bladder (252-3337) Membership is $15 annually. The address is P.O. Box 544, Union, South Carolina 29379. They can provide you and the patient with information on the latest information about the causes of and solutions for incontinence. They can also help find a specialist in your area for the patient.

Contact the local social services organizations — There are many agencies that will provide information and listings of resources available in your area. Agencies such as the offices on aging, local health agencies as well as religious-affiliated service groups also provide information, training and support. There are also associations and companies that provide care management services to serve as the link between you and community-based services. They charge for their services, so be sure you understand what it will cost to have them provide assistance.

Incontinence Management

INCONTINENCE is a condition that is seldom discussed, yet affects a great many people of all ages. Many patients are embarrassed by incontinence, but the doctor will treat it as the common and treatable medical condition it is. Incontinence is a medical condition that can be cured and/or greatly improved with proper treatment.

Simple changes in diet, pelvic muscle exercises, timed toileting, prescription drugs, bladder retraining and other procedures have been used successfully to treat incontinence. The most important thing the patient can do is to start using products specifically designed for incontinence protection. There are many different brands and types of incontinence products on the market and choosing the right one can be confusing. The doctor and/or the pharmacist can help you and the patient choose the right product.

Normal urine does not have a foul smell. If the patient's urine smells bad, see the doctor. Many patients with incontinence problems will restrict the amount of liquids to reduce troublesome leakage. Make sure that the patient is drinking plenty of liquids (6 to 8 glasses of water per day). Odor in the urine can be caused by asparagus, coffee or a medicine. Cranberry juice helps reduce urine odor but the patient will need to drink 6 to 8 ounces a day. Cranberry juice has also been found to reduce urinary tract infections. If you are diabetic or overweight be careful – cranberry juice is high in sugar.

Described below are the four levels of incontinence and the recommended products for each level. We can work with you to make sure the patient has the right product. Once the patient and you are comfortable that they have the right product, and everything is going well, LeBoeuf's Incontinence Service can set up a delivery schedule for all of the needed incontinence products until notified to stop. There is no extra cost for providing this service.

Choosing the Right Incontinence Product:

Symptoms — *Light*

- Small loss of urine, especially when laughing, coughing, sneezing or straining. The patient usually stays dry at night.

Recommended products:

- Poise Pads for Women. One size fits all. Wear with snug-fitting underwear.
- Depend Shields for Men and Women. Regular size and Extra size. Wear with snug fitting underwear.

Symptoms — *Light to moderate*

- Temporary or long-term loss of bladder control after surgery. Inability to prevent urine leakage after feeling strong urge to urinate. Leakage occurs on way to bathroom.

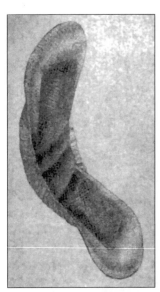

Le 270-2330 / Le 270-2439

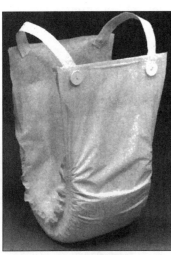

Le 148-6869

Recommended Products:

- Poise Guards for Women
- Depend Guards for Men

Symptoms — **Moderate**

- Frequent leakage — usually small amounts. Moderate loss of urine, especially when laughing, coughing, sneezing or straining. The patient usually stays dry at night.

Recommended Products:

- Depend Undergarments with Button Straps for Men and Women
- Depend EasyFit Undergarments for Men and Women

Symptoms — **Heavy**

- Heavy or continuous urine leakage. Heavy leakage at night or when lying down.

Recommended Products:

- Depend Fitted Briefs
- Depend Overnight Fitted Briefs

Products

Depend, Poise Pads. Discreet size. Dryness Plus™ layer pulls liquid away from surface. Super absorbent material locks liquid into a gel to help prevent leaks. Gentle elastic gathers designed to fit a woman's body.

Le 270-2330	Regular	Pack of 22	$6.95
Le 270-2439	Extra Long	Pack of 20	$6.95

Poise Pad Extra Plus Absorbent. Super absorbent material. Locks liquid into a gel that won't leak. Dryness Plus, layer pulls fluid away from skin for outstanding dryness.

Le 163-1621	Pack of 60	$31.95
Le 163-2140	Pack of 16	$6.95

Depend Undergarments. Double layer system, top layer absorbs fluid, second layer locks it away. Thin, form fitting shape. Elastic straps for secure, comfortable fit. Elastic leg gathers.

Le 148-6869	Regular absorbency	Pack of 12	$10.95
Le 147-9948	Regular absorbency	Pack of 36	$31.95
Le 340-1734	Regular absorbency	Pack of 72	$57.95
Le 165-3013	Regular absorbency	Pack of 144	$109.95
Le 164-9201	Regular absorbency, adjustable strap	Pack of 34	$31.95
Le 165-0035	Extra absorbency, adjustable strap	Pack of 28	$31.95
Le 169-2664	Extra absorbency	Pack of 10	$10.95
Le 161-7299	Extra absorbency	Pack of 30	$31.95
Le 340-2294	Extra absorbency	Pack of 60	$57.95

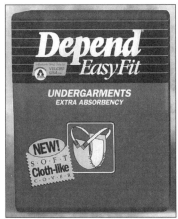

Le 164-9201 / Le 165-0035

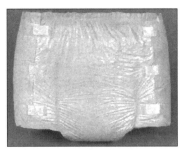

Le 116-9184

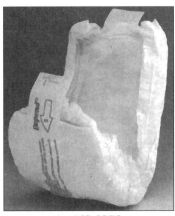

Le 163-0276

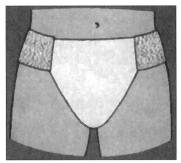

Le 133-5496 / Le 133-5660 /
Le 133-5579 / Le 133-5348

Depend Easy Fit Undergarments. Double layer system, top layer absorbs fluid, second layer locks it away. Thin, form fitting shape. Elastic leg gathers. Comes with adjustable Velcro strap tabs.

Le 164-9201	Regular absorbency	Pack of 34	$31.95
Le 165-0035	Extra absorbency	Pack of 28	$31.95

Depend Nonelastic Leg Undergarments. Same as Depend Undergarments but with nonelastic leg openings.

Le 342-2516	Extra absorbency	Pack of 30	$31.95

Depend Fitted Briefs. Double layer system, top layer absorbs fluid, second layer locks it away. Easy Grip™ tapes for better hold, easier use. Elastic at legs and waist for better fit. Fitted briefs come in:

Small	Hip 22″ to 32″
Medium	Hip 33″ to 41″
Large	Hips over 42″

Le 116-9184	Small	Pack of 26	$31.95
Le 165-7212	Small	Pack of 104	$109.95
Le 147-9955	Medium	Pack of 8	$10.95
Le 116-8723	Medium	Pack of 22	$31.95
Le 340-2963	Medium	Pack of 44	$57.95
Le 165-8681	Medium	Pack of 88	$109.95
Le 147-9963	Large	Pack of 6	$10.95
Le 116-7246	Large	Pack of 18	$31.95
Le 340-2658	Large	Pack of 36	$57.95
Le 166-2931	Large	Pack of 72	$109.95
Le 163-1217	Medium Overnight	Pack of 20	$31.95

Depend Shields. Double layer system, top layer absorbs fluid, second layer locks it away. Designed for discreet, comfortable fit. Adhesive tabs for secure hold.

Le 325-4596	Regular absorbency	Pack of 12	$4.95
Le 116-9374	Extra absorbency	Pack of 14	$10.95

Depend Guards for Men. Discreet, comfortable protection. Super absorbent material quickly locks liquid in get to prevent leaks. Comes with elasticized pouch that provides a cup-like fit for comfort. Wide adhesive strip to hold guard securely in place.

Le 163-0276	Super absorbency	Pack of 18	$11.95

Duro-Med Men's Incontinent Supporter. Designed for light incontinent problems. Pouch snaps out for washing and replacement. 3-inch wide elastic band. Pouch lined with flannel and quick-drying olefin.

Le 133-5496	Small	$8.95
Le 133-5660	Medium	$8.95
Le 133-5579	Large	$8.95
Le 133-5348	Extra large	$8.95

Depend Underpads. Stay-dry liner. Waterproof backing with sealed edges for leakage protection.

Le 116-6644	Chair size	17½″ × 24″	Pack of 36	$10.95
Le 116-6438	Bed size	23″ × 36″	Pack of 18	$10.95
Le 164-7874	Bed size	23″ × 36″	Pack of 108	$57.95

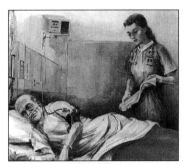

Ba 190015

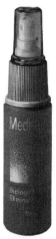

Ba 7012A

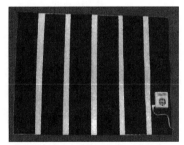

Le 175-9307

Attends Washcloths. Patented two-ply, textured wipes gently clean and apply lotion in one step. Folded design helps protect hand and allows for easy, one-hand use. Low profile tub for easy storage.

Le 227-7051	Pack of 68	$10.95

Viscot Disposable Wash Cloths. Rayon blue-white. 10″ × 13″ Nice big size.

Vi W1013-500	100 per bag	$10.95

Bard Fecal Containment Device. Self-adhesive fecal containment designed to minimize the time and backbreaking effort to manage a recurring problem. Simple to apply. Patient can walk about without fear of losing pouch or suffering pain from disconnection. Odor is contained and patients are spared the distress of soiling themselves. Adhesive is gentle enough to be used on a daily basis without breakdown of the skin. Each kit comes with latex collection pouch, powder adhesive, closure clip, drainage bag adapter and adhesive remover.

Ba 190015	Product is for one time use and is disposable	$18.95

Bard Medi-aire, Odor Eliminator. A spray or two of the odor eliminator's concentrated formula terminates unpleasant odors. Medi-aire chemically combines with foul smelling odors to eliminate them — not just cover them up.

Ba 7012A	Fresh air scent sprayer	1 oz.	$4.95
Ba 7008A	Refill bottle for sprayer	8 oz.	$14.95

Hy Tape Sani-Garm Washable Incontinence Brief. Designed for men and women with moderate to severe bladder control problems. Available in two types, pull-on or with front closing rustproof snaps. Highly absorbent, lightweight, quiet (no rustling sound), and reusable. The perfect cover for pads, panties, liners or adult diapers. Elastic waist and leg bands.

Small	20″ to 28″
Medium	30″ to 36″
Large	38″ to 44″
Extra large	46″ to 52″

Hy 210	Pull on with closed sides	$11.95
Hy 205	With snaps for patients confined to bed	$12.95

Burney Products Disposable Underwear. Unisex brief is full-cut and designed to be comfortable when worn the entire day. Each brief has an elastic waistband and lightweight, non-binding leg bands.

Bu 140-650	Small	Bag of 24	$15.95
Bu 140-651	Medium	Bag of 24	$15.95
Bu 140-652	Large	Bag of 24	$15.95
Bu 140-653	Extra large	Bag of 24	$15.95

Koregan Bedcheck, Bed Pad, and Alarm. For habitual bedwetters. Moisture sensing pad and easy to use alarm device. For adults or children.

Le 175-9307	$85.95

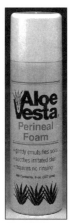

Co 6280-46

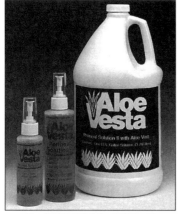

Co 6985-K6 / Co 6985-48

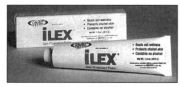

Co 6987-Y9

ConvaTec Aloe Vesta, Perineal Foam. Easy-to-use perineal thick foam cleaner won't run while cleaning the patient and clings to the patient at any angle. Cleans and deodorizes. No-rinse formula leaves behind moisturizers to alleviate dryness and a refreshing fragrance to help minimize odors.

Co 6280-46   8 oz. spray can $9.95

ConvaTec Aloe Vesta Perineal Solution II. Contains special formula for superior odor control. Gently emulsifies soil and brings soothing relief to perineal care. No-rinse formula leaves behind moisturizers and a refreshing fragrance.

Co 6985-K6   4 oz. spray bottle $3.95
Co 6985-48   8 oz. spray bottle $5.95

ConvaTec iLEX. Used for treatment of severe diaper rash and on weepy, denuded skin. Seals out wetness. When all else fails this may be the answer. Petroleum-based product.

Co 6987-Y9   1.5 oz. tube $6.95

Care-Tech Laboratories Incont-Aid Kit. Each incont-Aid Kit contains a 4-ounce spray bottle of Orchid Fresh perineal cleanser with odor control, a 1-ounce tube of Care-Creme containing natural aloe vera and a 1-ounce tube of Barri-Care ointment. A complete skin care system for incontinent patients. Great kit for traveling.

Ca C212 ID $14.95

Baxter Enema Administration Unit with Flexible Bag. Includes attached tube, soap, and underpad.

Le 220-7413   Medical grade plastic tubing $2.95

Chlorofresh Gel Caps. Natural chlorophyll. Reduces odors originating in the digestive tract.

Le 357-8432   30 Capsules $8.95

Nullo Tablets. Effective in helping to reduce the odors associated with incontinence.

Le 114-9913   60 Tablets $8.95
Le 241-9604   135 Tablets $16.95

Derifil Tablets. One of the more effective odor reducing products.

Le 143-4570   30 Tablets $24.95
Le 143-4588   100 Tablets $44.95

LeBoeuf's Services

Call **LeBoeuf's** ☎ 1-800-546-5559 for the following services. Please have ready the patient's name, address, zip code, age, telephone number and physical circumstances (Alzheimer's, heart problem, arthritis, etc.) when you call.

- Consulting Service
    - Wheelchairs (design, ultra-light, sports chairs, etc.)
    - Van Conversions
    - Electronics
        - Hearing
        - Vision
        - Security
        - Communication (TTY, Call Buttons, Telephones, etc.)
        - Television, VCR's, Radio, Stereo
        - Computers and Software

- Home Healthcare Workshops

- Caregivers Speakers Bureau

- Incontinent Supply Service

- Respite Network

- Home Modification Planning Service

- Assistive Travel Agency

- Employment Screening Service

- Referral Service for:
    - Hospitals
    - Nursing homes
    - Hospice
    - Visiting nurse associations
    - Adult day care programs
    - Respite care (nursing homes, support groups,)
    - Social services case workers
    - Household help

Incontinent Supply Service

We will track your orders for incontinent supplies over five to six weeks to ascertain quantity and type of product your patient requires.

To save you time and to insure that you will never run out of incontinent products, we can set up an automatic reorder and shipping service.

Once the service is established, we will ship to you on a regular schedule until you notify us to discontinue the service.

Lung Disorders

LUNGS ARE VERY COMPLEX and contain at least three dozen types of cells. They provide the body with its supply of oxygen, remove waste and are the first line of defense against the dusts, viruses, bacteria and other alien substances that invade the body each time a person breathes. Affecting people of all ages, over 26 million Americans are now living with chronic lung disease. There is no single cause for lung disease. While the death rate from heart disease and cancer has been dropping, the lung disease death rate is increasing at about 19 percent. Lung disease is the number three cause of death in the United States.

Lung disease includes lung cancer, emphysema, chronic bronchitis, asthma, pneumonia, flu, tuberculosis, respiratory distress syndrome (RDS), cystic fibrosis, sudden infant death syndrome, AIDS-related lung disease, occupation lung disease (black lung, silicosis, etc.), saroidosis, sleep disorder breathing (sleep apnea) and many others.

Lung Cancer

Lung cancer is the most common fatal cancer in the United States. The incidence of lung cancer peaks at 65 years old for men and 70 years old for women. Lung cancer accounts for about 15 percent of all cancer cases. It has been increasing faster than any other cancer, with cigarette smoking being the number one cause (87 percent). The outlook for the successful treatment of lung cancer is not good. Early intervention may help but, normally, by the time the disease is discovered, it has spread to other parts of the body. Overall, less than 10 percent of lung cancer patients live for five years after the disease is diagnosed. If surgery can be performed, the five-year survival rate goes up to between 15 and 30 percent.

Symptoms include coughing (80 percent), coughing up blood, chest pain and shortness of breath (wheezing). Lung cancer is usually discovered from taking a chest X-ray. Other tests include a check of the sputum and a biopsy (surgery or using a needle to take part of the suspected tumor).

If the cancer is found at an early stage, the surgeon may remove part or all of the lung. Drugs and radiation may also be used to prevent the spread of the cancer or to treat a small cell lung cancer.

Chronic Obstructive Pulmonary Disease (COPD)

Emphysema, chronic bronchitis and asthma are part of what people in the medical field call Chronic Obstructive Pulmonary Disease (COPD). Doctors who specialize in these diseases are called pulmonologists. In simple terms, it is an increased resistance to exhaling. COPD is second only to heart disease as a cause of disability in the United States, due mainly to the aging population. Over 82 percent of all COPD deaths are caused by smoking.

Many patients living with chronic obstructive pulmonary disease (COPD) can benefit from medications. They can open airways, fight lung infections, reduce coughing, thin mucous, decrease anxiety and relieve pain. In addition, learning to breath easier will also help.

Patients on oxygen therapy can experience extreme anxiety and become very frightened if they experience airflow obstruction (dyspnea). Education and training in oxygen therapy allow the patient to remain calm and under control. Patients must learn to exercise properly, not to exert themselves, how to use their standby oxygen and fill their portable oxygen tanks (if they can walk). Many patients on oxygen therapy remain hooked up to the concentrator 24 hours a day, 7 days a week. They will be on oxygen even when taking a bath or shower. For those patients able to walk, a hose can be attached to the concentrator that will enable them to move about the home and still be hooked to the concentrator. If the patient is capable of assisting in the kitchen, a rolling stool is a great help.

Emphysema

Emphysema is a disease of the lungs in which the small air sacs (alveoli) in the lungs become damaged. In most cases, emphysema is caused by smoking cigarettes. Rarely does atmospheric pollution cause emphysema. Oxygen is inhaled and passed into the blood stream through the air sacs. When these become damaged, the level of oxygen begins to fall and can lead to raised blood pressure in the pulmonary artery, which leads to an enlargement of the right side of the heart. Emphysema often goes hand in hand with chronic bronchitis. Emphysema affects about 1.65 million Americans.

Symptoms:

- Shortness of breath.
- Chronic cough with a slight wheeze.
- Barrel-shaped chest caused by air being trapped in the outer part of the lungs.
- Turns purple-blue, due to lack of oxygen (blue bloaters).
- Breathe rapidly, but retain normal coloring (pink puffers).
- Swelling in the legs because of an abnormal accumulation of fluids.
- Frequent depression or marked anxiety.

The doctor will take a blood test from an artery to determine oxygen and carbon dioxide levels. Chest x-rays are also taken to exclude the possibility of another lung disease. The doctor will also perform a pulmonary function test to determine the breathing capacity of the patient.

Treatment:

- Drugs to widen the airways that link the windpipe to the lungs. These drugs are taken by an aerosol inhaler or a nebulizer that produces a fine spray.
- Corticosteroid drugs taken by inhaler.
- Salt restricted diet.
- Oxygen by mask or a tube in the nose.
- Breathing training to treat anxious patients who have developed a rapid breathing rate (see Breathing Easier, below).
- Increase physical activity.

As long as there is no severe heart disease, a regular exercise program prescribed by the doctor will prevent excessive disability that results from prolonged inactivity.

Bronchitis

Bronchitis is the inflammation of the airways that connect the windpipe to the lungs. Acute bronchitis happens suddenly and does not last long. Chronic bronchitis is persistent over a long time and recurs. Both are more common in smokers and for those who live in areas of high air pollution.

Acute bronchitis is usually caused by a viral infection such as a cold. The inflammation of the windpipe causes swelling and pus to form. When the patient coughs, yellow or green sputum comes out. The patient may also have pain behind the breastbone and a higher than normal temperature.

Treatment:

- Use a humidifier– do not breathe hot steam – it can be very harmful.
- Drink plenty of fluids.
- Use antibiotics prescribed by a doctor if there is a bacterial infection. If it is a virus, antibiotics will not work.
- Increase physical activity.

Bronchitis is considered chronic if a person coughs up yellow or green sputum for three consecutive months in two or more consecutive years. Chronic bronchitis results from the obstruction of the airways in the lungs and is mainly caused by smoking cigarettes. Most patients are over 40 and male sufferers outnumber females by a 2 to 1 ratio.

The doctor may decide to investigate the patient's condition by taking x-rays, blood tests, sputum analysis and breathing function tests. Symptoms and treatment is the same as acute bronchitis

Asthma

There are about 10 million asthmatics in the United States. Asthma usually starts in childhood and tends to clear up and become less severe in early adulthood. More than half of the children who have asthma outgrow the problem by the time they are 21. There are two main types of asthma:

- Extrinsic — external cause of an attack by pollen, house dust, animal hair, dander or feathers.
- Intrinsic — where there is no apparent external cause.

Most asthma attacks occur early in the morning. Heredity is the major factor in the development of extrinsic asthma. However, asthma seems to becoming more common in the United States. During an asthma attack which may last from a few minutes to hours, the airways contract and mucus clogs the airway.

Prevention of asthma attacks can be enhanced by avoiding foods that trigger attacks. Other triggers include overexertion, common cold, flu, viruses, fear, anger, laughing too hard, crying and smoke from cigarettes. The doctor can run tests to identify asthma attack triggers. It is important to avoid those areas, foods or exposures to hot or cold that the doctor has identified as a cause of an asthma attack if at all possible.

Symptoms:

- Breathlessness.
- Dry cough.
- Wheezing.
- Chest feels tight.
- Hyperventilation.

Treatment for an asthma attack:

- Give the medicine prescribed by the doctor with an oral inhaler. If it does not seem to work and the doctor has said that two doses is okay, wait a couple of minutes before repeating.
- Help the patient to relax. It is extremely important that the patient remain calm. One way to reassure the patient is to speak calmly and softly while gently and tenderly massaging the shoulders.
- Have the patient sit upright in a chair.
- Tell the patient to breath slowly (see Breathing Easier, below).
- Have the patient close their eyes.
- If coughing starts, try to control the cough so that the coughing brings up mucus by having the patient lean forward slightly with the patient's feet still on the floor.
- Have the patient breath in deeply and hold it for a second or two.
- Have the patient cough twice. First cough is to loosen the mucus and the second cough to bring the mucus up.
- Cough into a tissue.
- If the attack gets worse, call the doctor or take the patient to the hospital.

Many of the available drugs have proved to be very helpful, but the drugs do not work for all patients. Make sure that the medicine the doctor has prescribed is not out of date. Outdated medicine loses its effectiveness.

How to Breath Easier

Abdominal breathing exercise for deeper breathing. Deep breathing promotes coughing and keeps the lungs clear.

- Have the patient place one hand on their chest. This hand should remain still as the patient breathes.
- Place the patient's other hand on their abdomen (thumb should be just below the navel. This hand should be rising and falling as the patient breathes.
- The patient should inhale through the nose to a count of 3. Exhale to a count of 6.
- Repeat this exercise for about 15 minutes.
- The patient should practice this exercise often. Learning to coordinate abdominal movements and breathing takes time.

Pursed-Lip Breathing:

- Have the patient inhale slowly through the nose.
- The patient should pucker the lips and exhale slowly making a soft hissing sound.

What to do:

Contact a doctor — Have the patient make and keep the appointment. There is no single or simple test for Chronic Airways Obstructive Disorders (COPD). Testing may include blood tests, x-rays, sputum analysis and breathing function. If the diagnosis determines that the patient has COPD, the following will provide the caregiver with information, support and services to assist the patient to cope with breathing problems.

Contact the Allergy and Asthma Association — Call 1-202-466-7643 or toll free 1-800-7 ASTHMA (1-800-727-8462) for their information line. A free information kit is available. They are located at 1125 15th Street, NW, Suite 502, Washington, DC 20005. The personnel are very responsive and understanding.

Contact the American Lung Association — 1-800-586-4872 or write to them at 1740 Broadway, New York City, NY 10019-4374. Information and literature on various problems of the lungs is available. Founded in 1904 to fight tuberculosis, there are 116 constituent and affiliate associations and thousands of volunteers and staff to assist in providing information and research. For a listing of the nearest American Lung Association office to you, call their 800 number or **LeBoeuf's ☎ 1-800-546-5559.**

When you call the American Lung Association 800 number, you will be automatically directed to the closest office.

Contact local social services organizations — There are many agencies that will provide information and listings of resources that are available in your area. Agencies such as the offices on aging, local health agencies as well as religious-affiliated service groups also provide information, training and support. There are also associations and companies that provide care management services to serve as the link between you and community-based services. They charge for their services — so be sure you understand what it will cost to have them provide assistance.

Contact a lawyer — It is very important to act appropriately to protect the future security of the patient. There are lawyers who specialize in elder law. You will need to execute a Durable Power of Attorney for Health Care or a Living Will. Better yet, have your lawyer prepare a Living Trust. **LeBoeuf's ☎ 1-800-546-5559** has a listing of lawyers in your area.

Communication — Tell family and friends how they can help the patient cope with emphysema and asthma. If the patient has cancer of the lung, be sure that you call a family meeting to discuss the prognosis. The patient will need a lot of understanding and TLC. While it is natural to become upset, someone has to keep things under control.

LeBoeuf's Services

Call **LeBoeuf's** ☎ 1-800-546-5559 for the following services. Please have ready the patient's name, address, zip code, age, telephone number and physical circumstances (Alzheimer's, heart problem, arthritis, etc.) when you call.

- Consulting Service
    - Wheelchairs (design, ultra-light, sports chairs, etc.)
    - Van Conversions
    - Electronics
        - Hearing
        - Vision
        - Security
        - Communication (TTY, Call Buttons, Telephones, etc.)
        - Television, VCR's, Radio, Stereo
        - Computers and Software

- Home Healthcare Workshops

- Caregivers Speakers Bureau

- Incontinent Supply Service

- Respite Network

- Home Modification Planning Service

- Assistive Travel Agency

- Employment Screening Service

- Referral Service for:
    - Hospitals
    - Nursing homes
    - Hospice
    - Visiting nurse associations
    - Adult day care programs
    - Respite care (nursing homes, support groups,)
    - Social services case workers
    - Household help

Respiratory Therapy

The best way to keep a heart healthy is to keep the lungs healthy.

Relaxation therapy is critical. Meditation, yoga and Tai Chi are some of the ways that patients have been able to gain control of their emotions and reduce anxiety from the fear of oxygen being cut off. Alcohol and medications do not mix. Hot spicy foods can cause coughing. Learning to cough under control takes years of experience and patients will learn to develop their own methods. Many close their eyes and concentrate on something that is relaxing to try and control the coughing.

The caregiver must have patience — and even more patience is required when caring for a patient on oxygen. Most patients start the day out very slowly and build up energy during the day. If you have outings planned, make them in the early afternoon. Encourage patients to get out if they can. When patients are trying to do something new, you must keep encouraging them. One or two tries is not enough. There are portable oxygen units that allow patients to go just about anywhere. Always buy a cart to go with a portable oxygen unit. For most patients, the weight of a portable oxygen unit is too much for them to carry around for any length of time.

Patients with chronic bronchitis, emphysema, lung cancer, congestive heart failure, cystic fibrosis or an occupational lung disease such as black lung may need oxygen therapy. Oxygen is used to treat patients who have inadequate oxygen in their tissues.

Oxygen makes up 21 percent of the earth's atmosphere.

There are two ways to obtain respiratory therapy in the home. You can call providers who will rent oxygen concentrators and/or deliver oxygen to the home or, for those patients who do not have local oxygen service companies, you can purchase the oxygen concentrators to provide your own oxygen for the patient. Look in the yellow pages under oxygen for a vendor who will provide home oxygen service. The home oxygen vendor should offer:

- 24 hour service.
- Trained personnel who will instruct the patient and you on how to use the equipment and what maintenance to the equipment should be performed.
- Regular visits to check equipment and make sure the patient is getting what has been ordered by the doctor.
- Continuing cost review to insure that the system is the most cost effective.

If patients complain that they are not getting enough oxygen, call the vendor and have them check both the flow of oxygen and the concentration.

A patient's normal breathing rate is 12 to 20 breaths per minute and has an arterial blood gas reading of 80-100 mm Hg for level of oxygen and 35-45 mm Hg for level of carbon dioxide. The level of carbon dioxide in the blood is what stimulates a normal person to breath.

There are three main components to an oxygen system: the regulator which releases oxygen at a safe rate; a humidifier (that prevents the mucous membranes from drying out), and the oxygen itself. The oxygen can be supplied in cylinders (either liquid or compressed gas) or can be supplied by oxygen concentrators. Oxygen concentrators separate oxygen from the air and remix it in a higher than normal concentration. Most patients will have oxygen delivered to them from the oxygen tanks or the concentrator via tubing and by either a cannula (nose prongs that fit into the nostrils) or a face mask that covers the patient's nose and mouth. The flow rate and the concentration of oxygen determines what delivery system will be recommended by the doctor. If the flow rate is more than 6 liters per minute and oxygen concentration is over 50 percent, a face mask will probably be required. The cannula is the easiest to use and the most comfortable for the patient.

If the cannula is not comfortable, keep trying different types. Many of the cannulas have nose prongs that may be too big for the patient and are very uncomfortable. If the patient complains, have the patient try what is called a "low flow" cannula, which has smaller nose prongs. Cannulas that are being used on a continuous basis should be changed at least once a week to prevent the build-up of bacteria. According to many patients who use oxygen, changing once a week results in fewer colds and other problems. For those patients who are able to walk, the hose to the cannula probably should be at the back of the head to keep it from being in the way. For those in bed, the cannula would be best positioned over the head or in a stethoscope type configuration.

Tips for using oxygen equipment:

- Don't change the flow rate without consulting the doctor.
- Avoid alcohol and other sedatives when using oxygen. They can slow the patient's breathing.
- Prevent skin irritation from tubing by tucking gauze pads behind the patient's ears and against the cheeks and/or use a cannula support.
- Use water-based lubricants to moisten lips or nostrils. Never use oil-based products.
- Order a supply of oxygen from your supplier 2 to 3 days before the patient will need it. Make sure you have the phone number written where you can find it. Write the number on the inside of the front cover of the *Handbook* so you don't lose it.
- Check the level of the sterile or distilled water in the humidifier bottle often. When refilling the humidifier, pour out what is left and refill with new water.
- To see if the patient is getting oxygen, take the nasal cannula and invert it in a glass of water. If bubbles appear, oxygen is flowing through the system. Shake off excess water before reinserting the cannula in the patient's nose.

Caring for oxygen equipment:

- For the cannula or mask, wipe with a damp cloth every 8 hours. Wash nasal prongs with liquid soap 1 to 2 times a week and rinse well. Change cannula once a week and throw out the old one.
- For the oxygen concentrator, wipe the cabinet with a damp cloth and towel dry each day. Clean air filter at least once a week and clean the compressor filter as directed by the manufacturer.
- For the humidifier, wash the bottle daily in warm, soapy water, rinse well and air dry. Disinfect the bottle and top 1 to 2 times a week. Use distilled or filtered water.
- For the metered dose inhaler or nebulizer, rinse mouthpiece with warm water after each use. Separate plastic parts and disinfect daily as directed. Some parts may be dishwasher safe. Be sure to read the manufacturer's instructions.

Using oxygen safely requires that you, the patient and visitors must follow certain rules. Oxygen is odorless, colorless and tasteless. While not explosive by itself, oxygen can facilitate combustion. The greater the concentration of oxygen, the more quickly fires can start and the harder they are to put out.

Safety Tips

- Do not smoke in the room or let others smoke. Put " No Smoking" signs on door and in the room.
- Make sure that any electrical equipment such as razors, hearing aids, television, heating pads, etc. are in good condition and cannot cause a spark.
- Use the nonsmoking sections of restaurants.
- Do not use flammable products such as aerosols, rubbing alcohol, paint thinners, nail polish remover, or oil-based lubricants.
- Make sure that the cylinder is secure and will not fall over. It can go like a rocket if it is knocked over and the gas escapes.
- Turn the oxygen off when not in use.
- Inform the electric company that the patient is on an oxygen concentrator.
- Let visitors know that there are tubes (usually clear plastic and hard to see) running from the concentrator to the patient so that they can avoid tripping over them. Use utility grips to organize the tubing. Do not run the tubing under clothing, bedcovers, carpet or furniture. You will not be able to see if the tubing is kinked or has a cut.
- Clothing worn by both you and the patient should be cotton. Use cotton blankets and sheets to avoid static sparks.

- Make sure all electrical equipment is grounded.
- Alert the fire department that you have oxygen in the home. Make sure everyone knows how to use the fire extinguisher. If a fire does occur, turn off the oxygen and get everyone out of the house.
- If the patient can walk around, do not let the patient into the kitchen with the oxygen if a gas stove is on.

The patient will need to obtain a doctor's order and have the doctor provide the blood gasses/blood saturation count before you call a provider of oxygen rental equipment. The type of oxygen therapy the doctor has prescribed has a lot do with what equipment is appropriate.

You can rent a concentrator for about $370 per month and the provider will usually provide an emergency tank of oxygen at no charge, just in case the power goes off.

Remember, if in doubt about what to do, call the doctor or ask the nurse. If the patient experiences any of the following symptoms, call the doctor at once.

Signs of not enough oxygen:
- Fast breathing (more than 24 breaths a minute), irregular breathing.
- Restlessness.
- Anxiety and/or confusion.
- Tiredness or drowsiness (patient starts leaning on everything).
- Blue fingernails or lips.

Signs of too much oxygen:
- Headaches.
- Slurred speech.
- Difficulty waking the patient.
- Shallow, slow breathing.

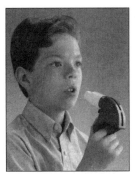

Mc 162-7256

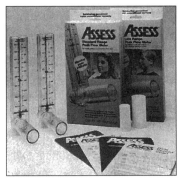

Mc 195-4866, . . ., Mc 195-3769

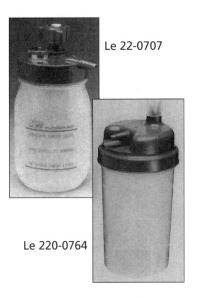

Le 22-0707

Le 220-0764

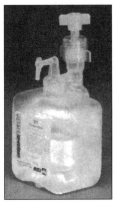

Le 211-6838

Peak Flow Meters

Peak Flow Meters are a device that measures the force of air expelled from the lungs. This measurement is called a peak expiratory flow rate (PEFR). It helps determine the amount of patient airflow obstruction. The PEFR is important because it can detect subtle changes in lung function before the patient is aware of them. Based on the reading from the flow meter, the doctor may adjust medication. If the peak flow meters are used correctly, the patient will tend to require less medication and enjoy a better quality of life. Usually, the flow meter is used by asthma patients. Keeping a daily record of the patient's PEFR scores is very important to establish a pattern that will assist the patient and the doctor in managing asthma better.

DeVilbiss Pocketpeak Low-Range Flow Meter. Reusable mouthpiece attaches for secure storage. Meets or exceeds National Asthma Education Program (NEAP) and National Heart, Lung, Blood Institute (NHLBI) standards. Plastic housing and stainless steel vane are dishwasher safe. Fits in shirt pocket and easy to use. Accuracy within 10 percent of reading.

Le 162-7256	3.4″ × 3.2″, Weight 1.4 ounces	$23.95
Le 163-3015	Universal Flow Meter	$23.95

HealthScan Products Assess, Peak Flow Meters. Patented flow-sampling technology. Easy-to-read scale. Tough polycarbonate body. Includes molded plastic case with 1 adult and 1 pediatric mouthpiece, 14-week patient record chart and instructions. Accuracy plus or minus 5 percent.

Le 195-4866	Standard Range 60 to 880 LPM	$32.95
Le 195-4494	Low Range 30 to 390 LPM	$36.95
Le 195-3769	Assess Disposable Mouthpieces, adult. Case of 100	$38.95

Oxygen Equipment

Most oxygen equipment is available only by prescription. Check with the doctor before ordering.

Hudson Reusable Humidifier. Features a shatter-proof dishwasher safe polypropylene jar, 2 psi pressure relief valve, chromed brass connectors, and removable diffuser head. Leak-proof jar with maximum and minimum water markings.

Le 220-0707		$49.95

Hudson Disposable Humidifier. Disposable, durable plastic with preset audible alarm at 4 psi pressure relief. Maximum and minimum water level lines. Recessed nipple helps reduce possibility of breaking off outlet connection.

Le 220-0764	Each	$2.95

Hudson AQUAPAK. Sterile water. Comes with sterile humidifier adapter 040.

Le 211-6838	Each	$4.95

B & F Large Cylinder Base. Used for H-type cylinder. Fiberglass.

Le 220-7942	White	$48.95

B & F Medium Cylinder Base. Used for M-type cylinder.

Le 220-7777	White	$47.95

B& F Small Cylinder Base. Used for D- and E-type cylinders.

Le 220-7124	White	$20.95

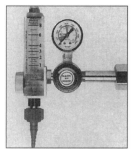

Le 171-6026

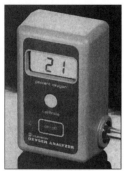

Le 147-7769

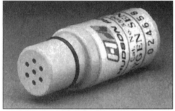

Le 147-7752

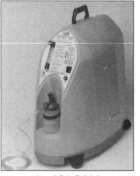

Le 161-9444

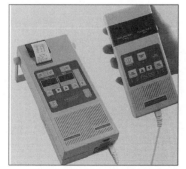

Pa 010-340, Pa 010-400

Erie Liter Meter. Zero to 8 liter range.

Le 220-3321 $19.95

Mada Regulator. Flowmeter type. Shatter free acrylic flowmeter. Back-pressure compensated, with built-in safety release valve. Accurate to plus or minus .2 liter. Easy-to-read scale with .5 liter increments, marked from 0 to 2 liters. 1/4 to 8 liters per minute (LPM) flow rate. Lifetime warranty on internal parts.

Le 171-6026   For cylinders H,KM,S,T $139.95

Mada Regulator. Gauge type. Diaphragm-free construction. Fingertip control knob for flow rate. Contents gauge with pressure relief device. Accurate to plus or minus .2 liter, with .5 liter increments. Easy-to-read scale. 1/4 to 8 liters per minute (LPM) flow rate.

Le 171-5952   For small cylinder D & E $115.95

Hudson Oxygen Analyzer and Sensor. For use with oxygen concentrators, tanks and liquid oxygen systems. Auto-off feature turns analyzer off after 5 minutes. Comes with 9-volt battery, oxygen tubing, nipple and nut. Accuracy of plus or minus 2% of full scale after calibration. Maintenance-free sensor.

Le 147-7769   Analyzer $368.95
Le 147-7652   Sensor $193.95

DeVilbiss Keystone™ Oxygen Concentrators. Microprocessor controlled. Provide continuous low-flow oxygen to meet needs of home oxygen patient. Self-diagnostic system. Extended life intake bacterial filter. Humidifier bottle not included. 5 liter unit.
Concentration: 90% at 1/4 LPM; 93% at 1/2 to 5 LPM plus or minus 3%.

Le 161-9444   4 year parts warranty $3175.95
Le 161-8388   With oxygen sensing device $3525.95

DeVilbiss Service Kit. Contains assorted tools and supplies needed to repair and maintain the DeVilbiss oxygen concerator. Sturdy gray plastic tool kit. You will need both kits to service the Keystone oxygen concentrators.

Le 221-2066 $285.95
Le 378-9500   Keystone upgrade kit $65.95

Palco Labs Model 300 Oximeter. Over 1,000 readings on one set of 6 "AA" alkaline batteries. Nicad rechargeable version also available. Bright LED display for saturation and pulse rate. Rugged, water-resistant case withstands shock and vibration. Used for "spot checks". Can be used for continuous monitoring and batteries should last for about 4-6 hours.

Pa 010-300 $895.95

Palco Labs Model 340 and 400 Pulse Oximeter. Model 340 has Ni-cad rechargeable battery and has high and low alarm features for the percent of oxygen saturation and pulse/heart rate. Has a "pulse-tone-pitch-change" to alert the caregiver or the nurse if a change occurs in the percent of oxygen saturation.

Pa 010-340   Handheld $1,395.95
Pa 010-400   Same as 340 but has printing capability $1,495.95

All Palco oximeters come with six-foot extension cable and operators manual. Models 340 and 400 have AC power adapter.

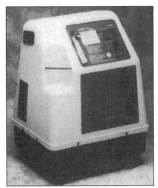

Le 225-0587

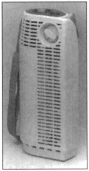

Le 271-2693

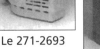

Le 225-6733

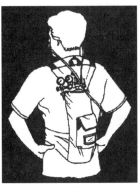

Ro 5003

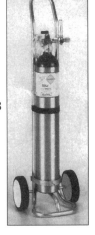

Le 219-7838

Invacare Mobilaire V 5 Liter Oxygen. Concentrator. Battery-Free™ power loss alarm sounds audible signal if flow is blocked or power fails. Consistent oxygen delivery. Internal ventilation for cooler operation. Performance of 95% plus 2% at 1 to 3 LPM, 94% plus 3% at 4 LPM, 91% plus 4% at 5 LPM.

Le 225-0587   Microcomputer checks performance continuously $2885.95

LeBoeuf's can also supply other DeVilbiss model concentrators as well as Healthdyne, Caire Pioneer, Puritan-Bennett Companion, and other models of Invacare. Whatever the patient's doctor recommends, we will be able to assist you in locating the equipment.

Puritan-Bennett Companions 31A Stationary Liquid Oxygen System. 31 liquid liters capacity. Weighs 125 pounds full; 50 pounds empty. Mode of operation is continuous. Flow range from .25 to 6 LPM. Nominal use time at 2 LPM: 213 hours.

Le 225-6733 $2695.95
Le 271-1919   Roller base 20 inches x 20 inches x 24 inches $ 84.95

Puritan-Bennett Companion 1000 Portable Liquid Oxygen System. Small, lightweight and portable. No batteries required. Sleek, modern appearance with recessed controls and indicators. Continuous mode operation. Flow range .25 to 6 LPM. Nominal use time at 2 LPM: 8.5 hours. Capacity is 1.23 liquid liters. Height is 13.8 inches. Compatible with Companion stationary units.

Le 271-2693   Weighs 8 pounds full $1290.95

Hudson RCI 4000 Small Cart for D or E Cylinders. 6-inch heavy duty wheels. Chrome-plated tubular steel.

Le 340-2161 $84.95

Roo Express Portable Cylinder Cases. Come with adjustable shoulder strap, clear visibility to gauges and dials. Tough, handwashable material. Personal identification card holder.

Ro 5000	"D" Cylinder L-Top	$41.95
Ro 5001	"D" Cylinder Dome Top	$41.95
Ro 5002	"C" Cylinder L-Top	$41.95
Ro 5003	"C/D" Cylinder Back Pack , waist belt	$67.95
Ro 5006	Mini-Slim Cylinder Waist Pack fits M-6 cylinders	$54.95

Roo Express Universal Concentrator Cover. Made of lightweight, handwashable material. Fits most concentrators, easy access to handles. Wraps around unit and Velcros in place.

Ro 5022   Comes in gray or navy $59.95

Custom covers are available for all makes of concentrators, wheelchairs, mattresses, CPAP carrying cases, and cylinders. Call LeBoeuf's ☎ 1-800-546-5559 for information and pricing.

Erie E Cart System. For either ambulatory use or as a concentrator back-up system. Filled E-cylinder with adjustable flow 0 to 8 LPM regulator. 7 foot tube with cannula. 3-position aluminum cart with adjustable handle.

Le 219-7838   Weighs 14 pounds $315.95

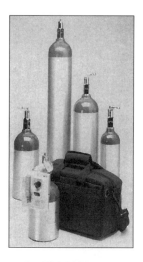

Le 327-5880, . . .,
Le 328-1862

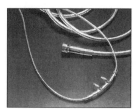

Le 224-8706

Le 364-5256

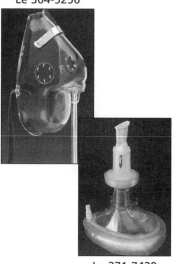

Le 271-7429

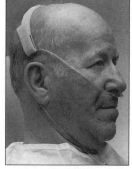

Da 250

Erie Travelers. Lightweight aluminum cylinders with sturdy carrying case. 0 to LPM variable flow regulator. Contents gauge. On/off lever handle with interchangeable yokes that fit all standard oxygen tanks. Cannula included.

Le 220-4691	406 liter capacity. Weighs 9 1/2 pounds	$355.95

DeVilbiss Walkabout Portable Gaseous Oxygen Systems. Patented Pulse-Dose technology. 11 selectable Pulse Dose flow rates. Pulse interruption alarms; both audible and visual. Low battery indicator. Continuous flow backup to a set flow rate available through toggle switch. Includes battery charger.

Le 327-5880	Mini 164 Liter, 4.1 hours at 2 LPM, 20 breaths per minute	$1,195.95
Le 327-5427	248 Liter 6.3 hours at 2 LPM, 20 breaths per minute	$1,155.95
Le 327-4925	415 Liter 10.5 hours at 2 LPM, 20 breaths per minute	$1,175.95
Le 328-1862	682 Liter 17.2 hours at 2 LPM, 20 breaths per minute	$1,195.95

Mada OCD-50 Oxygen Conserving Device. Senses inhalation and instantly releases a programmed dose of oxygen. No oxygen release during exhalation; extends cylinder life by up to 300%. Easily adaptable to any cylinder design. Built-in safety features. Power source AC, DC. Nicad battery. 11-position flow selector. 1 year warranty

Le 247-9640		$895.95
Le 179-6838	Regulator for use with OCD-50	$108.95
Le 179-7463	Elbow to use with OCD-50	$16.95

Salter Adult Cannulas with Tubing. Unique anatomical design prevents irritation. Over-the-ear styling provides secure positioning. 3-channel safety tubing helps percent occlusion.

Le 224-8706	Salter 1600 With 7 feet of tubing	$1.95
Le 224-8961	Salter 1600-25 With 25 feet of tubing	$3.95
Le 224-9258	Salter 1600-50 With 50 feet of tubing	$6.95

Hudson Adult Elongated See-Thru, Medium Concentration Mask. Clear, soft vinyl for patient comfort and visual assessment of patient. Adjustable nose clip for comfortable fit. Includes 7 foot oxygen supply tubing.

Le 364-5256		$3.95

Hudson Adult Lifesaver Filtered Isolation Valve Kit. Complete with valve, mouthpiece and disposable resuscitation mask.

Le 271-7429		$14.95

Dale Medical Products Oxygen Cannula Support. Prevents irritation to ears and helps insure proper positioning of the cannula in the nostrils. Helps to prevent accidental dislodgment of cannula.

Da 250	One size fits all	$2.95

Dale Medical Hospital Utility Grip. Secures tubing, cords and other devices to bed linens. Holds tubing and cords securely in place. Stainless steel grip will not puncture or tear bed linens. Velcro fastener holds the cords and tubing. Washable and reusable.

Da 1120	Each	$2.95

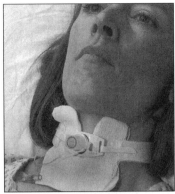

Da 240

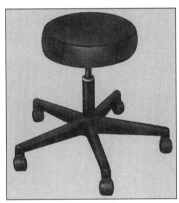

Br 13111

Dale Medical Tracheostomy Tube Holder. Increases patient comfort. Quickly and easily applied and saves nursing time. Infinitely adjustable. Will not irritate the skin. Inclusion of stretch material allows for cough reflex and ensures a snug comfortable fit.

| Da 240 | Box of 10 | $42.95 |

Brandt Revolving Stools. Professional quality. Five legs provide better stability when rolling about. Composite base. Height adjustable.

Br 13111	17½" to 23" height adjustment	$145.95
Br 13112	17½" to 23" height adjustment, 2-position backrest	$202.95
Br 13131	20½" to 28" height adjustment	$155.95
Br 13132	20½" to 28" height adjustment, 2-position backrest	$215.95

Nebulizers

Nebulizers are used to provide the patient with a fine spray of medication or moisture to assist in the removal of accumulated lung secretions and to relieve difficult or labored breathing. Nebulized drug delivery offers quicker drug action and lower therapeutic dose. To ensure that the drug is delivered to the correct part of the lung, it is important that you choose the correct nebulizer. The doctor will tell you what particle size the patient will require. Normally, a particle size of 5 microns or larger would be for deposition in pharynx, larynx and upper respiratory airways. A 2-5 micron particle size is optimal for tracheobronchial deposition and .5 to 2 micron particle size would be optimal for alveolar (tiny air sacs in the lung) deposition. A micron is one millionth of a meter (human hair is 75 to 100 microns in diameter).

You should look for a nebulizer that will minimize the amount of medication left in the nebulizer, will work effectively when the patient is in a horizontal position, has an anti-spill feature that will prevent waste if tipped in use, and that will prevent the drug from spilling into the mask or mouthpiece and being swallowed by the patient. The nebulizer should be easy to clean and simple to operate.

Using the nebulizer (treatment time usually takes 10 to 25 minutes):

- Do not schedule treatment one hour before or one hour after eating.
- Take pulse before and after each treatment.
- Make sure tubing is connected tightly to machine.
- Add medication to nebulizer, being careful not to touch the inside of the nebulizer cup (use a clean medicine dropper with easy-to-read calibration to be sure of dosage).
- Store opened medication bottles in the refrigerator.
- Have a glass of water and tissues handy to use during and after treatment.
- Turn on compressor and have the patient exhale completely. Place the mouthpiece between the teeth and close lips. Try and hold nebulizer straight to minimize any spilling and to obtain the best mist.
- Have the patient breathe (inhale) deeply through the mouth, hold breath for two seconds and exhale slowly

through pursed lips. Have the patient take an occasional deep breath during the treatment.

- Tap side of nebulizer every couple of minutes.
- Carefully clean the equipment after each treatment. When cleaning the compressor, be sure to unplug it first.
- Be sure that you and the patient are absolutely clear on the doctor's instructions before using the nebulizer. If the medication takes longer than 15 minutes to nebulize and/or if misting is poor, check to see if the tube is blocked or if the pump is not working right. If the patient becomes tired and wants to remove the mouthpiece or mask, be sure to turn off the compressor to prevent wasting the medication. It is normal to have a small amount of medication left in the nebulizer after treatment.

Cleaning the nebulizer cup:

Daily

- Prepare a weak solution of dishwashing detergent and hot water.
- Disassemble the cup and allow to soak for a few minutes.
- Remove and rinse thoroughly and air dry.

Weekly

- Soak the nebulizer cup and tube for 10 minutes in a solution of 1 cup of white vinegar to 3 cups of water.
- Rinse thoroughly under running warm water.
- Air dry.

Always clean the nebulizer in a pan and not the sink. The sink usually has a residue of grease and the grease can easily clog the nebulizer. Keep a few spare nebulizer cups on hand so you will always have one that's clean and dry and ready to use. Do not use a cloth for drying the nebulizer cup. Cloths may contaminate the nebulizer with bacteria and/or lint. When cleaning the compressor, always follow the manufacturer's instructions that come with the unit.

SunMark Compressor/Nebulizer. Compact and lightweight; weighs just 4.8 pounds. Operating pressure is 15 psi. Flow rate: 13 LPM; 8.5 LPM at the nebulizer. Particle size range: .5 to 5 microns. Percent of drug nebulized is 90 percent. Compressor requires no lubrication. Automatic shut-off prevents overheating. Includes nebulizer, mouthpiece, tube, and tubing.

Le 193-5147	5 year warranty		$149.95
Le 119-9531	Filter	Box of 50	$20.95

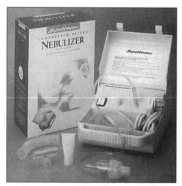

Le 193-5147

DeVilbiss Pulmo-Aide Traveler. 3 sources of power — AC, DC or rechargeable gel-cell battery. High-output pump designed to power all types of nebulizers effectively. Compact and portable comes with a Pulmo-Neb disposable nebulizer. Weighs 6.4 pounds including battery. Operating pressure 11-13 psi. Liter flow at 6-8 LPM. Particle size .5 to 5 microns.

Le 247-1613	Rugged nylon carrying case		$425.95
Le 168-4638	Filters for Traveler	Pack of 12	$3.95

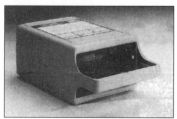

Le 247-1613

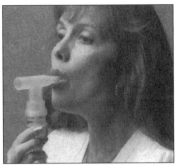

Le 275-8555

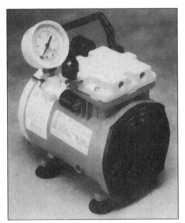

Le 114-4393

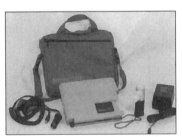

Le 195-0088

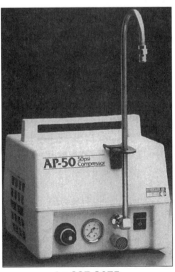

Le 327-3075

DeVilbiss Pulmonary Nebulizer. Advanced medical nebulizer for deep deposition of aerosols in the respiratory system. Hand powered. Mist density may be controlled by adjusting vent. Break-resistant tough clear plastic. Disassembles into cleanable parts.

Le 226-5031 $25.95

DeVilbiss Pulo-Neb Disposable Nebulizer. 60 day, single-patient, multiuse nebulizer. Complete with 7 feet of tubing and mouthpiece. Has 10 ml capacity.

Le 275-8555   Bag of 12 $42.95

Schuco-Mist Heavy-Duty AIDS Compressor/Nebulizer. Operates from 0 to 50 psi. For aerosolization of Pentamidine for treatment of AIDS. 11 liters per minute at maximum psi. High pressure relief valve.

Le 114-4393   Weighs 11 pounds $427.95

DeVilbiss AeroSonic Ultrasonic Nebulizer. Produces .3 ml per minute; reservoir capacity 9 ml. Portable. Operates very quietly on AC, DC or built-in battery. Includes controlling unit, chamber assembly, adapter/charger, power cord, and mouthpiece with check valve and adapter. 1-3 micron particle size range. Nebulizer capacity 9 ml.

Le 195-0088   Weighs 2.7 pounds $425.95

DeVilbiss Ultra-Neb, Ultrasonic Nebulizer. Output up to 6 ml minimum to meet all aerosol needs. Variable fan output control and aerosol output control. Visual alert for empty chamber. Optional filter removes bacteria from air supply. Easy to clean.

Le 142-4076   Weighs 9.5 pounds $797.95

DeVilbiss 50 PSI Compressor with Goose Neck. Operates from 5 to 50 psi. Optimal operating pressure 26 psi at 7 LPM. Compact and portable. Meets needs of tracheostomy patients. Includes regulator and tubing connector for nebulizer hook-up. Designed to hold 1000 ml bottle of sterile water without tipping.

Le 327-3075   Weighs 12.1 pounds $487.95

Continuous Positive Airway Pressure Systems

Continuous Positive Airway Pressure (CPAP) systems are designed to provide relief to patients with sleep apnea (cessation of breathing). Depending on the severity of the apnea, treatment will vary. Treatment can be as simple as changing the position the patient sleeps in. Surgery may be another option for those who cannot be helped with a home CPAP system.

The CPAP system is usually prescribed by a doctor after admitting the patient to a sleep laboratory. A technologist (polysomnographic) will monitor the patient's sleep and will be checking for breathing abnormalities, oxygen desaturations and abnormal heart beat rhythm or rate (cardiac arrhythmia). This process is called a polysomnogram.

The CPAP system consists of a mask that is placed over the nose and mouth of the patient and connected by hose to a compressor which supplies a constant flow of air, set at the highest pressure required to get air into the patient's upper airway. Since the systems must be properly adjusted, the doctor and/or the technologist will usually perform another polysomnogram to make sure everything is working as it should and that the patient is

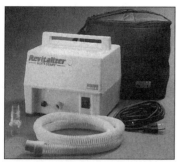

Le 379-5713

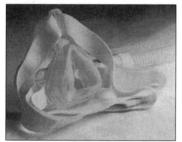

Le 379-5838

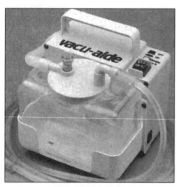

Le 149-5613

oriented to the unit. The appropriate pressure is called "an optimal CPAP triation."

There are two other procedures available for patients who cannot tolerate CPAP — BiPAP which decreases the air pressure during exhaling and is much more comfortable for patients requiring higher air pressures and DPAP (Demand Positive Airway Pressure) which senses the patient's demand and responds breath-by-breath. DPAP equipment is about twice as expensive as BiPAP and CPAP equipment.

Normally, the patient will be provided the equipment and service for CPAP treatment by companies that specialize in oxygen equipment rental.

DeVilbiss Revitalizer, Soft-Start Nasal CPAP System. Soft-Start technology gradually increases pressure to prescribed level. Exhalation port for low CO_2 retention. Pressure comes from variable fan speed and electronic components. Pressure range from 5 to 25 cm H20. Portable, includes carrying case and CPAP adjustment tool.

| Le 379-5713 | Weighs 9½ pounds | | $1207.95 |
| Le 247-9764 | DeVilbiss CPAP Filter | Pack of 6 | $36.95 |

DeVilbiss CPAP Mask. C-Flex material provides greater comfort for increased patient compliance. Mask adapts to all 22mm tubing. Comes with two Seal-Ring cushions.

Le 379-5838	Small	$65.95
Le 379-5895	Medium	$65.95
Le 379-5960	Large	$65.95

Aspirator

DeVilbiss Vacu-Aide Suction Pump. Oral, nasal, and pulmonary aspirator for homecare. Portable and lightweight. Wired for both AC and DC with built-in battery charging circuit. Reusable 1000 ml bottle. Maximum flow rate 22 LPM. Includes battery and DC cord.

| Le 149-5613 | Carrying case included | $419.95 |

Air Cleaning Equipment

High Efficiency Particulate Air (HEPA) is a technology developed during the early days of atomic research to clean the air of radioactive particles that may have been a health hazard. Today, HEPA filters are used in applications where totally clean air environments are required for human health and safety.

To obtain a 70 percent reduction in contaminants you need to change the air in a room at least six times an hour. To obtain an 85 percent reduction in contaminants, you need to change the air in the room eight or more times per hour.

We have Honeywell air cleaners that will meet just about any air cleaner need. Call for assistance in choosing the right size air cleaner for your patient. The patient's nose and throat will normally filter out any dust or particles larger than 10 microns and little gets into the lungs — it is the smaller particles that you cannot see that get into the lungs and cause problems.

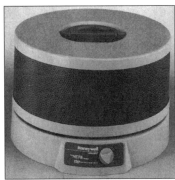

Le 219-9305

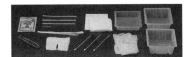

Le 220-3511

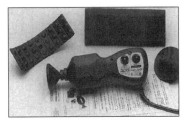

Le 215-2593

Honeywell/Enviracaire Portable Air Cleaner. (True HEPA filtration) Two-speed, 150 CFM. Recirculates and cleans 12 foot × 14 foot room six times an hour. Removes, 99.97% of airborne contaminants. 360 degree intake and discharge pattern. Highly efficient, unique design utilizes true HEPA filtration.

| Le 219-9305 | Weighs 11.5 pounds | $189.95 |
| Le 219-8737 | Replacement charcoal filter (one) | $79.95 |

Baxter Tracheostomy Cleaning Tray, with Gloves. Includes pre-cut, pre-sewn dressings, a specially designed brush, gloves, three separate basins, gauze sponges, pipe cleaners and 32 inch twill tape.

| Le 220-3511 | | Each | $5.95 |

Percussor

Percussion (clapping) is the forceful striking of the skin with cupped hands to assist in dislodging secretions from the bronchial walls. The cupped hand traps air against the chest and the trapped air causes vibrations through the chest. Done correctly, the percussion action should sound like a hollow, popping sound. Care has to be exercised to insure that easily injured areas such as the breasts, kidneys, sternum or spinal column are avoided. Don't try this on your own — be sure to have the doctor or nurse teach you how to perform this technique correctly.

Puritan-Bennett Vibrator/Percussor Home Care Kit. Portable, electrically powered device for use in postural drainage and muscle relaxation or stimulation. Adjustable intensity control to accommodate patient size and weight. Kit includes small 2-inch cup applicator, softer 3-inch cup applicator, 6-inch U-shaped vibration applicator arc, foam pad, and self-care instruction sheet.

| Le 215-2593 | | | $355.95 |

Menopause

MENOPAUSE (refers to the end of menstruation) is the end of a long slow process, typically occurring over a 15-year time span. When a woman is in her mid-thirties, the ovaries begin to make less of two female hormones, estrogen and progesterone. Then, about three to five years before her final menstrual period, the pattern of hormone production changes. For many women, periods change and become less regular and, in many cases, lighter. In other cases, some women have heavy bleeding. On average, periods stop altogether around age 50. However, menopause can occur anytime between the thirties to the mid-fifties.

At least 75 percent of women experience hot flashes. This symptom is the earliest and most common sign of menopause and can be as mild as a light blush or severe enough to wake her up from a sound sleep. They can occur rarely or as often as every hour. Most last only two to five minutes but some can go on for 30 minutes or more.

Suggestions on how to cope with hot flashes include:

- Sleep in a cool room.
- Dress in layers easily removed.
- Drink cold water or juice at the beginning of a hot flash.
- Use sheets and clothing that lets the skin breathe.
- Use medications prescribed by the doctor.
- Avoid alcohol, caffeine, hot/spicy foods.
- Use exercise to increase energy and reduce the risks of osteoporosis.

Lower estrogen levels cause the tissues of the vagina to become thinner, drier and less elastic, which can make sexual intercourse uncomfortable. Some women feel less interest in sex while others feel relieved that pregnancy is no longer a worry. Doctors recommend that women keep on using birth control until they have not had a period for one year.

Suggestions on how to cope with loss of vaginal lubrication:

- Ask your doctor about estrogen creams or other vaginal lubricants if discomfort during intercourse is a problem.
- Avoid petroleum jelly — it may contribute to infection and damage condoms.
- Get plenty of calcium and vitamin D before menopause.

Mood swings and depression around the time of menopause may affect some while others will not experience any emotional changes. Insomnia, as a result of hot flashes, can make even the most even-tempered woman tired and cranky. Changes in the home — such as children leaving or moving back in, responsibility for aging parents, change in sex drive or the illness of a loved one — all contribute to changes in emotions. Emotional changes are not necessarily due to menopause

Estrogen Replacement Therapy (ERT) is used by some women to replace the natural estrogen lost during and after menopause. Estrogen loss is the leading cause of bone loss in older women. A lowered estrogen level increases the calcium lost and contributes to osteoporosis. Women at high risk of developing osteoporosis should talk with their doctors about the pros and cons of ERT (see Osteoporosis in next section).

For many women the risks of ERT may be slight and many experts now believe that the benefits of estrogen replacement outweigh the dangers for persons at high risk of developing osteoporosis. Studies show that about 10 percent of women who take ERT experience some side effects such as headaches, nausea, vaginal discharge, fluid retention, swollen breasts or weight gain. Other possible problems include endometrial cancer (cancer of the uterine lining) which has been found to occur more often in women who use ERT containing estrogen as the only ingredient. The form of ERT usually prescribed today combines estrogen and progestin, another female hormone. This combined treatment appears to reduce or eliminate the risk of endometrial cancer. Women who have had a hysterectomy have no risk of endometrial cancer.

With respect to heart disease and ERT, studies show contradictory findings. To resolve this controversy, the National Heart, Lung and Blood Institute and the National Institute on Aging soon will begin a study on the effects of estrogen on the cardiovascular system.

What to do:

Contact the National Institute on Aging (NIA) for a more detailed booklet on menopause as well as information on exercise, nutrition, and other health topics related to aging. Write or call NIA Information Center, P.O. Box 8057, Gaithersburg, MD 20892-8057; 1-800-222-2225.

Contact the American College of Obstetricians and Gynecologists, 409 12th Street, S.W., Washington, D.C. 20024-2188; 1-202-638-5577.

Osteoporosis

OSTEOPOROSIS is a natural part of aging. Nearly one in four women over the age of 60, and nearly half of all people over the age of 75, suffer from osteoporosis. Osteoporosis is often called the "silent disease" because it occurs without symptoms. White and Asian women most often develop osteoporosis. Those women who have had an early menopause, or who have a family history of osteoporosis, are at highest risk. Women with fair skin or small frames are also at greater risk than other people.

Other factors that may mean the patient is at greater risk for osteoporosis include:

- Avoided diary products as a child.
- Smoker.
- Drinks alcohol every day.
- Diet high in salt, caffeine or fat.
- Little or no exercise.
- Fractured or lost teeth recently.

Through a process called remodeling, small amounts of old bone are removed and new bone is formed in its place.

Bones naturally become thinner as a person ages. Beginning at about the age of 30 or so, a little more bone is lost than is formed. In women, bone loss speeds-up around menopause, particularly when caused by the surgical removal of the ovaries. By the age of 70, the density of the skeleton has been reduced by one third. Osteoporosis is a major cause of fractures in the hip, spine, wrist and other bones.

Currently, the only drug approved by the U. S. Food and Drug Administration as a calcium supplement is calcitonin. However, a recent study has shown that there are other medicines that reduce fractures of the hip, wrist, spine and other bones. Check with the patient's doctor on the latest advances in treating osteoporosis.

Diet and exercise can both help prevent osteoporosis. Weight lifting increases the strength of bones and muscles. Foods that are high in calcium such as lowfat cheese, yogurt and milk should be a regular part of the diet. In middle age, bone mass can stay at a peak if the patient continues to exercise and get enough calcium. An 8-ounce serving of milk or fortified fruit juice contains about 300 mg of calcium according to the U. S. Department of Agriculture. Regular exercise is another important preventive measure. Walking (at least 3 miles at a brisk pace, three times a week), jogging, dancing and bicycle riding are good because they put stress on the spine and the long bones of the body.

According to the latest study by the National Institutes for Health in 1994, the current recommended dietary allowance for calcium is 1000 mg daily for premenopausal women 25-49 and women 50-64 years old who are taking estrogen. For women who are past menopause and over 65, 1,500 mg of calcium per day is now recommended. If diet alone does not provide enough calcium, check with the pharmacist or doctor for a recommended calcium supplement. People who are susceptible to kidney stones need to be careful about suddenly increasing their calcium intake.

Other than diet and exercise, treatment of osteoporosis consists of orthopedic support, analgesics, heat and massage when muscle spasm is present.

Vitamins D and B$_6$ are also needed because they help the body absorb the calcium. Fifteen minutes of mid-day sunshine may meet the daily need for vitamin D. Saltwater fish, tofu, oysters, dark green leafy vegetables, whole wheat bread, vitamin fortified milk and cereals as well as liver are also high in Vitamin D.

Symptoms:

- Fracture after a fall that wouldn't cause an injury in a younger person.
- Bones of spine collapse (vertebrae).
- Loss of height.
- Aching pain in the bones, especially the back (crush fractures).

What to do:

Contact the doctor — There are many new and exciting advances being made with medications that will help reduce the incidence of bone fractures. If you or the patient suspect that the patient has osteoporosis, make an appointment with the doctor. The most common tests are single and dual-photon absorptiometry and dual-energy x-ray absorptiometry. Prior to going to the doctor, contact one or more of the organizations shown below to be sure you have the most up-to-date information. If the doctor is not aware of the latest advancements in treating patients with osteoporosis, tell them of your research. The doctor will investigate and, if they believe that the new medication is appropriate, it will be prescribed.

Contact the National Osteoporosis Foundation — (202) 223-2226. They have nationwide programs to educate the public on osteoporosis and related research. You can also write for information to the National Osteoporosis Foundation, P.O. Box 96616, Washington, DC 20077.

The American Society for Bone and Mineral Research — (202) 857-1161. They have information on the latest research in new medications. You can write to them at 1200 19th Street, NW, Suite 300, Washington, DC 20036.

Contact the Older Women's League — 1-800-825-3695. The League has a free fact sheet on osteoporosis. Their address is 666 11th Street NW, Suite 700, Washington, DC 20001.

Contact the National Institute on Aging — 1-800-222-2225, which offers information on estrogen therapy, preventing falls and other information.

Multiple Sclerosis

MULTIPLE SCLEROSIS (multiple scars) usually will strike people between the ages of 20 and 40 and strikes about twice as many women as men. Multiple sclerosis (MS) occurrence is between 5 to 10 cases per 10,000 people. In a family that has the illness, the chances of a brother or sister developing multiple sclerosis is 20 times higher than these statistics. Multiple sclerosis is not contagious.

Multiple sclerosis is a progressive disease caused by the inflammation and scarring of tissue in the brain and spinal cord. The inflammation breaks down and destroys the myelin, a white fatty material that provides the covering for nerves in the central nervous system. Healthy myelin covering allows the nerves to send an electrical impulse at high velocity. When the myelin covering is inflamed or destroyed, the electrical impulses slow down. Sclerosis is the hardening of the nervous system and can be located at various sites in the brain or spinal cord. The severity of multiple sclerosis is unpredictable in most cases.

The severe forms of multiple sclerosis can shorten a person's life expectancy by about five years. Excess heat may accentuate symptoms and signs because heat slows the conduction of electrical impulses in the nerve fibers. A cold bath can sometimes temporarily relieve symptoms and/or reduce some of the fatigue that patients often have.

The medical profession has not yet discovered the causes for multiple sclerosis but the thinking is that a virus may trigger the disease. Also, genetic factors may predispose a patient to the disease. The disease is more common in colder climates than in warmer. Some researchers believe that measles and mumps may be linked to multiple sclerosis.

Doctors have divided multiple sclerosis in two types:
- **Exacerbating-remitting** — Periods of deteriorating ability are followed by periods of recovery. As time passes, recovery often becomes less and less frequent.
- **Chronic progressive** — A steady downhill progression without periods of recovery. People who start out with the exacerbating-remitting form of multiple sclerosis frequently go on to develop the chronic form.

Visual problems tend to clear up in the later stages of the disease.

Symptoms:
- Tingling, numbness of the arms or legs.
- Unsteady walk.
- Impaired speech
- Blurred or double vision.
- Partial blindness in one eye, dimness of vision.
- Numbness or pain on one side of the face.
- Fatigue and loss of strength.
- Muscle stiffness.
- Memory loss and depression.

From a list of drugs and treatments provided by the Multiple Sclerosis Association of America ("Motivator Newsletter," Spring, 1995).

Aminopyridine
  Increases energy.

Bee Venom Therapy
  Used for chronic progressive and relapsing/remitting MS.

Bataseron (beta interferon)
  Used for relapsing/remitting MS. Helps delay or halt progression. Is expensive and has side effects.

Bovine Myelin
  May assist the immune system. Currently under clinical study.

Cladribine
  Potent chemotherapy agent used for leukemia. Given intravenously for chronic progressive MS.

Copolymer 1 (copaxone)
  Under study. FDA may approve in a year. Very expensive. For reducing flareups for those with relapsing/remitting MS.

Methotrexate
  Used for slowing the progression of MS.

Prednisone
  A steroid which decreases inflammation. Taken orally, inexpensive; taken by I.V., expensive.

There is no single test for determining if a patient has multiple sclerosis. Magnetic resonance imaging and spinal fluid analysis, along with the doctor checking the patient's mental state, motor reflexes, sensory changes (especially feeling) and whether or not the patient has problems with incontinence and sexual impotence are all used to make a diagnosis.

There is no specific treatment therapy. There are two basic strategies for treating MS: one attempts to reduce the inflammation and the immune system's attack against the nervous system; the other is to provide relief by treating the symptoms.

Medications are being studied that will help to relieve stiffness, provide strength and reduce fatigue. Many doctors will prescribe a pituitary hormone know as ACTH to reduce inflammation. Synthetic steroids such as prednisone or methylprednisolone may be given to reduce inflammation in the nervous system.

An experimental treatment for severe and milder forms of multiple sclerosis is plasma exchange. In this procedure, blood is removed and the plasma portion of the blood is discarded before the red and white blood cells are returned to the body.

To date, the treatment of symptoms has been more successful than treating the root causes of MS. Drugs such as Lioresal treats symptoms of painful spasms and stiffness and Symmetrel reduces fatigue. For those patients experiencing problems controlling bladder function, Ditropan helps.

The amount of exercise and how the patient exercises is very important for keeping fit. Care must be taken so that the patient will not overdo it. Swimming in cold water will temporarily relieve symptoms. If severe pain persists, doctors may surgically remove or block a section of the nerve. For some patients, the loss of feeling may be as disturbing as the pain before surgery. Massage makes the patient more comfortable.

Cooling the body's core temperature with a cool suit helps control some of the distressing symptoms of multiple sclerosis. A cool suit consists of a lightweight vest and a head cap that circulates cool liquid. Many patients temporarily enjoy improved speech, vision and mobility. The cool suit is usually used for about two hours, three or more times a day. The Multiple Sclerosis Association of America has spent over $1 million on cool suit research, which is a NASA spin-off.

Assistive devices such as a motorized wheelchair or a motor scooter help patients who can no longer walk or those who tire easily. There are also a number of products that assist patients with dressing and eating.

What to do:

Contact a doctor — Have the patient make and keep the appointment. There is no single or simple test for multiple sclerosis. It will take a lot of testing to be sure that the patient has the disease. It is important to have this diagnosis done as soon as the first signs of multiple sclerosis appear. A family doctor may recommend that you take the patient to see a neurologist. If the diagnosis determines that the patient has multiple sclerosis, the following steps will provide the caregiver with information, support and services to assist in coping with the initial onset of the disease.

Contact the Multiple Sclerosis Association of America — Call 1-800-883-4MSA (1-800-883-4672) or write to The Multiple Sclerosis Association of America, 601-05 White Horse Pike, Oaklyn, NJ 08107. For over 20 years MSAA has supported and helped MS sufferers. They have a 24-hour hotline, equipment loan program, volunteer support and many other services. During the last 10 years there has been more research than in the previous 20 to 30 years.

Contact the local social services organizations — There are many agencies that will provide information and listings of resources available in your area. Agencies such as the offices on aging, local health agencies as well as religious-affiliated service groups also provide information, training and support. There are also associations and companies that provide care management services to serve as the link between you and community-based services. They charge for their services — so be sure you understand what it will cost to have them provide assistance.

Contact a lawyer — It is very important to act quickly to protect the future security of the patient. There are lawyers who specialize in elder law. You will need to execute a durable power of attorney, a living will and/or a living trust. Living trusts appear to be the best way to handle an estate because you can avoid probate and not have the estate's assets tied up by the courts. Contact LeBoeuf's at ☎ 1-800-546-5559 for a listing of lawyers in your area.

Safety — Organize the home to permit the patient to carry on as many of their normal routines as possible. Other tips and items that make for a safer home are listed below and in the "Home Modification and Safety Products" section.

Communication — Explain to the patient what is happening. Tell family and friends. Explain the symptoms and tell family and friends that you and the patient will be needing their support and love. Tell them how and when they can help. Be specific about your caregiving needs. Draw up a plan of action that allows everyone to understand the roles that can (and must) be played.

Parkinson's Disease

PARKINSON'S DISEASE is caused by the degeneration or damage to nerve cells located at the top of the brain stem (basal ganglia). It is estimated that one million people have Parkinson's in the U.S. and each year about 50,000 learn that they have the disease. Parkinson's affects both men and women, but men are more likely to be stricken. Usually the disease affects patients starting at about 40 years of age and older. Strangely, those who smoke have a lower incidence of Parkinson's.

There is no cure for Parkinson's disease. However, much can be done to improve morale and mobility through exercise, special aids in the home and lots of TLC (Tender Loving Care). Parkinson's can also be treated with drugs such as levodopa, which converts into dopamine and is usually the most effective. An operation on the brain can also be performed to reduce tremor and rigidity. This operation is usually reserved for those who are relatively young, in good health otherwise and in the early stages of the illness.

About one third of patients who have Parkinson's eventually show signs of a general decline in all areas of mental ability (dementia). Science is continuing to make strides in the treatment of Parkinson's and the outlook is promising.

Parkinson's usually begins with a slight tremor of one hand, arm or leg. In the early stages, the tremor is worse when the hand, arm or leg is at rest or when there is emotional stress. Generally, the tremor decreases or disappears when the patient exercises and normally disappears when sleeping. Muscle stiffness is another early symptom. Patients find it hard to get out of a chair, to turn and perform such movements as buttoning clothes. As the disease progresses, the patient may find it difficult to walk and speech may become affected. You have to pay particular attention to the patient and provide a lot of TLC and encouragement to help prevent anger, depression or dependency. Keep the patient involved in family activities as much as possible. There are a number of support groups that will assist both the patient and the caregiver.

The National Parkinson Foundation has provided helpful hints and exercises to assist the patient. Before doing any of the exercises, be sure to check with the doctor.

Symptoms appear slowly and in no sequence.

Hints

Safer Walking For the Patient

- Wear leather-soled shoes. Rubber-soled or crepe-soled shoes grip the floor and may cause falling. Take as large a step as possible, bringing the toes up with each step. Try and keep the feet 9 to 12 inches apart to provide a wider base and prevent falling.
- Try to keep the head high, looking straight ahead.
- Swing the arms — right arm with left leg, left arm with right leg.

- If the legs feel frozen or "glued to the floor, relax back on the heels and raise the toes. It may help to tap the hip of the leg to be moved; rock side to side; bend the knees and straighten up; or raise the arms in a sudden short motion.
- If help is needed to move from room to room, to the car, etc. the caregiver can assist by holding the arms and both rock side to side. The caregiver will be moving backward so be very careful and move slowly. The caregiver should provide support and not drag the patient.

Turning Safely

- For greater safety in turning, try to take short steps with the feet widely separated (9 to 12 inches apart).
- Avoid crossing one leg over the other when turning.

Practical Dressing

- Getting dressed and undressed is easier if the clothing is fastened by zippers or self-adhering Velcro strips.
- Avoid garments that fasten in the back or have small buttons or tight buttonholes.
- Patients should always try to dress themselves completely.
- Use a shoehorn, elastic shoelaces or extra-long shoelaces to help with shoes.
- Dress in the most comfortable and safe position, whether sitting or standing.
- Patients should practice buttoning and unbuttoning clothes.

Chair Advice

- Approach a chair as closely as possible, then back up. As it is reached, bend forward and sit down slowly.
- To get up, put one foot forward and keep the other back under the chair. Bend forward and push up vigorously, using the arms. Try counting "1,2,3, Go" before getting up or try rocking forward two or three times before getting up.
- In the case of a favorite armchair, raise the back legs with four-inch blocks to assist in getting up from the chair.
- Do not let people drag the patient up by the arms; a slight push up on the back is okay.

Getting In and Out of Bed

- Rock to a sitting position by extending the legs toward the side of the bed and using the arms.
- Some people will use a knotted rope tied to the foot of the bed to help pull themselves up. Blocks may also be placed under the legs of the head of the bed.

Bathroom Safety

- If it is difficult to sit down in the bathtub for bathing, use a stool or a transfer bench. Soap and rinse by using the shower or a hand held shower head.
- Buy bathtub grab bars and make sure that they are attached securely .
- Buy a raised toilet seat and/or install toilet grab bars.

Eating Carefully

- When chewing food, chew hard and move the food around; avoid just swallowing. The patient should practice cutting food.

Speech Exercise

- Practice singing and reading aloud with forceful lip and tongue motions.
- Practice making faces in front of a mirror, reciting the alphabet and counting numbers with exaggerated facial motions.

Physical Exercises

- Remember to check with the doctor before doing any of the following exercises. You may want to have the doctor review the exercises in *LeBoeuf's Handbook* and have the doctor check those that are appropriate for you.
- Try to perform the exercises twice a day.
- Depending on how the patient feels, increase the repetitions of each exercise from 5 times to a maximum of 10 times.

For tight muscles and poor posture

- Have the patient stand with back against the wall, lifting arms over head until they touch the wall. Look up to ceiling. Hold for count of 5. Lower head and arms, rest for count of 10. Repeat 5 times. Next, still standing with back against the wall, march in place, lifting legs as high as possible. Lift each leg 5 times.
- Holding onto something that is secure, squat down as far as possible, then straighten up. Repeat 5 times.
- Sitting in a straight-backed chair, put the arms behind the chair and bring the shoulders back as far as possible. Then raise the head and look up at the ceiling. Hold for a count of 5, then return to normal position and rest for a count of 10. Repeat 5 times.
- Sitting in a straight-backed chair, place one leg at a time on another chair directly in front and press the knee straight. Alternate legs, doing each leg 5 times.
- Sitting in a straight-backed chair, alternately raise each arm up and across the body in a diagonal pattern. As the arm is raised, keep the eyes on the hand, following its action by moving the head. Repeat 5 times with each arm.

- Lie on the back on the bed or on the floor. Try to press the back down as flat as you can. Hold for a count of 5, rest for a count of 10. Repeat 5 times. Move the head from right to left as far as possible. Repeat 5 times. Still lying on the back, bend and straighten the legs, as if riding a bicycle. Repeat 5 times with each leg.
- Lie on the stomach and do the following in order: Put the hands behind the back and look up, trying to raise the chest, pressing the shoulder blades together. Hold for a count of 5, return to resting position for a count of 10. Repeat 5 times. With knees straight, kick the legs from the hips alternately, as if swimming. Kick each leg 5 times. Turn head from right to left. Repeat 5 times.

For balance difficulty

- Stand with hands on hips and feet apart, or hold on to a support if necessary, to do the following:
Alternate raising each leg out to the side, keeping the knees straight. Repeat 5 times for each leg. Alternate drawing a circle with each leg. Keep the knees straight and avoid touching the feet to the floor. Repeat 5 times for each leg.
- Standing with the hands at the side and the feet spread apart: Lean forward and back. Repeat 5 times. Lean to right and left, bending at waist. Repeat 5 times. Rotate top half of body from waist, first moving forward, right, back, and left in a circular motion, then reversing the motion. Repeat 5 times. Do the same with head. Repeat 5 times.

The benefits of exercise are an important way to help the patient handle depression, stress, anxiety and to improve self image. Hospital-affiliated exercise programs, reputable gyms, senior citizen centers, YWCAs, YMCAs, and universities are places where you can find a good exercise program. To keep exercise routines enjoyable, keep a written record of progress, exercise to music, set realistic goals, pay attention to the patient's body. Forget the saying: No pain no gain. Make patient exercise part of a daily routine.

What to do:

Contact The National Parkinson Foundation. 1-800-327-4545. You can write it at 1501 N.W. 9th Avenue, Bob Hope Road, Miami, FL 33136. It provides clinical services, speechdrug tests, informaion, education, occupational therapy and other support.

Contact the American Parkinson Disease Association. 1-800-223-2732 (APDA). You can write it at 60 Bay Street, Suite 401, Staten Island, NY 10301. It has over 80 chapters and over 350 support groups.

Stress and Headaches

STRESS is anything that disturbs a person's mental and physical well-being. Stress is a natural part of life. Changes such as getting married, illness, changing jobs are but a few of the sources of stress. The body responds to stress by increasing the production of certain hormones. These hormone changes lead to changes in the heart rate, changes in blood pressure, changes in metabolism and physical activity. At certain levels, stress can disrupt an individual's ability to cope.

Continuous exposure to stress often leads to mental and physical symptoms such as anxiety, depression, palpitations and muscular aches and pains. Learning to read the signs is a way for the patient to determine stress. Cold hands, rapid breathing, rapid heartbeat, forgetfulness, shakiness, headaches are all signs of stress.

Have the patient talk things out with friends and family. Obtain professional help if necessary. Sometimes the patient has to tough it out and face the challenge. Suggest to the patient: take deep slow breaths to help relax, listen to music, take a walk in the rain and laugh at themselves. Drugs (illegal) and alcohol should never be used. A good prayer to repeat when things seem to be getting out of control: "God grant me the serenity to accept the things I cannot change, courage to change the things I can, and the wisdom to know the difference."

The patient can help prevent stress by doing such simple things as eating right, exercising, managing time better, getting proper rest and sleep. The patient should get at least seven or eight hours of sleep three or four times a week. Taking a nap may help. "Remember you only go around once — you have to learn to stop and smell the roses."

Sometimes medications are helpful. Tranquilizers or anti-anxiety drugs, recommended by a therapist and prescribed by a doctor might be used. Tranquilizers are central nervous system depressants. Tranquilizers can cause drowsiness. Older people can become sleepy, dizzy, unsteady on their feet and confused when taking these drugs. Be sure to inform the doctor what other medications the patient is taking before using tranquilizers and give only the amount of tranquilizers the doctor prescribed. If the patient forgets to take the tranquilizer medication, do not double the dose next time. Caffeine found in coffee, tea, soft drinks and chocolate can counteract the effects of the tranquilizer.

Once the patient begins taking a tranquilizer, do not stop the medication suddenly. This can cause withdrawal symptoms including convulsions, muscle cramps, sweating and vomiting. When it is time to stop the medication, the doctor will probably reduce the dose slowly to prevent these symptoms.

Headaches

The pain from headaches comes from outside the brain. The brain tissue itself does not have sensory nerves. The pain comes from the the outlying lining of the brain (meninges), the scalp and its blood vessels and muscles. Pain may be felt all over or just in one area such as the back of the neck, the

Warning!!!

Over the counter (OTC) analgesics should be used only for 48 hours before seeking medical advice. If pain persists, becomes more severe, recurs, or differs from pain previously experienced, call the doctor right away.

Cancer Warning!!!!

If the headache is recurrent, is present on waking and is accompanied by nausea or vomiting, it may indicate a brain tumor. See the doctor without delay!

Taking more than five pain relievers a day, more than twice a week can cause "rebound" headaches, requiring more and more pain relievers.

Warning!

Do not give aspirin or any aspirin-containing combination of products to children because of the risk of Reye's syndrome, a rare but serious disorder that is characterized by brain and liver damage.

forehead or on one side of the head. In some cases, the pain will move from one part of the head to another part. It is hard for doctor's to pinpoint the cause of headaches. They do know that stress worsens any kind of headache.

Tension headaches are the result of stress (the leading headache trigger) and/or poor posture and are caused by the tightening of the muscles of the face, neck and scalp. Tension headaches may last from a few hours to days and sometimes will last for weeks.

Migraine headaches can be severe and incapacitating. Migraines can be associated with upset stomachs and visual disturbances. Migraine headaches are often accompanied by sensitivity to light, sound, temperature and odors. They are caused by abnormal contraction and expansion of blood vessels in the head. Women are three times more likely to have migraine headaches and the migraine headaches often occur during hormonal changes.

Cluster headaches are headaches that cause intense pain behind an eye, usually at night, and may keep the patient awake nightly for weeks or months.

Factors that can trigger headaches are:
- Alcohol.
- Missed meals.
- Missed sleep or excessive sleep.
- Sleeping on stomach.
- Prolonged travel.
- Stress (tension).
- Noise.
- Tumors.
- Certain foods such as cheese, chocolate and red wine.
- Fevers.
- Colds.
- Teeth clenching.
- More or less caffeine than the patient is used to.

Treatment of headaches includes avoiding them if at all possible by controlling the factors that can cause headaches. If a headache has started, the patient can obtain relief by doing one or more of the following:
- Taking a hot bath.
- Lying down.
- Avoiding noise.
- Massaging the neck and scalp.
- Sleeping.
- Taking a mild analgesic (painkiller) drug (aspirin, acetaminophen, ibuprofen or naproxen). They are all equally effective in stopping head pain and all reduce fever. Aspirin is hardest on the patient's stomach; ibuprofen and naproxen can cause gastrointestinal discomfort too. You can minimize the patient's discomfort by giving food or milk.
- In some cases, the doctor may prescribe dihydroergotamine (DHE). The doctor may inject it or may provide the patient with a nasal spray. DHE has been especially effective for treating migraines.

What to do:

Contact the doctor if the headache:

- Disrupts the patient's life for more than a few days.
- Is accompanied by blurred vision, confusion or convulsions.
- If the patient loses consciousness.
- Follows a head injury.
- Occurs with a fever.
- Affects the same areas such as the eyes, ears, face or jaw.
- If the patient has pain when touching the chin to their chest (see the doctor right away — it may be that the patient has a brain injury or irritation of the meninges).
- If the patient has a dull pain and tenderness around the eyes and the pain gets worse when bending forward, the patient may have an infection of the sinuses.

Contact the National Headache Foundation. 1-800-843-2256. They provide information and literature on headaches and their treatment.

To receive information regarding headache causes and treatments, as well as a newsletter subscription form, send a self addressed business size envelope with three first-class stamps to the following address:

National Headache Foundation
428 West Saint James
2nd Floor
Chicago, IL 60614

Include a brief description of headache type or symptoms. Also available at your request is a list of physician members in your state.

Brain Tumors

BRAIN TUMORS (Intracranial Neoplasms) are common and frequently mis-diagnosed. They may occur at any age but are more common in early to middle adulthood. Brain tumors are an abnormal mass of tissue in which the cells multiply without hindrance. The main adult brain tumors occur in the membrane of the brain (meningliomas), cranial nerves (gliomas of the brainstem and optic nerves), pituitary, and tumors resulting from the spreading of tumors from skin, breast and lung cancer (metastatic tumors). Occurrence of brain tumors in men and women is about the same.

How lethal a brain tumor is will depend upon the size, location and rate of growth. Benign brain tumors grow slowly, while malignant brain tumors typically grow rapidly. The most common form of secondary brain tumor is metastatic (a tumor that originates in another part of the body) and there are about 100,000 metastatic brain tumors diagnosed a year. Benign tumors can be as lethal as a malignant tumors if they are located in an area of the brain that cannot be operated on to remove the entire tumor. Malignant brain tumors seldom spread cancer cells throughout the body and usually cause death by relentless growth within the brain.

Brain tumors are divided into six classes:

- **Skull** (bony tissue).
- **Membrane** that envelopes the brain and spinal cord (meninges).
- **Cranial nerves** such as glioma of the optic nerve (glioma is the tissue that forms the supporting structure of the nerves).
- **Neurolgila** (connective tissue that binds together and supports the nerve tissue of the central nervous system).
- **Pituitary** (small oval gland attached to the base of the brain — it secretes hormones that influence body growth, metabolism and other glands whose secretions are introduced directly into the blood stream, such as the thyroid gland).
- **Congenital origin** (such as a cyst of the outer layer of cells from which the nervous system, skin, hair and teeth are developed).

Symptoms of brain tumors usually provide a clue as to the location of the tumor in the brain:

- Headaches.
- Vomiting.
- Paralysis.
- Personality changes.
- Loss of vision.
- Speech problems.

Diagnosis of a brain tumor can be made by surgery, CT scans (computerized tomography), magnetic resonance imaging (MRI), X-rays, electroencephalogram (EEG) or radioisotopic brain scans. Magnetic resonance imaging is the most accurate and does not use radiation. The doctor will determine which is the best test for the patient. Patients having metal pins or metal plates in the body should not take an MRI test. Tell the doctor about any metal in the patient's body before any testing. Dental fillings are not magnetic and will not cause a problem. Chest X-rays may be taken to discover the source of metastases.

Treatment of brain tumors includes surgery, radiation and chemotherapy. For malignant brain tumors, the goal of treatment is to control growth as long as possible with the least number of side effects. Many malignant brain tumors are curable. When a brain tumor is in remission, it means that the tumor has stopped growing or multiplying. If the brain tumor has been completely destroyed, the area in the brain that had the tumor will be composed of only dead tissue.

Surgery is the primary treatment for brain tumors. The goal of surgery is to remove the entire tumor whenever possible — any tumor cells left after surgery will result in the tumor growing again. In many cases, radiation therapy and chemotherapy are used in conjunction with surgery. One of the most important advances in surgery has been the surgical microscope which gives the surgeon a much better view of the tissue and allows for greater precision when performing delicate procedures.

Radiation therapy is used after surgery for tumors that have not been removed completely or when surgery would be too risky. Radiation treatments vary from once a day for about 30 days, to two or more doses daily. Interstitial irradiation is the surgical implantation of radioactive pellets into the brain tumor. These pellets usually remain inside the tumor for 6 to 7 days and are then removed. Radiosurgery is a finely focused radiation beam that is used to treat tumors deep within the brain.

Chemotherapy works to destroy tumor cells with drugs. Chemotherapy is normally given by mouth or injected in the vein. The difficulty with chemotherapy is the problem of delivering sufficient amounts of the drug to the tumor without destroying healthy brain cells.

Recurrent brain tumors are the term for three conditions:

- A tumor that persists after treatment.
- A tumor that grows back after treatment that supposedly eradicated it.
- A new tumor that grows in the same place in the brain.

Anticonvulsant drugs can keep the patient free from seizures. Some patients may have to take the anticonvulsants for the rest of their lives. Side effects of the drugs are usually minor. The patient may experience drowsiness, unsteady gait and blurred vision (may have slurred speech and confusion, but it is rare). It seems that the most common side effect over a long period of time (years) is problems with the gums. Patients on these drugs should practice good oral hygiene and have their teeth professionally cleaned and checked at least two times a year. Let the doctor know if the patient has experienced any seizures, no matter how mild. In case of an emergency, it is a good idea for the patient to carry a card on which the doctor has written the ideal blood level of the anticonvulsant

The National Brain Tumor Foundation suggests that patients who have been diagnosed as having brain tumors focus on those things that they can control. It is okay to grieve and to seek psychological help to deal with the fear of not knowing the final outcome. It is also helpful for the patient to learn as much as possible about the disease and to join a support group to share concerns. It is very important for the patient not to lose touch with family and friends. Encourage the patient to socialize and have as much fun as possible. Last, but not least, suggest that the patient develop the spiritual self.

What to do:

Contact the doctor — The doctor will work with a team of other doctors, each of whom is a specialist. The patient may have a neurosurgeon, radiation oncologist, neuro-oncologist or chemotherapist on the team. One of the key issues is fully understanding what the course of treatment will be. Meetings should be held regularly to discuss the patient's condition and what changes may be needed in therapy.

Contact the American Brain Tumor Association — 1-800-886-2282. They are located at 2720 River Road, Suite 146, Des Plaines, IL 60018.

Contact the National Brain Tumor Foundation — 1-800-934-CURE (2873). Or write to them at 785 Market Street, Suite 1600, San Francisco, CA 94103. They can provide you and the patient with materials that discuss brain tumors in great detail. They also have a magazine that provides up-to-date information on new treatments and other topics of interest to those who may have or have had a brain tumor.

Contact the Brain Tumor Information Services, University of Chicago Hospitals — 1-312-684-1400. They are located at Box 405, Room J341, 5841 S. Maryland Avenue, Chicago, IL 60637.

Contact the Wellness Community, National Headquarters — 1-310-453-2300. They are located at 2190 Colorado Avenue, Santa Monica, CA 90404.

Contact the National Neurofibromatosis Foundation, Inc. — 1-800-323-7938. They are located at 147 Fifth Avenue, Suite 7F, New York, NY 10010.

Contact the National Familial Brain Tumor Registry, The Johns Hopkins Oncology Center — 1-410-955-0227. They are located at 600 North Wolfe Street, Room 132, Baltimore, MD 21287.

Stroke

A STROKE IS THE SUDDEN DISRUPTION IN THE FLOW OF BLOOD to an area of the brain. When the brain is deprived of blood, the affected brain cells become damaged or die. While cell damage can often be repaired by the body and lost function regained, the death of brain cells is permanent and results in disability. The loss of feeling, movement or function controlled by the damaged area of the brain is impaired. Strokes are fatal in about one-third of the cases and are a leading cause of death in developed countries. About one-third of major strokes result in permanent handicap and about one-third result in no lasting ill effects.

There are three major types of stroke:

- **Thrombotic** — Most common. Fatty deposits build up in the arteries to the brain until a clot or clump (thrombus) forms in an artery and entirely blocks the blood flow.
- **Embolic** — Results when a blood clot forms somewhere else in the body and moves to the brain. The traveling clot is called an embolus.
- **Hemorrhagic** — Most severe. It occurs when a blood vessel in the brain bursts or develops leakage and blood pours into the brain.

The warning signs of a stroke include:

- Sudden weakness or numbness of the face, arm and leg on one side.
- Sudden dimness or loss of vision — particularly in one eye.
- Loss of speech, trouble talking.
- Sudden severe headaches with no apparent cause.
- Dizziness, unsteadiness or a sudden fall, especially along with the previous symptoms.
- Pupils of the eye differ in size.
- Loss of bladder and/or bowel control.
- Strong, slow pulse.

A stroke requires immediate medical attention in a hospital. Patients may be treated by a family doctor, internist or a geriatrician and may be referred to a neurologist. The neurologist is a doctor specializing in diagnosis and treatment of problems with the brain and nervous system. A stroke can last from minutes to days (rarely). The neurologist will first determine if a stroke in process has been completed. Treatment will begin as soon as the stroke is diagnosed to ensure that no further damage to the brain cells occur. Anti-coagulant drugs may prescribed to prevent blood clots from becoming large; or, in the case of a hemorrhagic stroke, drugs may be prescribed to lower blood pressure.

Transient Ischemic Attack (TIA):

Sometimes people experience "little strokes" called TIAs, which are a warning that the brain is not receiving enough oxygen and that a stroke may occur. TIAs have the same symptoms of a stroke such as a headache, dizziness and confusion, visual disturbance, slurred speech or loss of speech, and difficulty swallowing, but usually last only a few moments and then disappear. If the patient is experiencing TIA's, see the doctor immediately!

Early diagnosis can be made by evaluating symptoms, reviewing the patient's medical history and performing routine tests. Tests may include a blood test, an electrocardiogram (measures electrical activity of the heart), an electroencephalogram (measures nerve cell activity in the brain), a computerized tomography scan (3-dimensional x-ray), and a magnetic resonance imager (can show where the blockage to the brain cells is occurring).

To lessen the risk of strokes, these steps may be taken:

- **Control blood pressure** — Check blood pressure regularly and follow the doctor's advice on how to lower it.
- **Stop smoking**.
- **Eat healthy** by choosing foods that contain lower amounts of fat, saturated fatty acids and cholesterol.
- **Exercise regularly** and keep weight under control.
- **Control diabetes** — If untreated, diabetes can cause destructive changes in the blood vessels throughout the body.
- **Promptly report warning signs** to the doctor. Sometimes people experience "little strokes" called TIA's which are a warning that a stroke may occur. A "little stroke" has the same symptoms of a stroke such as a headache, dizziness and confusion, visual disturbance, slurred speech or loss of speech and difficulty swallowing.

Possible complications of major stroke include pneumonia and the formation of blood clots in the veins of the leg which may travel to the artery supplying the lungs and cause a potentially fatal pulmonary embolism.

Therapy after a stroke will begin as soon as the patient is stable. If needed, the patient will receive speech and language therapy to develop communication skills; swallowing therapy (which affects about 50 percent of all stroke victims) to get patients off feeding tubes; and occupational therapy to teach the patient how to perform activities of daily living such as dressing, bathing, grooming, etc.

What to do:

Contact The National High Blood Pressure Education Program — 4733 Bethesda Avenue, Suite 530, Bethesda, MD 20814-4820 for information on high blood pressure or other stroke risk factors.

Contact The National Institute of Neurological Disorders and Stroke (NINDS) — 1-800-352-9424. Office of Scientific and Health Reports, Building 31, Room 8A-16, Bethesda, MD 20892. This office provides listings of stroke research centers around the United States and current research findings on stroke.

Contact the National Stroke Association — 1-800-787-6537. 8480 E. Orchard Road, Suite 1000, Englewood, CO 80111-5015. This organization provides a wide variety of publications and offers guidance to people interested in forming stroke support groups.

Contact the National Rehabilitation Information Center (NARIC) — 1-800-347-2742. 8455 Colesville Road, Suite 935, Silver Spring, MD 20910-3319.

Mental Illness

THE FOLLOWING IS FROM THE AUTHOR'S EXPERIENCE. It is important for you as a caregiver to understand that your loved one with a mental illness is not at fault. Also, you are not at fault, regardless of what the professionals, social workers, and others tell you. There is no cure for mental illness. The best hope is for a medication that will allow the patient to live a reasonably normal life and allow you to function as usual. It will not be easy and you will have many sleepless nights but you will learn to cope with the problem.

Mental illness is a general term that describes any form of psychiatric disorder. Usually, mental illness is divided into two categories:

- **Psychoses** — most severe, probably caused by biochemical brain disease.
- **Neuroses** — less severe, most likely related to upbringing and personality.

Psychiatry is the study, diagnosis, treatment and prevention of behavior disorders. The psychiatrist masters the skills of objective observation as well as subjective, participant and self observation.

There is no real understanding of the basic causes of mental illness. Classification of mental disease is an ever-changing, never-ending process. Techniques for measuring the brain and evaluating its functions are limited. Basically, it is a wide open field without definitive and meaningful standardization. Without standardization, there can be no measurement of success or of failure. Without a standardized diagnosis, there can be no prediction of the course of the disease. Without prediction, there can be no meaningful therapy. In other words, it is what it is because it is. While many professionals practicing psychiatry consider themselves successful in the treatment of a patient (regardless of the outcome), many family members associated with a mentally ill patient may consider the treatment a complete failure.

For the patient who cannot adjust to make social, family and work relationships successful, it is important that you maintain control and support good behavior and continue to confront bad behavior.

Many severely psychotic patients have been deinstitutionalized because of measures implemented to protect their civil rights. Of those patients who have been released, many have no continuing treatment and have become part of the homeless population. The rest are now struggling on their own, being cared for in monitored group homes or by their families.

Because of this deinstitutionalization, and the inability to individually commit a patient, the patient's family and the family physician have become more involved with therapy and rehabilitation. Many patients are not capable of understanding that they are sick and may need both drugs and an institutionally-controlled environment (hospitalization). The protection of the patient's civil rights has resulted in families becoming involved in a situation where there are no answers and no solutions. Patients can become very irrational and cause an untold amount of anxiety and anguish to all those who come in contact with them.

Many psychiatrists, psychologists and social workers address only the patient's needs and fail to understand that a family is involved which has needs also. Without the family's complete understanding and involvement, a successful relationship between family and patient will never happen. It is not enough for the family to be told that they need to understand that the patient is sick and to try and ignore the disruption in their lives. The family already knows this. Professionals should never convey to family members, intentionally or unintentionally, that it is their fault if the patient continues to get out of control. The professionals know, or should know, that they cannot cure the incurable. Mental illness is nobody's fault.

You have to be extremely careful that the psychiatrist or psychologist does not make suggestive remarks to the patient. Such suggestions to the patient are, in many cases, a reason for the patient to gain attention. An example of this is when professionals tell a patients to be sure and telephone if they feel like they want to harm themselves. In most cases, the patient will tell the caregiver that they want to harm themselves and will insist on talking with the psychiatrist or psychologist. The next thing you know, the patient is committed to some facility where the patient can be "observed" at a cost that can run up to hundreds of dollars a day.

Mental health care for the elderly is difficult to find and harder to afford. The emphasis is on outpatient care — yet Medicare Part B only pays $250 per year for outpatient psychiatric services.

Costs associated with mental illness are extremely high and, in most cases, the patient and the insurance company (if the patient has one) will pay and pay until the money runs out. At that time, the patient will be considered cured and sent home. There are no answers for families who have a mentally ill member, other than to know that whatever you do, it will not be enough. All you can do is try and section off a part of your brain to cope with the mentally ill person as needs dictate and let the rest of your mind attempt to concentrate on making life as full and enjoyable as possible.

Professionals who work with the mentally ill need to help the family and the patient become part of a self-help network that will provide support and acceptance. The professionals should be assisting the self-help groups to set goals that are realistic and help to instill hope.

Symptoms of mental illness:

- Can't sleep.
- Loss of appetite.
- Deep mood swings.
- Constantly depressed.
- Hears voices.
- Has unrealistic beliefs (think they are Jesus Christ, God, etc.).
- Always anxious without reason.
- Shuns social contacts unreasonably.
- Has extreme anger, aggression or excitement.

There are a number of antipsychotic drugs now in the marketplace that seem to help either singularly or in combination. They include Clozaril, Haldol, Navine, Prolixin, Thorazine, Lithium, Tegretol, Valium, Librium, Xanax, Prozac, Anafranil, Luvox and many others. There are numerous other drugs undergoing testing and the prospect for new and effective drugs looks promising. It is a good idea to read up on the medicines that the doctor may prescribe and understand the possible side effects of each. You can find information about drugs from books such as *The Merck Manual* and other medical reference books in your local library. If you notice that the patient is developing signs of an adverse reaction to a drug, contact the doctor immediately. Remember, the doctor is only human and may not be up-to-date on all the drugs and combinations of drugs being prescribed. This is another reason that it is important to use only one pharmacist. Your pharmacist should be able to tell you if the drugs prescribed can be taken in combination with other drugs and provide information on possible side-effects. The use of antipsychotic drugs seems to run in cycles and many professionals believe that their use is now entering a conservative phase. This change results from a heightened awareness of serious toxic side effects caused by some drugs.

What to do:

Contact the doctor — If the patient is out of control, you may have to call 911 for help. Calm words may not stop the patient's anger or violence but getting angry will only make the situation worse. Your doctor will probably recommend that you take the patient to a psychologist or a psychiatrist for a diagnosis.

Contact the National Alliance for the Mentally Ill — 1-800-950-NAMI (6264). You can write them at 200 North Glebe Road, Dept. P, Arlington, VA 22203. They have information on the symptoms and treatments for mental illness.

Contact the American Mental Health Fund — 1-800-433-5959 or, if in Illinois, 1-800-826-2336. They make available general information about organizations, mental health and warning signs of mental illness.

Depression

DEPRESSION CAN BE VERY HARD TO RECOGNIZE. Only about one-third to one-half of those with major depressive disorders are properly recognized by practitioners. Up to one in eight people may require treatment for depression during their lifetimes. Depression seems to be more prevalent in women, with about one in six seeking help for depression at some time in their lives. Only one in nine men may seek help. It has been estimated that as many as 30 percent of the elderly suffer from depression serious enough to interfere with daily function. The stereotype that depression and forgetfulness are a natural part of aging is simply not true.

Mental health care for the elderly is difficult to find and harder to afford. The emphasis is on outpatient care, yet Medicare Part B only pays $250 per year for outpatient psychiatric services.

Major depressive disorder may begin at any age but it most commonly begins in the 20s to 30s. Symptoms begin over days to weeks. More than 50 percent of those who suffer a single major depressive episode will eventually develop another. In some patients, the episodes of depression are separated by years of normal functioning without symptoms. For others, the episodes become increasingly more frequent with greater age. Major depressive episodes nearly always impact social, work and interpersonal relations.

Everyone gets the blues and is "down in the dumps" once in awhile, but if a depressed mood persists for more than two weeks, the patient should see a doctor. Talk therapy, drugs or other methods of treatment can ease the pain of depression. Depression can be treated successfully — the aim of treatment is complete remission. Depression is a medical illness, not a character defect or weakness. There is no reason to suffer.

Families, friends and health professionals should look carefully for signs of depression. Don't ignore the warning signs. At its worst, serious depression can lead to suicide. Statistics show that the rate of completed suicides, about 25 percent of those attempted, is higher for older people than that of the general population. You should pay attention and listen carefully when an older friend or relative complains about being depressed or of people not caring. They may be crying out for help.

The risk factors for depression include:

- Prior episodes of depression.
- Family history of depressive disorder.
- Prior suicide attempts.
- Being a female.
- Current substance abuse.
- After childbirth. (postnatal depression)
- Lack of social support.
- Stressful life events.
- Tendency to dwell on gruesome or gloomy matters.
- Under age 40 at onset of depression.

A clinical interview is the most effective method for detecting depression, which is the most treatable of all mental illness. About 60 to 80 percent of depressed people can be treated successfully outside a hospital with psychotherapy alone or with special drugs. Medical research has made great progress in devising treatments. There are doctors who specialize in the diagnosis and relief of depression late in life (geriatric psychiatry).

In some cases, major depressive illness can be avoided. Fostering and maintaining relationships with people over the years can help lessen the effects of losing a spouse. Interest in hobbies, staying involved in activities that keep the mind and body active, and keeping in touch with family and friends are ways to keep major depression at bay.

Treatments such as psychotherapy and support groups help people deal with major changes in life, such as retirement, moving, health problems that require new coping skills and social support. A doctor may recommend that an older patient use community-based programs such as senior centers, volunteer services or nutrition programs as a means to focus the patient's attention away from feelings of despair or depression.

Antidepressant drugs can also help. These medications can improve mood, sleep, appetite and concentration. Drug therapies often take from 6 to 12 weeks before there are signs of progress. The therapy may need to be continued for six months or longer after depression symptoms disappear.

"Shock" therapy can also help. Shock therapy can work well as a short-term treatment but its long-term benefits need more study. New techniques in "shock" therapy are safe and effective when properly used, unlike the scary movie versions of years ago.

Symptoms:

- An empty feeling, ongoing sadness and anxiety.
- Tiredness and lack of energy.
- Loss of interest or pleasure in ordinary activities, including sex.
- Sleep problems, including very early morning waking.
- Problems with eating and weight (gain or loss).
- A lot of crying.
- Problems with sexual functioning or desire.
- Aches and pains that won't go away.
- Difficulty concentrating, remembering, or making decisions.
- Feelings that the future looks grim.
- Feeling guilty, helpless or worthless.
- Irritability.
- Thoughts of death or suicide.

What to do:

See a doctor — The doctor will determine if there are medical or drug-related reasons for the symptoms of depression. The doctor may recommend that the patient see a mental health specialist for further treatment and therapy.

Contact the American Psychiatric Associaton. 1-(202) 682-6220. You can write it at Division of Public Affairs/Code P-H, 1400 K Street, NW, Washington, DC 20005. It conducts a nationwide mental illness awareness campaign for improving public understanding of mental illness. It also has many books on mental illness.

Contact the National Depressive and Manic-Depressive Association — 1-800-826-3632. They have over 200 chapters in the U.S. and Canada which offer support to people with depression and their families.

Contact the National Alliance for the Mentally Ill (NAMI) — 1 800-950-6264. You can write it at 2101 Wilson Boulevard, Suite 302, Arlington, VA 22201. They have a medical information series that provides patients and their families with information on several mental illnesses and their treatment. NAMI groups in all states provide emotional support and can help people find appropriate local services. There are over 1,000 local affiliates throughout the United States.

Contact the National Mental Health Association — 1 800-969-6642. You can write it at 1021 Prince Street, Alexandria, VA 22314. They have special information on depression and its treatment and provide referrals and support.

Dementia

DEMENTIA CAN OCCUR AT ANY AGE and more than one million Americans are incapacitated by it.

Dementia is grouped into two types:

- **Static dementia** — Normally the result of severe head trauma, heart attack or hemorrhaging in the brain (stroke).
- **Progressive dementia** — Can accompany brain disorders such as Huntington's disease, brain tumor, drug and alcohol abuse, syphilis and can also accompany degenerative diseases such as Parkinson's disease, Alzheimer's disease, multiple sclerosis and Wilson's disease.

Symptoms of dementia include:

- Personality and intellect breakdown, with the patient losing intuitive thinking and judgement.
- Depression.
- Paranoia.
- Becoming easily distracted.
- Exaggerated personality traits (periods of extreme anger, irritability and even violence).
- Becomes careless, dirty and incontinent (may urinate in public).

Causes of dementia include:
- *Head injury.*
- *Pernicious anemia (failure to absorb vitamin B12).*
- *Encephalitis (inflamation of the brain, usually caused by a viral infection).*
- *Myxedema (thicking and coarsening of the skin and other body tissues).*
- *Syphilis.*
- *Brain Tumor.*
- *Alcoholism.*

Accurate diagnosis of dementia is extremely difficult. Because depression and other psychiatric problems are often misdiagnosed as dementia, a second medical opinion is highly recommended. CT scans alone will not provide a reliable indication of dementia. Tests should include a complete blood count, blood electrolyte screen, serum vitamin B_{12} level, thyroid function test, chest X-rays, CT scans and STS. For those patients who may be at high-risk of AIDS, a test for HIV antibodies should also be given.

While there is a great deal of research into alleviating memory loss, no effective treatment is currently available.

Treatment for symptoms of dementia includes:

- Reducing and withdrawing drugs that affect brain metabolism.
- Providing a bright cheerful living area.
- Providing radio and TV to assist in focusing attention.
- Providing clear, simple and concise instructions.
- Developing routine activities.
- Wearing name tags with the name in large letters.
- Working with and encouraging the patient to perform simple tasks.

Sickle Cell Anemia

IN THE UNITED STATES, sickle cell disease affects more than 72,000 persons, primarily those of African heritage. Americans of Mediterranean, Caribbean, South and Central American, Arabian or East Indian descent can also be affected. It is estimated that eight percent of the African-American population carries the sickle cell trait and about one in 375 African-American children is affected by the sickle cell disease. There is no cure for sickle cell anemia but early detection and regular medical care can prevent the onset of serious infections and the severe attacks of pain associated with this disease.

Sickle cell disease comprises a group of genetic disorders characterized by the inheritance of sickle cell hemoglobin from both parents or sickle cell hemoglobin from one parent and a gene for an abnormal hemoglobin or beta-thalassemia from the other parent. The disease changes the structure of hemoglobin, the molecule that carries oxygen in the blood, causing the molecules to clump together at times and warp red blood cells into a "sickle" shape. The deformed cells become wedged in the tiny blood vessels, blocking the transport of oxygen and producing pain and tissue damage. It is a chronic disease that makes the body subject to infections. Many victims suffer sudden attacks of pain because of interrupted blood flow in the abdomen, back and joints. Some of the attacks are so painful that hospitalization and powerful painkillers are necessary.

Universal screening is the only way to ensure that all infants benefit from early diagnosis and lessen the risk of early death. Reliable results can be obtained from a blood test that is performed by licensed laboratories that meet the requirements of the Clinical Laboratory Improvement Act of 1988.

About one in 12 blacks has the sickle cell trait. The symptoms first appear after 6 months of age.

Symptoms:

- Fatigue, breathlessness, and rapid heartbeat.
- Severe attacks of pain.
- Drastic decrease in red blood cells.
- Light-headedness, particularly when standing.
- Susceptibility to infections.
- Skin ulcers in lower legs.

Treatment of sickle cell anemia includes:

- Folic acid supplements.
- Intravenous infusion of fluids to combat dehydration.
- Antibiotic drugs to combat infections; especially pneumonia.
- Oxygen therapy.
- Analgesic drugs to relive severe pain.
- Blood transfusions to temporarily replace hemoglobin

What to do:

Contact the American Medication Association — (312) 464-5000.

Contact the U.S. Department of Health and Human Services, Public Health Service, Agency for Health Care Policy and Research — (301) 443-2403. Or write to them at Executive Office Center, Suite 501, 2101 East Jefferson Street, Rockville, MD 20852

Contact the National Association for Sickle Cell Disease. 1-800-421-8453. You can write it at 4221 Wilshire Boulevard, Suite 360, Los Angeles, CA 90010-3505.

Sleep Disorders

About 40 million Americans have a chronic sleep disorder and another 20 million experience occasional or intermittent sleep disturbances. At least 95 percent of all people who have a sleep disorder remain undiagnosed. Symptoms range from depression to high blood pressure. Rarely does the patient or the doctor know enough about sleep disorders to provide proper diagnosis or treatment. However, there are hospitals and doctors that specialize in the diagnosis and treatment of sleep disorders.

A person's total health can be assured only if waking and sleeping health are good. Most sleep disorders can be lessened with early diagnosis and treatment. Basically, healthy sleep is the amount of sleep a person requires in order to retain optimal alertness during desired waking hours. In a study by the California State Department of Health, those who slept six hours or less a night had a 70 percent higher mortality rate than those who slept eight or more hours. This difference remained the same regardless of age, sex, race, health status and physical activity.

Sleep is divided into two categories: non-rapid eye movement (non-REM) sleep; and rapid eye movement (REM) sleep. In adults, non-REM sleep alternates with REM sleep about every 90-100 minutes throughout the night. Non-REM sleep usually occurs first and will be about 75 to 80 percent of sleep time. In REM sleep, a high level of brain activity takes place; there are bursts of rapid eye movement, increased heart and respiration rates and the paralysis of many muscles.

Everyone experiences occasional nights of insomnia and this lack of sleep usually results in diminished judgment and coordination, irritability and sometimes getting sick to the stomach. These problems go away after successive nights of good sleep.

Some of the more common sleep disorders include:

- **Sleep Apnea** — characterized by snoring and other breathing abnormalities during sleep and is the most serious sleep disorder. Apnea means "without breath." The most serious levels are characterized by the total collapse of the upper airway and extreme reduction of blood oxygen levels during sleep. Over 18 million people in the United States have this problem. The most typical patient suffering from this disorder is a middle-aged overweight male. Other risk factors include thyroid deficiencies, alcohol, tobacco, drug use, obesity and in children, enlarged tonsils and adenoids. The most successful and commonly used medical treatment is nasal continuous positive airway pressure (CPAP), a mask-like device and pump work together to keep the airway open. Improvement is immediate in most patients. Even though very effective, CPAP therapy can be likened to sleeping with a vacuum cleaner running in your ears with a scuba mask on your face.

- **Narcolepsy** is a disabling neurological disorder of unknown cause. It typically occurs between the ages of 15 and 30 and is often inherited. Nationwide, it is estimated that between 250,000 and 375,000 people have this disorder. The symptoms are excessive daytime sleepiness; brief episodes of muscle weakness or paralysis precipitated by strong emotions such as laughter or anger; paralysis upon falling asleep; and hallucinations that occur at the onset of sleep. Usually, excessive sleepiness is the most prominent symptom and the first sign of narcolepsy. Patients will fall asleep during business meetings, at social events, while eating or driving and even during conversations. There is no cure for narcolepsy. Medications can reduce the symptoms and provide the patient with an alertness level approximating 70 percent of normal without stimulants. However, government regulations regarding stimulant medication restrict their use and most doctors are reluctant to treat patients who require long-term use. There are some drugs under development or used in other countries (not yet approved by the Food and Drug Administration) that provide some relief.

- **Insomnia** is the most common sleep disorder. If a patient takes more than 30 to 45 minutes to fall asleep at night, wakes up many times during the night, wakes up early and can't get back to sleep, the patient probably has insomnia. Insomnia is 1½ times more common in the elderly. Women are more likely to suffer from insomnia than men. Insomnia can be caused by chronic medical problems, poor sleep habits or routines (drinking coffee just before bedtime), stress and life changing situations (loss of spouse, moving, etc.).

To overcome insomnia in patients, these suggestions have proven helpful:

- Follow a regular schedule.
- Exercise at regular times each day (2 to 4 hours before bedtime).
- Get some exposure to natural light in the afternoon each day.
- Watch what is eaten and drunk. No caffeine.
- No alcohol or smoking. Nicotine is a stimulant.
- Develop a bedtime routine and follow it each night.
- Use the bedroom only for sleeping. If doesn't come in 15 minutes, get up and go to another room until sleepy.
- Don't worry about sleep.

If your patient is so tired during the day that normal function is impossible, and this situation lasts for more than 2 or 3 weeks, take the patient to the doctor.

For information on a variety of sleep problems, contact:

National Sleep Foundation
1367 Connecticut Avenue, N.W.
Suite 200
Washington, D.C. 20036
(202) 785-2300

Sleep Disorders Center
Alexandria Hospital
4320 Seminary Road
Alexandria, VA 22304
(703) 504-3220

Vision

I<small>N THE</small> U<small>NITED</small> S<small>TATES</small>, more than 5 million people are legally blind. Blindness can result from injury, disease, degeneration of the eyeball, degeneration of the optic nerve or nerves connecting the eye to the brain or the brain itself. The Department of Health and Human Services reports that 13 percent of Americans over the age of 65 have some form of visual impairment, with eight percent having a severe disability. Half the population of blind Americans is over age 65 with 55 percent of new cases of blindness occur among older people. Of those who are over age 85, one in 20 is legally blind.

It may be more difficult for the older patient to see objects clearly because the lens of the eye can become opaque and yellow, making it harder to tell the difference in closely related colors. This is especially true in the blue-green color spectrum. Generally, older persons need two to three times as much light as younger persons. It also takes an older person longer to focus when they move from a dark to a light area or vice versa. To avoid nasty falls for patients who cannot see clearly, instruct them to take it easy and move slowly. Color blindness affects about five percent of the population and they have difficulty with the blues, greens and violets, also.

In the United States, blindness is usually defined as corrected visual acuity of 20/200 or less in the better eye or a visual field of no more than 20 degrees for the better eye. Loss of vision impacts quality of life and isolates individuals and limits their activities.

Common eye complaints include:

- **Presbyopia** — a gradual decline in the ability to focus on close objects or to see small print. It is not uncommon after the age of 40. There is no known prevention for presbyopia, but the problem can be relieved with eyeglasses.

- **Floaters** — tiny spots or specks that float across the field of vision. Most people notice them in well-lighted rooms or outdoors on a bright day. Floaters are normal and usually harmless. However, they may be a warning of certain eye problems, especially when occurring with light flashes. If your patient notices a sudden change in the type or number of spots or flashes, call the doctor.

- **Dry eyes** — occurs when the tear glands produce too few tears. The result is itching, burning or in some cases reduced vision. An eye specialist can prescribe special eyedrop solutions to correct the problem.

- **Excessive tears** — may be a sign of increased sensitivity to light, wind or temperature changes. In these cases, protective measures such as sun glasses may solve the problem. Tearing may also indicate more serious problems such as an eye infection or a blocked tear duct, both of which can be treated and corrected.

- **Cataracts** — are cloudy or opaque areas in part or all of the transparent lens located inside the eye. When a cataract forms, light cannot easily pass through the lens and this will affect vision. Cataracts usually develop gradually and without pain, redness or tearing in the eye. If the cataract becomes too big or too dense, it can be surgically removed. Cataract surgery is a safe procedure and is almost always successful. After surgery, vision is restored by using special glasses, or contact lenses. Sometimes an intraocular lens is implanted during the eye surgery.

- **Glaucoma** — occurs when there is too much fluid pressure in the eye, causing internal eye damage and gradually destroying vision. The basic cause of glaucoma is unknown but with early diagnosis and treatment it can usually be controlled and blindness prevented. Treatment consists of prescription eyedrops, oral medications, laser treatments or, in some cases, surgery. Glaucoma seldom produces early symptoms, and usually there is no pain from the increased pressure.

- **Retinal disorders** — are a leading cause of blindness in the United States. The retina is a thin lining on the back of the eye made up of nerves that receive visual images and pass them on to the brain.

- **Macular degeneration** — a condition in which the macula (a part of the retina responsible for sharp central and reading vision) stops functioning efficiently. First signs may include blurring of vision, distortion or loss of central vision. Early detection is important since some cases may be handled well with laser treatments.

- **Retinopathy** — one of the possible results of diabetes or hypertension occurs when the small blood vessels that feed the retina fail to do so properly. In the early stages of the condition, the blood vessels may leak fluid, which distorts vision. In later stages, new vessels may grow and release blood in the center of the eye, resulting in serious loss of vision.

- **Retinal detachment** — is a separation between the inner and outer layers of the retina. Detached retina can usually be surgically reattached with good or partial renewal of vision. New surgical and laser treatments are being used with increasing success.

Many people with visual impairments are being helped by using low-vision aids. These aids are special devices that provide more power than regular eyeglasses. Low vision aids include telescopic lenses and magnifying glasses, along with a variety of electronic devices.

Symptoms:

- Loss, distortion or dimness of vision.
- Pain in or around the eyes.
- Excessive tearing or discharge from the eye.
- Swelling of the eyelids or protrusion of the eye.
- Double vision.
- Flashes of light, floating spots or halos around lights.
- Changes in vision or movement of one eye.
- Changes in the color of an eye.

If your patient is visually impaired, there are a number of things you can do to enable adaptation:

- Clearly mark with white or reflective tape (tape that is both is preferred) changes in floor levels and the edges of steps.
- Mark the first and last step differently from the others.
- Arrange furniture so the walkway is not an obstacle course.
- Use higher wattage lightbulbs. Be sure not to overload electrical circuits or lamp fixtures.
- Avoid shiny surfaces to prevent glare.
- Buy furniture, dishes, and other items for the home that are red or yellow-orange because they are easier to distinguish.
- Use contrasting colors as much as possible (e.g. white dishes on a red tablecloth).
- Use night lights that come on automatically when it becomes dark.
- Keep light levels between the bedroom and the hallway the same or as close to the same as possible.
- Use indirect lighting as much as possible because it is much easier on patient's eyes, especially if they wear glasses.

What to do:

Contact the doctor — See the family doctor, an ophthalmologist (can do surgery) or an optometrist for a check up. Most eye problems can be corrected or improved with early detection. An optician is trained to fit, adjust and dispense eyeglasses and other devices.

Contact the American Foundation for the Blind — 1-800-232-5463. The Foundation will provide information on programs and services that help the blind keep their independence. They have lots of material and a number of regional offices.

Contact the National Society to Prevent Blindness — 1-800-221-3004. They have a "Home Eye Test for Adults" which is available for $1.25. You can write the Society at 500 East Remington Road, Schaumburg, IL 60173.

Contact the Library of Congress National Library Services for the Blind and Physically Handicapped — 1-800-424-8567, (202) 287-5100 if in Washington, DC. Provides audio and Braille formats for the blind through a network of state libraries.

Cataracts

CATARACTS affect about 50 percent of Americans between the ages of 65 and 74. About 70 percent of those age 75 and over have cataracts. Most people will have a cataract in both eyes but because each cataract develops at a different rate, one eye may be worse than the other. About 1.35 million cataract operations (extractions) are performed annually in the United States.

Currently, there is no medical treatment to prevent the formation or progression of cataracts in an otherwise healthy adult. A number of factors influence the risk of cataracts:

- Ultraviolet-B radiation
- Diabetes
- Drugs
- Smoking
- Diarrhea
- Alcohol
- Low antioxidant vitamin status

The way to surgically treat a cataract is to remove all or part of the lens and replace it with an artificial lens. There are three types of cataract surgery.

- **Extracapsular surgery** — The surgeon removes the lens, leaving the outer covering of the lens.
- **Phacoemulsification** — The surgeon will soften the lens with sound waves and remove it through a needle.
- **Intracapsular surgery** — The surgeon will remove the entire lens, including the capsule. This surgery is rarely used.

The success rate for cataract surgery is 95 percent in otherwise healthy patients. If your patient has cataracts in both eyes, it is best to wait until the first eye heals before having surgery on the second eye.

A patient who has cataract surgery usually gets an artificial lens at the same time. A plastic disc, called an intraocular lens, is placed in the lens capsule inside the eye. Other choices are contact lenses and cataract glasses. The doctor will decide what is best for the patient.

Cataracts cannot return because all or part of the lens has been removed. However, in about half of all patients who have extracapsular surgery or phacoemulsification, the lens capsule becomes cloudy. This cloudiness of the lens capsule usually develops a year or more after surgery and will cause the same vision problems as a cataract. To correct this problem, the doctor will use a laser beam to make a tiny hole in the capsule to let light pass through. The surgery is painless and does not require a hospital stay.

Symptoms:

- Cloudy, fuzzy or filmy vision
- Changes in the way colors are seen
- Problems driving at night because headlights seem too bright
- Problems with glare from lamps or the sun
- Frequent changes in eyeglass prescription
- Double vision
- Better near vision for awhile in farsighted people

What to do:

See a doctor — A regular eye exam is all that is needed to find a cataract. The doctor will ask the patient to read an eye chart and will probably dilate the eye to enable the doctor to see inside the eyes. If the patient is scheduled for an eye operation, be sure that you have the doctor teach you and the patient how to administer eye drops and apply an eye patch. Make sure that this is done before the operation as most patients will be discharged a few hours after surgery.

Contact the American Optometric Association — (314) 991-4100. You can write them at 243 North Lindberg Boulevard, St. Louis, MO 63121. They have a number of free publications.

Contact the National Eye Care Project Helpline — 1-800-222-EYES (3937). They offer information on free eye examinations. To qualify for this program, the patient must be financially disadvantaged, at least 65 years old, a U. S. citizen and must not have seen an ophthalmologist in three years.

Products for the Visually Impaired

Magnifying Glasses

A magnifying glass is a lens where both sides of the lens are usually curved to form a double convex (curving outward). The power of magnification is directly related to the field of view. The higher the power of magnification, the smaller the field. The distance between the object being viewed and the center of the lens (focal length) also plays an important role. The greater the curve of a lens, the shorter its focal length. For example, a 10× lens must be placed much closer to the object being viewed than a 2× lens. If you and/or the patient want to work on something with your hands, a lower magnification will be needed to allow for room for the hands (sewing, building models, etc.) It may be that you will want to buy two lenses – one for reading and one for close work.

Diopter is a word used by eye care professionals to refer to the power of a lens to refract (bend) the rays of light. The relationship between diopter and magnification is usually calculated by dividing diopter by 4 and then adding the number 1 (one). 4 diopter is equivalent to 2× and 8 diopter is equivalent to 3×. Check with your eye care professional for help in making the right choice of magnifier.

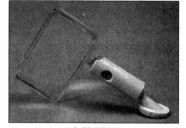

Li 690705

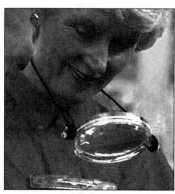

Li 454430

Brandt Spring Arm Halogen Magnifier. Professional quality magnifier provides undistorted magnification, wide viewing area and glare-free light. High intensity illumination (600-foot candles). Comes with 3 or 5 diopter, 5-inch magnification lens. Arm has 45-inch reach.

Br 43133	3 Diopter halogen, pedestal base	$289.95
Br 43233	5 Diopter halogen, pedestal base	$315.95

Brandt Circline Magnifiers. Available with either a 3 diopter (+75 percent magnification — 13-inch focal length) or a 5 diopter (+125 percent magnification — 8-inch focal length). 5-inch diameter, bi-convex lens. 22-watt cool white circline fluorescent tube. 45-inch reach.

Br 43143	3 Diopter, pedestal base	$255.95
Br 43243	5 Diopter, pedestal base	$285.95

LILA Deluxe Sewing Machine Magnifier. Flexible plastic device that attaches with adhesive to a sewing machine. Helps threading the needle.

Li 690705	Lens measures 2 × 3 inches	$10.95

LILA Around-the-Neck Hands Free Magnifier. Large 4-inch lens. Neck cord for holding in any desired position. Great for work that requires the use of both hands.

Li 454430	Bifocal insert provides extra hi-power viewing	$6.95

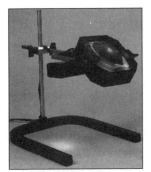

Li 714433

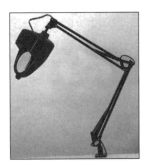

Li 275925

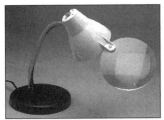

Li 275974

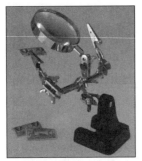

Li 366174

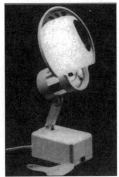

Li 452728

LILA Stereoptic Magnifier with Light. Precision-ground 2.75× acrylic lens that is 6 inches by 6 inches. Two 7-watt fluorescent bulbs concentrate the light where it is needed. Additional lens can be attached (not included) to increase total magnification to 5.5×.

Li 714433	Heavyweight steel tubing base	$239.95
Li 714434	Additional lens	$139.95

LILA Economy Model Magnifying Lamp. Affordable answer to illuminated magnification. 4-inch optically fine ground 3 diopter (1.75×) lens provides excellent magnification. Lamp head will reach 36 inches. Requires one 60-watt bulb (not included). Comes in black.

Li 275925	4-way mounting clamp.	$29.95

LILA Economy Fluorescent Magnifying Lamp. Low priced fluorescent magnifying lamp with a 5-inch three diopter (1.75×) magnifying lens. Comes with a 22-watt circline fluorescent bulb and a heavy duty clamp. Black

Li 275974	Has a 5″ reach.	$99.95

LILA Multi-power Magnifier. Pocket magnifier with 5 magnifications. (2×, 3×, 4×, 5× and 8×) in 2 lenses that slide into a sturdy carrying case. Perfect for reading menus in restaurants, telephone directories, etc.

Li 502981	Fits in pocket or purse. 3 × 1½ × ¾ inches	$4.95

LILA Home and Hobby Round Magnifiers. High quality 2× magnifiers with a 5× bifocal insert. Great for reading small print. Ultra clear shatterproof lens and comfortable handles.

Li 370348	2″ lens	$3.95
Li 370351	3″ lens	$5.95
Li 370355	4″ lens	$9.95

LILA Round Magnifier with 3″ Lens. All purpose magnifier with high quality lens made of optical scratch-resistant glass. Features a wide field of view.

Li 666345	Easily carried in pocket or purse	$9.95

LILA 2× Rectangular Magnifier. Comes with 5× bifocal lens. High quality optical plastic.

Li 454440	2″ × 4″	$8.95

LILA E-Z Pickens Magnifier Tweezer.

Li 331555	$3.95

LILA "Helping Hand" Magnifier. Hands-free concept comes with heavy duty alligator clips for holding items to be magnified. Optically ground 2× lens. Base is heavy cast iron and fittings are nickel-plated steel. Great for hobbies and crafts.

Li 366174	7″ × 7″ × 3″	$13.95

LILA Magnifying Mirror with Light. A focused bright beam with a 5× magnification mirror allows for precise views of the tiniest details. Originally designed for dental and medical use. Great for eyebrow tweezing, applying makeup, etc. Mirror is 5 inches in diameter and 10 inches high. Weighted base keeps it from tipping. Hinged arm allows the patient to swivel the mirror for the best view and folds flat for travel. Off-white color. Works on normal house current.

Li 452728	2¼″ × 3½″ × 1¾″ base	$57.95

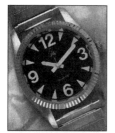

Li 856819

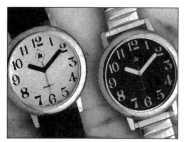

Li 856774, Li 856777

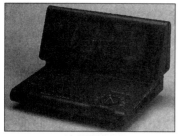

Li 247525

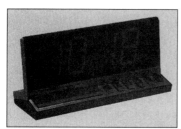

Li 835900

LILA Low-Vision Quartz Watches. Inexpensive and easy to read. Gold color cases with large numerals at the 3, 6, 9 and 12 positions for maximum visibility. Choose white or black face with either leather strap or metal expansion band.

Li 856819	Gold expansion band, black face	$29.95
Li 856821	Gold expansion band, white face	$29.95
Li 856820	Leather band, black face	$29.95
Li 856822	Leather band, white face	$29.95

LILA Unisex Low-Vision Watches for Him and Her. New "Slimline" watches can be worn by both men and women. Big face and extra wide hand for extra visibility and ease of reading. These are the widest hands on any watch. Gold color and black or white face.

Li 856774	Leather strap, black numbers on white face	$29.95
Li 856775	Leather strap, white numbers on black face	$29.95
Li 856776	Gold expansion band, white face, black numbers	$29.95
Li 856777	Hold expansion band, black face, white numbers	$29.95

LILA Low-Vision LED Alarm Clock. Red LED numbers are nearly 2 inches high. Bright/dim switch allows patient to set the brightness they prefer. 24-hour electronic alarm can be reset right after it goes off. Snoozer sounds every 9 minutes. Has a.m./p.m. indicator. Takes 9 volt battery for back-up if power fails (not included).

Li 247500	100% solid state circuitry	$25.95

LILA Low Vision LED Alarm Clock with Green Numbers. For those patients who find that green illuminated numbers are easier to read. Numbers are almost an inch high (.9"). Snooze function repeats alarm every 9 minutes. Battery back-up (9V battery not included).

Li 247548	Built-in night light	$21.95

LILA Low Vision LED Alarm Clock with AM/FM Radio. Large 1.8-inch red LED numbers. Snooze function included. Has PM and Alarm-on indicators. Battery back-up (9V battery not included).

Li 247525	Black	$30.95

LILA Vox Clock-4 Talking Electric Alarm Clock. Easy to operate with battery back-up. Clear female voice announces the time at the touch of a button. Has large .9 inch red LED display. 9V battery for back-up not included.

Li 835900	6" × 5" × 2"	$54.95

LILA Big Bold Timer. 8 inches across and extra easy to read. Set for any interval from 5 to 60 minutes. Black numbers on white background. Great for cooking and exercise.

Li 790790	Can be wall mounted too	$14.95

LILA Low Vision Playing Cards. 2-inch numbers. Spades are black, hearts are red, diamonds are green and clubs are blue.

Li 308605	Cards measure 2½" × 3½"	$2.95

LILA Super Jumbo Number Playing Cards. Patented by a doctor for people who have impaired vision. The 1-inch high bold numbers and designs are in black or red on a white background. Large numbers are in the corners so you can see your hand.

Li 733427	Cards measure 2¼" × 3½"	$3.95

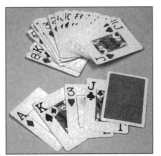

Li 126777

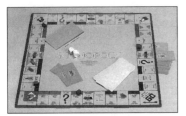

Li 126736

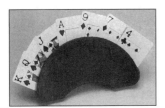

Li 147622

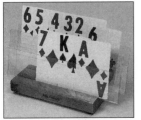

Li 614600

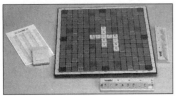

Li 126822

LILA Jumbo Index Playing Cards with Braille. Comes in bridge and pinochle decks.

| Li 126777 | Bridge or poker | $6.95 |
| Li 126780 | Pinochle | $6.95 |

LILA Uno Game with Brailled Cards. Bright colors make the cards easily visible.

| Li 817346 | Uno game with cards (not brailled) | $10.95 |
| Li 127505 | Brailled Uno cards | $10.95 |

LILA Brailled Monopoly. British version offers fun and education. Boardwalk and Park Place become Mayfair and Park Lane. Prices are in English pounds and not US dollars. Large print with brailled dice and playing cards.

| Li 126736 | Brailled instructions | $59.95 |

LILA Card Player, Card Holder. Solid, light, easy to hold, yet built to stand up. Self adjusting action inner liner lets the patient space cards farther apart and hold them even when the hand is turned down. ABS plastic. Great for those patients with arthritis.

| Li 147622 | Weighs 5 ounces | $9.95 |

LILA Disc Card Holder. Simple device allows those without finger strength or dexterity to hold a hand of cards. Single cards can be added or removed without disturbing the other cards.

| Li 257418 | Weighs only ½ ounce | $2.95 |

LILA Playing Card Holder. Unique tension device holds up to 13 cards. Metal with a walnut wood grain finish. Weighted to stay on the table without tipping.

| Li 614600 | Card holder is 10¾" long | $6.95 |

LILA Playing Card Shuffler. Shuffles two decks of cards at the touch of the lever. Two "C" batteries are required and are not included.

| Li 151400 | Unit is 8" × 4¼" × 3½" | $14.95 |

LILA Brailled Scrabble. Made in England and modified with braille by the Royal National Institute for the Blind. Each tile has the point and letter values in both print and braille.

| Li 126822 | Board squares have a raised outline to prevent slipping | $105.95 |

LILA Brailled Cluedo. All the written information on the board is in braille. All pieces are plastic and fit neatly in each square. Cards are also in braille. All squares on the board have raised borders and the outer edges of the rooms are marked by a raised line.

| Li GB-50 | Tactile dice included | $55.95 |

LILA Chess and Checker Board Set. Beautifully made plastic board in orange and white for easy visibility. White sections lower than orange sections for tactual differentiation. All sections have a hole drilled in the center to match corresponding pegs in the chess pieces. Red and black checkers are shaped differently for tactual identification.

| Li 375000 | Complete set | $37.95 |

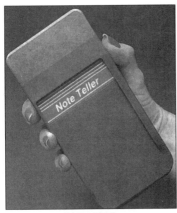

Li 541600

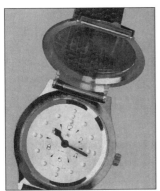

Li 856799

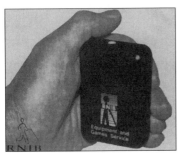

Li CV-03

LILA Note Teller™ Talking Money Identifier. Compact 6 inches by 3 inches by 1 inch and lightweight (8 oz.). Verbally announces the denomination of all bills from one dollar to one hundred dollars. Automatically turns on when bill is inserted and off when the bill is removed. Powered by a 9-volt battery which is included. Battery is good for about 3,000 bills.

Li 541600 $525.95

LILA Enhanced Note Teller™. Designed for people who are deaf or have a hearing deficit. Has a tactile output instead of an audio output for identifying bills. Will identify bills from one dollar to and including one hundred dollar bills.

Li 550550 $615.95

LILA Marktime Timer with "Touch-Time" Markings. Reliable 60-minute timer with a brailled face so the patient can set without seeing it. Three raised dots at 15, 30, and 45 minutes – two raised dots at remaining 5 minute intervals, with one raised dot at remaining 2½ minute intervals.

Li 459600 $20.95

LILA Braille "TouchTime" Watches. Silver dial, with black numerals and hands. Crystal is hinged at 12 o'clock, flips up at 6 o'clock for tactual time-telling. The face is 1½ inches in diameter.

Li 856799	Men's quartz with leather band	$56.95
Li 856798	Men's quartz with stainless steel expansion band	$56.95
Li 856800	Men's gold plated with expansion band	$68.95
Li 856801	Men's gold plated with leather band	$68.95

LILA Braille "Touch-Time" Watches. Smaller version of the "Touch-Time" for men. The face is ¾ inch in diameter.

Li 856805	Black leather band	$56.95
Li 856803	Stainless steel expansion band	$56.95
Li 856806	Gold plated with expansion band	$68.95
Li 856807	Gold plated with leather band	$68.95

LILA Tactiwatch. Can be used by deaf-blind patients. Time can be determined by pulses of varying duration which vibrate the unit. Time is read by pressing the recessed switch on the top of the unit. Powered by two AAA batteries which are included.

Li CV-03 $106.95

LILA Brynolf Pocket Counter. Can be used to count up to 99.99. Comes with wrist strap.

Li DH-23 $8.95

LILA Walkmate. Puts out a signal that is two feet wide and runs from about two feet off the ground to about eight feet off the ground. Use for detecting tables and other indoor and outdoor hazards that might otherwise be missed during the normal "sweep" of a cane. Will warn wearer within 7 feet of an object by beeping intermittently. The sound of the beep changes when the patient is within 4 feet of an object. A vibrator also comes with the unit to warn those who are also hard of hearing. *The Walkmate should always be used with a cane and not alone.*

Li 868800 $178.95

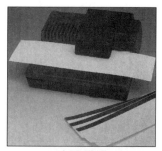

Li 836742

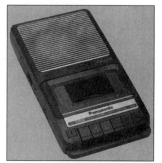

Li 153253

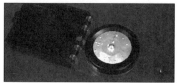

Li 254900

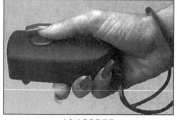

Li 182355

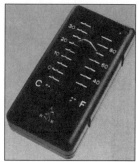

Li DH-87

LILA Voxcom® Recorder Kit. Inexpensive and convenient way to record messages on cards or tape. The recorder measures 5 inches by 5 inches and weighs just 15 ounces. Uses magnetically pre-striped cards which pass through the recorder and then serve as message reminders. A recorded card can be taped to food to identify its contents later. Cards can be used over and over. For a permanent record, a talk/tape with adhesive can be pasted on the backs of checks, and other important papers. Comes with four AA batteries, 50 cards and 180-inch roll of talk/tape.

Li 836742	Recorder kit	$69.95
Li 836745	50 Extra cards	$7.95
Li 836748	180" Roll of Talk/Tape	$3.95

LILA 4-Track "Talking Books" Cassette Player. Plays Library of Congress formatted four-track cassette recordings, as well as regular tapes. Auto-stop shuts off at end of tape (Not auto-reversible). Uses 4 "C" batteries which are not included. An AC adapter is included.

Li 153253 $115.95

LILA Braille Directional Compass. Made by Silva of Sweden. It is held steady in the palm of the hand with cover open. Cover is then closed for about 8 seconds. When the cover is opened, the directional disc locks in place for a tactual reading of direction.

Li 254900 $49.95

LILA "Columbus" Talking Compass. Verbally announces the major compass points as well as the interim points of North-East, North-West, South-East and South-West. Measures 4 inches by 2 inches wide and weighs less than 4 ounces. Speaks in either English or Spanish at the flip of a switch. Requires 2 N batteries (included).

Li 182355 $165.95

LILA 12" Metal Rule. Each inch is marked with 3 raised dots and by braille numerals. Every ½ inch is indicated by 2 dots . . . every ¼ inch by 1 dot.

Li 127500 $11.95

LILA Tactile Meat Thermometer. Ensures properly cooked meat. Fahrenheit demarcations have been marked for easy tactile identification. Temperature range is from 120 to 200 degrees and is marked in 20 degree intervals. Made of stainless steel, Dishwasher safe.

Li 755908 $17.95

LILA Audible Room Thermometer. Reads indoor room temperatures between 23 and 95 degrees Fahrenheit. Can be hand-held or mounted on the wall. Sliding pointer is pushed up until an audible noise is heard and a vibration is also felt. Temperature is read from scale with tactile dots. 4 AAA batteries are included.

Li DH-87 $76.95

LILA Aluminum Clothing Color Identification Tags. Provided by the Telephone Pioneers of America. Rust proof tags are braille marked with a color identification and can be sewn into clothing. Packed in envelopes of 28 tags with 2 tags each of 14 colors. Provided by the folks at the phone company.

Li 061000   FREE

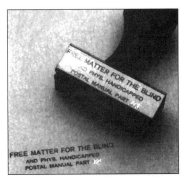

Li 336777

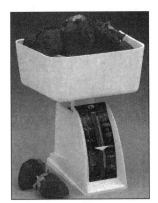

Li 755912

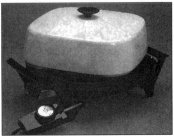

Li 664385

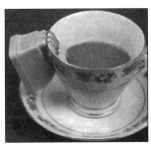

Li 765444

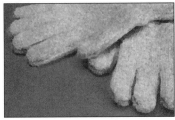

Li 786939

LILA "Free Matter for the Blind" Rubber Stamp. Blind persons can mail recorded or brailled letters free — if the wording appears on the envelope.
Li 336777 — $2.95

LILA Tactile Portion Control Scale. Ounces are marked with one dot and each four-ounce location has three dots. Can be used for mail too. Food container is removable for easy washing. A calorie counter book is included. Weighs in ½ oz. increments (5 gram).
Li 755912 — $23.95

LILA West Bend Electric Fry Pan with Brailled Controls. Temperature control has been brailled. There are two raised dots at 200 degrees, three dots at 300 degrees and four dots at 400 degrees. One raised dot at every 50 degree interval. 11 inches across.
Li 664385 — $43.95

LILA Automatic Egg Cooker. Fool-proof. Just add the pre-determined amount of water, put the eggs into the contoured slots and push the "on" button. Automatic shut-off. Cooks up to eight eggs at a time.
Li 276200 — $42.95

LILA Liquid Level Indicator. Tells when liquid reaches two different levels. When filling a cup, an intermittent tone indicates that the cup is nearly full and a continuous tone indicated that the cup is full. Indicator also produces vibrations for those people with hearing impairments.
Li DK-31 — $18.95

LILA Liquid Level Indicator. For the blind and deaf-blind to determine when a glass or cup is filled within a half inch of the top. Buzzer sounds and vibrates. Easy to carry. Comes with 9-volt battery.
Li 765444 — $15.95

LILA Jar Opener. Strong and compact opener which attaches permanently to the underside of any table, counter or cabinet. Opens any screw lid from ⅜ of an inch to 3⅜ of an inch in diameter. Operates with one hand and is especially good for those bigger and heavier jars that require two hands to open. Comes with mounting screws.
Li 400660 — $5.95

LILA Thick Terry Gloves. Allow for maximum finger movement when handling pots, pans or foods that are either hot or cold. Made of heavyweight knit cotton. Machine washable. 14 inches length.
Li 786939 — $5.95

LILA Credit Card Guide and Magnifier. Small credit card size magnifier plus a special signature guide. Magnifier can be used as an aid in reading menus and reviewing the bill.
Li 198653 — $1.95

LILA Full Page String Writing Guide. Stringed frame holds 8½ inches by 11 inches sheet of paper firmly against a wood blackboard. For letters that dip below the line such as "g," "j," etc. the string has enough give so perfect letters can be formed. Each string has a bead on it to mark your place when writing.
Li 275749 — $22.95

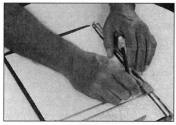

Li 682700

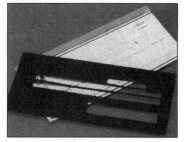

Li 163733

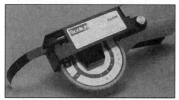

Li 430700

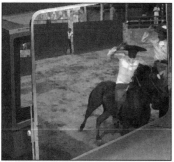

Li 107092

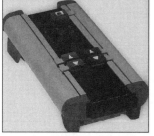

Li 657500

LILA Marks Script Guide. Clipboard takes 8½-inch by 11-inch paper. Left edge of board has a notched guide along which a carriage with a clicking device carries a ¾-inch slot formed of two thin metal rods 8 inches long. A metal block slides on the rods to serve as a margin stop.

Li 682700   **$29.95**

LILA Check Writing Guide. A template for filling in information on a standard 3¾-inch by 6-inch check.

Li 163733   **$1.95**

LILA Signature Guide. Sturdy plastic mask with aperture to correspond with standard signature area. Fits in wallet (2⅛ inches × 3⅜ inches)

Li 692222   **$.95**

LILA Deluxe Signature Guide. Two rubber blocks support two 4¼-inch lengths of metal rod 9/16 of an inch apart. Rubber tips reduce slipping.

Li 224850   **$1.95**

LILA Envelope Writing Guide. Sturdy plastic mask with apertures corresponding to standard "address to" and "address from" areas on envelopes.

Li 291355   **$1.95**

LILA 3M Large Print Labeler. Large sharp letters and numbers ½-inch high on a ¾-inch wide tape. One roll of tape included with labeler.

Li 430700		**$139.95**
Li 830060	Black vinyl labeling tape ¾" × 288"	**$9.95**
Li 454358	Magnetic labeling tape ¾" × 197"	**$15.95**

LILA Sock Clips. Pack of twelve sock clips to help keep socks in matching pairs. Tactile coloring code to identify sock clips. Machine washable.

Li DH-71   **$7.95**

LILA TV Screen Enlarger. Optometrically tested and approved screen that more than doubles the size of a TV screen. Provides exceptional color, brightness and clarity. Durable acrylic is easy to keep clean. Simply slide the braces under the TV set for mounting. Not for consoles.

Li 107092	For 10" to 15" TV screens	**$77.95**
Li 107095	For 17" to 23" TV screens	**$82.95**

LILA "Remote Idea" Large Button Adapter for TV Remote. Slide the patient's remote into the attractive holder, position the large button keys over the basic functions keys. Large buttons can be operated with the patient's fist for those who have arthritis. Basic functions include: On-Off, Up Channel, Down Channel and Up-Down Volume.

Li 657500   **$11.95**

LILA Large Button Universal Remote. Easily programmable — has only five buttons. On-Off, Up channel, Down channel, Up volume and Down volume.

Li 434350   **$13.95**

LILA Tray Mate®. Clamps on any chair, including wheelchairs — any chair or couch with a solid side panel. Sturdy, no-wobble surface. Made of durable plastic and can be left outdoors all season.

Li 804517   **$13.95**

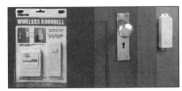

Li 852673

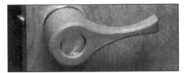

Li 436755

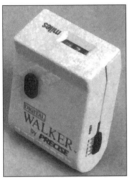

LI 583176

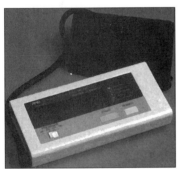

Li 151443

LILA Automatic Seat Lifter. Gives the patient a gentle lift of about 5 inches up. Weighs only 9 pounds. Made of padded, deluxe vinyl. Measures 13 inches by 15 inches. Not for use on easy chairs.

| Li 097041 | 2 springs for people up to 150 pounds | $132.95 |
| Li 097042 | 3 springs for people up to 250 pounds | $144.95 |

LILA Ease In — Ease Out. For those patients who have difficulty swiveling to get in and out of a chair. Base constructed of durable plastic which will not leave indentation marks on leather seats. Built-in carrying handle.

| Li 273440 | | $20.95 |

LILA Wireless Door Chime. Electronic doorbell easily mounts on door. Chime unit is plugged into any AC wall outlet within 50 feet of the doorbell button. Doorbell button uses a 9 volt battery (not included).

| Li 852673 | | $15.95 |

LILA Leveron Easy Touch Door Handle. Easy to install over any standard door knob. Comes with clear instructions and a custom wrench for easy installation. Glows in the dark.

| Li 436755 | | $11.95 |

LILA Soft Grip Doorknob Turner. Rubber ribbed cover fits over a standard doorknob to give the patient a firmer grasp of the knob. Comes in brown or white. White glows in the dark. Washable. Packed two to a bag (one color).

| Li 700325 | Brown | $2.95 |
| Li 700331 | White (Glows in the dark) | $2.95 |

LILA Fanny Pack. Roomy pack with an adjustable waist belt and three pockets. Made of durable nylon and is waterproof.

| Li 310655 | | $8.95 |

LILA Pedometer "Walker." Can be hooked to waistband or belt. Records how far the patient has walked. Long life lithium batteries are included.

| LI 583176 | | $13.95 |

LILA Talking Blood Pressure Meter. Designed to meet the needs of those with low vision who must regularly check blood pressure. Unit announces blood pressure and pulse rate. Arm cuff inflates and deflates automatically. Kit includes meter with standard adult size arm cuff (fits 7½ to 12½ inches in arm circumference). Large print and audio cassette instructions included. Requires 4 AA batteries (not included).

Li 151443		$228.95
Li 151448	Large arm cuff (11" to 14")	$33.95
Li 151451	AC adapter for blood pressure meter	$22.95

LILA Talking Thermometer. Lightweight (1.4 oz.) talking thermometer is accurate to within 0.3 to 0.4 degrees in clinical range of 89.6 to 107.6 degrees Fahrenheit. Can be used orally or rectally. Thermometer will beep and then announce temperature 4 times. Has digital display for optical reading. Comes with carrying case. Operates on two lithium batteries which are included.

| Li 756224 | | $64.95 |

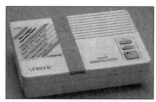

Li 764287

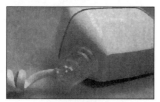

Li 603537

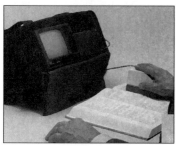

Li 451520

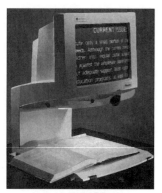

Li 289000

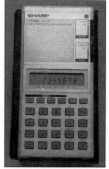

Li 756000

LILA Autodrop Eyedrop Dispenser. Developed in England in collaboration with the Royal National Institute for the Blind. Clip the Autodrop to the top of the eyedrop container after the cap has been removed. The Autodrop will then fit right over the eye, a special lip holds the lower eye lid down to prevent blinking.

Li 089733 $4.95

LILA Telephone Answering Machine. Easy to operate. Comes with call screening function. You will know who is calling you and skip those unwanted calls. Has only four buttons. Compact size only 4½ inches by 6½ inches.

Li 764287 $57.95

LILA Phone Coil Twisstop. A snap to install. Keeps the telephone cord from twisting and getting tangled.

Li 603537 $5.95

LILA LV-105 Portable Electronic Magnifying Viewer. Self-contained and weighs under 10 pounds. Has advanced model CCD camera and 5-inch monitor. Plugs into standard wall socket. Hand-held scanner weighs just 12 ounces and has its own built-in LED light for optimal imaging control.

The LV-105 can be connected to a desk-top CCTV or to your own home TV. All cables and accessories needed are included. Three lens options are available. When the medium lens is used, ordinary newspaper print will be almost ⅝ inches high on the portable built-in monitor and will be approximately 2¾ inches high on a standard 19-inch home TV screen.

Li 451520 $2,145.95

LILA "Aladdin"™ Electronic Magnifier. Black and white monitor. 14-inch screen permits a range of magnification form 4× to 25×. Reading matter can be viewed in black on white or reversed for viewing in white on black.

Unusually large depth of field permits curved surfaces, such as cans and bottles, as well as books with pronounced valleys at their bindings to be read with minimal need for refocusing.

Just plug it in. Measures 14 inches by 19 inches by 21.3 inches and weighs 37 pounds. Call for full color brochure.

Li 289000 $2,235.95

LILA Sharp Talking Clock-Calculator. Automatically announces time every hour on the hour. Can be set for use as an alarm clock, countdown timer and will tell you the day, month, day of the week and year on command. When used as a calculator, it will announce each use of the buttons (add,subtract, etc.), the number input and the results. 8-digit LCD readout. Uses 4 AA batteries (included). Measures 6 inches by 3 inches by ¾ inches.

Li 756000 $123.95
Li 756001   AC adapter $9.95

LILA Postal Wallets. Heavy vinyl with a Velcro® seal and clear vinyl pocket to insert the address. Small size holds one cassette; large size holds up to three cassettes.

Li 624735   Small $3.95
Li 624737   Large $4.95

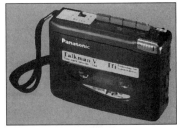

Li 757810

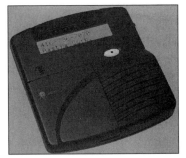

Li 756490

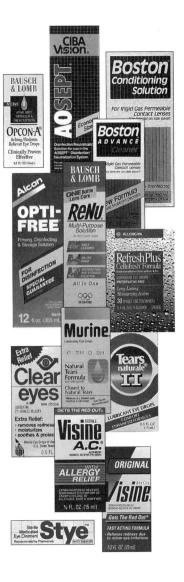

LILA Classmate 4-Track Cassette Player/Recorder. Specially modified player/recorder will play 4-track "Talking Books" formatted tapes as well as standard 2-track tapes. Will also record 4-track and 2-track at either speed. Built-in microphone and speaker. Operates on 4 C batteries (not included) or regular household current. Rechargeable C batteries are available. AC adapter is included. (Note: Classmate will recharge special batteries while running on AC.).

Li 540320		$270.95
Li 540325	Rechargeable batteries (4)	$29.95

LILA Panasonic Talkman IV by TFI. Pocket-sized for "Talking Books." Specially adapted to play the 4-track slow speed Library of Congress format tapes. Weighs only 8 ounces. Has 2 track, monaural, slow speed recording, which allows for twice as much material on each tape. Will also play music on standard cassettes. Built-in speaker, voice activated recording. Uses 2 AA batteries (included) or AC adapter (included).

Li 757810	$240.95

LILA Talking Caller ID. Announces as well as displays on an LCD screen the phone number of all incoming calls. In addition, up to nine messages can be pre-recorded and linked to specific phone numbers so that the caller's name or other information will also be spoken. Up to 30 numbers can be stored in memory. Date and time also given. Operates on household current with battery backup. Requires one 9 volt battery (not included). Must be used in conjunction with phone company's Caller ID service.

Li 756490		$165.95
Li 756955	90 Number memory	$185.95

Eyecare Products

Le 361-5622	Aosept Disinfectant Solution	12 oz	$10.45
Le 110-4736	B&L Opcon-A Eye Drops	0.5 oz	$6.85
Le 118-3912	B&L Saline Solution Sens Eyes	12 oz	$3.85
Le 248-0457	Boston Advance Cleaner	30 ml	$12.45
Le 193-0007	Boston Adv Cond Solution	4 oz	$12.85
Le 168-8548	Boston Cond Solution	4 oz	$10.35
Le 222-6140	Celluvisc Ophth/S 1%	.01oz	$12.85
Le 221-6240	Clear Eyes Drops	0.5 oz	$3.95
Le 163-9897	Collyrium Fresh Eye Wash	4 oz	$5.45
Le 221-8766	Hypotears Lub Drop	0.5 oz	$9.85
Le 120-3488	Hypotears Lub Drop	1 oz	$14.65
Le 136-6517	Murine Eye Drop	0.5 oz	$4.65
Le 349-7070	Opti-Free Chem Disinfectant	12 oz	$10.35
Le 136-4074	Refresh Plus Oph Sol .5% UD	30 ml	$9.85
Le 147-1697	Renu Multi-Purpose Solution	8 oz	$8.65
Le 141-3319	Renu Multi-Purpose Solution	12 oz	$10.95
Le 121-7819	Stye Ophth Ointment 7660	1/8 oz	$7.65
Le 243-9784	Tears Naturale II	15 ml	$10.35
Le 188-6274	Tears Naturale DT	1/2 oz	$9.85
Le 132-4573	Visine Eye Drop Plast	1/2 oz	$4.65
Le 120-1581	Visine A.C. Eye Drop	0.5 oz	$4.65
Le 341-9538	Visine Extra Eye Drop	0.5 oz	$4.65

LeBoeuf's
Home Healthcare
Handbook

Care &
Prevention
of Skin
Problems

Rain Sounds

BY ANNE KEITH

Yesterday we dug chrysanthemums.
Dug down in silent dust
That sifted from the roots.
We had grown used
To the smell of dryness—
Almost forgotten
The sound of rain.

But tonight there is music,
The music of rain sounds,
Not only drops
Ticking on glass,
But a murmuring beyond.
I find myself
Hoping
It may continue,
It may swell and flow
Till earth softens,
Till roots grow wet
And stretch
Deep into the rich, sweet,
        autumn darkness.

Skin Care

Skin care is one of the most important tasks you will be performing for your patient. Good skin care increases comfort and well being and prevents bed sores. There are many products and protocols that can be used to prevent skin breakdown. The nurse or doctor will tell you how to move the patient, give massages and prevent chafed skin.

There are a number of products such as sheepskins, powders, antiseptic creams and moisturizers that will prevent chafing, sweating and infection, but the most important thing you can do is keep the patient dry. If you are using a plastic mattress cover, make sure there is a sheet of cloth between the cover and the patient to prevent sweating. After a bath, dry the patient *thoroughly* and dust the body with powder (do not put powder on wet skin.). If the skin does become chafed (irritated from rubbing), exposure to air is the one of best ways for the skin to heal.

Bed Sores

Bed sores (pressure sores/decubitus ulcers) are caused by pressure on the skin that squeezes the blood vessels and cuts off the supply of oxygen and blood to the skin. When the skin is deprived of oxygen and blood for too long, the skin (tissue) dies. Bed sores range in severity from mild (minor skin reddening) to severe (deep holes down to the muscle and bone). Over two billion dollars are spent annually in the United States for the treatment of bed sores. The cost of treating each patient with serious bed sores can exceed $20,000. Skin reddening that disappears after pressure is removed is normal and is *not* a bed sore.

Symptoms:

- Cracked, blistered, scaly, broken skin.
- Red areas on skin that do not go away after pressure is removed.
- Open sore.
- Yellowish-colored stains on clothing, chair or sheets.
- Pain at "pressure points" (back or head, back of shoulders, elbows, buttocks, heels).

Most bed sores form where bone causes the greatest pressure on skin and tissue — usually on the lower back below the waist, the hip bone and on the heels. For those patients in chairs or wheelchairs, where bed sores form is dependent on the patient's sitting position. It is possible to get a bed sore in as little as 1-2 hours. Most companies that rent or sell wheelchairs will also sell cushions that help prevent bed sores and most insurance companies, including Medicare, will reimburse the patient for the cost of the cushion.

Inspect the patient's skin once a day. Pay special attention to any red areas that remain after the patient has been moved. A good-sized hand mirror

(8-10 inches) is helpful for looking at hard to see areas. Pay special attention to these places:

- Back of head.
- Shoulder blades.
- Spine.
- Elbows.
- Lower back.
- Hip bone.
- Knees.
- Ankles.
- Heels.

Other procedures you should follow to prevent bed sores:

- Clean skin as soon as possible if soiled from loss of bladder control or bowels. Use a soft cloth or sponge. Do not rub hard to remove waste. There are products you can spray on that will reduce the waste to an easily removed semi-liquid consistency and will eliminate or reduce odors.
- Have the patient take a bath or a shower when needed for comfort and cleanliness. If this is not possible, see the section on Bathing.
- When giving the patient a bath or shower, use warm (not hot) water and a mild soap to reduce skin dryness.
- Use creams or oils after each shower or bath to moisten and help protect the skin.
- Avoid cold or dry air.
- Maintain room temperature at a comfortable level to reduce sweating.
- Pads or underwear that absorb urine and have a quick drying surface that keeps moisture away from the skin should be used. A cream or an ointment to protect the skin from urine or bowel movements should also be used.
- Avoid massaging skin over bony areas or on reddened areas.
- Change position of the patient at least every two hours. Reduce rubbing by lifting (not dragging) the patient when changing position. There are several types of equipment that will allow you to move the patient without a great deal of effort. See page 48 for some of the lifting equipment available from LeBoeuf's.
- If the patient is in a chair or a wheelchair, change their position every hour or less. For those patients able to shift themselves, have them shift their weight every 15 to 30 minutes.
- A thin film of corn starch can be used on the skin to help reduce damage from friction. You can also sprinkle corn starch on the sheets.
- For those confined to bed, use a special mattress that contains air, foam, gel or water.

- Use pillows or wedges to keep knees or ankles from touching each other.
- Place a pillow between the knees and the ankles to keep heels off the bed. Be careful not to put the pillow behind the knees; you may cut off circulation to the lower legs.
- Have the patient eat a balanced diet with foods high in protein (e.g., fish, cheese, tuna, milk, peanut butter). If not possible, find out about nutritional supplements from the doctor.
- Patient's bed should be raised as little as possible. If the bed is raised over 30 degrees, the patient's skin may slide over the bed surface, damaging the skin and blood vessels
- Have the patient participate in a rehabilitation program.
- Clean pressure sores daily. A whirlpool bath is the preferred method.

Be sure to ask questions if you are uncertain about what needs to be done. The doctor or nurse will instruct you what to do. You can prevent most bed sores — the extra effort you make will mean that the patient is more comfortable and will have better health.

If a bed sore does develop, it is important to care for the sore as soon as possible to prevent infection and to promote healing. *Contact the doctor or nurse immediately and let them provide the treatment protocol necessary to cure the pressure sore.*

Bed sores are grouped into four stages.

Stage I	Skin is red but unbroken.
Stage II	Partial skin loss similar to an abrasion, blister or shallow crater.
Stage III	Full thickness skin loss resembling a deep crater.
Stage IV	Full thickness skin loss with extensive destruction.

The doctor or nurse will provide instructions about how to care for the bed sores. The following procedure is usually followed for bed sores in Stages I and II:

- Relieve pressure and prevent further friction and shearing.
- Prevent build-up of surface moisture by using moisture barrier creams.
- Cleanse and lightly lubricate skin.
- Apply protective ointment to surrounding skin.
- If needed, apply a protective dressing.
- Be alert to infection (as drainage levels increase, odor may be present).
- Have the patient exercise as much as possible. If not able to walk, move arms and legs up and down and back and forth.

If the pressure sores are in stage III and IV, it is very important that the doctor or nurse closely monitor the treatment to prevent infection and to treat the sore to insure new skin growth.

Skin Care Products

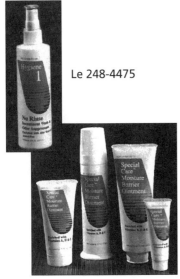

Le 248-4475

Le 271-3824

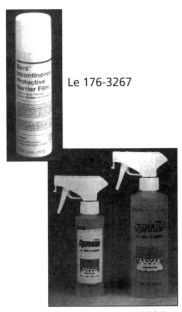

Le 176-3267

Le 145-6896,
Le 117-0174

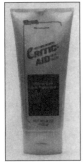

Le 120-0005

Bard Hygiene 1, No Rinse Wash. Rapidly deodorizes, moisturizes and cleanses skin of emesis, urine and feces. Can be diluted 50/50 for minor incontinent episodes. Alcohol-free formula enriched with aloe vera gel.

Le 271-4061	4-ounce spray bottle	$2.95
Le 248-4475	8-ounce spray bottle	$4.95
Le 112-3108	Foam 4-ounce squeeze bottle	$6.95
Le 112-1110	Foam 8-ounce squeeze bottle	$9.95

Bard Special Care, Moisture Barrier Ointment. Protects denuded skin from irritants associated with incontinence. Moisturizes and is enriched with vitamins A, D, and E. Encourages healing of skin. Lanolin free and non-greasy. Provides quick relief.

Le 248-6074	1.75-ounce tube	$6.95
Le 271-3824	2.7-ounce pump	$6.95

Bard Incontinence Protective Barrier Film. Waterproof, yet breathable. Promotes rapid healing. Inhibits growth of staphylococcus aureus and escherichia coli.

Le 176-3267	5.5-ounce spray can	$11.95

3M No Sting Incontinence Barrier Film. Completely alcohol free. Forms a barrier to protect against the damaging effects of moisture, urine or feces. One application works for 24 hours. Sterile, unit-dose, foam applicator.

Le 210-7704	Box of 50	$50.95

IGI Apply and Dry Shaving Gel. Ultrasponge leaves standup coating on hair shafts. Hydrogel allows for smooth, close shave.

Le 121-7488	4-ounce bottle	$5.95

Sween Sproam™ All-Body Cleanser. A spray and a foam in one nonaerosol container. An all-inclusive body cleaner for incontinence cleanup and bedside or routine shampooing and bathing. Nonrinsing, moisturizing. Mild formula free of dyes and perfumes. Antiseptic and deodorizing.

Le 145-6896	6-ounce bottle	$7.95
Le 117-0174	12-ounce bottle	$10.95

Sween Peri-Wash, II. Medicated, antiseptic cleaner/odor control for incontinence management. Moisturizing, no-rinse formula.

Le 143-1717	8 ounces	$5.95

Sween Critic-Aid, Skin Care Pack. Cleanses inflamed, denuded perineal or peristomal skin. No-rinse, nonstinging formulation. Paste adheres to, protects and conditions skin damaged by caustic diarrhea. Contains one Peri-Wash II (8 oz.) and one Critic-Aid (6 oz.)

Le 120-0005	$18.95

Smith & Nephew United Uni-Wash Skin Cleanser. Soapless cleanser for daily cleansing and deodorizing of irritated skin.

Le 127-7367	8.1-ounce bottle	$9.95

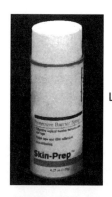

Le 146-8495

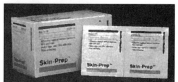

Le 146-8701

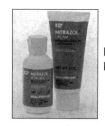

Le 198-8187
Le 198-7551

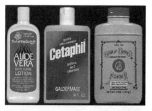

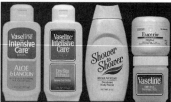

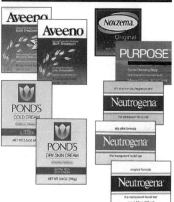

Smith & Nephew United Skin-Prep™ Protective Dressing. Helps protect skin from adhesive trauma. Also for use with TENS electrodes, adhesive tapes and dressings, and elastic products.

Le 146-8701	Wipes	Box of 50	$9.95
Le 146-8495	Aerosol can, 4.25 ounces		$18.95
Le 277-6649	Brush-on liquid with applicator brush	2 ounces	$13.95

Healthpoint, Mitrazol™ Cream and Powder. Greaseless and fragrance free. Helps treat superficial skin infections caused by yeast. Soothes itches, burning and irritation due to fungal infections such as athlete's foot, ringworm and jock itch. 2% miconazole nitrate.

Le 198-7551	2-ounce tube	$5.95
Le 198-8187	Powder in 1-ounce bottle (non-caking)	$9.95

Care-Tech Velvet Fresh. A (non-caking) nursing lubricant powder formulated of premium grade, super-soft cornstarch. Creates a fine, protective barrier against friction and moisture to eliminate irritation. Eliminates skin tears.

Ca C204	4-ounce bottle	$2.95
Ca C204	10-ounce bottle	$4.95

Popular Skin Care Products

Le 122-3718	Aveeno Bath Trt Itchy 8pk	12 oz	$7.95
Le 122-3759	Aveeno Bath Trt Dry 8pk	6 oz	$7.95
Le 148-3494	Cetaphil Skin Cleanser	16 oz	$13.35
Le 161-6846	Corn Huskers Lotion	7 oz	$3.95
Le 172-1141	Eucerin Creme	4 oz	$9.35
Le 185-9891	Eucerin Moist Lotion	8 oz	$9.35
Le 174-8771	Fruit of Earth Aloe Lotion	12 oz	$3.25
Le 127-6773	Gold Bond Med Bdy Pwd	4 oz	$4.85
Le 168-3515	Lubriderm Lot Uns Pump	16 oz	$11.85
Le 137-4446	Neutrogena Soap Orig	3.5 oz	$3.25
Le 214-5449	Neutrogena Soap Dry Unsc	3.5 oz	$3.25
Le 167-3151	Neutrogena Soap Oily	3.5 oz	$3.25
Le 125-1370	Neutrogena Hand Cream	2 oz	$5.65
Le 137-8231	Noxzema Skin Cream Original	10 oz	$4.65
Le 1684133	Oil of Olay Bty Fld Org	4 oz	$10.65
Le 120-2217	Ponds Cold Cream	3.5 oz	$5.25
Le 120-2357	Ponds Dry Skin Cream	3.9 oz	$5.25
Le 166-0034	Purpose Gentle Clns Soap	3.6 oz	$2.95
Le 130-1373	Shower To Shower Original	8 oz	$3.85
Le 182-6494	Vaseline IC Lot Dry Tube	2.5 oz	$2.65
Le 241-1817	Vaseline IC Lot Dry	6 oz	$3.45
Le 241-1791	Vaseline IC Lot Dry	10 oz	$4.85
Le 275-3010	Vaseline IC Lot Dry	15 oz	$6.95
Le 131-2305	Vaseline IC Lot X-Strength	6 oz	$3.45
Le 162-5516	Vaseline IC Lot Aloe/Lan	6 oz	$3.45

Wound Management Products

SPECIAL CARE MUST BE TAKEN when caring for an injury to the patient's body that has caused the skin and other tissue to become cut (*surgery, accident*), torn (*shearing, friction*), or infected (*pressure sores*). This injured area is called a wound.

There are three major types of wound drainage (exudate):

- A watery, clear drainage called *serous*. This consists of the clear liquid part of blood.
- A sticky fluid consistency called *purulent*. Its color can be blue, white, green. This consists of white blood corpuscles (leukocytes), liquefied dead tissue, and dead and/or living bacteria.
- A dark or bright red liquid called *sanguineous*. This consists of red blood cells.

Most of the wound problems you will be facing are from either surgery or from bed sores (pressure sores or sometimes called decubitus ulcers). The doctor and/or nurse will explain how to take care of the wounds and it is important that you follow their instructions carefully. Ask to be shown how to change dressings (bandages), clean the wound, inspect for infections (what to look for) and how to maintain a sterile environment for both yourself and the patient.

In 1988, Marion Laboratories, Inc. developed a color code for wounds that gives some guidance on the severity of the wound:

- Red — Protect the wound
- Yellow — Clean the wound
- Black — Remove the infected and dead (necrotic) tissue

If your patient develops any type of wound, call the doctor or nurse. Wounds not treated properly can lead to very serious consequences such as gangrene. Indications of a possible infection are redness, swelling, pain, hardening of the tissue and fever. Signs that the patient is hemorrhaging (heavy bleeding) are an increased pulse rate, increased breathing rate, lower blood pressure, thirst and cold, clammy skin.

Normally, a wound caused by surgery will be inflamed for one to three days. During the next seven to 10 days, the skin will start to heal and inflammation will subside (if the inflammation increases, this is a sign of infection, and the doctor should be called at once). Scar formation starts in about four days and will continue for six months or longer. The patient will experience severe to moderate pain for three to five days after surgery. Make sure that prior to the patient having surgery, you and the patient work with the doctor and the medical team to develop a pain control plan.

Bed sores (pressure sores) are a very serious problem. You and the patient should do everything possible to prevent them. If you even suspect that the patient is getting a bed sore, call the doctor or nurse. The doctor and/or nurse will tell you what product or treatment will be needed to stop the development of bed sores.

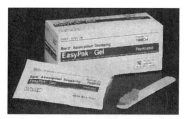

Le 140-1033

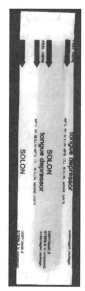

So FBL00-369

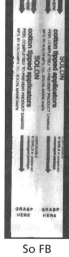

So FB
100-367 1WC

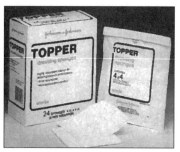

Le 139-6316

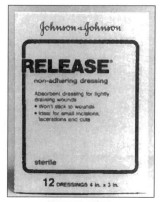

Le 245-6382

To treat a bed sore (pressure sore) the doctor and/or nurse must either perform the following or train you to perform or use the following:

- Clean the sore daily, preferably in a whirlpool bath.
- Dress (bandage) the sore.
- Develop a schedule for positioning the patient so the cause of the bed sore is relieved or not made worse.
- Reduce friction in the bed by using cornstarch.
- Provide a special mattress that keeps the pressure off the bed sore.

Wound Care Products

Bard Absorption Dressing EasyPak™ Gel. Ready-to-use, pre-mixed packet. Saves nursing time. Superior absorption means fewer dressing changes. Provides a cool, moist environment to promote healing. Non-adherent gel molds to the wound to provide complete coverage of exposed tissue. Continually absorbs odor generated by the wound.

Le 140-1033	Carton of 10	$39.95

Solon Medical Individually Wrapped Tongue Depressors. Sterile. Can be also used for application of dressings. 6 inches.

So FBL00-369	Packed 100 to the package	$5.95

Solon Medical Individually Wrapped Cotton Tip Applicator. Sterile. 6-inch wood with cotton tip.

So FBI00-367 1WC	Packed 100 to the box	$6.95

Johnson & Johnson MIRASORB™ Gauze Sponges. Made of nonwoven cotton/polyester MIRATEC™ fabric. For wound cleansing and applying medication. Greater absorbency than 100% cotton gauze.

Le 139-6704	4 × 4 inch 2-ply, 2 per envelope	50 per box	$8.95

Johnson & Johnson ADAPTIC, Non-Adhering Dressing. Coated mesh dressing allows free flow of fluids to overlying absorbent dressing. Will not stick to wound.

Le 139-6993	3″ × 3″	12 per box	$11.95

Johnson & Johnson TOPPER, Dressing Sponges. Specifically designed for dressing wounds and incisions. Highly absorbent for a drier wound site. For moderately to heavily draining wounds.

Le 139-6316	4″ × 4″, 2 per envelope	24 per box	$4.95

Johnson & Johnson RELEASE, Non-Adhering Dressing. Non-adhering absorbent dressing for very lightly draining wounds. Easy to remove. May be used with or without additional dressings.

Le 245-6382	4″ × 4 ″	12 per box	$3.95

Johnson & Johnson SOF-WICK, Dressing Sponges. Superior absorbent dressing for heavily draining wound sites. Fast wicking.

Le 139-6571	4″ × 4″, 2 per envelope	24 per box	$8.95

Johnson & Johnson SOF-WICK, Drain Sponges. Superior absorbent sponge pre-cut to fit around drains, catheters and I.V.s. Makes dressing changes faster and more convenient.

Le 139-6449	4″ × 4″, 6-ply, 2 per envelope	24 per box	$11.95

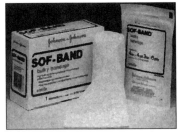

Le 220-7207

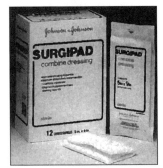

Li 757810

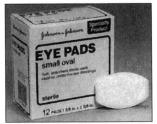

Le 128-7218

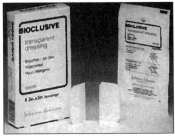

Le 220-7207

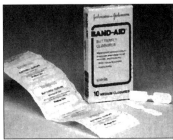

Le 139-5946

Johnson & Johnson SOF-BAND, Bulky Bandage. Excellent stretch for difficult-to-bandage areas. Excellent absorbency for wrapping heavily draining wounds.

| Le 220-7207 | 4" × 84", 6-ply | 1 per box | $3.95 |

Johnson & Johnson SURGIPAD, Combine Dressing. For use as a highly absorbent secondary dressing over primary dressings. Provides maximum absorbency and cushions the wound site.

| Le 139-6852 | 5" × 9" | 12 per box | $6.95 |

Johnson & Johnson Eye Pads, Small Oval. Protective eye dressings made with non-fraying fabric. Highly absorbent cotton with sealed edges. Rapidly absorbs drainage.

| Le 128-7218 | 1⁵/₈" × 2⁵/₈" | 12 per box | $4.95 |

Johnson & Johnson BIOCLUSIVE, Transparent Dressing. Thin film dressing applies directly over a non-draining wound. Adheres to dry skin but not the moist wound area. Keeps germs out. Helps prevent skin breakdown.

| Le 177-3969 | 2" × 3" | 8 per box | $7.95 |
| Le 128-9834 | 4" × 5" | 4 per box | $12.95 |

Johnson & Johnson BAND-AID Brand, Butterfly Closures. Waterproof closures that hold small wounds and incisions together. They will not stick to the wound.

| Le 139-5946 | 1³/₄" × ³/₈" (medium) | 10 per box | $1.95 |

Johnson & Johnson Industrial First Aid Kit. General use first aid kit for the home and auto. First aid booklet included.

| Le 275-4752 | Steel container | | $60.95 |

Johnson & Johnson DERMICEL Hypo-allergenic Cloth Tape. Holds dressings securely in place for maximum wound protection. Hypo-allergenic to reduce chance of skin irritation. Tears easily without shredding.

| Le 116-7349 | 1" wide × 10 yards | | $3.95 |
| Le 116-7501 | 2" wide × 10 yards | | $6.95 |

Johnson & Johnson DERMICLEAR, Transparent Tape. Ideal for securing catheters, tubing and I.V.s. Clear to allow wound inspection.

| Le 129-8520 | 1" × 5 yards | | $2.95 |
| Le 129-9668 | 2" × 5 yards | | $4.95 |

Johnson & Johnson STERI-PAD, Gauze Pads. Individually wrapped cotton pads. Ideal for almost any setting. 12-ply cotton gauze.

Le 130-2710	2" × 2"	100 per box	$13.95
Le 130-2728	3" × 3"	100 per box	$16.95
Le 130-2736	4" × 4"	100 per box	$28.95

Johnson & Johnson Nu-Gel, Wound Dressing. Occlusive hydrogel dressing. Helps cool and soothe. Absorbs light-to-moderate wound exudate. Bacterial barrier.

| Le 247-3437 | 3³/₄" × 3³/₄" | 5 per box | $27.95 |
| Le 247-3635 | 6" × 8" | 5 per box | $57.95 |

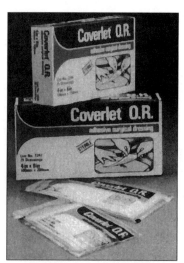

Le 364-5173, Le 364-5231

Beiersdorf Medical Coverlet O.R. Dressings. All-in-one dressing provides sterility, high absorbency, a non-adhering pad and hypoallergenic tape. Designed for patient comfort and user convenience. Ready-to-use single units packed in peel packages.

| Le 364-5173 | 4″ × 4″ | 25 per box | $25.95 |
| Le 364-5231 | 4″ × 6″ | 25 per box | $37.95 |

Carrington Cara-Klenz™. Gentle wound and skin cleaner for preparing wounds for application of wound dressing. Assists in softening scabs and dead tissue. Contains moisturizers. Helps break down blood clots.

| Le 176-1949 | 16-ounce spray bottle | $20.95 |

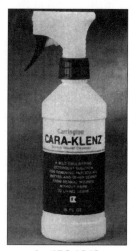

Le 176-1949

Humidifiers & Vaporizers

To help maintain good health and comfort, the patient's skin and respiratory system depend on the proper level of moisture in the air (humidity). When the humidity is too low, the patient's body cannot easily rid itself of infections. Also, the patient's skin can dry and crack, which can lead to problems with bed sores and other infections.

There are several options for increasing the humidity in the home:

- **Vaporizer** — Moisturizes the air with a warm steam. Normally used to assist in the treatment of coughs and colds. They can be used to dispense medicated vapor.
- **Humidifier** — Creates moisture in the air in the form of a cool mist. Because the humidifier does not have to heat the water, it can begin to work at once.
- **Evaporative humidifier** — Using the latest technology to create a vapor so clean that it is invisible. The moisture released is free of bacteria due to a special built-in filtering system that eliminates dust and odors.

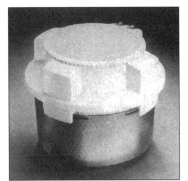

Mc 184-1782

SunMark 502 Evaporative Humidifier. Operates up to 28 hours per filling. On/off switch; high/low output switch. Collapsible circular wick for most efficient operation. Bacteria-free moist air — no rain-out, no white dust. Snap-off directional air flow grill. Water level indicator. Circular design for easy cleaning.

| Mc 184-1782 | 2.5 gallon capacity | $55.95 |
| Mc 278-5384 | Wicking filter replacement | $4.95 |

SunMark 901 Cool Mist Humidifier. Operates 18 to 20 hours per filling. Removable tube and disk. Dust-trap charcoal filter. On/off switch. Directional spout.

| Mc 185-2144 | 2 gallon capacity | $29.95 |
| Mc 278-1086 | Charcoal filter replacement | $2.95 |

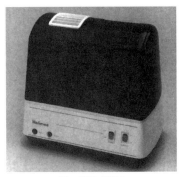

Mc 174-1271

Holmes Cool Mist Humidifier. Operates 24 hours per filling. Water purification filters out impurities. Efficient propeller for low cost operation. Two speeds; mist control. Will humidify an area up to 850 sq. feet.

| Mc 174-0513 | 2.3 gallon capacity | $69.95 |

Holmes High Output Humidifier. Operates 16 hours on one filling. Auto safety shut-off; refill light. Distributes warm medication. No white dust. Two speeds with mist control. Portable with carrying handle. Dupont Silverstone coating for easy cleaning.

| Mc 174-1271 | 2.2 gallon capacity | $69.95 |

SunMark Warm Steam Vaporizer. Operates 8 to 10 hours per filling. Safe-to-touch design with automatic shut off. Medicine cap.

| Mc 185-2433 | 1.2 gallon capacity | $12.95 |

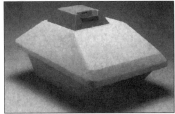

Mc 185-2433

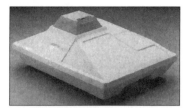

Mc 184-1576

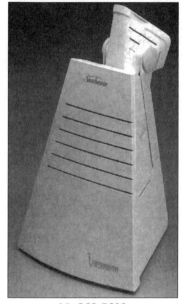

Mc 368-5609

SunMark Warm Steam Vaporizer. Operates 18 to 20 hours per filling. Safe-to-touch design with automatic shutoff. Medicine cap.

Mc 184-1576   3 gallon capacity $18.95

Sunbeam Virotherm. Provides moist air heated to 109°F for 30 minutes to help relieve symptoms and nasal congestion of colds, sinusitis and allergies. Uses plain tap water — no drugs or chemical additives. Moist air is available in four minutes. Produces approximately 10 gallons of air per minute.

Mc 368-5609   Simple to use $75.95

SunMark Vaporizer Tablets. Shortens vaporizer start-up time. Cleans vaporizer heating element as it steams.

Mc 278-1029   24 tablets per package $1.95

SunMark Vaporizer Inhalant. Enhances effects of a vaporizer to help relieve symptoms of colds, coughs and chest congestion. Soothing eucalyptus scent.

Mc 278-0856   6 oz bottle $3.95

LeBoeuf's
Home Healthcare
Handbook

Personal Care

The Forester

BY ANNE KEITH

The squirrel digs.
Small shoulder muscles
Dance beneath gray fur.
He plants the nut—
Then careful, paw by paw,
He covers it,
Thinking perhaps
It will taste good next year.
But, little does he know,
Forgetfulness upon his part
May help a forest grow.

Bathing

BATHING IS RELAXING and makes the patient feel better by improving morale and appearance. Bathing also removes dead skin cells, oils and eliminates unpleasant odors and bacteria. Bathing is the best time to inspect the patient's skin for signs of bed sores or other changes in skin condition. Any changes should be reported to the doctor or nurse. They will assist you in developing a skin care plan.

Patients should be encouraged to bathe themselves, if at all possible, in order to maintain personal dignity and independence. However, you must protect the patient's health and safety at all times. If the patient will not or cannot perform the task, the caregiver must provide the appropriate care. The bath should be a pleasant and relaxing experience.

It is not set in stone that the patient should have a bath every day. For many patients, two or three times a week may be best. It all depends on the condition of the patient. Try not to rush bathing and make sure that you have everything ready before you start. Make sure the bath water is warm and, if it cools, change it. If giving a bed bath, always make sure that the patient cannot roll off the bed. Raise the bed rails, even if you will be leaving the patient unattended for only a few seconds. If you leave the patient in the tub or shower alone, make sure that there is some way of calling for help.

Do not let the patient become chilled. Have plenty of towels on hand and cover the patient. Don't worry about getting too many towels wet. A few wet towels to insure that the patient is comfortable is well worth an extra load of towels in the laundry. Nothing is more uncomfortable to the patient than becoming chilled.

Safety in the bathroom is very important. Loose rugs, electrical outlets without GFI protection (ground fault interrupter), scalding water, no hand rails and not having non-skid protection in the bath or shower can all lead to serious injury and even death. Towel racks are not a substitute for hand rails. A little time spent doing a safety check in the bathroom can save you and the patient a lot of grief.

Bed Bath Protocol

Assemble Equipment and Supplies:
- Wash basin (a plastic dish pan would be fine).
- Mild soap .
- Shampoo.
- Skin lotion, powder, deodorant.
- Soft towels (two or three smaller towels are better then a big bath towel).
- Bed pan or urinal.
- Gloves (if performing perineal care or working with an HIV positive patient).
- Clean linen.
- Clean gown or pajamas.
- Water temperature gauge.

Wash your hands, remove bed linen (top sheet and blankets) and assist the patient to a flat position and as close to you as possible. Suggest that the patient use the bedpan or toilet before starting. The bed should have a flannel-lined waterproof cover over the mattress. It is not a good idea to use an unlined plastic sheet as it will feel cold to the patient.

- Raise the bed to a height comfortable for you to work, remove patient's clothes and cover patient with a sheet.

- Fill wash basin with 1/2 gallon water and adjust water temperature to between 105 and 115 degrees for adults or between 100 degrees and 105 degrees for children. Add mild soap. Use a water temperature gauge. If you don't have a gauge, use your elbow to test the water temperature. Because your hand is probably used to hot water, it is not a good temperature indicator. If the patient has dry skin, a capful of baby oil in the water will help.

- Place a towel across the patient's chest. Make a mitt with the wash cloth and wash patient's face, starting with the eyes. A bath mitt can be made by laying the hand palm up on a wash cloth. Wrap the wash cloth around the hand and then double the wash cloth toward your wrist and tuck it under the cloth on the palm side. The thumb of the hand will be on the outside and will help hold the mitt on the hand.

- Place a towel under the patient's arm, supporting the elbow. Wash the entire arm, then place the hand in basin and wash. Repeat with the other arm and hand.

- Fold sheet down to patient's stomach (just below the rib cage). Wash ears, neck and chest. Cover chest with towel, fold sheet to above pubic areas and wash stomach. Recover the patient with the sheet and remove the towel.

- Change the bath water. Expose the patient's leg and wash. Place the foot in basin if possible and wash. Inspect toes. Repeat with the other leg.

- Change the bath water. Assist the patient to their side, placing the towel near the back. Wash the neck and back, remove towel and assist the patient to lie flat.

- If the patient has soiled and the feces has partially dried, you will need to use a product that will emulsify (liquefy) the fecal soil and make clean-up much easier. These products usually come in a spray type container to make application easy. Spray directly on the soiled area. Many of the products will control odors at the same time. Keep spraying the area as you clean and use a damp cloth. Make sure that you dry the area thoroughly.

- Wash the perineal area or encourage the patient to do so if possible. Carefully dry the patient. Apply skin cream and protective ointment liberally to appropriate areas.

- Assist the patient to dress, tidy area, change bed linen, wash hands. Report any skin changes to doctor or nurse. Again, encourage the patient to dress on their own if possible.

There are products available that allow you to give the patient a bath in bed without the need for patient lifts or heavy lifting. The EZ-Bathe inflatable tub is made of heavy-duty vinyl and comes with a 25-foot shower hose, hand-held shower with push button control, 25-foot drain hose, inflatable pillow, and a wet-and-dry vacuum. The vinyl tub itself is 80-inches long, 32-inches wide and 10-inches deep to prevent splashing and spilling. The wet-and-dry vacuum allows you to completely drain the tub. The drain hose has an on-off switch to allow for constant draining or full bathing and soaking. Inflation only takes 30 seconds. See the Bath & Toilet Aids section.

Inflatable Bed Bath Tub Protocol

- Assemble equipment and supplies as above, except for the wash basin.
- Move the patient to one edge of the bed, being sure that the bed rail is up to prevent the patient from falling out of bed.
- Place the inflatable vinyl bath on the bed.
- Position the patient in the center of the inflatable bath.
- Inflate the bath.
- Fill the tub with water that is between 110 and 115 degrees. The hand-held shower can be connected to a sink. Run the water until temperature is right and *then* fill the bath. Otherwise, you may get a lot of cold or very hot water.
- Patient can soak for awhile or you can begin the bath. If possible, the patient should bathe on own.
- After the bath, rinse the patient well.
- Drain the tub and deflate.
- Dry the patient well.
- Move the patient off the bath making sure that the guard rail is up.
- Change bed linens and dress the patient in clean gown or pajamas.

Bath & Toilet Aids

WARM SHOWERS OR BATHS are a good way to relax the patient. A whirlpool bath also helps in relaxation by its massaging action. Whirlpool baths are especially good for relieving pain associated with stiff or aching joints and hemorrhoids. Multiple baths or showers are more beneficial than a single long bath or shower. Four showers or baths a day will help relax the patient and minimize stiffness.

A comfortable water temperature for the patient is 105°F to 110°F. Always check the water with a bath thermometer. Fill the tub from 1/3 to 1/2 full. The perineal area should be covered. Cover all intravenous catheters or wound dressings with plastic coverings. If your patient needs help getting in and out of the tub, be sure that you take your time and don't rush. Instruct the patient to hold onto the rails when getting in and out of the tub. Allow adults three to five minutes for private bathing but make sure that there is a way for the patient to signal for help. Drain the water before the patient gets out to lessen the risk of slipping and falling. Be sure that the patient does not get a chill by placing a bath towel over the body as soon as the bath is completed. Be sure that the patient is dry before dressing.

The patient or you should check the skin each time the patient bathes. Look for:

- Cracked, blistered, scaly, broken skin.
- Red areas on skin that do not go away after pressure is removed.
- Open sores.
- Yellowish-colored stains on clothing, chair or sheets.
- Pain at "pressure points" (back or head, back of shoulders, elbows, buttocks, heels).

If there appears to be a bed sore, contact the doctor or nurse right away. Bed sores can be a very serious problem and should not be ignored.

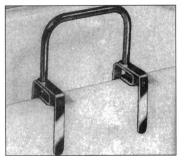

Le 141-2592

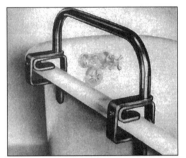

Le 221-1977

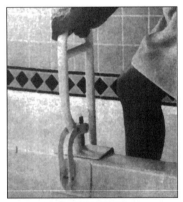

Le 351-7281

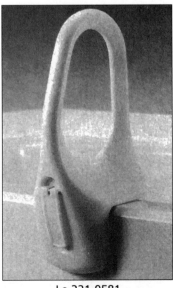

Le 321-9581

Selecting Bath and Toileting Aids

Bathtub rails provide security and convenience when the patient is getting in or out of the tub. The rails help eliminate stooping and are a great way to improve safety.

SunMark Bathtub Security Rails. Chrome plated flexible steel construction, 1″ diameter or soft-touch vinyl gripping area. Preassembled, ready for installation. Mounting wrench included. Rubber lined clamps adjust from 3¾ inches to 6 inches to fit most tubs, including molded plastic types.

Le 141-2592	8.5″ high and 11″ wide	Chrome	$33.95
Le 162-4303	7″ high and 18″ wide	Chrome	$41.95
Le 345-7488	15″ high and 7″ wide	Vinyl	$46.95
Le 162-4360	18″ high and 12″ wide	Chrome	$45.95

SunMark Bathtub Rail For the older style cast iron tub with a curved lip.

| Le 221-1977 | 7″ high and 18″ wide | Chrome | $44.95 |

Futuro Hi-Lo Bathtub Safety Rail. Dual heights for use when standing or sitting. Corrosion proof anodized aluminum. Fits most standard bathtub sizes. Large plastic locking knobs with pivoting clamp.

| Le 351-7281 | 16.5″ and 6″ height, 17.75″ wide | Aluminum | $106.95 |

Lumex Tub-Guard Safety Rail. Ergonomic handle designed with textured surface for comfortable, secure grip. Attaches easily without tools. Ideal for travel. Rubber pads prevent slippage and will not scratch tub. Rustproof molded plastic. Weights only 2½ pounds. Cam-action mechanism holds securely to all bathtubs. Fits tubs 2½ inches to 6½ inches wide.

| Le 321-9581 | White | | $58.95 |

Grab Bars

Grab bars must be strong enough to withstand the stress that will be placed on them. They must be long enough and wide enough to grab easily.

Grab bars must be attached to a stud. The more grab bars the better. Remember, grab bars are not towel bars. Remove towels or laundry (nylon stockings, etc.) prior to using the tub or shower — it will do your patient no good to grab for the bar to prevent a fall and come away with a handful of towel.

To insure that you have installed the grab bars into a stud, you will need to use a stud finder. Assemble the grab bar unit and have someone help you place it on the wall while you use the level to be sure the grab bar is straight and the mounting brackets are over the studs. Mark wall with a pencil through the holes in the mounting hardware.

If in doubt of your ability to install the grab bars, ask for help. Most everyone knows of a neighbor who is handy and has the right tools. It is always better to measure twice and drill once. You will also need a variable speed electric drill, screwdriver (Phillips and/or straight tip), oil, ruler, level, safety goggles and a pencil for marking where to drill. To drill through tile you will need to purchase a special masonry drill bit. Take the screws that come with the grab bar to your hardware store or lumber yard to be sure you will be buying the right size drill bit. Put a drop of oil on the tile and drill at a slow speed — keep oiling as you go.

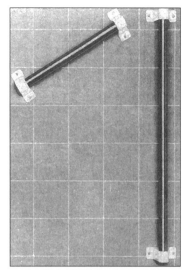

Le 220-5771, Le 220-5839

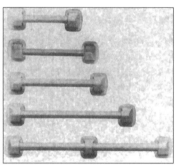

Le 247-7842, . . .,Le 165-6966

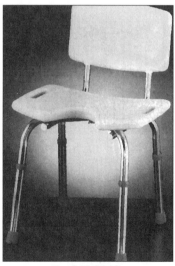

Le 141-2949

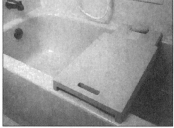

Le 216-5728

SunMark Grab Bars. Chrome plated steel tubing 1¼″ O.D. Mounting brackets of high impact white plastic. Easily assembled with mounting hardware and instructions included. 250 pound capacity.

| Le 220-5771 | 16″ straight bar | Chrome | $20.95 |
| Le 220-5839 | 32″ straight bar | Chrome | $24.95 |

SunMark 90 Degree Angle Grab Bar. Mounts as left or right hand corner. Can mount around inside or outside corners. Units can be used in combination to provide "safety surround" combination. 250 pound capacity.

| Le 220-5789 | 25″ × 20″ | Chrome | $36.95 |

Lumex Tub-Guard Safety Rails. Rounded square shape ergonomically designed for safer grip. VersaGuard coating is warm to the touch. Mounting hardware included. Rustproof and easy to clean. 250 pound capacity.

Le 247-7842	12″ long	White	$39.95
Le 247-8006	16″ long	White	$40.95
Le 247-8105	18″ long	White	$41.95
Le 247-8212	24″ long	White	$45.95
Le 165-6966	32″ long	White	$48.95

Safety 1st Sof'Spout™ Bathtub Spout Cover. Used to cover tub faucet to prevent injury to patient in the event of a fall. Inflatable.

| Sa 103 | | | $3.95 |

Safety 1st Bath Pal Safety Thermometer. Monitors the temperature of the bath water. Easy to read temperature display.

| Sa 162 | | | $3.95 |

Resources Conservation Scald Safe Tub Hot Water Sensor. Automatically shuts off hot water before scalding occurs. Restart water flow with the touch of a finger. Easy to install. Shuts off water at 114 degrees. Solid brass.

| Ho 920-073 | | | $34.95 |

Resources Conservation Scald Safe Shower Hot Water Sensor. Automatically shuts off hot water before scalding occurs. Restart water flow with a touch of a finger. Easy to install. Shuts off water at 114 degrees. Solid brass.

| Ho 555-054 | | | $16.95 |

Bath Seats & Boards, Shower Seats & Stools

SunMark Hygienic Adjustable Bath Bench with Back. Designed for improved hygiene with cut-away open front seat. Blow molded polyethylene plastic with steel inserts in seat for added strength. One inch aluminum legs. Nonslip rubber tips. Height adjusts from 14 inches to 21 inches. Patient can remain seated while cleansing the perineal area. 250 pound capacity

| Le 141-2949 | Seat dimensions, 19″ wide and 13″ deep | $70.95 |
| Le 140-0431 | Bench. Same as above but has no back | $48.95 |

Frohock-Stewart Bath Board. Adjustable seat; double locking device holds board in place. Fits standard tub widths up to 31 inches. Compact and portable. Weights 6.5 pounds. Nonslip, nonskid surface. Sets up in seconds and has a built-in soap dish. 300 pound capacity.

| Le 216-5728 | Seat dimensions 19¾″ long × 11¾″ wide | $90.95 |

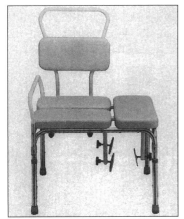

Le 341-6286

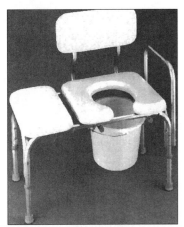

Le 224-2931

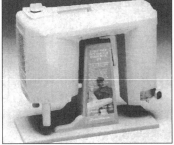

Le 218-7177

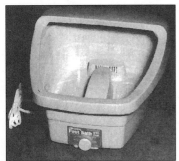

Le 220-1887

SunMark Round Shower Stool. White polyethylene plastic top. Bright, chrome plated steel legs with nonslip rubber feet. Designed for use in the bath or as a vanity stool. Rust-proof. 250 pound capacity.

Le 321-3790	16″ high and 13″ diameter	$32.95

Invacare Shower Seat. Durable plastic seat with drain holes and handles. Nonslip textured finish with contours. Flared legs and rubber tips for stability. Sturdy, lightweight aluminum, frame. Almond color seat back. Adjustable from 14″ to 18″.

Le 113-7496	Seat width 20″	$68.95
Le 113-7314	Same as above, but without back	$50.95

Transfer Seats

Guardian Deluxe Transfer Bench with Tub Clamps. Large 27″ × 17″ seat is constructed of marine plywood base and 2½″ thick foam pad and durable textured vinyl. Unique design of backrest and side rail ensure safe transfer. 250 pound capacity.

Le 341-6286	Patented tub clamps for extra security	$276.95

Guardian Economy Nonpadded Transfer Bench. Height adjustable in ½-inch increments. Splayed legs for added stability. Textured seat and backrest. Side arm for easy transfer. Reversible backrest and side are for use on either side of the bench. 250 pound capacity.

Le 229-5053	Easy to assemble	$104.95
Le 140-4623	Same as above, but padded	$139.95

Carex Vinyl Padded Transfer Bench with Commode Seat Opening and Pail. 1″ aluminum. Comfortable, waterproof vinyl padded seat and back. Interchangeable back brackets for left- or right-hand shower faucet. Seat height adjusts from 17″ to 22″ in ½ inch increments. 300 pound capacity.

Le 224-2931	29″ long × 16″ wide	$185.95
Le 211-8065	Same as above, but without commode opening	$135.95

Whirlpools and Massagers

Dazey Whirlpool Bath. Help speed recovery from fractures and sprains. Alleviate chronic pain and relieve tension and fatigue. 180 degree directional flow control, up to 50 gallons per minute. 60 minute automatic timer. Adjusts to any bathtub securely. UL listed.

Le 218-7177	13″ high × 4⅞″ wide × 17¾″ length	$179.95

SunMark Foot Massager with Heat and Aeration. 284 Vibra-Nodes stimulate tired muscles. Wet heat soothes aching feet, hands, wrists and elbows. Raised foot pads. Top mounted, four-way controls. Carrying handle

Le 220-8924	1½ gallon capacity	$59.95

SunMark Vibrating Foot Bath with Heat. 474 Vibra-Nodes stimulate tired muscles. Heat retaining hood. Full depth tub and four way switch. Use hot or cold, wet or dry.

Le 220-1887	1 gallon capacity	$47.95

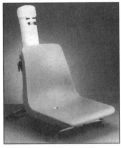

Le 348-9887

Fully one third of all the falls that happen in and around the home occur in the bathroom.

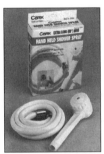

Le 149-5217

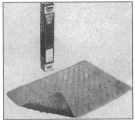

Le 222-0648

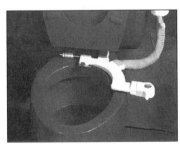

Lu 311

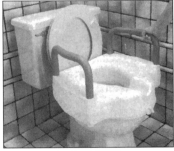

Le 119-2897

Guardian Nolan Tub Lift. 21″ seat height. Sturdy H-frame adheres snugly to tub bottom. Shower or tub spout diverter included. Operates with household water pressure as low as 20 PSI. Lowers any person up to 200 pounds to within 2″ of tub bottom. Arms and headrest can be special ordered.

Le 348-9887   Weighs only 19 pounds $722.95

Shower Units & Bath Mats

Carex Hand Held Shower Spray. Easily attaches to existing shower arm. Fits all ½-inch shower arms. Extra-long 80-inch nylon reinforced hose. On/Off valve on shower spray controls water flow.

Le 149-5217   Comes with wall mounting bracket $24.95

LILA Wooden Bath/Hand Bath or Shower Brush. 16-inch long. Brush detaches and can be held with strap on brush head.

Li 858216   Made of natural bristles $6.95

Carex Diverter Valve. Attaches easily to shower arm. Offers option to use existing shower head spray or hand held shower spray.

Le 168-4687   Convenience is well worth the money $10.95

Carex Safety Bath Mats. For added safety in bath or shower. Helps prevent slipping. Suction cups prevent mat from sliding. 100% cushioned vinyl. Size 28″ × 17½″.

Le 222-0648   Blue $15.95
Le 149-8443   White $15.95

Homecare Sof-Sitz Bath. For treatment of rectal and postpartum discomfort. Allows patient to sit comfortably without compression while applying moist heat and medication. Fits all standard toilet seats.

Le 119-8134   Portable and inflatable $9.95

SunMark Sitz Bath. Fits any toilet. Comfortable contoured extra-sturdy polyethylene supports even the heaviest patient. 200cc bags with "Seat-Tite" filler valve prevents spillage without having to hold or hang bag. 60″. Tube clamps to front of bowl to promote front-to-rear water flow.

Le 130-7719   Glossy, non-porous finish cleans easily $12.95

Lubidet USA, Inc. Makes essential personal cleaning more simple and pleasant than ever before. Mounts right on your toilet to deliver warm-water wash and warm air drying. More effective than a sitz bath and is especially helpful when the patient is incontinent or has hemorrhoids. Easy to operate.

Lu 311   Installs in less than an hour $399.95

Raised Toilet Seats & Guard Rails

Guardian Locking Elevated Toilet Seat with Arms. Wraparound, foam padded armrests. Orthopedically designed for special toileting needs. Easy-to-use locking system requires no tools. Contoured seating surface for comfort. Underside handles for extra stability. 250 pound capacity.

Le 119-2897   Height above toilet 5″ $75.95
Le 118-9943   Same as above, but without arms $66.95

Guardian Easy Care Toilet Safety Frame. Cant-I-Levered arm design for easy transfer. Foam covered arm rests for secure handgrip. Height adjusts from 26″ to 31″.

Le 113-0509   Width adjusts from 18″ to 24″ $48.95

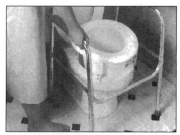
Le 351-7034

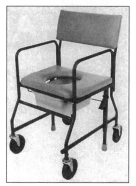
AC 450

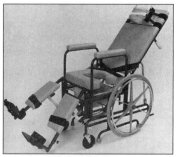
AC 462-20

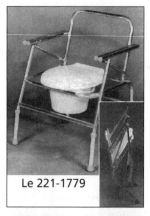
Le 221-1779

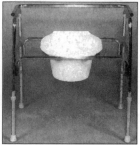
Le 348-0845

Futuro Adjustable Elevated Toilet Seat. Height adjustable from 3″ to 6″ above toilet bowel. Rear bracket acts as anti-tipping mechanism. Full protection splash guard. (Chrome frame shown in picture extra see page 439).

| Le 351-7034 | Fits most standard toilet bowels | $79.95 |

Commodes

Note: All Activeaid products can be customized to meet the needs of the patient. Call LeBoeuf's for information, pricing and free Activeaid catalog. You will work direct with the factory to design a chair that will meet your patient's requirements.

Activeaid Shower Commode Chair. Use as bedside commode, over toilet commode, showerchair, and "get about" chair. Safe, secure steel construction with sturdy plunger brakes (not caster brakes), easy on easy off. Removable arms, padded seat and removable back rest. Comes with pail.

| AC 450 | Seat height 20 inches, Seat width 17½ inches | $456.95 |

Activeaid Shower Commode Chair. Rolling, folding wheelchair shower/commode. 20″ rear wheels with hand rim allow patient to move the chair. Removable arms and cushioned removable back. Comes with pail.

| AC 462-20 | Adjustable, removable swing under footrests | $945.95 |

Activeaid Traum-Aid Shower Commode Wheelchairs. Reclining back 15 degrees from vertical to 25 degrees from horizontal. Elevating leg and foot rests. Leg straps, head positioning wedge and restraint belt for chest or pelvic areas. Plunger foot brakes. Floor to top of seat measures 23″. 24″ mag wheels with safety-sealed bearings. Can be ordered with 5″ caster wheels that swivel for easy maneuvering. Comes with pail.

| AC 494 | Narrow profile for easy accessibility | $1785.95 |

SunMark Drop Arm Commode. Constructed of sturdy chrome plated steel tubing with white plastic seat and lid. Push-button seat height adjustment from 18″ to 22″. Usable as a commode and over-toilet seat. Arms drop below seat height for easy transfer. Plastic armrests adjust from 26″ to 30″. 21¼″ wide × 17″ deep. 250 pound capacity

| Le 220-2885 | 18½″ between arms | $174.95 |

SunMark Folding Commode. Folds easily for transport or storage. 1″ bright aluminum thick-wall aluminum tubing with rubber tips. 6-quart plastic pail with seat and lid. Seat height adjustments from 17¼″ to 21¼″ in 1″ increments. 23″ wide and 25″ deep. 250 pound capacity

| Le 221-1779 | 18⅓″ between arms | $134.95 |

SunMark Extra Wide Commode. Sturdy steel construction with white plastic seat and lid. Push button seat height adjustment from 19″ to 23″. 27″ wide × 21″ deep. 250 pound capacity.

| Le 348-0845 | 24″ width between arms | $128.95 |

Guardian Heavy Duty Commode. Reinforced steel braces front and back. Gray powder coated. Extra wide 24″ seat. Comes with pail. Can serve as toilet seat, toilet safety rail and portable commode.

| Le 139-3792 | Supports 400 pounds | $153.95 |

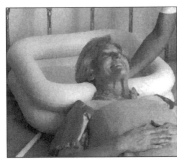
Le 365-3136

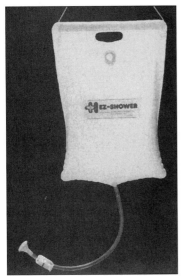
Le 2214617

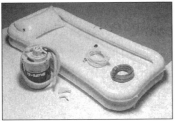
Le 119-8662

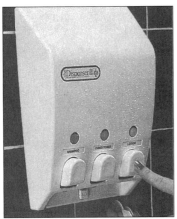
Li 258714

Homecare EZ-Shampoo Hairwashing Basin. Form-fitted basin cushions neck and shoulders. 6″ deep, no-spill basin with attached drain hose. Made from heavy duty vinyl.

Le 365-3136   28″ wide and 24″ long $29.95

Homecare EZ-Shower Shampoo. Hangs on bedpost or I.V. stand. Holds 2½ gallons of water. Flexible 4-foot shower hose for through rinsing.

Le 2214617   Made of mildew-resistant vinyl $16.95

Homecare EZ-Bathe. Sets up in minutes. Inflates in 30 seconds around patient. Can take a patient up to 6′ 2″. Heavy-duty vinyl is formulated to resist bacteria, mold and mildew. Includes 25-foot drain hose and 25-foot shower hose. Portable wet and dry vacuum inflates, deflates and dries tub and pillow. Hand-held shower with push-button operation.

Le 119-8662   80″ × 32″ × 10″ high $359.95

LILA Dispenser™. Perfect way to eliminate all the bottles in the shower and bath. Three 16-ounce chambers can be filled with soap, shampoo and conditioner. Ideal for patients who have arthritis.

Li 258714   Mounts on wall using tape or screws,
                 which are included $31.95

Personal Care Products

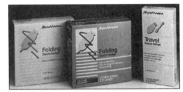

Le 114-2934

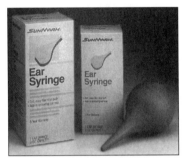

Le 114-3072, Le 241-6626

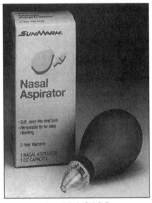

Le 114-3106

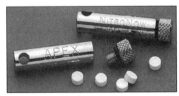

Ap 70020

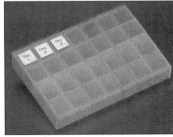

Ap 70014L

SunMark Feminine Folding Douche Syringe.

| Le 114-2959 | 2 quart | **$9.95** |

SunMark Combination Syringe. Textured surface for added strength and style. Water bottle, douche and enema application.

| Le 114-2934 | 2 quart | **$11.95** |

SunMark Ear Syringe.

| Le 114-3072 | 1 ounce | **$3.95** |
| Le 241-6626 | 2 ounce | **$4.95** |

SunMark Nasal Aspirator.

| Le 114-3106 | 1 ounce | **$3.95** |

Medication and Pill Organizers.

According to a recent Mayo Clinic Study, Apex Pill Organizers boosted patient compliance from 22 percent to over 95 percent.

Apex Seven-Day Pill Organizer. Seven compartment weekly organizer. Raised, highlighted letters and Braille markings for the sight impaired. Dishwasher safe on top shelf.

| Ap 70010 | Medium | $4^{1}/2'' \times 1^{1}/4'' \times {3}/4''$ | **$1.95** |
| Ap 70011 | Large | $5^{1}/2'' \times 1^{1}/4'' \times {7}/8''$ | **$2.25** |

Apex Dayplanner. Easy to carry in pocket or purse. Dishwasher safe on top shelf.

| Ap 70016 | $3^{7}/8'' \times {3}/4'' \times {3}/4''$ | **$1.95** |

Apex Cloisonné Pillcase. Stylish pill container.

| Ap 70009 | **$6.95** |

Apex Nitronow Pill Vial. Holds 6 to 7 Nitroglycerin tablets. Allows quick and easy access. Waterproof, heat resistant metal. Comes with 24″ chain.

| Ap 70020 | **$5.95** |

Apex Mediplanner. Allows for dispensing medication 7 days a week, up to 4 times a day (marked morning, noon, bedtime, evening). Translucent bottom and top enables user to see if medication has been taken.

| Ap 70012 | $5^{7}/8'' \times 4^{1}/8'' \times {3}/4''$ | **$6.95** |

Apex Mediplanner II. Each compartment holds up to 27 aspirin tablets. Features extra large, easy access compartments.

| Ap 70013 | $8^{3}/8'' \times 5^{5}/8'' \times 1^{1}/8''$ | **$7.95** |

Apex Fla Top Mediplanner II. Fla Top comes with two sets of labels for individual marking of compartments. Ideal for patients with irregular schedules.

| Ap 70014L | $8^{3}/8'' \times 5^{5}/8'' \times 1^{1}/8''$ | **$7.95** |

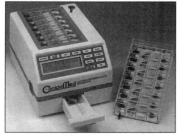
Ap 70015

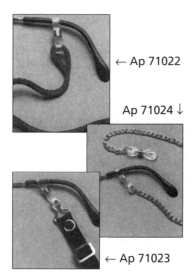
← Ap 71022

Ap 71024 ↓

← Ap 71023

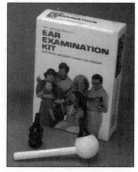
Ap 05002

Apex MediChest. Comprised of 7 Dayplanners in an organizer tray. The Dayplanners can be removed for convenience when traveling or used with the tray to organize a whole week's medication.

Ap 70015	6⁷/₈″ × 4¹/₂″ × ⁷/₈″	$7.95

CompuMed, Automated Medication Dispenser. CompuMed dispenses dry oral medications and displays important instructions for all the patient's medications up to 4 times a day for a week. Two week battery backup, is lockable, tamper-proof, portable and has a one year warranty. Dispenses pills into an easily removed drawer.

Co Auto		$795.95
Co Strobe	Flashing strobe light when time to take pill	$59.95

Apex Eyeglass Fix-It-Kit. Complete home eyeglass repair kit includes a screw driver, 4 hinge screws, a screwstarter, magnifier, temple pads and nose pads.

Ap 71014	$2.95

Apex Economate Contact Lens Cases. Suitable for all types of lenses.

Ap 71016	$1.95

Apex Eyeglass Cords. Keeps eyewear handy and prevents loss. Fits all eyeglasses.

Ap 71022	Fashion Cord	$1.95
Ap 71023	Sports band	$1.95
Ap 71024	Fashion Chain Silver	$1.95
Ap 71025	Fashion Chain Gold	$1.95

Apex Medical Alert Wallet Cards, Necklace or Bracelet.

Ap 73001	Necklace	Diabetic	$5.95
Ap 73005	Necklace	Heart Patient	$5.95
Ap 73012	Necklace	Penicillin Allergy	$5.95
Ap 73017	Necklace, Blank to be engraved		$5.95
Ap 74001	Bracelet	Diabetic	$5.95
Ap 74005	Bracelet	Heart	$5.95
Ap 74012	Bracelet	Penicillin Allergy	$5.95
Ap 74017	Bracelet, Blank to be engraved		$5.95
Ap 76001	Card	Diabetic	$1.95
Ap 76005	Card	Heart	$1.95
Ap 76006	Card	High Blood Pressure	$1.95
Ap 76009	Card	Bee Sting	$1.95
Ap 76010	Card	Hard of Hearing	$1.95
Ap 76011	Card	Tetanus Allergy	$1.95
Ap 76012	Card	Penicillin Allergy	$1.95
Ap 76013	Card	Contacts	$1.95
Ap 76014	Card	Hemophiliac	$1.95
Ap 76015	Card	Alzheimer's	$1.95
Ap 76016	Card	Thyroid	$1.95
Ap 76017	Card Blank (see other side)		$1.95

Apex Ear Examination Kit. Kit includes earlight Otoscope, disposable alkaline battery penlight, 4 viewing tips, 24-page guide book with easy to follow instructions.

Ap 05002	Ear Exam Kit	$29.95
Ap 05005	4 viewing tips	$3.95
Ap 05006	2 penlight replacements	$9.95

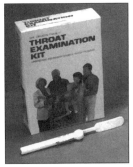

Ap 05007

Ap 00508

Ap 00508

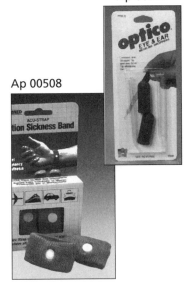

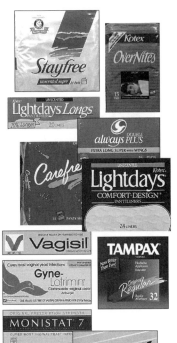

Apex Throat Exam Kit. Kit includes tongue depressor, disposable alkaline battery penlight and easy to follow instructions.

Ap 05007	Throat Exam Kit	$25.95
Ap 05009	Tongue depressor replacements (2)	$8.95

Apex Eye & Ear Medicine Dropper. Glass droppers. Contains one straight tip and one bent tip dropper. Dishwasher safe.

Ap 00508	Kit	$1.95

Apex Acu-Strap Motion Sickness Band. Applies mild pressure to an acupuncture point on both wrists to alleviate the symptoms of motion sickness. Relief of motion sickness without pills!

Ap 01000	Set	$7.95

Feminine Hygiene Products

Le 142-2302	Always + Thin Sup 20 66151	20s	$4.15
Le 123-7106	Always + Xlng Sup W/W	16s	$4.15
Le 142-3268	Always + Maxi Reg 20 66171	20s	$4.15
Le 142-2013	Always + Nght Sup 20 66251	20s	$4.15
Le 124-0043	Always Max Reg N/D 24 66381	12s	$4.15
Le 117-5215	Carefree P/Shld Orig	22s	$1.85
Le 181-0183	Gyne-Lotrimin Vag Crm+App	45 gm	$17.85
Le 271-1026	Kotex Litda Pad Unsc	22s	$1.85
Le 180-6645	Kotex Overnite Pad	14s	$4.15
Le 340-3334	Kotex Litda Long Unsc	18s	$1.65
Le 196-9450	Monistat-7 Crm (Otc)	1.59 oz	$17.65
Le 196-9575	Monistat-7 Supp (Otc)	7 ct	$18.25
Le 117-5330	Monistat-7 W/Appli Disp	1.59 oz	$18.25
Le 121-8734	Playtex Tamp Sup Deod	22s	$6.35
Le 121-8700	Playtex Tamp Reg Deod	22s	$6.35
Le 211-5145	Stayfree Max Sup	24s	$4.15
Le 146-7125	Stayfree Max Reg	24s	$4.15
Le 174-0216	Tampax Tampon Orig Reg	32s	$7.55
Le 270-4260	Tampax Tampon Orig Reg	8s	$2.15
Le 147-9872	Tampax Tampon Slender Reg	8s	$2.15
Le 147-9922	Tampax Tampon Super	8s	$2.15
Le 147-9930	Tampax Tampon Super	32s	$7.55
Le 192-0354	Tampax Tampon Super Plus	8s	$2.15
Le 192-0362	Tampax Tampon Super Plus	32s	$7.55
Le 248-5472	Vagisil Feminine Cream	1 oz	$4.15

Deodorant

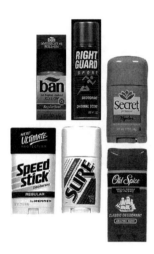

Le 118-3276	Ban A/P R-O Reg	1.5 oz	$3.15
Le 168-8035	Cool/W A/P Clear Gel	3 oz	$3.85
Le 361-9376	Degree A/P Solid Reg	1.75 oz	$2.65
Le 367-9636	Degree A/P Solid Pwd Fr	1.75 oz	$2.65
Le 368-0170	Degree A/P Solid Sport	1.75 oz	$2.65
Le 127-5452	Lady Spd Stk A/P Scen	1.5 oz	$2.35
Le 179-6945	Lady Spd Stk A/P Pwd/F	1.5 oz	$2.35
Le 145-4883	Old Spice Rnd Stick Orig	2.5 oz	$2.55
Le 211-2605	Old Spice Wide Stick Orig	3.25 oz	$3.65
Le 171-7040	Old Spice A/P Sol Orig	2 oz	$2.65
Le 166-6593	Old Spice Wide Stick Frsh	2.25	$2.65
Le 365-7426	Right Guard A/P Stk Spt Frsh	2 oz	$3.35
Le 144-1872	Right Guard Aero Original	5 oz	$3.95
Le 144-1880	Right Guard Aero Original	10 oz	$5.45
Le 197-9491	Secret Wide Solid Reg	1.7 oz	$2.65
Le 197-9293	Secret Wide Solid P/Frsh	1.7 oz	$2.65
Le 197-9418	Secret Wide Solid P/Frsh	2.7 oz	$3.95
Le 179-4791	Secret Wide Solid S/Brez	1.7 oz	$2.65
Le 131-8724	Secret Wide Solid Shwr Frs	1.7 oz	$2.65
Le 197-9574	Secret Wide Solid Unsc	1.7 oz	$2.65
Le 134-6949	Speed Stick Deod Reg	2.25 oz	$2.85
Le 124-9853	Speed Stick A/P Fresh	2.25 oz	$2.95
Le 277-0840	Suave A/P Solid Baby Pwd	1.75 oz	$1.95
Le 197-9830	Sure Wide Solid Unsc	1.7 oz	$2.65
Le 197-9764	Sure Wide Solid Reg	1.7 oz	$2.65

Hair Care

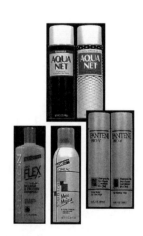

Le 137-8454	Aqua Net Hair Spray Aer Ex Super	7 oz	$1.75
Le 229-9204	Aqua Net Hair Spray Aer Ex Sup Uns	7 oz	$1.75
Le 168-0560	Aqua Net Hair Spray Aer Super	7 oz	$1.75
Le 168-0552	Aqua Net Hair Spray Aer All Purp	7 oz	$1.75
Le 131-4152	Flex Shampoo, Oily	15 oz	$3.35
Le 353-6083	Frizz-Ease Hair Serum	2 x .25oz	$2.15
Le 363-5158	LA Looks Gel Ex Super	16 oz	$2.55
Le 274-9398	L'Oreal Studio Mousse Mega	6.9 oz	$3.95
Le 244-2432	L'Oreal Studio Pmpcrl Hypchg	8 oz	$3.95
Le 133-4374	Neutrogena Shampoo T/Gel	4.4 oz	$6.15
Le 179-1656	Neutrogena Shampoo Xmild	6 oz	$6.65
Le 172-9227	Pantene Pro-V Shm/Cnd Norm	13 oz	$4.65
Le 172-9508	Pantene Pro-V Shm/Cnd Dry	13 oz	$4.65
Le 271-7965	Pert Plus Shmp/Cnd Norm	15 oz	$4.95
Le 365-3649	Rave Hair Spray Aer 3 Ultra Hold Uns	7 oz	$1.75

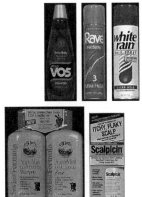

Le 162-4956	Rave Hair Spray N/A 3 Ultra Hold	7 oz	$1.75
Le 189-2991	St. Ives Twin Apple Mnt	2 x 16 oz	$5.35
Le 120-0369	Scalpicin Dandruff Shmp	1.5 oz	$6.55
Le 223-5018	VO5 Shampoo Extra-Body	15 oz	$1.75
Le 113-5698	VO5 Hairdress Regular Tube	1.5 oz	$3.95
Le 113-5979	VO5 Shampoo Normal	15 oz	$1.75
Le 212-2810	VO5 Cnd X-Body W/Collagen	15 oz	$1.75
Le 173-0001	Pantene Pro-V Shm/Cnd Exbdy	13 oz	$4.75
Le 172-9755	Pantene Pro-V Shm/Cnd Perm	13 oz	$4.75
Le 149-7023	White Rain Hair Spray Aer Extra	7 oz	$1.95

Shaving Cream & Razors

Le 129-2614	Atra Plus Blade Disp	5s	$5.55
Le 132-4359	Barbasol Shv/Crm Reg	11 oz	$1.75
Le 166-3962	Bic Shaver Reg	5s	$1.55
Le 273-9233	Bic Shaver S/S	5s	$1.55
Le 121-6068	Colgate Ins/Shv Reg	11 oz	$1.75
Le 163-3452	Edge Shave Gel Sns Skin	7 oz	$3.35
Le 223-3591	Edge Shave Gel Reg	7 oz	$3.35
Le 353-1332	Edge Shave Gel X/Prot	7 oz	$3.35
Le 172-9607	Foamy Shv/Crm Reg	11 oz	$2.35
Le 127-4331	Foamy Shv/Crm Reg	6.25 oz	$1.95
Le 198-0077	Gillette Sensor Razor	1 Ct	$5.95
Le 245-7943	Good News Razor Card	3s	$2.55
Le 216-8300	Good News Razor Card	5s	$3.55
Le 279-1283	Good News Plus Razor	5s	$3.55
Le 114-5549	Good News Plus Razor	10s	$5.95
Le 145-4685	Old Spc A/S Lotion Orig	4.25 oz	$6.95
Le 144-0627	Schick Inj+ Chro 00600	7s	$5.95
Le 344-4924	Schick Tracer Cartridges	5s	$6.55
Le 197-9723	Sensor Cartridge	5s	$6.95
Le 212-0632	Sensor Excel Refill 1544	5s	$7.95
Le 197-9921	Sensor Cartridge	10s	$12.95
Le 130-0862	Sensor Cartridge Wmn	5s	$6.95
Le 212-0459	Sensor Excell Razor 2603	1 ct	$6.85
Le 134-6865	Skin Bracer Reg	3.5 oz	$3.85
Le 116-0464	Trac-II Blades Disp	5s	$5.55

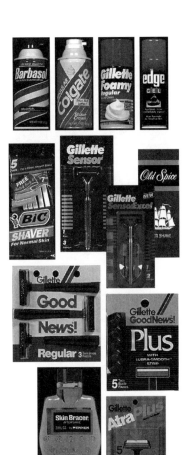

TO ORDER CALL TOLL FREE

LeBoeuf's

PHONE 1-800-546-5559

FAX 1-800-233-9692

Hearing Impaired with TDD
CALL 1-800-855-2880

Protect Your Skin in the Sun

Dermatologists who belong to the American Academy of Dermatology have begun a campaign to inform people of the dangers of cancer of the skin. People who have fair complexions, blond or red hair, blue, grey or green eyes, a history of blistering sunburns and a family history of melanoma have the highest risk of cancer of the skin.

Nearly all skin cancers are curable if caught early. The most common form of skin cancer is basal cell cancer which affects 750,000 Americans yearly.

Fun in the sun safety tips:

- Stay out of the sun between the hours of 10 a.m. and 2 p.m.
- Use a sunscreen with at least a Sun Protection Factor (SPF) of 15.
- Reapply sunscreen as needed. Buy a waterproof brand sunscreen.
- Wear dark colored clothes and a hat with a wide brim.
- Buy a sunscreen that protects against UVA and UVB rays.

Sun Care

Le 354-1059	Ban/B Ultr Sup Sunb SPF-30+	3 oz	$7.95
Le 222-9573	Ban/B Sunscreen Lotion SPF-8	3 oz	$5.55
Le 222-9482	Ban/B Sunblock Lotion SPF-15	3 oz	$6.45
Le 364-7146	Coppertone Sunb Lotion SPF-30+	4 oz	$9.95
Le 140-7089	Coppertone Lotion SPF-4	4 oz	$6.45
Le 224-7443	Coppertone Sport Lotion SPF-15	4 oz	$8.95
Le 123-6041	Coppertone Sunb Lotion SPF-15	4 oz	$6.55
Le 353-8741	Coppertone Sunl Tan Xms	3.75 oz	$9.95
Le 223-9937	Haw Trop Dark Tan Oil	8 oz	$9.45
Le 225-2922	Haw Trop Dark Tan Lotion SPF-4	8 oz	$9.45
Le 354-0101	Haw Trop Sunblk Lotion SPF-45+	4 oz	$9.95
Le 127-3218	Haw Trop Sunblk Lotion SPF-15+	4 oz	$9.45
Le 324-1221	L.A. Tan Greasels Oil Spr	8 oz	$5.45
Le 324-1890	L.A. Tan Out Tan Lotion SPF-15	8 oz	$5.45
Le 323-9837	L.A. Tan Pure Aloe Gel	8 oz	$5.45
Le 128-4645	Neut Sunb Stick	.42oz	$8.45
Le 244-6086	Neut Sunblock SPF-30	2.25 oz	$8.35
Le 128-5261	Neut Sunv Chem Free SPF-17	4 oz	$11.55
Le 144-3530	Neut Sunblock Tube 985	2.25 oz	$8.45
Le 276-1617	Presun Sens Skin SPF-29	4 oz	$7.75
Le 352-3610	Presun Active SPF-30	4 oz	$7.65
Le 199-2577	Shade Sunblock Lotion SPF-45	4 oz	$9.95
Le 145-2762	Solbar PF Ultra Cream SPF-50	4 oz	$10.85

LeBoeuf's
Home Healthcare
Handbook

Diet, Nutrition & Exercise

A Single Leaf

BY ANNE KEITH

The mind balks—refuses—
It cannot be aware of every leaf,
New silk of green on every tree.
One leaf must be enough,
One leaf to study
In its new perfection.
One single leaf speaks all
That this one mind
Can hold of wonder and creation.

Nutrition

The Surgeon General's Report on Nutrition and Health in 1988 documented the growing weight of evidence that diet plays a major role in five of the ten leading causes of death in the United States. These five are heart disease, some types of cancer, stroke, diabetes, and the narrowing of the arterial wall (atherosclerosis).

Nutrients are the organic and inorganic chemicals found in foods which nourish the body. Organic substances are those derived from living organisms. Inorganic substances are not derived from living organisms. Many elements present in food are essential for good health. Calcium, phosphorus and potassium occur in the body with concentration greater than 0.005 percent. Other elements, normally called trace elements, such as iron, zinc and iodine occur in much smaller concentrations. Some elements such as barium and strontium are suspected by the scientific community to be essential, but definite proof is lacking. Elements found in the body such as gold and silver have no known metabolic role.

Metabolism is the chemical reaction that makes it possible for the body cells to live. The energy in food maintains the basal metabolic rate of the body and provides energy for walking, swimming, running, etc. The basic metabolic rate (BMR) is the rate at which the body metabolizes food to maintain the energy requirements of a person who is awake and at rest.

Metabolic rates decrease with age and older people require fewer calories than when they were young adults. This is the reason older people gain weight more easily. However, the nutrient requirements remain unchanged. An older person's requirement for nutrients is not much different from that of a younger adult, but some older people do not eat enough food to supply the necessary nutrients.

Poor Diet

A poor diet can result in a lack of energy, malnutrition and bad health. Older people who live alone (especially men) are at risk of not eating because they have problems buying and preparing food. Other signals indicating that the patient may be at risk of poor nutrition are:

- Fad diets.
- Not eating for 10 or more days.
- No or inadequate food storage.
- No money to buy food.

Signs of poor nutrition and of not eating:

- Weakness or trembling.
- Excessive sweating.
- Loss of weight (weight loss and loss of appetite combined with abdominal pain could be a sign of cancer).
- Cheeks become sunken.
- Appearance has changed.
- Bouts of diarrhea.

- Dry, dull hair.
- Scaly, rough skin.
- Dry and reddened eyes.
- Swollen and red patchy tongue.
- Poor muscle tone.
- No energy.

Good Nutrition

A nutritious diet provides vitamins, minerals, carbohydrates, fat and calories from protein. The diet should include a variety of foods. Use the following guide to help you remember what foods and how much your patient needs to eat every day. Try and have at least the lowest number of suggested servings. The lowest number of servings, with modest amounts of fats and sweets, will provide your patient with about 1,600 calories. This is just about right for older women.

Suggested number of servings for older adults (women should have the lower number of servings and men the higher number of servings).

Food Group	Number of servings
Bread group (bread, pasta, cereal, rice)	6 to 9
Vegetable group	3 to 4
Fruit group	2 to 3
Milk group (milk, yogurt, cheese)	2
Meat group (poultry, meat, fish, dry beans, eggs, nuts)	2

One serving is equal to:

Bread, Cereals, Rice and Pasta
- 1 slice of bread
- ½ cup of cooked rice or pasta
- ½ cup of cooked cereal
- 1 ounce of ready-to-eat cereal

Fruits
- 1 piece of fruit or melon wedge
- ¾ cup of juice
- ½ cup of canned fruit
- ¼ cup of dried fruit

Vegetables
- ½ cup of chopped raw or cooked vegetables
- 1 cup of leafy raw vegetables

Milk, Yogurt and Cheese
- 1 cup of milk or yogurt
- 1½ to 2 ounces of cheese

Meat, Poultry, Fish, Dry Beans, Eggs and Nuts
- 2½ to 3 ounces of cooked lean meat, poultry or fish
- 1 egg or 2 tablespoons of peanut butter count as 1 ounce of lean meat

Fats, Oils and Sweets
- Limit butter, cream, margarine, candy, soft drinks, sweet deserts and alcohol

Coming up with a diet that meets the patient's requirements for good nutrition means working with the doctor, registered dietitian and nurse. Planning a schedule in advance with the patient's healthcare team insures that the patient will be receiving the right foods in the right amounts. Normally, if the patient is eating balanced meals, many nutrition problems can be avoided entirely. Be aware that "natural foods," "health foods" and "organic produce" are no better for the patient and no safer to eat than foods found in a regular grocery store and the regular grocery store will usually be much less expensive. Buy iodized salt. When buying snacks buy fruit, vegetable sticks, nuts, yogurt, cheese and crackers, bread and cereal and eat in moderate amounts. These snacks are much better than candy, cake, cookies, potato chips, pretzels, and other items with high sugar and salt content.

Food Supplements

Patients who are not getting the necessary vitamins and minerals in their diet because of digestive problems, chewing difficulty and/or the use of certain drugs can benefit from a dietary supplement. Make sure that you check with the doctor or a registered dietitian (R.D.) first to see if a dietary supplement for the patient is necessary.

The use of megavitamins and high-potency formulas are currently of concern to many scientists. Usually, these supplements contain 10 to 100 times the recommended daily allowances (RDA) of vitamins and minerals. Large doses of some nutrients can act like drugs and may have serious results. Large amounts of vitamin A or D are especially dangerous. Too much vitamin A can cause headaches, nausea, diarrhea, and eventually liver and bone damage. High doses of vitamin D can cause kidney damage and even death.

If the patient requires nutrition support because an adequate amount of food cannot be taken orally, the doctor will institute one of the following:

- Oral supplements with energy and protein-rich foods such as Compleat Regular Formula Liquid, Amin-Aid Instant Drink Powder, Ensure and others. The doctor or nutritionist will recommend what products the patient should use.

- Tube feeding is the feeding of nutrients directly through the gastrointestinal tract. This is the feeding of nutrients directly into the stomach or the middle of the small intestine — usually through a tube inserted through one of the nostrils, down the throat and into the stomach. To be effective, the patient must have a functioning gastrointestinal tract (GI), stomach and intestines.

- Total parenteral nutrition (intravenous (IV) feeding) is the IV administration of all the patient's daily nutrient needs. The nutrients are given directly into the blood stream via a catheter inserted into a large central vein near the heart. For many who have lost small bowel function, this procedure allows them to lead useful lives at home on home parenteral nutrition (HPN).

Some supplements have no value. According to scientists, Vitamin B$_{15}$ or pangamic acid and superoxide dismutase (SOD) have no medical usefulness. In fact SOD, when taken by mouth, breaks down into amino acids which are not reassembled and do not enter body cells.

No food or food product has been proven to cure a disease or reverse the aging process. If a product being promoted sounds too good to be true, it is. You should suspect a product that does not list ingredients, cites only one study or a preliminary study, does not give information on possible side effects, claims to be a secret formula, promises immediate or fast results and is available from only one source.

Feeding the Patient

The traditional three meals a day at set times is not for everyone. Tailor the patient's eating schedule to suit your own needs. It is not necessary to eat a big meal first thing in the morning — several smaller meals may be better. Meals should be enjoyed in a relaxed manner. Music can be very helpful in making the mealtime more enjoyable. Inviting a friend over for lunch or dinner can be fun. If possible eat in a different location, such as the porch or living room, from time to time. If the patient can get out, many communities have centers that provide free or low-cost meals and a chance to be with other people.

Often, the sense of taste and smell get duller with age. As a result, the patient may overload their food with salt and/or lose interest in food. By being creative with herbs, spices and lemon juice, it is possible to perk up the patient's appetite. Adding color and providing a variety of food textures may also increase the patient's appetite.

If the patient is confined to bed, he or she may find it embarrassing and difficult to accept the fact that help is required for eating. Often the patient becomes depressed. It is very important to make meal time a pleasant and unhurried experience for the patient. Attractive presentation of food is also important.

While normal eating utensils should be used whenever possible, special utensils may be needed to help the patient eat and drink. There are many assistive feeding aids available. Utensils with wide handles can be purchased, or a utensil can be modified by wrapping tape around the handle. Handles on forks and spoons can be bent to accommodate a patient who has limited motion. Bands can be attached that prevent utensils from being dropped. Plate guards, suction cups attached to the plate and no-spill mugs are useful when the patient has limited or impaired hand coordination.

If you have to help the patient eat:
- Ask if the patient needs to go to the bathroom.
- Assist in washing the patient's hands.
- If the patient has problems with oral hygiene, brushing their teeth or using a mouthwash can improve the taste of food and improve the appetite.
- Place the patient in a comfortable position.
- Position the bed table and tray so the patient can see the food.
- If the patient cannot sit up, assist him or her so they are lying on their side. It is much easier to swallow on your side than on your back.
- Sit beside the patient. This conveys a more relaxed situation.
- Encourage the patient to eat independently and do not take over the feeding process, unless necessary.

- Butter the bread, pour the coffee or tea and cut the meat if necessary.
- For those who are blind, tell the patient where the food is on the plate as you would tell the time on a clock. i.e. the potatoes are at 4 o'clock.
- Tell the patient which foods are hot.

If the patient is not eating, let the nurse and doctor know so that other measures can be taken.

There are hundreds of cookbooks, books on cancer diets, books on heart diets, books on almost any diet imaginable. LeBoeuf's has listed a number of books on nutrition, food preparation and presentation, cookbooks and special diet books. Many of these books provide daily menus that make it easy for you to serve the right foods in the right amount for needed nutritional values. Many also provide information on food content, such as how much salt, sugar, unsaturated fat, etc.

What to do:

Contact Human Nutrition Information Service — (301) 436-5724. Provides information on using the Dietary Guidelines and preparing foods. Write to them at U.S. Department of Agriculture, 6505 Belcrest Road, Hyattsville, MD 20782.

Contact National Institute on Aging — 1-800-222-2225 or (301) 496-1752. Provides information on health and other issues of interest to older people. Write to them at Public Information Office, Federal Building, Room 6C12, 9000 Rockville Pike, Bethesda, MD 20892.

Vitamins & Minerals

Le 216-9498	Caltrate 600 + Vitamin D	60s	$8.65
Le 143-1857	Centrum Silvr Multivitamin	100s	$13.85
Le 246-0491	Centrum Multivitamin	100s+30s	$14.45
Le 348-0274	Centrum Silver Mulitivit Tb	60s	$9.95
Le 362-9144	Centrum Adv Form Vit Liquid	8 oz	$10.35
Le 183-1379	Citracal 950 Cal Citrate	100s	$9.95
Le 342-2110	Citracal 1500+D Cal Citrate	60s	$9.95
Le 163-1654	Geritol Complete	40s	$5.95
Le 115-0341	Ginsana Gelcap	30s	$16.45
Le 275-2681	N-M Oy Sh Cl 500mgw/D	130s	$9.65
Le 117-9753	N-M C 500mg	100s	$3.85
Le 220-8346	N-M E 400IU	100s	$7.35
Le 136-0312	N-M Odorless Garlic	100s	$13.65
Le 198-6769	Ocuvite Vit Tabs	60s	$9.95
Le 218-4752	One-A-Day Women's Vitamins	60s	$7.65
Le 275-6336	Os-Cal 500 Calcium + D	60s	$10.65
Le 215-2932	Os-Cal 500 Calcium	60s	$10.75
Le 115-1299	Os-Cal 500 Tab	120s	$19.65
Le 341-8951	Slow-Mag Tab 500mg	60s	$12.65
Le 165-3831	Posture D	60s	$11.95
Le 229-4007	Protegra Vit Softgels	50s	$10.95
Le 127-0321	Slow Fe Tablets	30s	$9.95
Le 146-3652	Theragran M Tab	100s+30s	$15.65
Le 146-3595	Theragran Tab	100s+30s	$15.65
Le 186-2424	Z-Bec Vitamins	60s	$9.35

Popular Diet Aids

Le 364-0216	Nestle S/S Rtd Chocolate/Almond	10 Oz	$1.45
Le 173-5174	Sequester Tab	90s	$13.65
Le 192-2483	Slim Fast Shake Chocolate 1611	15 oz	$4.95
Le 179-8214	Slim-Fast Chocolate Malt Can	15 oz	$4.95
Le 227-1773	Slim-Fast Ultra Vanilla Can	15 oz	$9.35
Le 192-2491	Slim-Fast Vanilla Can	15 oz	$4.95
Le 179-8156	Slim-Fast Strawberry Can	15 oz	$4.95
Le 179-8271	Slim-Fast Bars Dutch Chocolate	8s	$5.95
Le 227-8505	Ultra Slim-Fast Choc Royal	15 oz	$9.35
Le 218-4745	Ultra Slim-Fast Liquid Chocolate	11 oz	$1.55
Le 213-3817	Ultra Slim-Fast Liquid Coffee	11 oz	$1.55
Le 213-3627	Ultra Slim-Fast Liquid Strawberry	11 oz	$1.55
Le 131-0762	Ultra Slim-Fast Liquid Vanilla	11 oz	$1.55
Le 180-8807	Ultra Slim-Fast Juice Mix	15 oz	$9.35

Enternal Feeding & Nutritionals

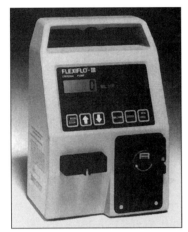

Le 220-8510

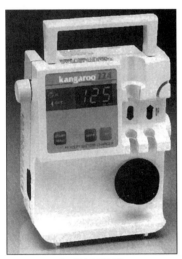

Le 219-7960

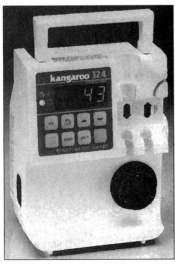

Le 148-2215 / Le 220-8205

THERE ARE a number of companies that provide home infusion therapy. Depending on the needs of the patient and the length of time enternal feeding may be required, renting equipment may be the best way to go. You will need a prescription from the patient's doctor to purchase the products shown on this page. Call **LeBoeuf's** ☎ 1 -800-546-5559 for the names of providers in your area.

Ross Flexiflo-III Enternal Pump. Computer controlled rotary peristaltic pump with electronic touch controls and easy-to-read display numbers. Flow rate variable from 1 to 300 ml per hour in 1 ml increments. Flow rate accuracy to plus or minus 5 percent. Battery life of 8 hours when fully charged. Displays volume fed and selected dose to be fed. Visual and audible alarms for tube occlusion or empty container, open cover, low battery and completed dose. Easy to clean — can be disassembled without tools. Easy to set up. UL approved.

Le 220-8510	Portable, lightweight design		$1,349.95

Ross Flexiflo Top-fill Enternal Nutrition Bag and Pump Set. Includes pre-attached Flexiflo Companion Pump set. Angled rigid neck for easy filling and handling. Lightweight and compact. Accuracy to plus or minus 10 percent. Flow rate 5 to 300 ml per hour in 1 ml increments.

Le 217-7897	100 ml bag	Case of 30	$579.95

Ross Flexiflo Gravity Enternal Feeding Set. Includes preattached gravity feeding set. No assembly necessary.

Le 340-1056	1 liter top-fill bag for easy filling	Case of 24	$355.95

Ross Flexitainer, Enternal Nutrition Container. Rigid neck and lip for ease of handling, with large opening for easy filling and cap for pre-use storage. Built-in hanging ring. Ready to use and disposable. May also be used with Flexiflo gravity gavage sets for gravity feedings. Large measurement graduations. Readily visible sight chamber. Seamless one-piece construction.

Le 118-2054	1 liter volume	Case of 24	$159.95

Sherwood Medical Kangaroo Feeding Pump. Wide flow range from 1 to 50 ml per hour in 1 ml increments; 50 to 300 ml per hour in 5 ml increments. Preset dose delivery capability. Volumetric infusion device with rotary peristaltic pumping mechanism. Exclusive safety feature safeguards against over-infusion. 24-hour battery, recharge time is approximately 15 hours. Built in IV pole clamp. Touch panel for easy cleaning. Audio and visual alarms displayed in message form on LED display. 12 PSI occlusion pressure. Weighs 3½ pounds.

Le 219-7960	Volume totalizer		$1,195.95

Sherwood Medical Kangaroo Pump Set. Includes tubing and container. For use with pumps or gravity feeding. Easy Cap closure with ice pouch. Sterile.

Le 148-2215	1000 ml bag	Case of 36	$519.95
Le 220-8205	1200 ml bag	Case of 36	$579.95

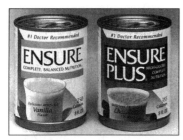

Le 227-2912 / Le 121-7678

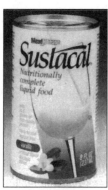

Le 351-8008

Ross Ensure. Provides protein, vitamins, and minerals to maintain good nutrition and proper weight levels. Ensure with fiber helps maintain normal bowel function. Ensure Plus, is concentrated for extra calories; good for those who fill up easily. All come in 8 oz. cans, 6 per pack. Can be used as supplement or primary source of nutrition.

Ross Ensure. 8 oz provides 250 calories and 8.8 g protein

Le 227-2912	Vanilla	$13.95
Le 121-7678	Chocolate	$13.95
Le 166-1347	Strawberry	$13.95
Le 166-1529	Coffee	$13.95
Le 174-8250	Egg Nog	$13.95
Le 120-3439	Black Walnut	$13.95
Le 162-8726	Butter Pecan	$13.95

Ross Ensure Plus. 8 oz provides 365 calories and 13 g protein

Le 180-7460	Vanilla	$14.95
Le 121-7777	Chocolate	$14.95
Le 166-1438	Strawberry	$14.95
Le 166-1636	Coffee	$14.95
Le 174-8268	Egg Nog	$14.95
Le 162-8452	Butter Pecan	$14.95

Ross Ensure with Fiber. 8 oz provides 260 calories and 9.4 g protein

Le 271-1851	Vanilla	$14.95
Le 214-3451	Chocolate	$14.95
Le 162-8221	Butter Pecan	$14.95

Ross Osmolite. 8 oz, 6 per pack

Le 243-1757		$12.95
Le 243-1773	32 oz size	$12.95

Ross Advera. Specialized, complete nutrition for dietary management of HIV infection or AIDS.

Le 149-4087	Chocolate, 8 oz can, 6 pack	$30.95
Le 149-3790	Orange Cream, 8 oz can, 6 pack	$30.95

Mead Johnson Sustacal Liquid. For use with geriatric patients, cancer patients and surgical patients. Persons with increased nutritional needs and those trying to control weight also use Sustacal. Lactose free; fiber free. 36 ounces will provide 100% of U.S. RDA/DV essential vitamins and minerals.

Le 351-8065	Chocolate, 8 oz can, 4 pack	$10.95
Le 351-8008	Vanilla, 8 oz can, 4 pack	$10.95
Le 116-4532	Strawberry, 8 oz can, 4 pack	$10.95

Mead Johnson Sustacal Plus Liquid. Sustacal Plus is intended for use with patients with volume restrictions and fluid restriction. Also good for patients trying to gain weight. Lactose free.

Le 123-2792	Chocolate, 8 oz can,	$2.95
Le 193-8331	Vanilla, 8 oz can,	$2.95

Mead Johnson Sustacal Pudding

Le 246-1697   Chocolate, 5 oz, 4 pack $10.95

Mead Johnson Sustacal Powder

Le 214-3972   Vanilla   16 oz $14.95

Milani Diafoods Thick-It. Instant health care food thickener. Modifies liquids and pureed foods for people with swallowing disorders.

Le 141-9738   8 oz can, regular strength $7.95

Milani Diafoods Thick-It 2. Low in sodium. Concentrated formula for maximum thickening.

Le 134-9620   8 oz can $11.95

Cookbooks

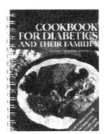

In 108730

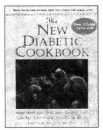

In 601458

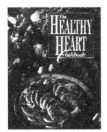

In 506916

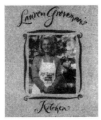

In 195748

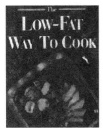

In 601568

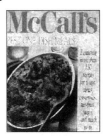

In 511245

If you want a book and we don't have it listed, we can get it for you as long as it's still in print.

All-New Cookbook for Diabetics and Their Families. *Sheila Lukins*
Guidebook for diabetics features over 200 delicious recipes. Included with each recipe is a nutritional analysis approved by registered dietitians. Spiral binding.
In 108730   Paper $14.95

The New Diabetic Cookbook. *Mabel Cavaiani*
More than 200 delicious recipes for a low-fat, low-sugar, low-cholesterol, low-salt, high-fiber diet. Author is a diabetic and a dietitian.
In 601458   Paper $14.95

The Healthy Heart Cookbook. *Sunset Publishing*
Reduce the risk of heart disease and stroke with these tempting, mouthwatering recipes low in fat, cholesterol and sodium. More than 350 kitchen-tested recipes and 16 menus follow guidelines established by the American Heart Association.
In 506916   Hardback $24.95

Lauren Groveman's Kitchen.
Nurturing Food for Family and Friends. *Laura Groveman*
Delicious, simple and comforting meals are possible again with a comprehensive book that reinvents cooking as a relaxing, creative activity. Tips on time management.
In 195748   Hardback $24.95

The Low-Fat Way to Cook. *Oxmoor House*
Cookbook/guide to healthy eating. A collection of recipes, menus, and helpful information designed to make low-fat cooking with everyday foods easier than ever. Over 450 recipes, 30 menus, substitution chart and more.
In 601568   Hardback $29.95

Linda McCartney's Home Cooking. *Linda McCartney*
Vegetarian cookbook stress freshness and nutrition. 200 meatless dishes that are quick, economical and sacrifice nothing in taste.
In 462707   Paper $17.95

McCall's Best One-Dish Meals *McCall's Magazine*
Lavishly illustrated cookbook features 152 recipes that reinvent the one-dish meal. 80 full-color photos. Practical and nutritious meals.
In 511245   Hardback $21.95

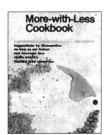

In 568932

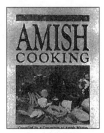

In 192177

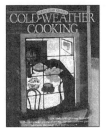

In 266803

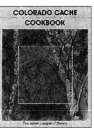

In 396655

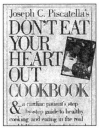

In 053974

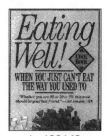

In 132142

More-With-Less Cookbook. *Doris Janzen Longacre*
500 recipes from Mennonite kitchens that tells us how to eat better. All recipes have been tested by home economists.

In 568932   Paper $15.95

**The Southern Living
Complete Do-Ahead Cookbook.** *Southern Living Magazine*
Takes the hassle out of meal planning with timesaving recipes and menus to make ahead and serve later. Over 300 delicious recipes. Includes over 90 color photos.

In 601750   Paper $14.95

Amish Cooking. *Amish Women*
More than 800 old-time recipes and hints from Amish country kitchens. Features simple instructions for making delicious food.

In 192177   Spiral bound $16.95

The California Cookbook. *Betty Evans*
More than 250 easy-to-follow recipes covering meals, snacks, and drinks make up this culinary collection.

In 514910   Hardback $21.95

Cold-Weather Cooking. *Sarah Leah Chase*
Over 300 eclectic, soul-warming intensely flavored recipes.

In 266803   Paper $13.95

Colorado Cache Cookbook. *Junior League of Denver*
Classic cookbook offers a treasure trove of recipes that reflect Colorado's casual style of living and natural bounty. Features 680 delicious triple-tested recipes.

In 396655   Spiral bound $15.95

Cooking for Two Today. *Jean Hewitt and Marjorie Page Blanchard*
More than 200 recipes, including 50 meals that can be made in 30 minutes or less. Emphasis is on healthful, easily prepared foods. Directions are clear and concise.

In 298513   Paper $10.95

Don't Eat Your Heart Out Cookbook. *Joseph C. Piscatella*
Now revised to feature 200 all-new and 200 revised and lower-in-fat recipes. Over 84,000 copies in print.

In 053974   Paper $6.95

Eating Well! *Jane W. Wilson*
Recipes, tips, techniques and philosophy for feasting lightly every day and cutting back on fat, cholesterol, salt, sugar and calories. Two-color illustrations throughout.

In 132142   Paper $12.95

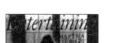

In 058296

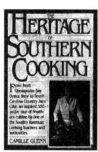

In 169804

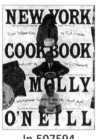

In 507594

Entertaining. *Martha Stewart*
Thousands of inspiring ideas. 300 original recipes. The most sumptuous book on entertaining ever published.

| In 058296 | Hardback | $39.95 |

The Heritage of Southern Cooking. *Camille Glenn*
Lavish collection of 550 delectable recipes including Sea Island Fish Chowder, Loin of Pork and Mushroom Stew. Photos throughout.

| In 169804 | Paper | $15.95 |

New York Cookbook. *Molly O'Neill*
Collected from all five boroughs by *New York Times* food writer Molly O'Neill. Over 400 recipes and 500 photos.

| In 507594 | Paper | $17.95 |

James Beard's American Cookery. *James Beard*
More than 1,500 recipes and advice on dozens of cooking questions. 144 illustrations. Beard's very best.

| In 052047 | Paper | $18.95 |

The Moderation Diet. *Renny Darling*
Simply the best diet book ever. More than 450 easy-to-prepare recipes with low fat, calories, cholesterol, sodium and sugar content. A masterpiece in combining eating for health and eating for pleasure.

| In 258602 | Paper | $14.95 |

Miami Spice. *Steven Raichlen*
Steven Raichlen, an award-winning food editor shares the best recipes from Florida. The book captures the irresistible convergence of Latin, Caribbean and Cuban influences with Florida's cornucopia of ingredients. Two-color.

| In 047950 | Paper | $12.95 |

Mennonite Country-Style Recipes and Kitchen Secrets. *Ester H. Shank*
Prized collection of over 1,100 recipes also includes hundreds of tips for success while baking bread, making pie crusts, etc., as well as microwave and quick-fix sections.

| In 346677 | Paper | $18.95 |

Quick and Healthy Recipes and Ideas. *Brenda J. Poichtera, R.D.*
For people who say they don't have time to cook healthy meals. Contains recipes that are quick to prepare, low-fat and tasty. Offers great time saving ideas, weight loss tips, nutritional analysis and recipes.

| In 277802 | Paper | $16.95 |

Exercise

I T'S NEVER TOO LATE TO EXERCISE. Getting started is the hard part. According to the President's Council on Physical Fitness and Sports, most physical frailty is actually the result of inactivity, disease or poor nutrition. The good news is that many problems can be reversed by exercising. You must encourage the patient to start a program to increase strength, lose fat, gain muscle and feel better emotionally. For exercise to be effective, the patient should understand that it involves some pushing beyond a comfortable limit. Ordinary household chores such as taking out the garbage and doing the wash don't count.

Exercise can have a beneficial impact on three of the most common chronic diseases: arthritis, hypertension and heart disease. Exercise can help control weight, blood pressure and blood sugar. It also helps improve flexibility and range of motion for those with arthritis. Based upon a study from the 1985 Health Interview Study by the National Center for Health Statistics, about 45 percent of older adults reported walking as a form of exercise within the previous two weeks. Only 30 percent claimed to exercise or play sports regularly.

Before starting, any exercise program, the patient should talk with the doctor or physical therapist to determine their current level of fitness and ask what level of exercise would be appropriate.

For safe and enjoyable exercise:

- Exercise with others — try and do this at the same time every day. Play music during the exercise period.
- Drink plenty of water before and after exercising to prevent dehydration.
- Stop exercising if severe pain, dizziness or other unpleasant symptoms such as feeling very hot, low abdominal pain, blue lips or fingers, lack of coordination.
- Sweating and breathing a little harder than normal are not unusual nor necessarily harmful reactions to exercise.

There are many seniors who have formed exercise clubs. Classes in water walking, yoga, dancing, weight training, bowling all are available and will probably appeal to the patient. Remember — the fun and socializing aspect of the classes will do wonders for the patient's physical and mental health. These groups can be found at hospitals, community recreation centers, senior citizen centers or you can start your own group. The important thing is to encourage the patient to get started — sign your patient up for a class.

Start the exercise program slowly. Find a friend for the patient to walk with on a regular basis. Find a route that is interesting and fits the goals for distance; 5 to 10 minutes of walking twice a day is a good start. Work up from there to half-hour walks several times a week. Set reasonable goals or the patient will become discouraged. Lifting weights can also be an effective exercise. It can be as simple as lifting a can of soup or a milk carton filled with sand. Whatever exercise is done, the patient should breathe deeply and evenly and not hold the breath. Encourage your patient to keep a daily record of what has been accomplished.

Swimming is another good exercise. If the patient has access to a pool, a 20 minute swim three times a week is very good exercise.

LeBoeuf's has a number of good books on fitness. There are also a number of good books and pamphlets available at little or no cost from AARP, National Institute on Aging and many other groups such as the Heart Association.

Fitness and Exercise Books

Listed below are a number of books on fitness and exercise. This is a small sample of the books we have available. If you have a special book that you would like to have, please call us and we will find it for you. As with the diet book section, we have numerous pamphlets from various associations on fitness and exercise that are free. Always check with the doctor before starting any fitness or exercise program.

Title	Author	Item	Price
Aerobic Walking	Myers	In 068492Q	$10.00
Arthritis — What Exercises Work	Sobel	In 026231R	$19.95
Complete Waterpower Workout Book	Huey	In 558132Q	$15.95
Complete Yoga Book	Hewitt	In 100673Q	$16.00
David Carradines Tai Chi	Carradin	In 111177Q	$11.95
Exercise for the Elderly	Jamieson	In 143342Q	$6.95
Faithfully Fit	Cloninge	In 339994Q	$10.99
Fitness Walking	Iknoian	In 149766Q	$14.95
Healing Touch of Massage	De Paoli	In 045119Q	$14.95
Healthy Heart Walking Book	American AMA	In 074912Q	$14.95
Pritikin Program of Diet and Exercise	Pritikin	In 207791P	$5.95
Royal Canadian Air Force Exercise Book	Royal Canadian AF	In 091127Q	$5.95
Six Week Fat to Muscle Making	Darden	In 087603Q	$10.95
Step by Step Tai Chi	Chuen	In 561145Q	$14.00
Total Fitness In 30 Minutes	Morehouse	In 268503P	$5.50
Fit For Life	Diamond	In 187028P	$6.99
Food Your Miracle Medicine	Carper	In 491347Q	$14.00
Ultimate Workout Log	Schlosbe	In 032941Q	$11.95
Walk Yourself Thin	Rives	In 291578Q	$12.95
Water Exercise	White	In 150862Q	$14.95
Yoga Made Easy	Kent	In 357885Q	$14.95
90 Day Fitness Walking Program	Fenton	In 486095Q	$10.00

Books, Videos & Tapes

Healing

BY ANNE KEITH

Many words from now,
Words spoken by the rising moon
And the setting sun
And the soundless flight of birds,
Words from hot tears
That sting behind the eyes
But must be held all day,
Words from the Word
That seep through crusts
Like snow melt
Sinking into earth.
These will I hear—
And cling to.

Joy will return.

Healing & Divine Health

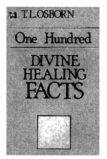

Ha HH-299

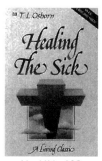

Ha HH- 403

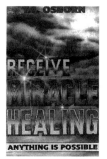

Ha TL-221

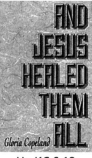

Ha KC-S 18

The following books and tapes are written by some of the best teachers in America. They all promote life and truth as revealed in the Bible. We are proud to provide this section to assist you in choosing inspirational messages from spirit-filled men and women. Learn how to live a peaceful life, renew your confidence, gain strength and practical advice for both the patient and the caregiver.

When things seem to be piling up, call LeBoeuf's for help. We have a network of intercessors who can assist you.

Book sizes are as follows:

- Little Hands   5¼″ × 5″
- Mass Market   (MM)   4½″ × 7″
- Syllabus   (Syll.)   11″ × 8½″
- Leather Bound   (LB)   3½″ × 5⅜″
- Minibook   (MB)   3½″ × 5⅜″
- Trade   (TD)   5⅜″ × 8⅜″
- Hardcover   (HC)   6″ × 9″
- Workbook   (WB)   8½″ × 11″

Minibooks are sold in packs of 10. Prices are subject to change without notice.

100 Divine Healing Facts   T. L. Osborn
Have at your fingertips in a pocket size book the Bible's message on healing.

Ha HH-299	10 Pack (MB)	$9.90

Healing the Sick   T.L. Osborn
With over one million copies in print, this new and enlarged edition has been acclaimed worldwide as a 20th century classic on divine healing. Thousands have been healed just by acting upon the truths in it.

Ha HH- 403	(TD)	$14.99

Receive Miracle Healing   T.L.Osborn
Inside are the basic truths which the Osborns have taught to millions. You will find the seven steps to receive the miracle you need from Christ.

Ha TL-221	(TD)	$8.99

And Jesus Healed Them All   Gloria Copeland
This book examines the overwhelming, scriptural evidence which proves that God's plan is to "heal them all."

Ha KC-S 18	(TD)	$2.50

God Wants You Well   Gloria Copeland
In two cassette tapes, Gloria shares with the listener God's Word for you to be well all the time.

Ha TKC -10	2 Tapes	$10.00

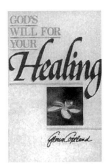

Ha KC-503

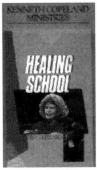

Ha KC-949

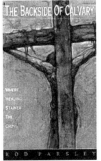

Ha TKC-06

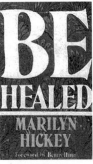

Ha MH-021

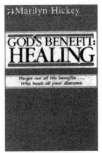

Ha HH-228

God's Will For Healing   Gloria Copeland
Gloria guides you through the Word of God and shows you scriptural answers to questions that may be standing between you and the healing power of God.

| Ha KC-503 | (TD) | $2.99 |

Healing Promises   Kenneth and Gloria Copeland
This hands-on healing manual is presented in a way to give you practical applications of God's healing Word in your life. Includes four translations of each Scripture, including King James Version, The Amplified Bible, The James Moffat Translation and The New English Bible.

Ha KC-949	(TD)	$6.99
Ha PM-007	Compact disc	$12.99
Ha PM-006	Cassette	$9.99

Healing School   Gloria Copeland
Gloria reviews the scripture passages on God's healing promises for your life in six cassette tapes. Join Gloria on a journey through the Word of God to explore the passageways of our Father's heart concerning healing for all of us. Also available in video.

| Ha TKC-06 | Six tape set | $30.00 |
| Ha VKC-203 | Video | $24.99 |

The Backside of Calvary   Rod Parsley
This book provides answers to questions that many have about healing and its availability today.

| Ha HH-897 | (TD) | $5.99 |

Be Healed   Marilyn Hickey
You will learn that the healing miracles of the Bible are readily available to you today!

| Ha MH-021 | (TD) | $8.99 |

Experience Long Life   Marilyn Hickey
In this pocket -size book learn what the Word of God says about living a long and healthy life.

| Ha MH-152 | 10 pack (MB) | $9.90 |

God's Benefit: Healing   Marilyn Hickey
Marilyn explains how God provides healing for us.

| Ha HH-228 | 10 pack (MB) | $9.90 |

Your Total Health Handbook: Spirit, Soul and Body   Marilyn Hickey
The Apostle Paul told us that our bodies were the temple of the Holy Spirit. That is why Marilyn complied this handbook filled with Scriptures and proven advice that will help you put your whole being under the authority of God's Word so you can truly experience "total health."

| Ha MH-024 | (TD) | $9.99 |

Bodily Healing and the Atonement   Kenneth Hagin
The T.J. McCrossan classic re-edited by Kenneth Hagin and Roy H. Hicks, D.D. This in-depth study proves beyond a doubt Christ died for our sickness just as He died for our sins.

| Ha KH-505 | (TD) | $3.99 |

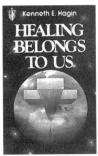

Ha KH-016

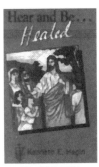

Ha KH-272

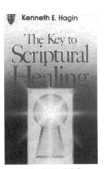

Ha KH-008

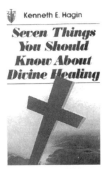

Ha KH-400

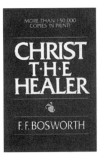

Ha FB-001

Como Retener Sue Sanidad   Kenneth Hagin
Reverend Hagin explains how to keep your healing according to the Word of God.

| Ha KH -159 | 10 pack (MB) | $7.50 |

God's Medicine   Kenneth Hagin
This pocket-size book lists God's prescription for your perfect health. Also available in Spanish.

| Ha KH -053 | 10 pack (MB) | $7.50 |
| Ha KH-153 | 10 pack (MB) Spanish | $7.50 |

Healing Belongs to Us   Kenneth Hagin
This important book shows that our healing is an accomplished fact and how we can possess the promise of healing in our life.

| Ha KH-016 | (TD) | $1.99 |

Healing Scriptures   Kenneth Hagin
Now the popular cassette tape is a book! This book contains Scriptures about healing as well as commentary on God's medicine.

| Ha KH -521 | (TD) | $3.99 |
| Ha TKH-63H03 | Cassette tape | $4.95 |

Hear and Be Healed   Kenneth Hagin
This pocket-size book contains God's Word on healing — perfect for quick reference and to give as gifts.

| Ha KH-272 | 10 pack (MB) | $7.50 |

How to Keep Your Healing   Kenneth Hagin
Learn how to keep your healing in this pocket-size book that is great as an easy reference guide to God's Word.

| Ha KH-059 | 10 pack (MB) | $7.50 |

The Key to Scriptural Healing   Kenneth Hagin
Scriptural truths in this book dispel common errors about healing and opens an important recipe for life and health form the Word of God.

| Ha KH-008 | (TD) | $1.99 |

Laying On of Hands   Kenneth Hagin
Learn what the Word of God says about the laying on of hands in this mini-book.

| Ha KH-250 | 10 pack (MB) | $7.50 |

Seven Things to Know About Divine Healing   Kenneth Hagin
Hagin shares the results of his lifelong study on the Scriptures that answer many common questions about divine healing.

| Ha KH-400 | (TD) | $3.99 |

Christ The Healer   F.F. Bosworth
The truths discussed in this book, together with "the prayer of faith, "have brought healing within the grasp of many thousands of sufferers who could not have recovered without the direct action of the Holy Spirit.

| Ha FB-001 | (TD) | $9.99 |

God's Creative Power for Healing   Charles Capps
This book is filled with God's Word on healing for you through His creative power.

| Ha HH-815 | 10 pack (MB) | $12.50 |

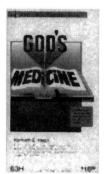

Ha TKH-63H

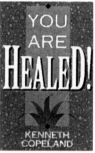

Ha KC-O13

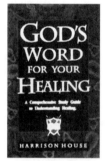

Ha HH-907

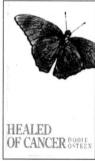

Ha J0-029

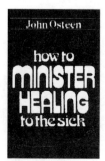

Ha J0-023

God's Medicine   Kenneth Hagin Ministries
In this four-cassette tape package, you'll learn by hearing God's Word for healing in your life.

| Ha TKH-63H | Four tape cassettes | $16.00 |

Redeemed from the Curse   Kenneth Hagin
In this three-cassette package, hear Reverend Hagin teach you about being redeemed from the curse of the law — and that includes being redeemed from sickness.

| Ha TKH-49H | Three tape cassettes | $12.00 |

You Are Healed   Kenneth Copeland
This book gives you God's Word on healing and how to receive it. Available in Spanish: Usted es Sanado.

| Ha KC-O13 | 10 pack (MB) | $7.50 |
| Ha KC-306 | Spanish 10 pack (MB) | $7.50 |

Y Jesus Sanaba a Todos (And Jesus Healed Them All)   Kenneth Copeland
Kenneth presents how Jesus went about healing all those who were afflicted and explains how healing is for you today.

| Ha KC-315 | | $1.99 |

God's Provision for Healing   Jerry Savelle
Jerry provides God's Word plainly on His provision for healing in your life.

| Ha HH-213 | 10 pack (MB) | $9.90 |

God's Provision for Healing Study Manual   A.L. & Joyce Gill
This manual lays a solid foundation that will release faith for effectively receiving or ministering healing.

| Ha ALG-04 | (WB) | $12.99 |

God's Word for Your Healing   Harrison House
This book has been designed to help Christians stand in faith and prepare to receive their healing. Combining a 31-day healing devotional, teaching and healing Scriptures from 10 different translations, this book is a powerful and complete healing handbook.

| Ha HH-907 | (TD) | 7.99 |

Healed of Cancer   Dodie Osteen
Read this powerful miracle healing testimony and your faith will be strengthened! The story of Dodie Osteen's miraculous healing of cancer. Also available in Spanish: Sanada de Cancer.

| Ha J0-029 | (MM) | $4.00 |
| Ha J0-129 | (MM) Spanish | $4.00 |

How to Minister Healing to the Sick   John Osteen
This mini-book gives you a simple way to share God's Word on healing.

| Ha J0-023 | 10 pack (MB) | $7.50 |

The Healing Heart of God   Malcolm Smith
You will learn to know Jesus, and the God who sent Him to us and for us, in a whole new way. You will have your broken heart healed!

| Ha MS-921 | (MM) | $3.99 |

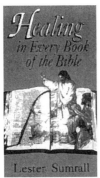

Ha LS-029

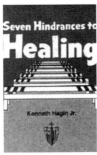

Ha KH-705

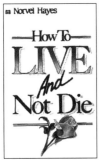

Ha HH-395

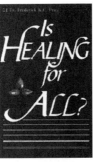

Ha HH-005

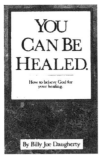

Ha HH-876

Healing in Every Book of the Bible   Lester Sumrall
Dr. Sumrall has chosen a Scripture from every book of the Bible which teaches that God wants man well in his total being — spirit, soul and body.
Ha LS-029   (MM) $2.99

Healing a Forever Settled Subject   Kenneth Hagin, Jr.
This book clearly presents that God's will to heal is forever settled because God's Word is forever settled.
Ha KH-723   (TD) $2.99

Seven Hindrances to Receiving Healing   Kenneth Hagin, Jr.
This mini-book presents clearly what will block you from receiving your healing. Available in Spanish: Siete Impedimentos Para Recibir Sanidad.
Ha KH-705   10 pack (MB) $7.50
Ha KH-175   10 pack (MB) Spanish $7.50

Health and Beauty   Cheryl Prewitt-Salem
The former Miss America 1980, Cheryl, a devout Christian, gives quick and easy steps to overall health and beauty.
Ha CS-479   10 pack (MB) $9.90

How to Live and Not Die   Norvel Hayes
This book explains to Christians how they can live as long as God intended them to if only they will truly live and obey God's Word in all areas of their lives. It is an anointed teaching to encourage and instruct those declared terminally ill and those who have no hope.
Ha HH-395   (TD) $6.99
Ha TNH-Ol   Cassette six tape set $30.00
Ha VNH-OOl   Video 60 minutes $24.99

What to Do for Healing   Norvel Hayes
This mini-book tells you in a simple manner how to receive your healing from God.
Ha HH-216   10 pack (MB) $9.90

Is Healing for All?   Fred Price
Dr. Price addresses the crucial question, "Is healing for all?" by relating his own testimony of healing.
Ha HH-005   (TD) $6.99

Jesus The Healer   E.W. Kenyon
This book has challenged and stirred Christians and has inspired multitudes to step out in faith and receive the healing that Christ purchased for us.
Ha EK-007   (TD) $7.99

There's a Healer in the House   Ed Dufresne
Jesus paid the price for your healing! Learn about the power and deliverance God has already purchased for us through Jesus' victory on the cross.
Ha ED-307   (TD) $5.99

You Can Be Healed   Billy Joe Daugherty
With a strong Scriptural foundation, this book contains necessary information that is needed to be healed.
Ha HH-876   (TD) $6.99

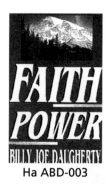

Ha ABD-003

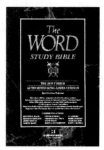

Ha HH-750

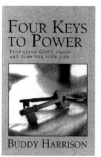

Ha HH-694

Faith Power   Billy Joe Daugherty

The purpose of this book is to help believers grow and mature in their relationship with the Father and the Son through the Holy Spirit.

Ha ABD-003	(TD)	$4.99

The Word Study Bible   Complete King James Version

More than 4,200 key Scriptures identified by special symbols. 31-day Bible study plan and a one-year Bible reading program. More than 20,000 Scripture reference in a Concordance of more than 90 pages.

Ha HH-750	Black Bonded Leather	$49.99
Ha HH-764	Burgundy Bonded Leather	$49.99
Ha HH-749	Paperback	$19.99

Four Keys to Power   Buddy Harrison

Harrison gives readers biblical principles that are essential for allowing God's power to function in every area of our lives. Readers will learn to unlock the dynamic power of God within them by putting into practice these four keys to power.

Ha HH-694	(TD)	$5.99

TO ORDER CALL TOLL FREE

LeBoeuf's

PHONE **1-800-546-5559**

FAX **1-800-233-9692**

Hearing Impaired with TDD
CALL **1-800-855-2880**

Useful Reference Material & Entertainment

LeBoeuf's has a complete collection of books for diet, health, fitness and just plain entertainment. Shown below are some of the books we have available. If you do not see the book you want, call us and we will try to find it for you. Books may not always be available for immediate shipment or may be out of print. LeBoeuf's will attempt to find the book for you, but if the book is not available, we will credit your account. In addition, we have free pamphlets from many associations and government agencies on diet and health. Remember, the patient's doctor, nurse, pharmacist, nutritionist and therapist are all ready to assist you in developing a proper diet. Be sure to ask them.

Diet and Nutrition Books

Beating Cancer with Nutrition	Quillin	In 162549Q	$14.95
Beyond the Food Game	Latimer	In 603167Q	$9.95
Cancer & Nutrition	Simone	In 379348Q	$12.95
Cancer Prevention Diet	Kushi	In 251575Q	$15.95
Chicken Soup & Other Folk	Wilen	In 144122O	$11.00
Cholesterol & Triglyceride	Moyer	In 092552Q	$10.95
Complete Vitamin Book	Lowe	In 477931P	$5.99
Complete Scarsdale Medical Diet	Tarnower	In 082336P	$6.50
Controlling Your Fat Tooth	Piscatel	In 266764Q	$15.95
Dick Gregory's Natural Diet	Gregory	In 097039Q	$6.50
Diet for All Seasons	Haas	In 125590Q	$12.95
Dine Out and Lose Weight	Montigna	In 562550Q	$19.95
Dr. Bruce Lowells Fat Finder	Lowell	In 291768Q	$9.00
Eat Away Illness	Wade	In 508739Q	$9.95
Eating Right to Live	Ketcham	In 150850P	$5.99
Fat to Muscle Diet	Zak	In 232395P	$4.99
Healing Foods	Hausman	In 289685Q	$13.95
Healing Yourself with Food	Prevention	In 356132R	$21.95
Low Blood Sugar Cookbook	Krimmel	In 150786Q	$12.95
Take It Off and Keep It Off	Ulene	In 341009Q	$9.95
Natural Energy Boosters	Wade	In 599408Q	$9.95
Recipes for Diabetics	Little	In 277023Q	$11.00
Zap the Fat	French	In 1333341Q	$14.95
Betty Crocker, Eat and Lose Weight	Crocker	In 098315R	$18.95

Medical Books

The following is a list of books was chosen to address a special problem, disease or interest. If you or your patient have come across other books that you believe may be especially helpful, please let us know and we can add them to the list.

General

AMA Family Medical Guide	Clayman	In 199719R	$37.50
AMA Guide to			
Your Family's Symptoms	AMA	In 460918Q	$15.00
Mayo Clinic Family Health	Mayo Clinic	In 266339R	$40.00
Book of Massage	Lidell	In 048574Q	$14.00
How To Survive Medical Treatment	Fulder	In 310479Q	$13.95
At Home With Terminal Illness	Appleton	In 356810Q	$14.00
Johns Hopkins Medical Handbook	Johns Hopkins	In 461328R	$39.95
Dying At Home	Sankar	In 352555Q	$12.95
Current Medical Diagnosis	Tierney	In 349029Q	$41.95
Healthy at 100	Willix	In 206542Q	$13.95
Freedom From Chronic Pain	Marcus	In 176093R	$20.00
Hands On Healing	Prevention	In 331400Q	$18.95
Prescription Drugs	Consumer	In 338914P	$7.99
Reader's Digest Live Longer	Readers Digest	In 004124R	$35.00
Safe In The Sun	Siegel	In 045059Q	$8.95
Complete Book of Dental Remedies	Parsa	In 471453Q	$10.95

Acupuncture

Acupressure For Health	Young	In 498867Q	$14.00
Acupuncture	Nighting	In 131889Q	$12.95
Acupuncture Without Needles	Cernery	In 008580Q	$8.95

AIDS

AIDS Care at Home	Grief	In 345394Q	$17.95
AIDS & Beyond	Kushi	In 278577Q	$5.95
AIDS and HIV In Perspective	Schoub	In 456900Q	$19.95

Alzheimer's

Alzheimer's Handbook for Caretakers	Driscoll	195870Q	$12.95
Beating Alzheimer's	Warren	In 370774Q	$12.95
Facing Alzheimer's	Coughlan	In 561091P	$4.99
36 Hour Day	Mace & Rabbins	In 543341P	$6.50

Arthritis

Arthritis Helpbook	Lorig	In 292929Q	$14.00
Arthritis Sourcebook	Brewer	In 343531Q	$12.95
Arthritis What Exercises Work	Sobel	In 426976Q	$10.95
Arthritis and Common Sense	Alexander	In 081448	$9.95

Cancer

After Cancer	Harpham	In 061186R	$23.00
Alpha Book on Cancer and Living	Ryder	In 562529R	$24.95
Answer Cancer Answer for Living	Parkhill	In 043697Q	$9.95
Breast Cancer	Baron	In 355658R	$23.00
Cancer Battle Plan	Frahm	In 564860Q	$12.00
Cancer Therapy	Moss	In 551436Q	$19.95
Prostate & Cancer	Marks	In 079389Q	$14.95

Diabetes

A Touch of Diabetes	Jovanovi	In 425572Q	$10.95
Diabetes Sourcebook	Guthrie	In 033875Q	$15.00
Diabetics Book	Bierman	In 137081Q	$12.95
Managing Type II Diabetes	Bergenst	In 191258Q	$9.95

Heart

American Heart Association, Your Heart	AHA	In 328932R	$27.95
Beat Heart Disease Without Surgery	Collins	In 240444Q	$9.00
High Blood Pressure Solutions	Moore	In 527331Q	$12.95
Living Heart Diet	DeBakey	In 142374Q	$13.00

Headache

Headache Book	Minirth	In 171046P	$5.99
Headache Help	Robbins	In 144575Q	$10.95
Managing Your Migraine	Burks	In 235628R	$22.50

Multiple Sclerosis

Multiple Sclerosis	Graham	In 247506Q	$12.95
Living With Multiple Sclerosis	Shuman	In 462696Q	$10.00
Multiple Sclerosis Diet Book	Swank	In 161562R	$29.95

Osteoporosis

Osteoporosis Handbook	Bonnick	In 356683Q	$14.95

Parkinson's

Living With Parkinson's	Carroll	In 573591Q	$11.00
Living Well With Parkinson's	Atwood	In 269863Q	$14.95
Parkinson's Handbook	McGoon	In 369321Q	$10.95

Stroke

After A Stroke	Donnan	In 500419Q	$9.95
Living With Stroke	Senelick	In 343705Q	$9.95
Stroke	Hay	In 092389Q	$10.95

Varicose Veins

Varicose Veins	Baron	In 031423R	$24.95

"How To" Videos

All videos are in color unless stated otherwise. LeBoeuf's has a complete collection of videos. If your favorite is not listed here, call us. If it is still in print, we can get it for you. None of the "How To" videos are rated.

Dixie Carter's Unworkout. Carter brings humor to this gentle routine to deliver a more relaxed, toned and energized body without the strain.

| MCA 81416 | 1992 | 80 Minutes | $19.98 |

Dr. Heimlich's Home First Aid Video. The creator of the "Heimlich Maneuver" uses easy-to-follow procedures on how to handle common household emergencies.

| MCA 80767 | 1987 | 36 Minutes | $19.98 |

Stop Thief! How To Protect Your Home From A Break-in. A former cat burglar and a veteran police officer expose the secrets of professional thieves while arming viewers with practical advice on how to beat the odds of becoming a victim.

| WKP 1192 | 1993 | 60 Minutes | $9.98 |

How to Stop the One You Love From Drinking and Using Drugs. Real solutions for people who face the day-to-day trauma of a loved one's alcohol or drug abuse.

| PAR 12587 | 1988 | 56 Minutes | $24.95 |

How to Have a Moneymaking Garage Sale. Phyllis Diller tells, in a light-hearted manner, how to have fun and make money at the same time. Learn what sells and what doesn't, how to advertise effectively and how to deal with shoplifters.

| JTC 0007 | 1987 | 30 Minutes | $9.95 |

Jody Watley — Dance to Fitness. A program of light aerobic dance.

| PPI 207 | 1990 | 45 Minutes | $19.98 |

Say Goodbye to High Blood Pressure. Learn how to control risk factors of high blood pressure through diet, nutrition, exercise and relaxation.

| WKP 1150 | | 45 Minutes | $19.95 |

TO ORDER CALL TOLL FREE

LeBoeuf's

PHONE **1-800-546-5559**
FAX **1-800-233-9692**

Hearing Impaired with TDD
CALL **1-800-855-2880**

Entertainment Videos

All ratings are shown next to the price. LeBoeuf's carries a full line of action videos. If you don't see what you would like, call us and if the video is still in print, we can get it for you.

20,000 Leagues Under the Sea. A fanatical submarine captain tries to stop warfare at sea by sinking all ships that come within range. Kirk Douglas, Jean Mason and Peter Lorre.

| DIS 15 | 1954 | 126 Minutes | Rated G | $19.99 |

48 Hours. A wise-cracking convict is given a 2-day furlough to help a street-smart detective track down a group of cop killers. Nick Nolte and Eddie Murphy star.

| PAR 1139 | 1982 | 71 Minutes | Rated R | $14.95 |

Airport. The original all-star airplane disaster movie. Burt Lancaster, Jacqueline Bisset, Helen Hayes and Dean Martin.

| MCA 55031 | 1970 | 137 Minutes | Rated G | $14.98 |

Company Business. A former CIA agent is reinstated to return a former Soviet mole to the Soviets, along with $2 million in drug money. Gene Hackman, Mikhail Varyshnikov.

| MGM M902356 | 1991 | 99 Minutes | Rated PG-13 | $14.95 |

Crocodile Dundee. A free-spirited Australian who hunts crocodiles with his bare hands is brought to the sophisticated urban jungles of Manhattan. Paul Hogan, Linda Kozlowski.

| PAR 32029 | 1986 | 98 Minutes | Rated PG-13 | $14.95 |

The Dirty Dozen. Twelve criminals are given a chance to redeem themselves by becoming a "suicide" squad in World War II. Lee Marvin, Ernest Borgnine, Charles Bronson, Donald Sutherland.

| MGM M700008 | 1969 | 149 Minutes | Not Rated | $19.98 |

The Emerald Forest. An American engineer searches for his son, who has been kidnapped by Indians in the Amazon rain forest. Based on a true story. Powers Boothe, Charley Boorman

| COL 2179 | 1985 | 113 Minutes | Rated R | $14.95 |

Romancing the Stone. A novelist ends up living an adventure better than any she's ever written when she goes to Columbia to rescue her sister. Michael Douglas, Kathleen Turner, Danny DeVito.

| FOX 1358 | 1984 | 106 Minutes | Rated PG | $14.98 |

The Jewel of the Nile. Sequel to *"Romancing the Stone."* Joan is kidnapped by an Arab political leader and Jack must come to her rescue.

| FOX 1491 | 1985 | 106 Minutes | Rated PG | $14.98 |

Jurassic Park. A wealthy entrepreneur creates a theme park featuring live dinosaurs, only to have his attraction turn into a nightmare. Sam Neill, Laura Dern. Directed by Steven Spielberg.

| MCA 81409 | 1993 | 127 Minutes | Rated PG-13 | $24.98 |

Patriot Games. Intrepid CIA analyst Jack Ryan is caught up in international intrigue when his family becomes the target of revenge seeking terrorists. Harrison Ford, Anne Archer. Based on a Tom Clancy novel.

| PAR 32530 | 1992 | 120 Minutes | Rated R | $19.95 |

Patton. A turbulent biography of the bold WW II hero who led American forces in Africa and Europe. George C. Scott, Karl Malden, Stephen Young

FOX 1005 | 1970 | 171 Minutes | Rated PG | $29.98

Raiders of the Lost Ark. Indiana Jones goes in search of the Lost Ark of the Covenant which holds the sacred Ten Commandments. Harrison Ford, Karen Allen. Directed by Steven Spielberg.

PAR 1376 | 1981 | 115 Minutes | Rated PG | $19.95

The Greatest Story Ever Told. Von Sydow, as Jesus, leads an all-star cast in this epic depicting the life of Christ. Charlton Heston, Claude Rains, John Wayne. Directed by George Stevens.

MGM M301658 | 1965 | 196 Minutes | Rated G | $29.98

King of Kings. The majestic sweep of the life and times of Jesus Christ fills the screen in this epic film. Jeffery Hunter, Slobhan McKenna, Robert Ryan.

MGM M700326 | 1961 | 164 Minutes | Not rated | $29.98

An American In Paris. A wonderful musical about an American painter's romantic adventures. Gene Kelly, Leslie Caron, Nina Foch, Oscar Levant.

MGM M60006 | 1951 | 113 Minutes | Not rated | $14.95

Annie. The comic strip cutie comes alive in this production as Annie dreams of a life outside the orphanage. Aileen Quinn, Carol Burnett, Albert Finney.

COL 60127 | 1982 | 128 Minutes | Rated PG | $19.95

Carousel. Experience the miraculous powers of love in the inspiring Rodgers and Hammerstein musical masterpiece. Gordon MacRae, Shirley Jones, Cameron Mitchell.

FOX 1713 | 1956 | 128 Minutes | Not rated | $19.98

Seven Brides For Seven Brothers. The oldest of seven brothers living in the mountains decides to get married, inspiring all his brothers to do the same. Howard Keel, Jane Powell, Julie Newmar.

MGM M700091 | 1954 | 103 Minutes | Rated G | $14.95

The Unsinkable Molly Brown. A spunky western girl is determined to break into Denver high society. Debbie Reynolds, Harve Presnell.

MGM M600578 | 1964 | 128 Minutes | Not rated | $19.98

Gunfight At The O.K. Corral. Doc Holiday and Wyatt Earp face off against the Clanton Gang in this landmark western film. Burt Lancaster, Kirk Douglas, Rhonda Fleming.

PAR 6218 | 1957 | 120 Minutes | Not rated | $14.95

The Man From Snowy River. A mountain youth comes of age on the untamed frontier of turn-of-the-century Australia. Kirk Douglas, Jack Thompson.

FOX 8135 | 1983 | 104 Minutes | Rated PG | $14.98

Nevada Smith. A highly-charged story of a young man who teams up with a sharpshooter to hunt down the gang that murdered his parents. Steve McQueen, Karl Malden, Brian Keith and Arthur Kennedy.

PAR 6532 | 1966 | 135 Minutes | Not rated | $14.95

Two Mules for Sister Sara. A tough gunslinger runs into a nun in the Mexican desert. Clint Eastwood, Shirley MacLaine.

MCA 66046 | 1970 | 105 Minutes | Rated PG | $19.98

TO ORDER CALL TOLL FREE

LeBoeuf's

PHONE 1-800-546-5559
FAX 1-800-233-9692

Hearing Impaired with TDD
CALL 1-800-855-2880

Northwest Passage. The true story of Major Robert Rogers who led his rangers on excursions to discover new territory in colonial America. Spencer Tracy, Robert Young, Walter Brennan and Ruth Hussey.

MGM M301132   1940   127 Minutes`   Not rated $19.98

Only Angels Have Wings. A hardened air freight service owner is faced with using an untrustworthy pilot to keep an ailing friend from flying. Cary Grant, Jean Arthur, Rita Hayworth. *Black & White.*

COL 60946   1939   121 Minutes   Not rated $19.95

A Star Is Born. A fading star helps a young singer get her start. Judy Garland, James Mason.

WAR 11335   1954   176 Minutes   Not rated $29.98

Illustrated Note Cards from Wolf Run Studio

Illustrated fold-over note cards feature beautifully detailed reproductions of black & white drawings by Clifton, Virginia artist Bill Harrah. The back of each wildlife card has a description of the animal or bird pictured on the front. Domestic animal note cards do not have descriptions. Each package includes eight cards and eight plain envelopes. Printed on acid-free recycled paper. All cards are blank inside. Other cards are available, including popular dog breeds and historic buildings in and around the Nation's capital. For a list of other note cards by the same artist, call 1-800-546-5559.

Wo 11718   Eight illustrated note cards w/ envelopes $6.00

Artist Bill Harrah works at his home in Clifton, Virginia. Inspiration for many of his drawings comes from the abundance of beautiful birds and small animals seen outside the windows of his spacious studio. Sometimes deer even venture out of the nearby woods to nibble on the azaleas or succulent grasses. His backyard pond is home to several pairs of Canada geese in summer and a stopover for small flocks during spring and fall migrations.

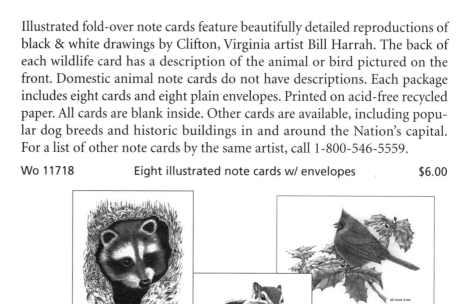

Raccoon

Eastern Chipmunk

Northern Cardinal

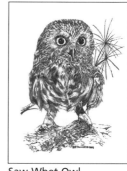

Saw-Whet Owl

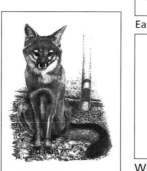

Gray Fox

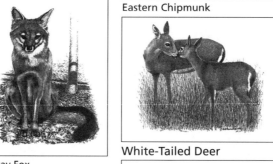

White-Tailed Deer

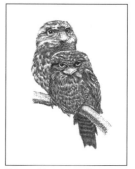

Tawny Frogmouths

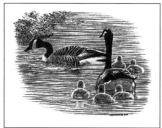

Canada Geese

Dorcas Gazelle

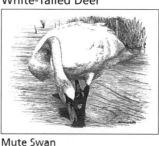

Mute Swan

Folded cards measure 5½ inches wide and 4¼ inches high. Blank area inside an opened card measures 8½ inches high.

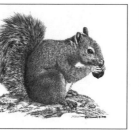

Gray Squirrel

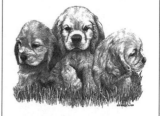

Cocker Puppies

LeBoeuf's
Home Healthcare
Handbook

Emergency Care

First Aid

The Universal Choke Sign

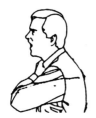

The Heimlich Maneuver:

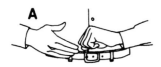

A. Correct placement of fist with thumb side against victim's stomach, slightly above the navel and below the ribs and breastbone.

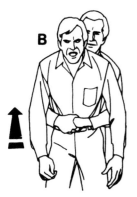

B. If victim is standing or sitting, stand behind victim with your arms around his or her waist. Place your fist as shown in the illustration. Hold your fist with your other hand and give four quick, forceful upward thrusts.

Illustrations courtesy, American Medical Association Handbook of First Aid and Emergency Care, Revised Edition, Random House, 1990

CHOKING

Heimlich Maneuver

When a person is choking, the Heimlich maneuver (abdominal thrust) appears to be the most effective way to clear a person's windpipe. If the Heimlich maneuver is not successful, hit the patient forcefully and repeatedly between the shoulder blades with the palm of the hand.

Symptoms:

- Patient begins gasping or breathing noisily
- Patient grabs his or her throat
- Patient is unable to talk
- Patient has difficulty in breathing and begins coughing; breathing may stop
- Patient's skin becomes pale, white, gray or blue
- Patient looks or acts panicked
- Patient becomes unconscious

Universal choking sign is the patient grabbing his or her throat.

What to do:

If the patient is conscious:

- If the patient can talk, cough or breath, do not interfere in any way with his or her efforts to cough out a swallowed or partially swallowed object.
- If the victim cannot breathe, stand behind them and place your fist with the thumb side against their stomach—slightly above the navel and below the ribs and breastbone. Hold your fist with your other hand and give four quick, forceful upward thrusts. Doing so increases pressure in the abdomen, which pushes up the diaphragm. This increases the air pressure in the lungs and will often force the object out from the windpipe.
- Do not squeeze on the patient's ribs with your arms. Just use your fist in their abdomen. It may necessary to repeat the Heimlich maneuver 6 to 10 times.
- If the patient is lying down, turn them on their back. Straddle the patient and put the heel of your hand on their stomach, slightly above the navel and below the ribs. Put your free hand on top of your other hand to provide additional force. Keep your elbows straight. Give four quick, forceful downward and forward thrusts toward the head of the patient in an attempt to dislodge the object. The forceful downward thrusts increase the pressure in the abdomen, forcing pressure into the lungs to expel the object out of the windpipe and into the

The Heimlich Maneuver on a Victim Lying Down:

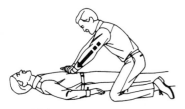

Straddle the victim and put the heel of your hand on the victim's stomach, slightly above the navel and below the ribs. Put your free hand on top of your other hand. Keep your elbows straight. Give four quick, forceful downward and forward thrusts toward the head.

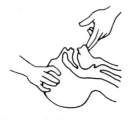

Opening the Patient's Airway

mouth. It may be necessary to repeat the Heimlich maneuver 6 to 10 times.

- If you cannot get results, repeat the Heimlich maneuver until the patient coughs up the object or becomes unconscious. Look to see if the object appears in the patient's mouth or the top of the throat. Use your fingers to pull the object out.

If the patient is unconscious or becomes unconscious:

- Place the patient on their back on a rigid surface such as the ground.

- Open the patient's airway by extending their head backward. To do this, place the palm of your hand on the patient's forehead, and the fingers of your other hand under the bony part of the chin. Attempt to restore breathing with mouth-to-mouth resuscitation.

- If still unsuccessful, and with the patient lying on their back, begin the Heimlich maneuver by putting the heel of one hand on the patient's stomach—slightly above the navel and below the ribs. Put your free hand on top of your other hand to provide additional force. Keep your elbows straight. Give four quick, forceful, downward and forward thrusts toward the patient's head.

- If these procedures fail, grasp the patient's lower jaw and tongue with one hand, and lift up to remove the tongue from the back of their throat. Place the index finger of your other hand inside the patient's mouth alongside the cheek. Slide your fingers down into the throat to the base of the patient's tongue.

- Carefully sweep your fingers along the back of the throat to dislodge the object. Bring your fingers out along the inside of the other cheek. Be careful not to push the object further down the patient's throat. If a foreign body comes within reach, grasp and remove it. Do not attempt to remove the foreign object with any type of instrument or forceps unless you are trained to do so.

- Repeat all of the above steps until the object is dislodged or medical assistance arrives.

- DO NOT GIVE UP!!!!

The Heimlich Maneuver on an Infant:

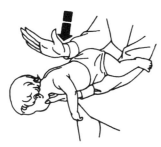

Rest your forearm on your thigh. Support the infant's head by firmly holding the jaw. Give four forceful back blows with the heel of your hand between the infant's shoulder blades.

If unsuccessful, turn the infant over and give four quick thrusts on the chest. To do this, place two fingers one finger-width below an imaginary line joining the nipples. Push downward and forward. Thrusts should be more gentle than those for an adult.

The Heimlich Maneuver on a Child:

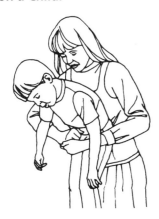

If necessary, repeat both procedures. Stand behind the child with your arms around his or her waist. Place the thumb side of your fist against the child's stomach, slightly above the navel and below the ribs and breastbone. Hold your fist with your other hand and give 4 quick, forceful upward thrusts. It may be necessary to repeat the procedure 6 to 10 times.

If the patient is an infant:

- Place the infant face down across your forearm with their head low. Support the head by firmly holding the jaw.
- Rest your forearm on your thigh. Support the infant's head by firmly holding the jaw. Give four forceful back blows with the heel of your hand between the infant's shoulder blades. The blows should be more gentle than those for an adult.
- If unsuccessful, turn the infant over and give four quick thrusts on their chest. To do this, place two fingers one finger-width below an imaginary line joining the nipples. Push downward and forward. Thrusts should be more gentle than those for an adult.
- If necessary, repeat both procedures.

If the patient is fat or pregnant:

- Stand behind the patient and place your fist on the middle of the breastbone in the chest, but not over the ribs. Put your other hand on top of your fist. Give four quick, forceful movements. Do not squeeze with your arms. Just use your fist.
- If this procedure does not work, stand behind the patient and support their chest with one hand. With the heel of the other hand, give four quick blows on the back between the patient's shoulder blades.

If you are alone and choking:

- Place your fist on your stomach slightly above the navel and below your ribs. Place your other hand on top of your fist. Give yourself four quick, forceful upward abdominal thrusts.
- If this procedure does not work, press your stomach forcefully over a chair, table, sink, or railing.

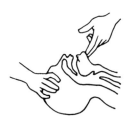

Opening the Patient's Airway

A simple way to remember the order of action to take if the patient is not breathing or their heart is not beating, is the use of the term "ABC."

These letters stand for
   Airway
      Breathing
         Circulation

They are the three basic steps in the procedure known as CPR.

CARDIOPULMONARY RESUSCITATION (CPR)

CPR is a basic life-support technique that is used when the patient is not breathing and it is possible that their heart has stopped beating. CPR allows you to perform manually the involuntary actions of the heart and lungs that provide vital blood and oxygen to all parts of the body.

CPR involves opening and clearing the patient's airway, restoring breathing and restoring blood circulation. Although opening the patient's airway and restoring breathing can be done effectively at the time of the crisis by following the instructions in this book, restoring circulation with manual chest compressions should be learned through classroom instruction taught by qualified personnel to be most effective. It is also recommended that regular refresher courses be taken.

Airway

The patient's airway must be clear and open in order to restore breathing.

To clear the airway:

- Lay the patient on their back on a firm, rigid surface such as the floor or the ground. For an infant, the hard surface may be the palm of your hand.
- Quickly clear the mouth and airway of foreign material with your fingers.
- If there does not appear to be any neck injury,* tilt the patient's head backward to open the airway. To do so, place your palm on the patient's forehead and the fingers of your other hand on the bony part of their chin. Doing this will elevate the tongue from the back of the throat. For an infant or small child, tilt the head back only slightly, so the airway does not become closed off.

Breathing

To restore breathing:

- Be sure the patient's head is tilted backward.
- With the hand that is placed on the patient's forehead, pinch their nostrils closed, using your thumb and index finger.
- Open your mouth widely and take a deep breath.
- Place your mouth tightly around the patient's mouth and give 2 full breaths — so that air enter their lungs — 1 to 1½ seconds per breath. Remove your mouth after each of your exhalations and take a deep breath between each of your breaths. For an infant or small child, place your mouth tightly over their mouth *and* nose. Use less air for an infant.
- If the patient's mouth cannot be used due to an injury, lift the lower jaw to close their mouth. Use one hand over the patient's mouth to keep it closed. Open your mouth wide and take a deep breath. Place your mouth tightly around the patient's nose and blow into it. After you exhale, remove your hand from the patient's mouth to allow air to escape.

*If you suspect a head or neck injury—especially if the patient has fallen from a height, or has been involved in an automobile accident— and the patient is unconscious, do not move them unless you and the patient are in imminent danger.

CPR Breathing:

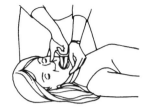

1. Make sure the victim is on a hard, flat surface. Quickly clear the mouth and airway of foreign material.

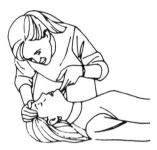

2. Tilt the victim's head backward by placing the palm of your hand on his or her forehead and the fingers of your other hand under the bony part of the chin.

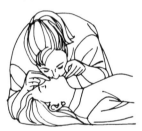

3. Pinch the victim's nostrils with your thumb and index finger. Take a deep breath. Place your mouth tightly over the victim's mouth (mouth and nose for an infant or small child). Give 2 quick breaths.

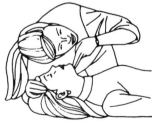

4. Stop blowing when the chest is expanding. Remove your mouth form the victim's mouth and turn your head toward the victim's chest, so that your ear is over his or her mouth. Listen for the air being exhaled. Watch for the victim's chest to fall. Repeat the breathing procedure.

- Moderate resistance will be felt when you blow. If you encounter marked resistance and the chest does not rise, the airway is not clear and more airway opening is needed. Place your hand under the patient's lower jaw and thrust the lower jaw forward so that it juts out farther.

- As you blow air into the patient's mouth, nose or mouth and nose, watch closely to see when their chest rises. Stop blowing when the chest is expanding.

- Remove your mouth from the patient's mouth, nose or mouth and nose and turn your head toward the patient's chest so that your ear is over his or her mouth. Listen for air leaving the patient's lungs and watch the chest fall. You may also feel air being exhaled from the patient's nose and mouth.

- Continue blowing into the patient's mouth, nose or mouth and nose at approximately 12 breaths per minute (1 breath every 5 seconds) for an adult; 15 breaths per minute (1 breath every 3 seconds) for an infant. Quantity is important, so provide plenty of air with each breath so that the patient's chest rises.

- Continue breathing for the patient until he or she begins breathing on their own or until medical assistance arrives.

- If the patient has drowned, and their stomach is bloated with swallowed water, put the patient on their stomach with the head turned to the side. To empty the water, place both hands under the patient's stomach and lift. After water is emptied, or if no water is emptied after approximately 10 seconds, return the patient to their back. Resume mouth-to-mouth breathing until the patient is breathing well on their own, or until medical assistance arrives.

Circulation:

The following procedure is best done by those who are professionally trained and must be done in conjunction with artificial breathing. In emergency situations, however, restoring circulation for the patient is essential for survival, and chest compressions, as outlined below, should be attempted. If you are performing CPR, have someone else call for paramedics or an ambulance.

For an adult:

- Assess the situation. Is the patient conscious? Gently shake them and shout "Are you okay?"

- If there is no response, call for someone to get help

- Look, listen and feel for breathing. Look for the patient's chest to rise and fall.

- Check for any foreign matter in the patient's mouth. If they are not breathing, tilt their head backward to open the airway. Do this by placing your palm on the patient's forehead and the fingers of your other hand under the bony part of their chin.

Checking for a Pulse:

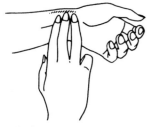

To find your pulse, place three fingertips at your wrist just below the thumb.

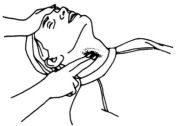

To check for a pulse on the victim's neck (carotid artery): move two fingers along the victim's throat to the Adam's apple. Then move these fingers off to the side of the victim's throat between the trachea (windpipe) and the muscles at the side of the neck. Press down gradually and firmly until you feel a pulse. A pulse means that the heart is beating.

Hand Position for CPR:

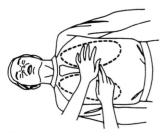

Move your fingers up the center of the victim's chest to the notch where the ribs meet the breastbone (sternum). With two fingers on this notch, place the heel of your hand two finger-widths above your fingers. Remove your fingers from the notch and place this hand on top of your other hand. The fingers may be interlaced. Do not allow your fingers to rest on the ribs.

- Pinch the patient's nose closed and blow two full breaths into his or her mouth so that the chest rises. Remove your mouth after each of your exhalations and take a deep breath between each of your breaths.
- With the palm of one hand on the patient's forehead (to ensure that the head is tilted backward and that the airway is open), use your other hand check for a pulse on the patient's neck (carotid artery). To find the pulse in the carotid artery, move two fingers along the patient's throat to the Adam's apple. Then move these fingers off to the side of the patient's throat between the trachea (windpipe) and the muscles at the side of the neck. Press down gradually and firmly until you feel a pulse. A pulse means that the heart is beating.
- If there is a pulse, but no breathing, perform mouth-to-mouth resuscitation at 12 breaths per minute — 1 breath every 5 seconds.
- If there is no pulse, begin chest compressions as well.

Proper position for chest compressions: (Maintain proper hand position to prevent damage to the patient's internal organs.)

- If possible, make sure the patient is lying on a hard, flat surface. The head should be at the same level as the rest of the body, or slightly lower, so that blood flow to the brain is not further reduced. If possible, slightly elevate the legs which will help blood flow back to the heart. MOVE QUICKLY, HOWEVER, SO THAT VALUABLE TIME IS NOT LOST.
- Kneel near the patient's chest. With two fingers, locate the patient's rib cage on the side closest to you.
- Move your fingers up the center of the patient's chest to the notch where the ribs meet the breastbone (sternum).
- With your fingers on this notch, place the heel of your other hand two finger-widths above your fingers.
- Remove your fingers from the notch and place this hand on top of your other hand. The fingers may be interlaced.
- Do not allow your fingers to rest on the ribs. Press down with the heel of your hand only.
- While kneeling, position your shoulders directly over the patient so that all of your weight is forced down, through the heel of your hand, onto the patient's chest. Straighten your arms and lock your elbows. Use your arms as pistons to exert pressure.
- Push down on the patient's chest 15 times. With each compression, push down quickly and forcefully to a depth of 1½ to 2 inches. Let the chest rise after each compression, but do not remove your hands from the chest.
- Perform this technique rhythmically by counting out loud: "one and, two and, three and, four and, etc. to fifteen and"
- Release your hand from the patient's chest and open the airway by tilting their head and chin backward.

To Perform Chest Compressions:

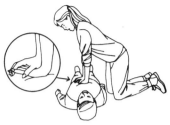

After finding the correct hand position for CPR (see previous page), push down on the chest 15 times. With each compression, push down quickly and forcefully to a depth of 1½ to 2 inches. Let the chest rise after each compression, but do not remove your hands from the chest.

- Pinch the patient's nostrils shut with your thumb and index finger. Blow two full breaths into the patient's mouth so that their chest rises.
- Reposition your hands on the patient's chest and repeat the 15 compressions and two breaths.
- Perform four complete cycles of 15 compressions and two breaths. Then, determine if the patient's pulse has returned. To do this, feel the patient's carotid artery in the neck. Do not interrupt CPR longer than 7 seconds.
- If there is a pulse but no breathing, perform mouth-to-mouth resuscitation at 12 breaths per minute (one breath every five seconds).
- If there is no pulse, repeat the 15 compressions and two breaths.
- Continue CPR until the patient begins breathing and their heart starts beating, until professional help arrives, or until you are too tired to continue.
- If vomiting occurs during CPR, turn the patient on their side (rolling the patient's whole body as a unit) and clear out the mouth with your fingers. Return the victim to their back and tilt the head backward to open the airway. Resume mouth-to-mouth resuscitation and CPR if necessary.

CPR Do's and Don'ts

- Do kneel alongside the patient to perform chest compressions. Straighten your arms and lock your elbows. Use your arms as pistons to exert pressure.
- Do perform quick, forceful compressions straight down on the patient's chest.
- Do keep your hands in place on the patient's chest while performing compressions.
- Do interlock your fingers and use the heel of one hand only for compressions.
- Don't rock back and forth or sit on your heels while performing compressions (blood will not be pumped out of the heart effectively).
- Don't roll your hand on the patient's chest.
- Don't lift your hands off the patient's chest or "bounce" your hands on their chest while performing compressions.
- Don't allow fingers to rest or exert pressure on the rib cage.

**Direct Pressure
for Bleeding:**

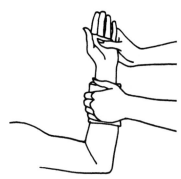

*Place a thick sterile or clean
compress directly over the entire
wound and press firmly with the
palm of your hand. If the wound is
bleeding severely, elevate the limb
above the victim's heart and
continue direct pressure.*

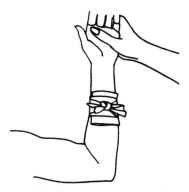

*Once bleeding stops or slows, apply
a pressure bandage to hold the
compress in place. Place the center
of the bandage directly over the
compress. Pull steadily while
wrapping both ends around the
injury. Tie a knot over the compress.
Do not tie so tightly that it cuts off
circulation. Keep the limb elevated.*

BLEEDING (External)

Direct pressure is the preferred treatment in bleeding injuries. Constant pressure (which may cause the patient some pain) is usually all that is necessary to stop the bleeding.

- Place a thick clean compress (sterile gauze or a soft clean cloth such as a handkerchief, towel, undershirt or strips from a sheet) directly over the entire wound and press firmly with the palm of your hand. If a cloth is not available, use bare hands or fingers (should be as clean as possible).
- Continue to apply steady pressure.
- Do not disturb any blood clots that form on the compress.
- If blood soaks through the compress, do not remove the compress. Apply another pad over it and continue with firmer hand pressure over a wider area.
- A limb that is bleeding severely should be raised above the level of the patient's heart and direct pressure continued.
- If bleeding stops or slows, apply a pressure bandage to hold the compress snugly in place.
- To apply a pressure bandage, place the center of the gauze, cloth strips, or necktie directly over the compress. Pull steadily while wrapping both ends around the injury. Tie a knot over the compress.
- Do not wrap the bandage so tightly that it cuts off arterial circulation. A pulse can be felt on an artery. You should feel a pulse below the bandage (below means at a point on an artery that is farthest away from the trunk of the body).
- Keep the limb elevated.

BLISTERS

If a blister is small and unopened, and will receive no further irritation, cover it with a sterile gauze pad and bandage in place. The fluid in the blister will eventually be absorbed by the skin and it will heal itself.

If a blister accidentally breaks, exposing raw skin, wash the area gently with soap and water and cover with a sterile bandage. The skin will regrow its outer layers.

Do not open a blister caused by a burn.

If a blister is large, and likely to be broken by routine activity, you should seek medical attention for treatment. Only if medical attention is not readily available should you try to open a blister.

To open a blister, gently clean the area with soap and water. Sterilize a needle by holding it over an open flame. Puncture the lower edge of the blister with the needle. Press the blister gently to force out the fluid. Cover the area with a sterile bandage.

Always look for signs of infection such as redness, pus, or red streaks leading from the wound. Seek medical attention promptly if these symptoms appear.

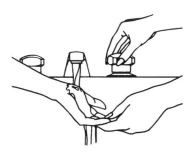

Immediately put the burned area under cold running water (as illustrated) or apply cold-water compresses until pain subsides.

Elevation Techniques:

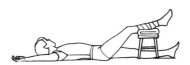

Elevate a foot or leg with second- or third-degree burns higher than the victim's heart.

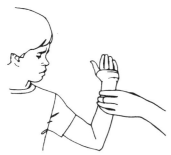

Cover the burn with a non-fluffy sterile or clean bandage to prevent infection. Elevate a hand or arm with second- or third-degree burns higher than the victim's heart.

BURNS

The objective of first aid for burns is to relieve pain, prevent infections and prevent or treat for shock.

First-Degree Burns

First-degree burns usually are the result of sunburn, hot water, steam or brief contact with a hot object. First degree burns are an injury to the outside layer of skin.

Symptoms may include any or all of the following: redness, mild swelling, pain and unbroken skin (no blisters).

What to do:

- Immediately put the burned area under cold running water or apply a cold-water compress (a clean towel, washcloth, or handkerchief soaked in cold water) until pain decreases.
- Cover burn with non-fluffy sterile or clean bandage.
- Never apply butter or grease to a burn. And do not apply other medications or home remedies without a doctor's recommendation.

Second-Degree Burns

Second-degree burns are burns that cause injury to the layers of skin beneath the surface of the body. Deep sunburn, hot liquids, and flash burns from gasoline and other substances are common causes of second-degree burns.

Symptoms may include any or all of the following: Redness or streaky appearance, sometimes marked with spots (blotchy), blisters, swelling that lasts for several days, moist oozy appearance of the surface of the skin and pain.

What to do:

- Put the burned area in cold water (not iced) or apply cold-water compresses until pain subsides.
- Gently pat the area dry with a clean towel or other soft material.
- Cover the burned area with a dry, non-fluffy sterile bandage or clean cloth to prevent infection.
- Elevate the burned arm or leg.
- Seek medical attention. If the victim has flash burns around the lips or nose, or has singed nasal hairs, breathing problems may develop. Seek medical attention immediately at the nearest hospital emergency room.
- Do not attempt to break blisters
- Do not apply ointments, sprays, antiseptics or home remedies.

Seek medical attention right away for any burn that covers more than 15 percent of the body of an adult or 10 percent of a child, or for burns of the face, hands, or feet. As a guide in determining the amount of burned area, your hand equals one percent of your body area. Also, if there has been smoke, the patient may have inhaled the smoke or other substances that can cause lung damage. When in doubt, always seek medical attention.

Elevation Techniques:

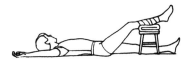

Elevate a foot or leg with second- or third-degree burns higher than the victim's heart.

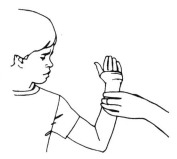

Cover the burn with a non-fluffy sterile or clean bandage to prevent infection. Elevate a hand or arm with second- or third-degree burns higher than the victim's heart.

TIP: Any cold liquid you can drink — such as water, iced tea, soft drinks, beer or a milk shake — can be poured on a burn. The purpose in pouring cold liquids on the burn is to decrease the temperature of the burned skin as quickly as possible to limit tissue damage.

Third-Degree Burns

Third-degree burns destroy all layers of the skin. Fire, prolonged contact with hot substances and electrical burns are the most common causes of third-degree burns.

Symptoms include: burned area that appears white or charred, destroyed skin and little pain because nerve endings have been destroyed.

Warning:

- Do not remove clothes that are stuck to a burn.
- Do not put ice or ice water on burns. This can intensify the shock reaction.
- Do not apply any ointments, sprays, antiseptics or home remedies.

What to do:

- If patient is on fire, smother the flames with a blanket, rug, bedspread or jacket.
- Breathing difficulties are common with burns, particularly with burns around the face, neck, mouth and with smoke inhalation. Check to be sure patient is breathing.
- Place a cold cloth or cool (not iced) water on burns of the face, hand, or feet to cool the burned areas.
- Cover burned areas with thick, sterile, non-fluffy dressings. Clean sheets, pillowcases, or disposable diapers can be used.
- Call for an ambulance immediately. It is very important that you take the patient to the doctor even if the burn is small.
- Elevate burned hand(s) higher than the patient's heart, if possible.
- Elevate burned legs or feet if possible. Do not let the patient walk.
- If the patient has face or neck burns, he or she should be propped up with pillows. Keep an eye on the patient to make sure they are not having trouble breathing.
- Treat for shock.

CHEMICAL BURNS

- Quickly flush burned areas with large quantities of running water for at least five minutes. Speed and quantity of water are both important in minimizing the extent of the injury. Use a garden hose, buckets of water, a shower or a tub. Do not use a strong stream of water if it can be avoided.
- Continue to flush with water while removing clothing from the burned area.
- After flushing, follow instructions on label of the chemical that caused the burn, if available.
- Cover the burn with a non-fluffy clean bandage or clean cloth.
- Seek medical attention. Do not apply any ointments, sprays, antiseptic or home remedies. Cool wet dressings are best for pain.

FAINTING

Fainting is the brief loss of consciousness due to a reduced blood supply reaching the brain. Recovery usually occurs within few minutes.

Symptoms may include any or all of the following: pale, cool and wet skin, lightheadedness and nausea.

What to do:

- Have the patient lie down with legs elevated 8 to 12 inches, or have the patient sit down and slowly bend the body forward so that their head is between their knees.
- Move any harmful objects out of the patient's way.
- Calm and reassure the patient.
- If the patient has fainted, keep them lying down and elevate their feet 8 to 12 inches unless a head injury is suspected.
- Maintain an open airway.
- Loosen tight clothing, particularly around the patient's neck.
- If the patient vomits, place them on their side. You want to prevent the patient from choking on their vomit.
- Gently bathe the patient's face with cool water. Do not pour water on the patient's face.
- Check for swelling or deformity that may have been caused by falling.
- Do not give the patient something to drink unless they seem fully recovered
- After the patient regains consciousness, keep an eye on them. Keep yourself and the patient calm.
- If recovery does not seem complete within a few minutes, seek medical attention.

LUMPS AND BUMPS

Lumps and bumps are common injuries. Any bump on the head resulting from an injury may be serious and requires medical attention.

As soon as an injury occurs, apply cold compresses or an ice pack to the affected area to decrease swelling and alleviate pain.

Seek medical attention promptly for a lump on the head if there is bleeding from the nose, mouth, unconsciousness, change in pulse, severe headache, difficulty in breathing, convulsions, severe vomiting, eye pupils of unequal size, slurred speech, a generally poor appearance, or a personality change.

If a bump is the result of a head injury, check or awaken the patient every half hour for the first two hours, every two hours for the next 24 hours, every four hours for the second 24 hour period and every eight hours for the third 24 hour period. By doing this, you are checking to be sure that the patient has not become unconscious.

Seek medical attention for any severe lump or bump on any part of the patient's body.

First Aid Products

Mc 130-1670	Band-Aid Sheer Band One Size	40s	$3.25
Mc 130-1431	Band-Aid Sheer Band Xlrg	10s	$3.65
Mc 130-1647	Band-Aid Sheer Band Assrt	60s	$3.25
Mc 160-2101	Band-Aid Flexible Assrt	30s	$3.65
Mc 223-1728	Band-Aid Plastic One Size	60s	$2.65
Mc 354-3832	Cortaid Max-Str Cream 1%	1oz	$6.45
Mc 351-6762	Cortizone 10 Crm Mx-Str Itch/R	1oz	$5.95
Mc 130-2587	J&J First Aid Rolled Gauze 2"	4 yds	$2.35
Mc 130-2595	J&J First Aid Rolled Gauze 3"	4 yds	$3.25
Mc 130-2603	J&J First Aid Rolled Gauze 4"	4 yds	$3.95
Mc 130-1761	J&J First Aid Tpe Waterprf 0.5"	5 yds	$1.75
Mc 274-1395	J&J First Aid Tape Paper 0.5"	5 yds	$2.35
Mc 211-9253	J&J First Aid Tape Paper 1"	5 yds	$3.95
Mc 130-1910	J&J First Aid Tape Cloth 0.5"	5 yds	$2.35
Mc 130-2652	J&J First Aid Strl Gauze Pd 2" × 2"	10s	$1.85
Mc 118-9893	Neosporin Ointment	0.5 oz	$5.45
Mc 118-9919	Neosporin Ointment	1 oz	$8.65
Mc 117-0265	Neosporin Plus Max-Str Oint	0.5 oz	$5.85
Mc 126-4696	Neosporin+ Crm Max/Str	0.5 oz	$5.85
Mc 241-7533	Nix Lice Treatment Crm Rns 2x2	2-2 oz	$23.45
Mc 241-7285	Nix Lice Treatmnt Crm Rns	2 oz	$14.45
Mc 118-9968	Polysporin	0.5 oz	$5.65
Mc 120-2738	Vaseline Petro Jelly	3.75 oz	$2.55
Mc 120-2712	Vaseline Petro Jelly	1.75 oz	$1.65
Mc 180-4764	Vaseline Petro Jelly Tube	1 oz	$2.05

LeBoeuf's
Home Healthcare
Handbook

Dying & Death

LeBoeuf's

Death

THE PATIENT WHO IS DYING has the right to refuse to stay in a hospital or nursing home and to return home. Many patients believe that dying at home or at the caregiver's home in comfortable and familiar surroundings gives them more control over their lives. However, the emotional stress of the situation may be too much for the caregiver and the family. Bringing the dying patient into the home should be carefully thought out. The best guidance for assisting the caregiver and the family can be obtained through hospice and the church (talk with both).

If the patient, support groups and family decide that it would be best for the patient to die at home, it is important for the patient to document their wishes in writing. If the patient doesn't document their wishes, organizations such as Adult Protective Services may intervene and obtain a court order to remove the patient from the home if a case worker believes that the patient is not receiving proper care.

Prior to the dying patient being discharged from the hospital, the caregiver should:

- Determine if health insurance will cover what Medicare and/or Medicaid does not.

- Contact the hospice, church and or a home health care agency that provides home care services and be sure that all arrangements for assistance are in place. It is a mistake for the caregiver to try and manage the dying patient's needs without help from experienced outside service providers.

- Obtain from the doctor a "To whom it may concern" letter that discusses the patient's condition and the desire to die at home. The letter should clearly state that the patient's death is expected. Keep a copy of the letter at home and tell family members where the letter is kept.

- Put in place a nonhospital "Do Not Resuscitate" (DNR) order. This is a document that is signed by the doctor directing paramedics not to perform CPR on the patient. Without this document, the paramedics will try and do everything possible to resuscitate the patient. Check with the doctor or hospital to see if your state allows a nonhospital DNR order. Some states do not have laws permitting nonhospital DNR orders.

- Make sure that you have all the equipment the patient will require prior to bringing them into the home.

- Develop a care plan which includes a medication schedule, who is on duty to assist and when professional assistance is needed (the doctor and nurse will help you with this).

- Develop a pain control plan with the doctor and nurse.

- Do not change the medical treatment of the patient unless the doctor provides written authorization to do so. Make sure the doctor signs and dates the authorization.
- Tell your friends and neighbors of the situation. They can help with running errands, cooking, visiting the patient, providing respite care and other routines.
- Know who, and in what sequence, to call when the patient dies.
- Work with the funeral home ahead of time so that arrangements can be made to move the body to the funeral home. The doctor and the funeral home should be in contact with each other to insure that the death certificate will be available without difficulty.

As patients near death, they become more tired and sleep more and more. They often become confused and restless. They may lose control of urine or bowels and breathing may become more difficult. When they are in a semi-coma or coma they may stop eating or drinking. A very deep sleep is called a coma. Even if the patient is in a coma, provide reassurance by letting them know you are near. Most doctors believe that a person in a coma is able to hear. They probably hear and understand even if they cannot talk back. If you have something to say to the patient, go ahead and say it. At this time, being with the patient is the most important thing you can do.

If the patient has problems breathing, raise the head of the bed and see if that helps. Do not force feed patients who do not want to eat or drink. Offer ice chips or sips of water if they want it. If you give the patient water with a straw, place the water toward their cheek to prevent choking. Moaning or restlessness may indicate the patient is in pain. It is not necessary for the patient to have any pain and the doctor and nurse will provide you with medications to control it.

Other signs of approaching death include a high fever, poor circulation which causes the legs and arms to become cool, periods of extreme perspiration, muscle twitching and the eyes stop blinking. If the patient runs a high fever, call the doctor or nurse for a fever reducing suppository. Muscle twitching is not painful to the patient.

Death occurs when:

The classic definition of death is the permanent cessation of the heart and lungs.

- Patient cannot be aroused.
- Patient stops breathing.
- Patient's heartbeat stops.
- Patient's eyelids are partially open with eyes in a fixed stare.
- Patient's mouth may fall open slightly.
- Bladder or rectum muscles relax and anything in them is released.

Call the nurse or doctor. You do not need to call 911 or the emergency number for your area if the doctor or nurse will offer an immediate visit. Most health care agencies such as hospice and visiting nurses will have someone on call 24-hours-a-day, 7-days-a-week and will send someone out right away. They will confirm that death has occurred and will call the doctor and the funeral home.

While the death of a loved one is painful, it is a natural part of life. It is important that you remain as calm as possible so that your loved one's final moments are calm and peaceful. If in doubt, calling 911 or the emergency number is appropriate and may be the best way to handle the situation. If you do call 911, the doctor should be called at once to direct the ambulance crew. If you cannot reach the doctor, have available for the ambulance crew the nonhospital DNR document stating that the patient wanted to die at home and the doctor's letter that describes the patient's condition.

The classic definition of death is the permanent cessation of the heart and lungs. Only a physician can pronounce death. By law, a death certificate must be completed when a person dies. The death certificate is usually signed by the attending doctor and filed with the local health office. Certified copies are issued by the local health office. You will need the certified copies of the death certificate to show the insurance companies, social security, etc. If a doctor cannot sign the death certificate because they are out of town, or you never had an attending doctor who knows the history of the patient, the funeral director will have to contact a medical examiner (sometimes called coroner).

Every state has laws stipulating when autopsies must be ordered. If the state does not require an autopsy, the hospital must obtain permission from next-of-kin to perform one. The medical examiner or coroner may or may not have an autopsy performed on the body and the decision to perform an autopsy is usually theirs alone. However, in some cases, they will perform an autopsy if the family requests one. The medical examiner (coroner) would then sign the death certificate after they are satisfied that the reasons for death have been determined.

Rigor mortis sets in about two to four hours after death. If the nurse or doctor cannot come right away, and because family members and others often want to view the body, it is important that the deceased appear natural and comfortable. Position the body, place the dentures in the mouth and close the eyes and mouth.

After your loved one has died, the following responsibilities should be taken care of as soon as possible:

- Contact your clergy (last rites).
- Contact the family and those closest to the deceased.
- Have the home care nurse or the hospital contact the doctor.
- Contact the mortuary or have the doctor or nurse contact the funeral home. If you are too upset, let the nurse or the doctor contact the funeral home.

Getting over the loss of a loved one is a difficult process — but grief is natural. Emotions will arise that are very painful and will come and go for weeks, months or even years. It is best to give into the pain of your loss and let it take precedence over other emotions. Forgive yourself for all the things that you feel you should have done or said. Make a special effort to eat and rest well. Grief is very exhausting. Do something different to distract yourself or something that you find gratifying — pamper yourself. Get help and support from a bereavement group. They can help you deal with feeling all alone. Give yourself as much time as you need to grieve. When you have found new energy, then it's time to start getting on with life.

Many caregivers find that reaching out to others in need provides them with a sense of belonging. Volunteering to help raise funds for a local charity, joining a community choral group, preparing meals for the homeless, working with hospice, etc. By filling your hours helping others, you have less time to brood about your loss and eventually you will be able to fully enjoy life again. Also, you will realize that your energy has returned and that your life has meaning and purpose to be shared with friends and family.

Preplanning for Funerals

PREPLANNING A FUNERAL avoids the necessity of making arrangements at an emotionally difficult time. It allows the patient and/or the family to make unhurried decisions and the time to think over the numerous details. Many patients want to plan their funerals and it is important to allow them to do so. It is definitely a relief to know that when death occurs, there are arrangements in place for the funeral services.

Costs will vary between funeral homes and you should remember that you are buying a service to meet the needs of the family and to respect the wishes of the deceased. While the funeral director may suggest various options, you are the boss and you should do what you believe to be best. Many times, considerable savings may be obtained by prepaying the funeral home for the funeral.

The national average for the cost of a funeral is over $3,500. The price of coffins alone can run from $1,200 to more than $4,000. Most funerals will cost thousands more and it is important that you carefully shop for the best price and service. Prices with funeral homes can be negotiated. If you have not planned ahead, however, you will probably be too emotional to haggle over prices.

You are not required to use the services of a funeral home. Some states have mortuary companies that perform only burials and/or cremations at a lower cost. Normally, cremation is less expensive than burial. All states have laws to insure that all burials will be carried out in a way that is consistent with local health requirements.

All cemeteries are regulated by agencies of the local, state or federal governments. Along with preplanning a funeral, you and the patient should decide on a cemetery plot. You may want to purchase a number of adjoining spaces for the eventual needs of the family. Aboveground interment in a mausoleum is another option. Arrangements for interment in a mausoleum are made in much the same way as arrangements for a cemetery lot. If the patient wishes to be cremated, a cemetery plot is not necessary.

Cemetery plots vary widely in price and custodial (maintenance) care and can be owned by any number of groups such as churches, fraternal organizations, public agencies, private companies, etc. You can make any choice you wish as long as the patient qualifies (usually military service or religious restrictions). It is important to find out if the cemetery will buy the plot back and at what price, if you or the patient change your mind. Some cemeteries allow one casket to be buried above another, which can substantially reduce the cost. It is worthwhile to find out if the cemetery offers this option.

Pricing a plot is not all there is to burial costs. Most cemeteries will require a special marker (brass, marble, granite, etc.) and the charge for a marker can range from about $1,000 to many thousands more. For opening the grave and closing it (interment), there will be a charge of about $650 or more. A grave liner (vault), which protects the casket from water and acids in the soil, can be as simple as a concrete box or as elaborate and expensive as stainless steel, copper, imitation marble, etc. The cost of a grave liner will range from a low of about $400 to more than $2,000. In addition, there is usually an additional fee for placing (installing) the liner (vault) in the grave. Usually this fee is in the range of $50 to $75.

Make sure that you visit the cemetery to check out how they care for the grounds. Ask about the maintenance fees. Some cemeteries will require a one-time fee for perpetual care while others will require an annual fee for upkeep of the plot. Make sure that you and the patient understand the maintenance fee schedule and that you can afford the fee before making any decision. You and the patient should also visit the site during wet weather, if possible, to make sure that the site is not under water when it rains.

If the patient is a veteran, burial in a national cemetery is possible. Some of the national cemeteries have limited space available and the assignment of space can be complex. You can ask the local Veterans Administration office what cemetery plots are available in your area. The burial will include all cemetery services and a grave marker but you will have to fill out a form for the grave marker. You will be responsible for the cost of having the grave marker installed. Ask the funeral home for assistance in obtaining the forms. Maintenance of veterans plots is paid for by the Veterans Administration.

After your loved one has died, the following responsibilities should be taken care of as soon as possible:

- Contact the family and those closest to the deceased.
- Have the home care nurse or the hospital contact the doctor.
- Contact the mortuary or have the doctor or nurse contact the mortuary (probably best if the nurse or the doctor contacted the funeral home).
- Contact your clergy.

The cost of all the funeral arrangements will be provided to you in a written memorandum by the funeral home. It is required by law that the funeral director present the General Price List at the start of the arrangements (including over the telephone). Services and products can be purchased separately and not just through a package deal.

Embalming is expensive and some states do not require it. If your state does not require embalming, you must be notified in writing. For all practical purposes, if the casket is to be open, embalming is necessary. Be aware that expenses incurred at the cemetery will not always be on the General Price List. Every funeral home will have its own General Price List and must provide an itemized statement for all goods and services purchased (Note: You are not obligated to pay for a casket if the patient has been cremated). There are no limits or standard prices set on any of the costs of caskets, burial vaults, etc., by the government. It is in your best interest to take the time to fully understand all the charges. If you are feeling too emotional to concentrate, back off and have a close and trusted friend help with the funeral home negotiations.

The funeral director will provide all the services needed for the funeral. The funeral director will ask for the following information to assist in preparation of the death certificate and the obituary or paid death notice. A death certificate is important because you will need it to file for Social Security, life insurance benefits, probate of the deceased's will, pension benefits and access to a safe-deposit box. The death certificate will state the time, place and cause of death. Make sure that the death certificate states the exact cause of death. The certificate is filled out by the doctor, medical examiner or the coroner and is the legal proof of death. It should be available to you within a matter of days unless an autopsy has to be performed. Additional copies can be obtained from the health department.

Provide the following personal information about the deceased to the funeral director:

- Name.
- Social Security number.
- Address.
- Date of birth.
- Birthplace.
- U.S. Armed services and Serial number.
- Occupation.
- Name of Father.
- Name of Mother.
- Name of Wife.
- Name of Wife's father and mother.
- Names of all children.
- Maiden name of wife, husband's mother's maiden name or wife's mother's maiden name.
- Place of birth of wife.

The funeral director will also want the names of organizations, clergy, relatives and friends that need to be contacted. In addition, if nothing has been planned ahead of time, the funeral director will want to know:

- What type of funeral — cremation, traditional service, restricted to family only, etc.?
- Who will be the pallbearers? Will there be any honorary pallbearers?
- What special readings, flowers, music, etc. are desired?
- Type of casket and burial vault?
- What clothing, jewelry the deceased should wear (family to provide)?
- If there is a family burial plot? If so, location, number of graves and which space?
- If there is no burial plot, where is burial preferred?

It has become customary to place a floral spray from the family on the casket. For veterans, a flag may drape the casket instead of flowers.

The funeral director will instruct the pallbearers, arrange transportation for the immediate family, perform the ushering at the funeral home, greet visitors, provide counseling to the family and a host of other services.

Funerals are often valuable for meeting the emotional and religious needs of the mourners. Family suffering is often lessened by the support of friends and loved ones.

A marker or monument can be installed at the grave site at any time. Check with the cemetery officials about any restrictions on size or style.

As soon as possible after the funeral, send notes to those who provided special help, sent flowers and/or made contributions. You can, if you wish, acknowledge letters or cards of sympathy but it is not necessary. Information about flowers will be on the back of each sender's card so you will know what was sent by whom. The funeral home will gather the senders' cards and give them to you.

After the funeral, the following should be done to settle the estate, change names and notify others of the death:

- Contact the Social Security Administration, Veterans Administration (if appropriate), retirement or pension fund, union membership benefits (if applicable) and life insurance companies.

Notify the following of the death and any name changes:

- Fraternal, civic and social organizations.
- Banking (savings account, safety deposit box, trust fund, titles and deeds to personal and real property).
- Insurance on the auto, health insurance, personal property, life insurance of your own (change beneficiaries).
- Stockbroker to find out about any stocks, bonds or mutual funds.
- CPA on estate taxes, current and/or delinquent taxes and inheritance taxes.
- Attorney if estate is to be probated, trust needs to be changed, administration of will.
- Vehicle registrations.
- Utilities if name change is needed.
- Medicare or Medicaid.
- Supplemental health insurance.

The following death benefits are free of federal income tax:

- Social Security death benefit ($225).
- Veterans' benefits.
- Life insurance.
- Health insurance.
- Employer's death benefits (up to $5,000).
- Gifts given as a gift to the survivors in memory of the deceased.

Your funeral director will help you attend to many of the chores listed above after the funeral. Do not hesitate to ask for help or advice if you are in doubt.

Getting over a loss is a hard, slow process. Emotions will arise that are very painful and will come and go for weeks, months or even years. It is best to give in to the pain and let it take precedence over other emotions. Forgive yourself for all the things that you feel you should have done or said. Eat and rest well. Grief is very exhausting. Do something different to distract yourself or something that you find gratifying — pamper yourself. Get help from a bereavement group. They can help you cope with the feeling that you are all alone. Give yourself as much time as you need to grieve. When you have found new energy, then it's time to start getting on with life.

LeBoeuf's
Home Healthcare
Handbook

Bibliography, Sources & Index

Bibliography

Accident Prevention and Safety

America Association of Retired Persons. *Product Report: PERS (Personal Emergency Response System.* 1992.

Breneman, Mary, and Brown, Colette. "Keeping Mobile and Independent." In *Our Aging Parents.* Ed. Colette Brown and Roberta-Onzuka-Anderson. Honolulu, HA: Univ. of Hawaii Press, 1985, p. 149.

Cahill, Matthew, ed. *Nurse's Reference Library.* Springhouse, PA: Springhouse Corp., 1987.

Clayman, C.B., ed. *The American Medical Association Encyclopedia of Medicine.* New York: Random House, 1989.

Deichman, Elizabeth S. "The Elderly and Their Environment." In *Working with the Elderly.* Ed. Elizabeth S. Deichman and Regina Kociecki. Buffalo, NY: Prometheus Books, 1989, p. 91.

"Fall Prevention Through Health Promotion." *Perspectives in Health Promotion and Aging.* 6, No. 3 (1991), p. 1.

Inger, Gustaf. "Old Hands at Driving." *The Washington Times*, May 3, 1995, Sec. C, p. 10.

Injury Control in the 1990's: A National Plan for Action. Report to the Second World Conference on Injury Control. May 1993.

Hansen, Leonard J. "Solving Physical Ailments." *The Washington Times*, May 3, 1995, Sec. C, p. 11.

Kozier, Barbara, et al. *Techniques in Clinical Nursing.* Redwood City, CA: Benjamin/Cummings Publishing Co., Inc., 1993.

"Making Life Easier for Older People at Home." *Work & Family Life*, 9, No. 4 (April 1995), p. 4.

Ramsey, Mildred. "Providing a Safe Home Environment." In *Our Aging Parents.* Ed. Colette Brown and Roberta-Onzuka-Anderson. Honolulu, HA: Univ. of Hawaii Press, 1985, p. 176.

"Study Suggests Ways to Reduce the Risk of Falling." *Work & Family Life*, 1995, p. 3.

U.S. Dept. of Health & Human Services. National Institute on Aging. *Accident Prevention.* 1991.

————. National Institute on Aging. *Preventing Falls and Fractures.* 1992.

U.S. Dept. of Transportation. National Highway Traffic Safety Administration. "Putting It Together: A Model for Integrating Injury Control System Elements." GPO, 1994.

U.S. Environmental Protection Agency. *Home Buyer's and Seller's Guide to Radon.* GPO, 1993.

Acquired Immunodeficiency Syndrome (Aids)

Berkow, Robert, ed. *The Merck Manual.* Rahway, NJ: Merck Research Laboratories, 1992.

Cahill, Matthew, ed. *Nurse's Reference Library.* Springhouse, PA: Springhouse Corp., 1987.

Centers for Disease Control National AIDS Clearinghouse. *Directory of National Organizations Providing HIV/AIDS Services; A Resource for Community-Based Organizations*, 1994.

Clayman, C.B., ed. *The American Medical Association Encyclopedia of Medicine.* New York: Random House, 1989.

Ed-Sadr W., et al. *Evaluation and Management of Early HIV Infection. Clinical Practice Guideline No. 7.* AHCPR Pub. No. 94-0572. Rockville, MD: Agency for Health Care Policy and Research, U.S. Dept. of Health and Human Services, Public Health Service, 1994.

————. *Managing Early HIV Infection: Quick Reference Guide for Clinicians.* AHCPR Pub. No. 94-0573. Rockville, MD: Agency for Health Care Policy and Research, U.S. Dept. of Health and Human Services, Public Health Service, 1994.

Hospice of Northern Virginia. *Hospice Care for Persons with AIDS.* Falls Church, VA: Hospice of Northern Virginia, n.d.

Kozier, Barbara, et al. *Techniques in Clinical Nursing.* Redwood City, CA: Benjamin/Cummings Publishing Co., Inc., 1993.

Tesini, David A. *Developing Dental Education Programs for Persons With Special Needs: A Training and Reference Guide.* 2nd ed. Boston, MA: MA Dept. of Public Health, 1988.

U.S. Department of Health & Human Services. National Institute on Aging. "HIV, AIDS, and Older Adults." 1994.

————. Public Health Service. *AIDS-Related CMV: How to Help Yourself.* NIH Pub. No. 94-3718. Bethesda, MD: National Institutes of Health, 1994.

————. Public Health Service. *AIDS-Related MAC: How to Help Yourself.* NIH Pub. No. 94-3719. Bethesda, MD: National Institutes of Health, 1994.

————. Public Health Service. *The Brain Infection Toxo: How to Help Yourself.* NIH Pub. No. 93-3326. Bethesda, MD: National Institutes of Health, 1993.

————. *Caring for Someone with AIDS.* 1993.

————. Public Health Service. *HIV-Related TB: How to Help Yourself.* NIH Pub. No. 93-3327. Bethesda, MD: National Institutes of Health, 1993.

————. Public Health Service. *Infections Linked to AIDS: How to Help Yourself.* NIH Pub. No. 92-2062. Bethesda, MD: National Institutes of Health, 1992.

————. Public Health Service. *The Lung Infection PCP: How to Help Yourself.* NIH Pub. No. 93-3325. Bethesda, MD: National Institutes of Health, 1993.

————. Public Health Service. *Taking the HIV (AIDS) Test: How to Help Yourself.* NIH Pub. No. 92-2060. Bethesda, MD: National Institutes of Health, 1992.

————. Public Health Service. *Testing Positive for HIV: How to Help Yourself.* NIH Pub. No. 92-2061. Bethesda, MD: National Institutes of Health, 1992.

————. Public Health Service. "Human Immunodeficiency Virus Transmission in Household Settings—United States." Reprinted from *Morbidity and Mortality Weekly Report*, 43, No. 19. (May 20, 1994), p. 347.

U.S. Dept. of Justice. Justice Management Division. *AIDS Awareness and Prevention Resource Book*, 1994.

U.S. GAO. *Report to the Ranking Minority Member, Committee on Commerce, House of Representatives. Tuberculosis. Costly and Preventable Cases Continue in Five Cities.* GAO/HEHS-95-11. Washington, D.C.: GAO, 1995.

Alcohol

"Alcohol and the Older Adult." *Perspectives in Health Promotion and Aging*, 4, No. 3 (May 1989), p. 1.

Berkow, Robert, ed. *The Merck Manual.* Rahway, NJ: Merck Research Laboratories, 1992.

Cahill, Matthew, ed. *Nurse's Reference Library.* Springhouse, PA: Springhouse Corp., 1987.

Clayman, C.B., ed. *The American Medical Association Encyclopedia of Medicine.* New York: Random House, 1989.

U.S. Dept. of Health & Human Services. National Institute of Aging. *Aging and Alcohol Abuse.* 1991.

————. Public Health Service. *Progress Report for: Alcohol and Other Drugs.* Oct. 11, 1994.

Alzheimer's Disease

"Alzheimer's Disease: A Health Promotion Approach to Caring for the Caregiver." *Perspectives in Health Promotion and Aging*, 8, No. 4 (1993), p. 1.

Alzheimer's Disease and Related Disorders, Inc. *"Alzheimer's Disease: An Overview.* 1994.

————. *Alzheimer's Disease: Fact Sheet.* 1994.

————. *Is It Alzheimer's? Ten Warning Signs.* n.d.

————. "Alzheimer's Costs to Families Staggering." *National Newsletter*, 14, No. 4 (1994).

————. *Safety.* 1990.

————. *Statistical Data on Alzheimer's Disease.* 1993.

————. *When the Diagnosis Is Alzheimer's.* 1990.

————. *A Checklist of Concerns/Resources for Caregivers.* 1987.

————. *Coping & Caring. Living with Alzheimer's Disease.* 1993.

Bach, Julie. "What to say when . . ." 1992.

Berkow, Robert, ed. *The Merck Manual.* Rahway, NJ: Merck Research Laboratories, 1992.

Blieszner, Rosemary, and Shifflett, Peggy A. "The Effects of Alzheimer's Disease on Close Relationships Between Patients and Caregivers." *Family Relations*, Jan. 1990, pp. 57-62.

Braudy Harris, Phyllis. "The Misunderstood Caregiver? A Qualitative Study of the Male Caregiver of Alzheimer's Disease Victims." *The Gerontologist*, 33, No. 4 (1993), pp. 551-556.

Cahill, Matthew, ed. *Nurse's Reference Library.* Springhouse, PA: Springhouse Corp., 1987.

Clayman, C.B., ed. *The American Medical Association Encyclopedia of Medicine.* New York: Random House, 1989.

Drickamer, Margaret A., and Lachs, Mark S. "Should Patients with Alzheimer's Disease Be Told Their Diagnosis?" *New England Journal of Medicine*, 326, No. 14 (April 2, 1992), pp. 947-951.

Eakes, M. Garey. *Lifetime Decision-Making and Estate Planning.* Part I of *Legal Issues for Persons with Alzheimer's Disease and Their Families in Virginia.* 1994.

————. *Planning to Pay for Long-Term Care.* Part II of *Legal Issues for Persons with Alzheimer's Disease and Their Families in Virginia.* 1995.

Farran, Carol J., et al. "Finding Meaning: An Alternative Paradigm for Alzheimer's Disease Family Caregivers." *The Gerontologist*, 31, No. 4 (1991), pp. 483-89.

Guiterrez-Mayka, Marcela. *Care to the Caregiver in Alzheimer's Disease: A Curriculum Guide.* 1991.

Hall, Cynthia. "The Great Tulip Project." *Guideposts.* June 1995, pp. 32-35.

Heilman Rattner, Joan. "The Good News About Alzheimer's." *Parade Magazine.* Aug. 13, 1995, p. 12.

Kamen, Al. "Former President Reagan Has Alzheimer's Disease." *The Washington Post*, Nov. 6, 1994, Sec. A, p. 1.

Kinney, Jennifer M., and Parris Stephens, Mary A. "Caregiving Hassles Scale: Assessing the Daily Hassles of Caring for a Family Member with Dementia." *The Gerontologist*, 29, No. 3 (1989), pp. 328-332.

Kozier, Barbara, et al. *Techniques in Clinical Nursing.* Redwood City, CA: Benjamin/Cummings Publishing Co., Inc., 1993.

McGrowder-Lin, Rachel, and Bhatt, Ashok. "A Wanderer's Lounge Program for Nursing Home Residents with Alzheimer's Disease." *The Gerontologist*, 28, No. 5 (1988), pp. 607-609.

Mace, Nancy L., et al. *The 36-Hour Day: A Family Guide to Caring for Persons with Alzheimer's Disease, Related Dementing Illnesses, and Memory Loss in Later Life.* Baltimore, MD: The Johns Hopkins Univ. Press, 1991.

Mittelman, Mary S., et al. "An Intervention that Delays Institutionalization of Alzheimer's Disease Patients: Treatment of Spouse-Caregivers." *The Gerontologist*, 33, No. 6 (1993), pp. 730-740.

Nash, Madeline J. "To Know Your Own Fate." *Time*, April 3, 1995, p. 62.

Nhu, T.T. "Daughter's Film Embraces Mother's Alzheimer's Life." *San Jose Mercury News*, June 8, 1995, Sec. C, p. 1.

Nicman, N.M. "Journey Into Alzheimer's." *The Washington Post*, Sept. 26, 1995, Sec. Health, p. 11.

Pruchno, Rachel A., and Resch, Nancy L. "Husbands and Wives as Caregivers: Antecedents of Depression and Burden." *The Gerontologist*, 29, No. 2 (1989), pp. 159-165.

Quayhagen, Mary P., and Quayhagen, Margaret. "Alzheimer's Stress: Coping with the Caregiving Role." *The Gerontologist*, 28, No. 3 (1988), pp. 391-396.

Skaff, Marilyn M., and Pearlin, Leonard I. "Caregiving: Role Engulfment and the Loss of Self." *The Gerontologist*, 32, No. 5 (1992), pp. 656-664.

Snyder, Lisa, et al. University of California, San Diego Medical Center. *Home Safety for the Alzheimer's Patient.* n.d.

Strahan, Genevieve W. "An Overview of Home Health and Hospice Care Patients: Preliminary Data from the 1993 National Home and Hospice Care Survey," *Advance Data*, July 22, 1994, p. 1.

Teri, Linda, and Logsdon, Rebecca G. "Identifying Pleasant Activities for Alzheimer's Disease Patients: The Pleasant Events Schedule-AD." *The Gerontologist*, 31, No. 1 (1991), pp. 124-127.

"Third Alzheimer's Gene Discovered," *The Washington Post*, Aug. 18, 1995, Sec. A, p. 6.

U.S. Dept. of Health & Human Services. National Institute on Aging, et al.. *Alzheimer's Disease—A Guide to Federal Programs.* 1993.

————. National Institute on Aging. *Alzheimer's Disease.* 1992.

————. National Institute on Aging. *Alzheimer's Disease and Related Dementias: Legal Issues in Care and Treatment.* 1994.

————. National Institute on Aging. *Caring and Sharing: A Catalog of Training Materials from Alzheimer's Disease Centers.* 1994.

————. National Institute on Aging. *Forgetfulness in Old Age: It's Not What You Think.* 1993.

————. National Institute on Aging. *Multi-Infarct Dementia.* 1993.

————. *Progress Report on Alzheimer's Disease 1994.* 1994.

————. *Research For a New Age.* 1993.

U.S. General Accounting Office. *Long-Term Care: Diverse Growing Population Includes Millions of Americans of All Ages.* Nov. 1994.

Webber, Pamela A., et al. "Living Alone With Alzheimer's Disease: Effects on Health and Social Service Utilization Patterns." *The Gerontologist*, 34, No. 1 (1994), pp. 8-14.

Winogrond, Iris R. "The Relationship of Caregiver Burden and Morale to Alzheimer's Disease Patient Function in a Therapeutic Setting." *The Gerontologist*, 27, No. 3 (1987), pp. 336-339.

Wright, Lore K. "The Impact of Alzheimer's Disease on the Marital Relationship." *The Gerontologist*, 31, No. 2 (1991), pp. 224-237.

Arthritis

ABLEDATA Database of Assistive Technology. *Assistive Devices for People With Arthritis.* ABLEDATA Fact Sheet, March 1992.

Berkow, Robert, ed. *The Merck Manual.* Rahway, NJ: Merck Research Laboratories, 1992.

Cahill, Matthew, ed. *Nurse's Reference Library.* Springhouse, PA: Springhouse Corp., 1987.

Clayman, C.B., ed. *The American Medical Association Encyclopedia of Medicine.* New York: Random House, 1989.

DeMello, Billie, et al. "Arthritis and Aging." In *Our Aging Parents.* Ed. Colette Brown and Roberta-Onzuka-Anderson. Honolulu, HA: Univ. of Hawaii Press, 1985, p. 100.

Galton, Lawrence. "Aches and Pains That Fool the Doctors." *Parade Magazine*, June 19, 1983.

Kozier, Barbara, et al. *Techniques in Clinical Nursing.* Redwood City, CA: Benjamin/Cummings Publishing Co., Inc., 1993.

Peterson, Margaret J. "The Elusive Syndrome Called Myofascial Pain." *New Jersey Rehab*, August 1989.

U.S. Department. of Health and Human Services. National Institute on Aging. *Arthritis Advice.* 1992.

——————. *Arthritis Medicines.* 1992.

Bathing

Cahill, Matthew, ed. *Nurse's Reference Library.* Springhouse, PA: Springhouse Corp., 1987.

Calgon Vestal Laboratories, Inc. *Patient Bathing: Would & Skin Care Protocols.* n.d.

Iowa Program for Assistive Technology. *Cleanliness Is Next To . . . .* n.d.

Kozier, Barbara, et al. *Techniques in Clinical Nursing.* Redwood City, CA: Benjamin/Cummings Publishing Co., Inc., 1993.

Bed Sores

Bates-Jensen, Barbara M., et al. "Validity and Reliability of the Pressure Sore Status Tool." *decubitus*, Nov. 1992.

Bergstrom, N., et al. *Pressure Ulcers in Adults: Prediction and Prevention. Clinical Practice Guideline, No. 3.* AHCPR Pub. No. 92-0047. Rockville, MD: Agency for Health Care Policy and Research, U.S. Dept. of Health & Human Services, Public Health Service, 1992.

——————. *Pressure Ulcers in Adults: Prediction and Prevention. Clinical Practice Guideline. Quick Reference Guide for Clinicians, No. 3.* AHCPR Pub. No. 92-0050. Rockville, MD: Agency for Health Care Policy and Research, U.S. Dept. of Health & Human Services, Public Health Service, 1992.

——————. *Pressure Ulcer Treatment. Clinical Practice Guideline. Quick Reference Guide for Clinicians, No. 15.* AHCPR Pub. No. 95-0653. Rockville, MD: Agency for Health Care Policy and Research, U.S. Dept. of Health and Human Services, Public Health Service, 1994.

——————. *Pressure Ulcer Treatment. Treating Pressure Sores. Consumer Guide, No. 15.* AHCPR Pub. No. 95-0654. Rockville, MD: Agency for Health Care Policy and Research, U.S. Dept. of Health and Human Services, Public Health Service, 1994.

Berkow, Robert, ed. *The Merck Manual.* Rahway, NJ: Merck Research Laboratories, 1992.

Cahill, Matthew, ed. *Nurse's Reference Library.* Springhouse, PA: Springhouse Corp., 1987.

Clayman, C.B., ed. *The American Medical Association Encyclopedia of Medicine.* New York: Random House, 1989.

Kozier, Barbara, et al. *Techniques in Clinical Nursing.* Redwood City, CA: Benjamin/Cummings Publishing Co., Inc., 1993.

Blind

American Foundation for the Blind, et al. *Aging and Vision: Making the Most of Impaired Vision*, 1987.

American Optometric Association. *Answers To Your Questions about Astigmatism.* n.d.

——————. *Answers To Your Questions about Conjunctivitis.* n.d.

——————. *Answers To Your Questions about Diabetes and Your Eyes.* n.d.

——————. *Answers To Your Questions about Farsightedness.* n.d.

——————. *Answers To Your Questions about Glaucoma.* n.d.

——————. *Answers To Your Questions about Nearsightedness.* n.d.

——————. *Answers To Your Questions about Presbyopia.* n.d.

——————. *Answers To Your Questions about Spots and Floaters.* n.d.

American Toy Institute, Inc., et al. *Guide to Toys for Children Who are Blind or Visually Impaired*, 1994.

Dickman, Irving R. *Making Life More Livable.* NY, NY: American Foundation for the Blind, 1985.

"Looking Out for Older Eyes." *Perspectives in Health Promotion and Aging*, 17, No. 2 (1990), p. 1.

U.S. Dept. of Health and Human Services. National Institute on Aging. *Aging and Your Eyes*, 1991.

Brain Tumor

Berkow, Robert, ed. *The Merck Manual.* Rahway, NJ: Merck Research Laboratories, 1992.

Clayman, C.B., ed. *The American Medical Association Encyclopedia of Medicine.* New York: Random House, 1989.

Eastwood, Susan, ed. *The Resource Guide.* National Brain Tumor Foundation. San Francisco, CA, 1994.

Cancer

American Cancer Society. *A Cancer Source Book for Nurses.* 1975.

——————. *Cancer Facts For Men.* 1990.

——————. *Danger—Cigarettes.* 1986.

——————. *Fry Now. Pay Later.* 1994.

——————. *Smart Move! A Stop Smoking Guide.* 1988.

——————. *The Decision Is Yours!* 1986.

——————. *Tick, Tick, Tick.* 1994.

——————. *Why Start a Life Under a Cloud?* 1986.

American Institute for Cancer Research. *Reducing Your Risk of Skin Cancer.* Washington, D.C.: American Institute for Cancer Research, 1992.

Berkow, Robert, ed. *The Merck Manual.* Rahway, NJ: Merck Research Laboratories, 1992.

Blakeman, Mary C. "Gamma Knife Offers Treatment Option To Some Tumor Patients." *Search*, Spring 1995, p. 1.

Bloch, Richard, and Bloch, Annette. *Cancer . . . there's hope.* Kansas City, MO: Bloch Cancer Foundation, Inc., 1981.

Cahill, Matthew, ed. *Nurse's Reference Library.* Springhouse, PA: Springhouse Corp., 1987.

Clayman, C.B., ed. *The American Medical Association Encyclopedia of Medicine.* New York: Random House, 1989.

Jacox, Ada, et al. *Management of Cancer Pain. Clinical Practice Guideline, No. 9.* AHCPR Pub. No. 94-0592. Rockville, MD: Agency for Health Care Policy and Research, U.S. Dept. of Health and Human Services, Public Health Service, 1994.

——————. *Management of Cancer Pain: Adults Quick Reference Guide, No. 9.* AHCPR Pub. No. 94-0593. Rockville, MD: Agency for Health Care Policy and Research, U.S. Dept. of Health and Human Services, Public Health Service, 1994.

——————. *Managing Cancer Pain. Consumer Version, No. 9.* AHCPR Pub. No. 94-0595. Rockville, MD: Agency for Health Care Policy and Research, U.S. Dept. of Health and Human Services, Public Health Service, 1994.

Kozier, Barbara, et al. *Techniques in Clinical Nursing.* Redwood City, CA: Benjamin/Cummings Publishing Co., Inc., 1993.

Morra, Marion, and Potts, Eve. *Choices: Realistic Alternatives in Cancer Treatment.* New York, NY: Avon Books, 1987.

Mullen, Fitzhugh. "Seasons of Survival: Reflections of Physician with Cancer." *New England Journal of Medicine*, 313 (July 25, 1985), pp. 270-273.

National Cancer Institute. National Institute of Dental Research. *What You Need To Know About Oral Cancer.* NIH Pub. No. 93-1574. Bethesda, MD: National Cancer Institute, 1993.

National Cancer Institute. *Testicular Self-Examination*, NIH Pub. No. 90-2636. 1990.

U.S. Dept. of Health and Human Services. National Institute on Aging. *Cancer Facts for People Over 50.* 1992.

——————. National Institute on Aging. *Skin Care and Aging.* 1992.

——————. National Institute on Aging. *Smoking: It's Never Too Late to Stop.* 1991.

Canes & Walkers

American Association of Retired Persons. *Product Report: Walkers*, 1, No. 7 (1991).

Kozier, Barbara, et al. *Techniques in Clinical Nursing.* Redwood City, CA: Benjamin/Cummings Publishing Co., Inc., 1993.

Caregivers

Albert, Steven M. "Caregiving Daughters' Perceptions of Their Own and Their Mothers' Personalities." *The Gerontologist*, 31, No. 4 (1991), pp. 476-482.

American Association of Retired Persons. *A Checklist of Concerns/Resources for Caregivers.* 1987.

——————. *Staying at Home: A Guide to Long-Term Care & Housing.* 1992.

——————. *A Path for Caregivers.* 1994.

Baum, Martha and Page, Mary. "Caregiving and Multigenerational Families." *The Gerontologist*, 31, No. 6 (Dec. 1991), pp. 762-69.

Berkow, Robert, ed. *The Merck Manual.* Rahway, NJ: Merck Research Laboratories, 1992.

Biegel, David E., et al. *Family Caregiving in Chronic Illness.* Newbury Park, CA: Sage Publications, Inc., 1991.

Cahill, Matthew, ed. *Nurse's Reference Library.* Springhouse, PA: Springhouse Corp., 1987.

Clayman, C.B., ed. *The American Medical Association Encyclopedia of Medicine.* New York: Random House, 1989.

Coberly, Sally. *An Employer's Guide to Eldercare.* 1991.

Collins, Clare, et al. "Assessment of the Attitudes of Family Caregivers Toward Community Services." *The Gerontologist*, 31, No. 6 (Dec. 1991), pp. 756-761.

Farran, Carol J., et al. "Finding Meaning: An Alternative Paradigm for Alzheimer's Disease Family Caregivers." *The Gerontologist*, 31, No. 4 (1991), pp. 483-89.

Fradkin, Louise, G., and Health, Angela. *Caregiving of Older Adults.* Santa Barbara: CA, ABC-CLIO, 1992.

Guiterrez-Mayka, Marcela. *Care to the Caregiver in Alzheimer's Disease: A Curriculum Guide.* 1991.

Kozier, Barbara, et al. *Techniques in Clinical Nursing.* Redwood City, CA: Benjamin/ Cummings Publishing Co., Inc., 1993.

Levin, Robert, et al. *Working With the Business Community on Eldercare: A Primer for the Aging Network.* 1990.

Lumsden, Kevin. "Home Care Prepares to Catch Wave of Managed Care, Networking." *Hospitals & Health Networks*, April 5, 1994, p. 58.

Mace, Nancy L., et al. *The 36-Hour Day: A Family Guide to Caring for Persons with Alzheimer's Disease, Related Dementing Illnesses, and Memory Loss in Later Life.* Baltimore, MD: The Johns Hopkins Univ. Press, 1991.

Miller, Baila, and McFall, Stephanie. "Stability and Change in the Informal Task Support Network of Frail Older Persons." *The Gerontologist*, 31, No. 6 (Dec. 1991), pp. 735-45.

Rodvik, Barbara. "Dealing with the Pain of Caregiving." *Nursing Homes*, March-April 1992, p. 39.

Scharlach, Andrew E. "Employment and Caregiver Strain: An Integrative Model." *The Gerontologist*, 31, No. 6 (Dec. 1991), pp. 778-87.

Strawbridge, William J., and Wallhagen, Margaret I. "Impact of Family Conflict on Adult Child Caregivers." *The Gerontologist*, 31, No. 6 (Dec. 1991), pp. 770-77.

Taking Care of Your Elderly Relatives. South Deerfield, MA: Channing L. Bete Co., Inc., 1987.

Watt, Jill, and Calder, Ann. *Taking Care.* North Vancouver, British Columbia: International Self-Counsel Press, Ltd., 1986.

Wheeler, Eugenie G. *Helping Someone Who Doesn't Want Help.* St. Meinrad, IN: Abbey Press, 1992.

Cataract

Berkow, Robert, ed. *The Merck Manual.* Rahway, NJ: Merck Research Laboratories, 1992.

Cahill, Matthew, ed. *Nurse's Reference Library.* Springhouse, PA: Springhouse Corp., 1987.

Cataract Management Guideline Panel. *Cataract in Adults: Management of Functional Impairment. Clinical Practice Guideline, No. 4.* AHCPR Pub. No. 93-0542. Rockville, MD: Agency for Health Care Policy and Research, U.S. Department of Health and Human Services, Public Health Service, 1993.

———. *Cataract in Adults: Management of Cataract in Adults. Clinical Practice Guideline, No. 4. Quick Reference Guide for Clinicians.* AHCPR Pub. No. 93-0543. Rockville, MD: Agency for Health Care Policy and Research, U.S. Department of Health and Human Services, Public Health Service, 1993.

———. *Cataract in Adults: Management of Cataract in Adults. Clinical Practice Guideline, No. 4. Patient's Guide.* AHCPR Pub. No. 93-0544. Rockville, MD: Agency for Health Care Policy and Research, U.S. Department of Health and Human Services, Public Health Service, 1993.

Clayman, C.B., ed. *The American Medical Association Encyclopedia of Medicine.* New York: Random House, 1989.

DiBacco, Thomas V. "The Long View of Cataract Surgery," *The Washington Post*, July 11, 1995, Sec. Health, p. 9.

Checklist

American Medical Association. Dept. of Geriatric Health. *Guidelines for the Use of Assistive Technology: Evaluation, Referral, Prescription.* 1994.

Death

Signs of Approaching Death: Information for the Family. Visiting Nurse's Association Community Hospice, Inc., 1994.

Dental

American Association of Retired Persons. "Program Memo—Hold That Smile!" *Healthy Older People*, 3, No. 1 (April-May 1988).

American Dental Association. *Dental Care for Special People.* 1991.

Clayman, C.B., ed. *The American Medical Association Encyclopedia of Medicine.* New York: Random House, 1989.

Cramer, Denise. "Oral Health Care and Older Adults." *Perspectives in Health Promotion and Aging*, 1, No. 9 (1994), p.1.

Kozier, Barbara, et al. *Techniques in Clinical Nursing.* Redwood City, CA: Benjamin/ Cummings Publishing Co., Inc., 1993.

National Cancer Institute. National Institute of Dental Research. *What You Need To Know About Oral Cancer.* NIH Pub. No. 93-1574. Bethesda, MD: National Cancer Institute, 1993.

National Oral Health Care Information Clearinghouse. *Oral Health Care of Older Adults and Residents in Long-term Care Facilities.* Bethesda, MD: National Institutes of Health, 1994.

———. *Oral Health Care for People with Developmental Disabilities.* Bethesda, MD: National Institutes of Health, 1994.

———. *Special Care in Oral Health.* 1994.

———. *Teaching Guides and Educational Resources on Special Care for the Professional.* Bethesda, MD: National Institutes of Health, 1994.

Rickey, Tom. "Treating Teeth with Laser Light Prevents Caries, Scientists Find." *NIDR Research Digest*, July 1995, p. 2.

Sheridan, Pat. "Financial Stress Linked to Periodontal Disease." *NIDR Research Digest*, July 1995, p. 2.

Tesini, David A. *Developing Dental Education Programs for Persons With Special Needs: A Daily Oral Health Guide for Parents and Staff.* 2nd ed. Boston, MA: MA Dept. of Public Health, 1988.

———. *Developing Dental Education Programs for Persons With Special Needs: A Training and Reference Guide.* 2nd ed. Boston, MA: MA Dept. of Public Health, 1988.

U.S. Department of Health and Human Services. National Institute on Aging. *Taking Care of Your Teeth and Mouth.* 1994.

———. National Institute of Dental Research. *Chemotherapy & Oral Health.* NIH Pub. No. 93-3583. 1993.

———. National Institute of Dental Research. *Diabetes & Periodontal Disease: A Guide for Patients.* NIH Pub. No. 94-2946. Bethesda, MD: National Institutes of Health, n.d.

———. National Institute of Dental Research. *Dry Mouth (Xerostomia).* NIH Pub. No. 91-3174. Bethesda, MD: National Institutes of Health, n.d.

———. National Institute of Dental Research. *Fever Blisters and Canker Sores.* NIH Pub. No. 87-247. Bethesda, MD: National Institutes of Health, 1987.

———. National Institute of Dental Research. *Fluoride to Protect the Teeth of Adults.* NIH Pub. No. 87-2329. Bethesda, MD: National Institutes of Health, 1987.

———. National Institute of Dental Research. *Radiation Therapy & Oral Health.* NIH Pub. No. 93-3584. 1993.

———. National Institute of Dental Research. *Rx for Sound Teeth; Plaque: What It Is and How to Get Rid of It.* NIH Pub. No. 91-3245. Washington, D.C.: GPO, 1991.

———. *What You Need to Know about Periodontal (Gum) Diseases.* NIH Pub. No. 94-1142, n.d.

Depression

Berkow, Robert, ed. *The Merck Manual.* Rahway, NJ: Merck Research Laboratories, 1992.

Cahill, Matthew, ed. *Nurse's Reference Library.* Springhouse, PA: Springhouse Corp., 1987.

Clayman, C.B., ed. *The American Medical Association Encyclopedia of Medicine.* New York: Random House, 1989.

Depression Guideline Panel. *Depression in Primary Care: Volume 1. Detection and Diagnosis. Clinical Practice Guideline, No. 5.* AHCPR Pub. No. 93-0550. Rockville, MD: U.S. Department of Health and Human Services, Public Health Service, Agency for Health Care Policy and Research, 1993.

———. *Depression in Primary Care: Volume 2. Treatment of Major Depression. Clinical Practice Guideline, No. 5.* AHCPR Pub. No. 93-0551. Rockville, MD: U.S. Department of Health and Human Services, Public Health Service, Agency for Health Care Policy and Research, 1993.

———. *Depression in Primary Care: Detection, Diagnosis, and Treatment. Quick Reference Guide for Clinicians, No. 5.* AHCPR Pub. No. 93-0552. Rockville, MD: U.S. Department of Health and Human Services, Public Health Service, Agency for Health Care Policy and Research, 1993.

————. *Depression in Primary Care: Depression Is A Treatable Illness. A Patient's Guide* AHCPR Pub. No. 93-0552. Rockville, MD: U.S. Department of Health and Human Services, Public Health Service, Agency for Health Care Policy and Research, 1993.

U.S. Department of Health and Human Services. National Institute on Aging. *Depression: A Serious but Treatable Illness.* 1992.

————. National Institute on Aging. *Special Report on Aging 1993. Older Americans Can Expect to Live Longer and Healthier Lives.* NIH Pub. No. 93-3409.

————. National Institute of Mental Health. *Depression: What You Need to Know.* Rockville, MD: Public Health Service; Alcohol, Drug Abuse, and Mental Health Administration.

————. Office of Disease Prevention and Health Promotion. "Mental Health Care for the Elderly: Why Bother?" *Program Memo,* 2, No. 5.

Diabetes

American Diabetes Association, Inc. *Balance: Food, Exercise, Medicines.* Basic Information Series No. 6. 1988.

————. *Complications of Diabetes.* 1989.

————. *Diabetes Forecast.* 1993.

————. "Diabetes in Seniors." *Diabetes Facts.* 1993.

————. *Right From the Start. How To Get Started Eating Well.* n.d.

————. *Seniors: Diabetes and You.* 1988.

————. *Standards of Care.* n.d.

————. *What is Non-Insulin-Dependent Diabetes?* 1992.

Berkow, Robert, ed. *The Merck Manual.* Rahway, NJ: Merck Research Laboratories, 1992.

Cahill, Matthew, ed. *Nurse's Reference Library.* Springhouse, PA: Springhouse Corp., 1987.

Clayman, C.B., ed. *The American Medical Association Encyclopedia of Medicine.* New York: Random House, 1989.

"Exercise and Diabetes." *Living Fit.* Parlay International, 1992.

"Diabetes: Health Promotion Can Help in Many Ways." *Perspectives in Health Promotion and Aging,* 7, No. 2 (1992), p. 1.

"Diabetes: Progress in Treatment Improves Patients' Lives." *Inova Regarding Health,* Fall 1995, p. 1.

McCarren, Marie. "Intensive Therapy: It Works." *Diabetes Forecast,* 1993, p. 1.

Novo Nordisk Pharmaceuticals, Inc. *The Glycated Hemoglobin Test.* 1990.

————. *Keeping Well With Diabetes.* 1994.

U.S. Department of Health and Human Services. National Institute on Aging. *Dealing With Diabetes.* 1991.

————. National Institute of Dental Research. *Diabetes & Periodontal Disease: A Guide for Patients.* NIH Pub. No. 94-2946. Bethesda, MD: National Institutes of Health, n.d.

Doctors

First Call. *Guide To Choosing A Physician and Preparing For An Office Visit.*

————. *How Do You Find The Right Doctor . . . Who Accepts Your Insurance?*

U.S. Department of Health and Human Services. National Institute on Aging. *Considering Surgery?* 1991.

————. National Institute on Aging. *Finding Good Medical Care for Older Americans.* 1992.

————. National Institute on Aging. *Talking with Your Doctor: A Guide for Older People.* NIH Pub. No. 94-3452. 1994.

————. National Institute on Aging. *Who's Who in Health Care.* 1991.

Emphysema, Bronchitis, Asthma

About Lungs and Lung Diseases. South Deerfield, MA: Channing L. Bete Co., Inc., 1987.

American Lung Association. *Air Pollution in Your Home?* 1993.

————. *Asthma . . . At My Age?* Washington, D.C.: The National Council on the Aging, Inc., 1993.

————. *The Asthma Handbook.* 1992.

————. *Childhood Asthma: A Matter of Control.* 1994.

————. *Facts about . . . AAT Deficiency-Related Emphysema.* 1989.

————. *Facts about . . . Air Pollution and Your Health.* 1992.

————. *Facts about . . . Asthma.* 1994.

————. *Facts about . . . Chronic Bronchitis.* 1992.

————. *Facts about . . . Dust Diseases.* 1988.

————. *Facts about . . . Emphysema.* 1990.

————. *Facts about . . . Fiberglass.* 1988.

————. *Facts about . . . Lung Cancer.* 1990.

————. *Facts about . . . Home Control of Allergies and Asthma.* 1995.

————. *Facts about . . . How to Keep Your Lungs Healthy.* 1993.

————. *Facts about . . . Occupational Asthma.* 1992.

————. *Facts about . . . Peak Flow Meters.* 1992.

————. *Facts about . . . Pneumonia.* 1992.

————. *Facts about . . . Pulmonary Fibrosis and Interstitial Lung Disease.* 1991.

————. *Facts about . . . Radon: The Health Risk Indoors.* 1989.

————. *Facts about . . . Sarcoidosis.* 1989.

————. *Facts about . . . Sleep Apnea.* 1991.

————. *Facts about . . . The TB Skin Test.* American Lung Association, 1992.

————. *Facts about . . . Tuberculosis.* American Lung Association, 1994.

————. *Pleurisy.* 1984.

————. *Sick Lungs Don't Show.* n.d.

————. *TB—What You Should Know.* 1993.

————. *Using Medicines Wisely.* 1994.

————. *What Everyone Should Know About Asthma.* 1989.

————. *What Everyone Should Know About Emphysema.* 1991.

————. *What You Should Know About Smoking and Cancer.* 1991.

American Lung Association of California, and California Thoracic Society. *What Parents Should Know About Tuberculosis.* n.d.

Berkow, Robert, ed. *The Merck Manual.* Rahway, NJ: Merck Research Laboratories, 1992.

Bowers, Margaret. *Help Yourself to Better Breathing.* American Lung Association, 1991.

Box, Jean, et al. *Helping Your Child with Asthma.* Timonium, MD: American Lung Association of Maryland, 1995.

Boyd, Carol W., et al. *Understanding Lung Medications: How They Work—How to Use Them.* American Lung Association, 1993.

Busse, William W. "What is Asthma?" *Asthma and Allergy Answers.* Washington, D.C. Asthma and Allergy Foundation of America, n.d.

Cahill, Matthew, ed. *Nurse's Reference Library.* Springhouse, PA: Springhouse Corp., 1987.

Clayman, C.B., ed. *The American Medical Association Encyclopedia of Medicine.* New York: Random House, 1989.

How to Use a Nebulizer. Rochester, NY: Fisons Corp., 1992.

Lockey, Richard F., et al. "What is Allergy?" *Asthma and Allergy Answers.* Washington, D.C.: Asthma and Allergy Foundation of America, n.d.

Luce, John M. *Lung Diseases of Adults.* American Lung Association, 1986.

Romanik, Katherine Meek. *Around the Clock with C.O.P.D.* American Lung Association, 1994.

Schultz, Dodi. *Lung Disease Data 1994.* New York, NY: American Lung Association, 1994.

U.S. Consumer Product Safety Commission, et al. *Biological Pollutants in Your Home.* 1993.

————. *What You Should Know About Combustion Appliances and Indoor Air Pollution.* Washington, D.C., 1993.

U.S. Department of Health and Human Services. Office of Disease Prevention and Health Promotion. "Smoking: It's Never Too Late to Quit." *Program Memo,* 4, No. 2 (Feb. 1989).

————. Office of Disease Prevention and Health Promotion. "Community Health Promotion: Where Ideas Become Action." *Program Memo,* 4, No. 1.

Using a Peak Flow Meter . . . What Every Asthma Patient Should Know. Rochester, NY: Fisons Corp., 1992.

Weiss, Jonathan H. *A Practical Approach to the Emotions and Asthma.* American Lung Association, 1990.

White, Martha. *What Everyone Needs to Know About Asthma.* Fairfax, VA: Allergy and Asthma Network/Mothers of Asthmatics, Inc., 1993.

Exercise & Health

Alexandria Hospital. *Two-Minute Hand Break: Stretching Exercises for People Who Work Hard at Their Desks and Computers.* n.d.

————. Department of Physical Medicine. *Bend and Stretch.* Parlay International, 1989.

————. Department of Physical Medicine. *Conditioning Exercise.* Parlay International, 1987.

American Association of Retired Persons. *Pep Up Your Life.* n.d.

American College of Obstetricians and Gynecologists. *Exercise and Fitness: A Guide for Women.* 1992.

———. *Weight Control: Eating Right and Keeping Fit.* 1993.

Clayman, C.B., ed. *The American Medical Association Encyclopedia of Medicine.* New York: Random House, 1989.

"Exercise Can Benefit Everyone." *Perspectives in Health Promotion and Aging,* 6, No. 2 (1991), p. 1.

"It's Never Too Late to Start Exercising—Really!" *Work for Life,* March 1995, p. 3.

Kozier, Barbara, et al. *Techniques in Clinical Nursing.* Redwood City, CA: Benjamin/Cummings Publishing Co., Inc., 1993.

"Making Health Promotion Programs Work." *Perspectives in Health Promotion and Aging,* 6, No. 4 (1991), p. 1.

"Making Health Promotion Work for Minority Elders." *Perspectives in Health Promotion and Aging,* 5, No. 5 (1990), p. 1.

National Dairy Council. *Get Out* There. 1992.

"Older Men: An Overlooked Minority." *Perspectives in Health Promotion and Aging,* 5, No. 4 (1990), p. 1.

"Older Women—Taking Action for Healthier Lives." *Perspectives in Health Promotion and Aging,* 4, No. 5 (Sept.-Oct. 1989), p. 1.

"Putting Prevention into Practice: Using Secondary Prevention for Reducing Disease and Disability." *Perspectives in Health Promotion and Aging,* 7, No. 3 (1992), p. 1.

Proulx, Lawrence G. "Rx Walking." *The Washington Post,* April 11, 1995, Sec. Health, p. 8.

Sharp, Deborah. "Pumping Iron is for Women (Yes, *Women*)." *The Herald,* April 11, 1995, p. 6HN.

"Tertiary Prevention: Essential to Health Promotion for Older Adults." *Perspectives in Health Promotion and Aging,* 7, No. 1 (1992), p. 1.

U.S. Dept. of Health and Human Services. National Institute on Aging. *Don't Take It Easy—Exercise!* 1992.

———. *Sexuality in Later Life.* 1994.

———. "Preventive Services—A Second Line of Defense." *Program Memo,* 3, No. 2 (June-July 1988).

———. Office of Disease Prevention and Health Promotion. "How Fit Are Older Americans?" *Program Memo,* 2, No. 3.

Feet

Clayman, C.B., ed. *The American Medical Association Encyclopedia of Medicine.* New York: Random House, 1989.

"Common Foot Problems: Prevention and Treatment." *Perspectives in Health Promotion and Aging,* 8, No. 2 (1993), p. 1.

"Healthy Feet." *Perspectives in Health Promotion and Aging,* 8, No. 2 (1993), p. 1.

U.S. Dept. of Health and Human Services. National Institute on Aging. *Foot Care.* 1994.

Fever

Alexandria Hospital. "Concerned About a Fever?" *Senior Health Access Newsletter,* Winter 1994-95, p. 4.

Berkow, Robert, ed. *The Merck Manual.* Rahway, NJ: Merck Research Laboratories, 1992.

Cahill, Matthew, ed. *Nurse's Reference Library.* Springhouse, PA: Springhouse Corp., 1987.

Clayman, C.B., ed. *The American Medical Association Encyclopedia of Medicine.* New York: Random House, 1989.

Kozier, Barbara, et al. *Techniques in Clinical Nursing.* Redwood City, CA: Benjamin/Cummings Publishing Co., Inc., 1993.

Financial

American Institute for Cancer Research. *Personal Family & Financial Record Book,* Washington, D.C.: American Institute for Cancer Research, n.d.

Anderson, Teri L. "How to Sell Property When the Owner Has Died." *Law & Realty Notes,* March-April 1995.

Clayman, C.B., ed. *The American Medical Association Encyclopedia of Medicine.* New York: Random House, 1989.

Gerson, David, and Cangro, Charles R. *10 Biggest Estate-Planning Mistakes . . . and How to Avoid Them.* New York, NY: Bottom Line/Personal, n.d.

Kirk, Juanda Morrison. *Caregiving: A Money Management Workbook.* American Association of Retired Persons, 1992.

U.S. Dept. of Health and Human Services. National Institute on Aging. *Getting Your Affairs in Order.* 1992.

Flu

Alexandria Hospital. *Flu & Earaches,* n.d.

Berkow, Robert, ed. *The Merck Manual.* Rahway, NJ: Merck Research Laboratories, 1992.

Clayman, C.B., ed. *The American Medical Association Encyclopedia of Medicine.* New York: Random House, 1989.

U.S. Dept. of Health and Human Services. National Institute on Aging. *What To Do About Flu.* 1994.

Funerals

Doka, Kenneth J. *Life Beyond Loss,* Stamford, NY: Guideline Publications, 1990.

Facts About Funerals Every Family Should Know. Forest Park, IL: Wilbert, Inc., 1989.

Guidelines at Time of Need. Stamford, NY: Guidelines Publications, 1994.

Hospice Council of Metropolitan Washington. *A Guide To Grief.* 1994.

Money & King Funeral Home. *Survivor's Guide,* Springfield, IL: OGR Service Corp., 1989.

Hearing Impaired

American Speech-Language-Hearing Association. *American Speech-Language-Hearing Association Answers Questions About Child Language,* n.p., n.d.

———. *American Speech-Language-Hearing Association Answers Questions About Articulation Problems,* n.p., n.d.

———. *How Does Your Child Hear and Talk?,* n.p., n.d.

———. *Recognizing Communication Disorders,* n.p., n.d.

Battat, Brenda. "Advocacy and Access: 'You Can't Have One Without the Other.'" *SHHH Journal,* Jan.–Feb. 1993, p. 11.

———. "Hard of Hearing People and the Telephone Relay Service." *SHHH Journal,* March-April 1993, p. 24.

———. "The Federal Communications Commission's Role in Regulating Telecommunications Relay Services." *SHHH Journal,* March-April 1993, p. 28.

Beck, L.B. "The 'T' Switch." *Shhh,* Jan.-Feb. 1989, p. 12.

Beck, Lucille. "Are You on the 'T'?" *SHHH Journal,* May–June 1991, p. 24.

Boone, Marjorie. "From Telephone Hate to TT Love." *SHHH Journal,* March-April 1993, p. 21.

———. "Equaling Access to Sound." *Your Church.* Jan.–Feb. 1993, p. 25.

Brown, Jerome D., et al. *Our Forgotten Children: Hard of Hearing Pupils in the School.* Ed. Julia Davis. 1990.

Clayman, C.B., ed. *The American Medical Association Encyclopedia of Medicine.* New York: Random House, 1989.

Compton, Cynthia L. "Comparison of Large-Area Assistive Listening Systems." *SHHH Journal,* Jan.-Feb. 1993, p. 16.

———. "Why Use Assistive Listening Devices?" *SHHH Journal,* Jan.-Feb. 1993, p. 14.

Cruzen, Lydia. "Hospitalized . . . AND Hard of Hearing." *SHHH Journal,* March-April 1991, p. 10.

Cutler, William B. *Audio Induction Loops—What, Why and How.* Bethesda, MD: Self Help for Hard of Hearing People, Inc., 1991.

———. *Large Room Listening Systems for Hard of Hearing People.* Bethesda, MD: Self Help for Hard of Hearing People, Inc., 1991.

———. *Set-Ups for Speeches: A Guide to Optimum Use of ALS and Interpreters.* Bethesda, MD: Self Help for Hard of Hearing People, Inc., 1991.

Davis, Julia, ed. *Our Forgotten Children: Hard-of-Hearing Pupils in the Schools.* Washington, D.C.: U.S. Dept. of Education, 1990.

Gilmore, Robert A. "What Do We Know About Telecoils in Hearing Aids?" *SHHH Journal,* March-April 1994, p. 24.

Harris, Paul M. "Let Them Hear—Communication Access in Houses of Worship." *SHHH Journal,* Jan.-Feb. 1995, p. 8.

Harvey, Michael A. "Dear Mom and Dad: If Only You Had Known." *SHHH Journal,* Sept.-Oct. 1992, p. 4.

Hatley, Ron. "Making a Connection: The Evolution of the Telecommunications Relay Service." *SHHH Journal,* March-April 1993, p. 4.

"Hearing Impairment: The Invisible Loss." *Perspectives in Health Promotion and Aging,* 5, No. 3 (1990), p. 1.

Hospitality for Guests with Hearing Loss: A Guide for Hotel/Motel Compliance with the Americans with Disabilities Act. Bethesda, MD: Self Help for Hard of Hearing People, Inc., 1992.

"How to Buy a Hearing Aid." *Consumer Reports*, Nov. 1992, p. 716.

Kisor, Henry. "Instruments of Freedom: Telephone Accessibility for All!" *SHHH Journal*, March-April 1993, p. 33.

Kozier, Barbara, et al. *Techniques in Clinical Nursing*. Redwood City, CA: Benjamin/ Cummings Publishing Co., Inc., 1993.

Johnson, Michael D., and Fawcett, Stephen B. "Consumer-Defined Standards for Courteous Treatment by Service Agencies." *SHHH*, July-August 1987, p. 6.

Onzuk-Anderson, Roberta. "Vision and Hearing Problems." In *Our Aging Parents*. Ed. Colette Brown and Roberta-Onzuka-Anderson. Honolulu, HA: Univ. of Hawaii Press, 1985, p. 52.

Preves, David A. "A Look at the Telecoil—Its Development and Potential." *SHHH Journal*, Sept.-Oct. 1994, p. 7.

Ross, Mark. "Hearing Aids." *SHHH Journal*, March-April 1994, p. 15.

————. "Update: Telecoils, Audio Loops and Hearing Aids." *SHHH Journal*, May-June 1994, p. 24.

————. "Update: Hearing Aids." *SHHH Journal*, July-August 1994, p. 31.

————. "More on Hearing Aids." *SHHH Journal*, Sept.-Oct. 1994, p. 17.

————. "Developments in Technology." *SHHH Journal*, Nov.-Dec. 1994., p. 25.

————. "Developments in Technology." *SHHH Journal*, Jan.-Fed. 1995, p. 25.

Scherer, Marcia J., and McKee, Barbara G. "What Employers Want to Know About Assistive Technology in the Workplace." *SHHH Journal*, Jan.-Feb. 1993, p. 23.

Self Help for Hard of Hearing People, Inc. "Be In the Know: Your Complete Guide to Terminology About Hearing Loss and Communication Access." *SHHH Journal*, Jan.-Feb. 1993, p. 18.

————. "Beyond the Hearing Aid With Assistive Devices." *SHHH Information Series #251*. Bethesda, MD: Self Help for Hard of Hearing People, Inc., 1994.

————. *Handyman Hints for Hard of Hearing Helps: A Compilation of Suggestions for Economical Assistive Devices*. Bethesda, MD: Self Help for Hard of Hearing People, Inc., 1993.

————. *Technical Assistance Resource Guide*. Bethesda, MD: Self Help for Hard of Hearing People, Inc., n.d.

————. *TV Listening: Some Do-it-Yourself Suggestions for Hard of Hearing People*. Bethesda, MD: Self Help for Hard of Hearing People, Inc., 1989.

Schwartz, Michael A. "State *Parens Patriae* Standing to Sue Under Federal Law: Where's the Beef?" *Net News*, Oct. 1994, p. 2.

Stone, Rocky. "Telecommunications Policy for the Future." *SHHH Journal*, March-April 1993, p. 10.

Stool, Sylvan E., et al. *Managing Otitis Media with Effusion in Young Children. Quick Reference Guide for Clinicians*. AHCPR Pub. No. 94-0623. Rockville, MD: U.S. Dept. of Health and Human Services, Agency for Health Care Policy and Research, Public Health Service, 1994.

————. *Middle Ear Fluid in Young Children. Parent Guide*. AHCPR Pub. No. 94-0624. Rockville, MD: U.S. Dept. of Health and Human Services, Agency for Health Care Policy and Research, Public Health Service, 1994.

"10 Facts About Children at Educational Risk with Hearing Problems." Petaluma, CA: Phonic Ear, Inc., 1994.

Trychel, Marc R. "If I've Heard It Once, I've Heard It A Thousand Times!" *SHHH Journal*, Sept.-Oct. 1990, p. 19.

Ubell, Earl. "New Devices Can Help You Hear." *Parade Magazine*, Jan. 15, 1995, p. 14.

U.S. Dept. of Health and Human Services. National Institute on Aging. National Institute on Deafness and Other Communication Disorders. *Hearing and Older People*. 1991.

Virvan, Barbara. "You Don't Have to Hate Meetings—Try Computer Assisted Notetaking." *SHHH* Journal, Jan.-Feb. 1991, p. 25.

Heart

Alexandria Hospital. *Cardiac Rehabilitation*. Alexandria, VA: Alexandria Hospital, n.d.

————. *Peripheral Vascular Exercise Program*. Alexandria, VA: Alexandria Hospital, 1994.

————. *Preparing for an Angioplasty (PTA) Procedure*. Alexandria, VA: Alexandria Hospital, n.d.

————. *Recognizing the Symptoms of Peripheral Vascular Disease*. Alexandria, VA: Alexandria, 1994.

American Heart Association. *About High Blood Pressure in African-Americans*. Dallas, TX: American Heart Association. 1990.

————. *Cardiopulmonary Resuscitation (CPR)*. Dallas, TX: American Heart Association, 1993.

————. *Controlling Your Risk Factors for Heart Attack*. Dallas, TX: American Heart Association, 1993.

————. *Heart Attack and Stroke: Signals and Action*. Dallas, TX: American Heart Association, 1992.

————. *Nutritious Nibbles*. Dallas, TX: American Heart Association, 1990.

————. *Shopping Smart Easier with New Food Label*. American Heart Association, 1994.

————. *Six Important Facts for a Healthy Heart*. Dallas, TX: American Heart Association, 1979.

————. *Smoking and Heart Disease*. Dallas, TX: American Heart Association, 1992.

————. *Test Your Cholesterol I.Q.* American Heart Association, 1991.

————. *Triglycerides*. Annandale, VA: American Heart Association, 1987.

————. *Weight Control Guidance in Smoking Cessation*. Dallas, TX: American Heart Association, 1985.

————. *Your Heart and Cholesterol*. Dallas, TX: American Heart Association, 1992.

Berkow, Robert, ed. *The Merck Manual*. Rahway, NJ: Merck Research Laboratories, 1992.

Braunwald, Eugene, et al. *Unstable Angina: Diagnosis and Management. Clinical Practice Guideline No. 10* (amended) AHCPR Pub. No. 94-0602. Rockville, MD: Agency for Health Care Policy and Research and the National Heart, Lung, and Blood Institute, Public Health Service, U.S. Dept. of Health and Human Services, 1994.

————. *Unstable Angina: Diagnosing and Managing Unstable Angina. Quick Reference Guide for Clinicians, No. 10* (amended) AHCPR Pub. No. 94-0603. Rockville, MD: Agency for Health Care Policy and Research and the National Heart, Lung, and Blood Institute, Public Health Service, U.S. Dept. of Health and Human Services, 1994.

————. *Unstable Angina: Managing Unstable Angina. Patient and Family Guide. Clinical Practice Guideline, No. 10*. AHCPR Pub. No. 94-0604. Rockville, MD: Agency for Health Care Policy and Research and the National Heart, Lung, and Blood Institute, Public Health Service, U.S. Dept. of Health and Human Services, 1994.

Cahill, Matthew, ed. *Nurse's Reference Library*. Springhouse, PA: Springhouse Corp., 1987.

"Cardiac Rehabilitation." *Rehab Brief*, 13, No. 3 (1990), p. 1.

"Cardiac Rehabilitation Is Often Overlooked, Federal Agency Says." *The Washington Post*, Oct. 11, 1995, Sec. A, p. 3.

Cigarettes and Heart Disease. Parlay International. 1990.

Clayman, C.B., ed. *The American Medical Association Encyclopedia of Medicine*. New York: Random House, 1989.

Controlling Your Cholesterol. Parlay International. 1990.

"Coronary Angioplasty Statistics Prompt Hospital Prescription." *The Washington Post*, Oct. 11, 1995, Sec. A, p. 16.

Coronary Artery Disease. Parlay International. 1990.

Hypertension and Heart Disease. Parlay International. 1990.

Konstam, Marvin A., et al. *Heart Failure: Evaluation and Care of Patients with Left-Ventricular Systolic Dysfunction. Clinical Practice Guideline No. 11*. AHCPR Pub. No. 94-0612. Rockville, MD: Agency for Health Care Policy and Research, Public Health Service, U.S. Dept. of Health and Human Services, 1994.

————. *Heart Failure: Management of Patients with Left-Ventricular Systolic Dysfunction. Quick Reference Guide for Clinicians No. 11*. AHCPR Pub. No. 94-0613. Rockville, MD: Agency for Health Care Policy and Research, Public Health Service, U.S. Dept. of Health and Human Services, 1994.

Kozier, Barbara, et al. *Techniques in Clinical Nursing*. Redwood City, CA: Benjamin/ Cummings Publishing Co., Inc., 1993.

Lancaster, Michael. *Women & Heart Disease*. Walla Walla, WA: Coffey Communications, Inc., 1994.

McNeil, Caroline. *Hearts & Arteries*. NIH Pub. No. 94-3738. National Institute on Aging, Public Health Service, U.S. Dept. of Health and Human Services, 1994.

The Mended Hearts, Inc. *Heart to Heart*. Dallas, TX: The Mended Hearts, Inc., n.d.

Providence Medical Center. *The Heart-Healthy Guide. Information and Recipes for Healthier Living.* Seattle, WA: Providence Medical Center, 1993.

Understanding Heart Attacks—What Can Happen . . . What You Should Do. Parlay International. 1990.

U.S. Dept. of Health and Human Services. *Emergency Department: Rapid Identification and Treatment of Patients with Acute Myocardial Infarction.* National Heart, Lung and Blood Institute, Public Health Service, 1993.

Weighing the Risk—What Excess Weight Does to Your Heart. Parlay International. 1990.

Hip Replacement

Berkow, Robert, ed. *The Merck Manual.* Rahway, NJ: Merck Research Laboratories, 1992.

Cahill, Matthew, ed. *Nurse's Reference Library.* Springhouse, PA: Springhouse Corp., 1987.

Clayman, C.B., ed. *The American Medical Association Encyclopedia of Medicine.* New York: Random House, 1989.

Engh, Charles A, Sr., and Engh, C. Anderson, Jr. *Porous-Coated Total Hip Replacement Patient Information.* n.p., 1994.

Kashner, T. Michael, et al. "Family Size and Caregiving of Aged Patients with Hip Fractures." In *Aging and Caregiving: Theory, Research and Policy.* Ed. David E. Giegel and Arthur Blum. Newbury Park, CA: Sage Publications, Inc., 1990, p. 184.

Kozier, Barbara, et al. *Techniques in Clinical Nursing.* Redwood City, CA: Benjamin/ Cummings Publishing Co., Inc., 1993.

Hiring

"Applicant Disclosure Affidavit." *School Safety,* Spring 1994, pp. 25-26.

Coberly, Sally. *An Employer's Guide to Eldercare.* Washington, D.C.: Washington Business Group on Health, Institute on Aging, Work & Health, 1991.

"Employer Disclosure Affidavit." *School Safety.* Spring 1994, pp. 28-29.

Fallon, Thomas J. "The Basic Do's & Don'ts of Interviewing." *NRCCSA News,* May-June 1995, 5.

Hall, Leonard. "ADA and Worker's Compensation." *Net News,* Oct. 1995, p. 4.

Internal Revenue Service. *Circular E, Employer's Tax Guide.* Pub. No. 15, 1994.

————. *Employee's Withholding Allowance Certificate.* Form W-4, 1995.

————. *Employer's Annual Federal Unemployment (FUTA) Tax Return.* Form 940, 1994.

————. *Instructions for Form 940, Employer's Annual Federal Unemployment (FUTA) Tax Return,* 1994.

————. *Employment Taxes for Household Employers.* Pub. No. 926, 1994.

McGahey, Richard. "Jobs and Crime." *National Institute of Justice Crime File.* Washington, D.C.: U.S. Dept. of Justice, n.d.

Nomani, Asra Q. "Limits Are Eased on Job Questions For the Disabled." *The Wall Street Journal,* Oct. 11, 1995, p. A5.

"Request for Information." *School Safety.* Spring 1994, p. 27.

Rubin, Paula N. "The Americans with Disabilities Act and Criminal Justice: Hiring New Employees." *National Institute of Justice,* Oct. 1994, p. 1.

Virginia State Police. "Criminal History Record Request." 1994.

Home

American Association of Retired Persons. *Staying at Home—A Guide to Long-Term Care and Housing.* 1992.

Belknap, Katherine. *Informed Consumer Guide to Accessible Housing.* Silver Spring, MD: ABLE-DATA Database of Assistive Technology, 1995.

Center for Accessible Housing. *Accessible Stock House Plans.* Raleigh, NC: North Carolina State University, 1993.

Delaware Assistive Technology Initiative and Maryland Technology Assistance Program. *Around the House—Independent Living Tips to Assist with Housecleaning and Storage.* n.p., n.d.

"Future Home is a Smart Idea." *Center for Accessible Housing News,* Dec. 1994, p. 1.

"Glossary: The Language of Home Comfort." *Comfort Zone,* Fall/Winter 1995, p. 15.

Mace, Ronald L. *The Accessible Housing Design File.* New York: Van Nostrand Reinhold, 1991.

National Rehabilitation Information Center. *Home Modification—A NARIC Resource Guide.* KRA Corp., 1994.

Pynoos, Jon, and Cohen, Evelyn. *The Perfect Fit: Creative Ideas for a Safe & Livable Home.* American Association of Retired Persons, 1992.

Rogers, Patricia Dane. "A Father's Gift." *The Washington Post,* March 16, 1995, Sec. Washington Home, p. 12.

————. "Design at Its Most Accommodating." *The Washington Post,* July 13, 1995, Sec. Washington Home, p. 12.

Salmen, John P.S. *The Do-Able Renewable Home.* American Association of Retired Persons, 1991.

"Stair Lifts." *ABLEDATA.* Feb. 1990, p. 1.

"Tune Up Your Home For Fall!" *Comfort Zone.* Fall/Winter 1995, p. 3.

U.S. Dept. of Veterans Affairs. *Handbook for Design: Specially Adapted Housing.* Washington, D.C., 1978.

"Van Lifts." *ABLEDATA.* Nov. 1991, p. 1.

Hospice

Hospice Association of America. *Hospice Facts & Statistics.* Washington, D.C.: Hospice Association of America, 1995.

————. *Information About Hospice.* Washington, D.C.: Hospice Association of America, 1995.

Hospice Council of Metropolitan Washington. *Grief in the Workplace: A Guide for Managers.* n.p., 1994.

————. *Grief in the Workplace: When a Co-Worker is Ill or Dies.* n.p., 1994.

————. *Grief in the Workplace: When a Co-Worker Suffers a Loss.* n.p., 1994.

Hospice of Northern Virginia. *Hope for Today— A Family-Centered Program for Children with Life-Threatening Illness.* Falls Church, VA: Hospice of Northern Virginia, n.d.

————. *Hospice Care for Persons with AIDS.* Falls Church, VA: Hospice of Northern Virginia, n.d.

————. *The Hospice Handbook.* SOC Enterprises, 1994.

————. *Patient Care Volunteer Training Manual.* n.p., n.d.

————. *Volunteer Opportunities.* Falls Church, VA: Hospice of Northern Virginia, n.d.

————. *What is Hospice?* Falls Church, VA: Hospice of Northern Virginia, n.d.

————. *What Will Happen to Me?* Falls Church, VA: Hospice of Northern Virginia, n.d.

National Hospice Organization. *Hospice Fact Sheet.* Arlington, VA: 1995.

Hospital

"America's Best Hospitals." *U.S. News & World Report,* July 18, 1994.

American Association of Retired Persons. *Knowing Your Rights.* Washington, D.C.: American Association of Retired Persons. 1989.

Liptack, Karen. *A Visit to the Emergency Center— An Educational Coloring and Activities Book.* n.p., 1988.

U.S. Dept. of Health and Human Services. *Hospital Hints.* National Institute on Aging, 1990.

U.S. GAO. *Report to Congressional Requesters. Health Care. Employers Urge Hospitals to Battle Costs Using Performance Data Systems.* GAO/HEHS-95-1. Washington, D.C., 1995.

————. *Report to the Ranking Minority Member, Committee on Labor and Human Resources, U.S. Senate. Health Care. Employers and Individual Consumers Want Additional Information on Quality.* GAO/HEHS-95-201. Washington, D.C.: GAO, 1995.

Hot & Cold

Kozier, Barbara, et al. *Techniques in Clinical Nursing.* Redwood City, CA: Benjamin/ Cummings Publishing Co., Inc., 1993.

U.S. Dept. of Health and Human Services. *Heat, Cold, and Being Old.* National Institute on Aging, 1985.

Hypertension

American Heart Association. *About High Blood Pressure.* Dallas, TX: American Heart Association, 1993.

————. *About High Blood Pressure in African-Americans.* Dallas, TX: American Heart Association, 1990.

Berkow, Robert, ed. *The Merck Manual.* Rahway, NJ: Merck Research Laboratories, 1992.

Cahill, Matthew, ed. *Nurse's Reference Library.* Springhouse, PA: Springhouse Corp., 1987.

Clayman, C.B., ed. *The American Medical Association Encyclopedia of Medicine.* New York: Random House, 1989.

"Hypertension and Heart Disease." Parlay International, 1990.

Kozier, Barbara, et al. *Techniques in Clinical Nursing*. Redwood City, CA: Benjamin/Cummings Publishing Co., Inc., 1993.

"Understanding Hypertension—Tips for Blood Pressure Management." Parlay International, 1987.

U.S. Dept. of Health and Human Services. *High Blood Pressure: A Common but Controllable Disorder*. National Institute on Aging, 1994.

Incontinence

Alliance for Aging Research. *Incontinence. Everything You Wanted to Know but Were Afraid to Ask*. n.d.

Berkow, Robert, ed. *The Merck Manual*. Rahway, NJ: Merck Research Laboratories, 1992.

Cahill, Matthew, ed. *Nurse's Reference Library*. Springhouse, PA: Springhouse Corp., 1987.

Clayman, C.B., ed. *The American Medical Association Encyclopedia of Medicine*. New York: Random House, 1989.

"Controlling Urinary Incontinence." *Clinical Bulletin*. National Institute on Aging, n.d.

Fantl, J. Andrew, et al. "Efficacy of Bladder Training in Older Women with Urinary Incontinence." *Journal of the American Medical Association*, 265, No. 5 (Feb. 6, 1991), pp. 609-613.

Kozier, Barbara, et al. *Techniques in Clinical Nursing*. Redwood City, CA: Benjamin/Cummings Publishing Co., Inc., 1993.

"Promoting Continence: Strategies for Success." *Perspectives in Health Promotion and Aging*, 8, No. 1 (1993), p. 1.

Sakado, Aileen, and Talbot, Alice. "Coping with Incontinence." In *Our Aging Parents*. Ed. Colette Brown and Roberta-Onzuka-Anderson. Honolulu, HA: Univ. of Hawaii Press, 1985, p. 134.

Trudeau, Susan Houff. "How to Take Care of Incontinence." *The Washington Times*, March 8, 1995, Sec. C, p. 15.

U.S. Dept. of Health and Human Services. *Constipation*. National Institute on Aging, 1994.

————. *Urinary Incontinence*. National Institute on Aging, 1992.

Urinary Incontinence Guideline Panel. *Urinary Incontinence in Adults: Clinical Practice Guideline*. AHCPR Pub. No. 92-0038. Rockville, MD: Agency for Health Care Policy and Research, Public Health Service, U.S. Dept. of Health and Human Services, 1992.

————. *Urinary Incontinence in Adults: Quick Reference Guide for Clinicians*. AHCPR Pub. No. 92-0041. Rockville, MD: Agency for Health Care Policy and Research, Public Health Service, U.S. Dept. of Health and Human Services, 1992.

————. *Urinary Incontinence in Adults: A Patient's Guide*. AHCPR Pub. No. 92-0040. Rockville, MD: Agency for Health Care Policy and Research, Public Health Service, U.S. Dept. of Health and Human Services, 1992.

"Urinary Incontinence—A Vocabulary." *Clinical Bulletin*. National Institute on Aging, 1992.

Urinary Incontinence in Adults. National Institutes of Health Consensus Development Conference Statement, 7, No. 5 (Oct. 3-5, 1988), p. 1.

Introduction

Cicirelli, Victor G. *Helping Elderly* Parents. Boston, MA: Auburn House Publishing Co. (1981).

Eisenhandler, Susan A. "The Asphalt Identikit: Old Age and the Driver's License." In *Growing Old in America*. Ed. Beth B. Hess and Elizabeth W. Markson. New Brunswick, NJ: Transaction Publishers, 1991, p. 107.

Kamo, Yoshinori. "A Note on Elderly Living Arrangements in Japan and the United States." In *Growing Old in America*. Ed. Beth B. Hess and Elizabeth W. Markson. New Brunswick, NJ: Transaction Publishers, 1991, p. 457.

Wagner, Donna L. "Eldercare: A Workplace Issue." In *Growing Old in America*. Ed. Beth B. Hess and Elizabeth W. Markson. New Brunswick, NJ: Transaction Publishers, 1991, p. 377.

Kidney

Berkow, Robert, ed. *The Merck Manual*. Rahway, NJ: Merck Research Laboratories, 1992.

Cahill, Matthew, ed. *Nurse's Reference Library*. Springhouse, PA: Springhouse Corp., 1987.

Clayman, C.B., ed. *The American Medical Association Encyclopedia of Medicine*. New York: Random House, 1989.

How Well Are Your Kidneys? Princeton, NJ: Bristol-Meyers Squibb, 1994.

Kozier, Barbara, et al. *Techniques in Clinical Nursing*. Redwood City, CA: Benjamin/Cummings Publishing Co., Inc., 1993.

National Kidney Foundation. *About Kidney Stones*. 1994.

————. *About Organ and Tissue Donation*. South Deerfield, MA: Channing L. Bete Co., 1985.

————. *Diabetes and Kidney Disease*. 1994.

————. *Facts About Kidney Disease, Organ Donation and Transplantation in the African American Community*. 1992.

————. *Urinary Tract Infections: A Guide for Women*. n.d.

————. *Your Kidneys: Mater Chemists of the Body*. 1994.

U.S. Dept. of Health and Human Services. *Medicare For People Who Have Permanent Kidney Failure*. Social Security Administration, SSA Pub. No. 05-10013, 1993.

"What Are Kidney Stones? Who Gets Them and Why?" *Healthy Decisions*, Spring 1995, p. 1.

Legal

Landers, Ann. "Dear Ann Landers." *The Washington Post*, July 27, 1995, Sec. D, p. 6.

Shellenbarger, Sue. "Planning Ahead For the Inevitable, An Elder's Illness." *The Wall Street Journal*, March 22, 1995, Sec. B, p. 1.

Tarnove, Lorraine. "Advance Directives: An Important Aspect of Self-Care." *Perspectives in Health Promotion and Aging*, 9, No. 2 (1994), p. 1.

U.S. GAO. *Report to the Ranking Minority Member, Subcommittee on Health, Committee on Ways and Means, House of Representatives. Patient Self-Determination Act. Providers Offer Information on Advance Directives but Effectiveness Uncertain*. GAO/HEHS-95-135. Washington, D.C.: GAO, 1995.

Virginia Hospital Association. *Virginia Advance Medical Directive*. 1992.

————. *Your Right To Decide*. 1993.

Virginia Hospital Association and Medical Society of Virginia. *Durable Power of Attorney for Health Care*. 1991.

————. *Natural Death Act Declaration ("Living Will")*. 1991.

Medicare

American Association of Retired Persons. *Medicare: What It Covers, What It Doesn't*. 1994.

Anderson, Jack and Binstein, Michael. "Medicare's Maddening Maze." *The Washington Post*, Nov. 9, 1992, Sec. D, p. 11.

"Filling Medicare's Gaps." *Car and Travel*, Sept./Oct. 1995, p. 18.

Georges, Christopher. "Republican Plans to Curb Medicaid Spending May Hit Purse Strings of Middle Class Families." *The Wall Street Journal*, Sept. 13, 1995, Sec. A, p. 14.

Hospice of Northern Virginia. *The Hospice Medicare Benefit*. n.p., n.d.

Jaggar, Sarah F. "Medicare. Modern Management Strategies Could Curb Fraud, Waste, and Abuse." Testimony before the Committee on Finance, U.S. Senate. July 31, 1995. GAO/T-HEHS-95-227. Washington, D.C.: GAO, 1995.

Joyner, Carlotta C. "Medicare. Enhancing Health Care Quality Assurance." Testimony before the Subcommittee on Health, Committee on Ways and Means, and the Subcommittee on Health and Environment, Committee on Commerce, House of Representatives. July 27, 1995. GAO/T-HEHS-95-224. Washington, D.C.: GAO, 1995.

Medicare Beneficiaries Defense Fund. *How to Receive the Medicare Home Health Benefit*. New York, NY: Medicare Beneficiaries Defense Fund, 1993.

Moon, Marilyn. "Health Reform." *The Washington Post*, June 27, 1995, Sec. Health, p. 15.

U.S. Dept. of Health and Human Services. *Medicare*. Social Security Administration, SSA Pub. No. 05-10043, 1993.

————. *Medicare For People Who Have Permanent Kidney Failure*. Social Security Administration, SSA Pub. No. 05-10013, 1993.

————. *Medicare Pays for Flu Shots*. Health Care Financing Administration, Pub. No. HCFA-10963, 1994.

————. *Your Medicare Handbook*. Health Care Financing Administration, Pub. No. HCFA-10050, 1995.

U.S. GAO. *High Risk Series. Medicare Claims*. GAO/HR-95-8. Washington, D.C.: GAO, 1995.

————. *Report to Congressional Requesters. Medicare Claims. Commercial Technology Could Save Billions Lost to Billing Abuse*. GAO/AIMD-95-135. Washington, D.C., 1995.

————. *Report to the Ranking Minority Member, Committee on Commerce, House of Representatives. Medicare. Tighter Rules Needed to Curtail Overcharges for Therapy in Nursing Homes*. GAO/HEHS-95-23. Washington, D.C., GAO, 1995.

Menopause

American College of Obstetricians and Gynecologists. *Hormone Replacement Therapy.* 1992.

———. *The Menopause Years.* 1992.

Berkow, Robert, ed. *The Merck Manual.* Rahway, NJ: Merck Research Laboratories, 1992.

Cahill, Matthew, ed. *Nurse's Reference Library.* Springhouse, PA: Springhouse Corp., 1987.

Clayman, C.B., ed. *The American Medical Association Encyclopedia of Medicine.* New York: Random House, 1989.

Hormone Replacement Therapy and Your Health. Philadelphia, PA: Wyeth-Ayerst Laboratories, 1995.

Kaiser, Fran E. "Coping with the Menopause Maze." *Perspectives in Health Promotion and Aging,* 8, No. 3 (1993), p. 4.

Kozier, Barbara, et al. *Techniques in Clinical Nursing.* Redwood City, CA: Benjamin/ Cummings Publishing Co., Inc., 1993.

Squires, Sally. "The Hormone Replacement Plot Thickens." *The Washington Post,* June 20, 1995, Sec. Health, p. 7.

Understanding Menopause. The Change of Life. Marietta, GA: Solvay Pharmaceuticals. n.d.

U.S. Dept. of Health and Human Services. National Institute on Aging. *Managing Menopause.* 1992.

———. *Should You Take Estrogen?* 1988.

What Women Should Know About . . . Menopause. Parlay International. 1989.

Mental Illness

Berkow, Robert, ed. *The Merck Manual.* Rahway, NJ: Merck Research Laboratories, 1992.

Cahill, Matthew, ed. *Nurse's Reference Library.* Springhouse, PA: Springhouse Corp., 1987.

Clayman, C.B., ed. *The American Medical Association Encyclopedia of Medicine.* New York: Random House, 1989.

Multiple Sclerosis

Berkow, Robert, ed. *The Merck Manual.* Rahway, NJ: Merck Research Laboratories, 1992.

Cahill, Matthew, ed. *Nurse's Reference Library.* Springhouse, PA: Springhouse Corp., 1987.

Clayman, C.B., ed. *The American Medical Association Encyclopedia of Medicine.* New York: Random House, 1989.

Schapiro, Randall T., and Multiple Sclerosis Association of America. *Understanding Multiple Sclerosis.* 1991.

U.S. Dept. of Health and Human Services. National Institutes of Health. *Multiple Sclerosis.* NIH Pub. No. 90-3015. 1990.

Wells, Susan. "When MS Enters the Family." *Motivator,* June 1995, p. 6.

Weinreb, Herman J. "Treating Spasticity with Intrathecal Baclofen." *Motivator,* Winter 1995, p. 7.

Nursing

Cahill, Matthew, ed. *Nurse's Reference Library.* Springhouse, PA: Springhouse Corp., 1987.

Kozier, Barbara, et al. *Techniques in Clinical Nursing.* Redwood City, CA: Benjamin/ Cummings Publishing Co., Inc., 1993.

What to Look for When You're Choosing an In-Home Health Agency. Alzheimer's Disease and Related Disorders Association, Inc., n.d.

Visiting Nurse Association of Northern Virginia. *Patient Information Guide.* 1994.

———. *Your Right To Decide—Communicating Your Health Care Choices.* 1991.

Nursing Home

Alternatives to Restraint Use. Washington, D.C.: National Citizens' Coalition for Nursing Home Reform, n.d.

American Association of Retired Persons. *Care Management: Arranging for Long Term Care.* 1992.

———. *Making Wise Decisions for Long-Term Care.* 1991.

———. *Nursing Home Life: A Guide for Residents and Families.* 1993.

How to Select a Nursing Center. Manor HealthCare, 1994.

Manning, Doug. *When Love Gets Tough.* Hereford, TX: In-Sight Books, Inc., 1983.

Reduction of Chemical and Physical Restraint Use. Washington, D.C.: National Citizens' Coalition for Nursing Home Reform, n.d.

Sharp, Anne. "For Easier and Happier Nursing Home Visits." *Work & Family Life,* June 1995, p. 3.

U.S. Dept. of Health and Human Services. National Institute on Aging. *When You Need a Nursing Home.* 1992.

———. National Institutes of Health. *Long-term Care for Older Adults.* Bethesda, MD: 1994.

U.S. GAO. *Report to the Ranking Minority Member, Committee on Commerce, House of Representatives. Medicare. Tighter Rules Needed to Curtail Overcharges for Therapy in Nursing Homes.* GAO/HEHS-95-23. Washington, D.C., GAO, 1995.

Wade-Farber, Farlee. "Activity Professionals: Not Just 'Fun and Games.'" *Quality Care Advocate.* March-April 1995, p. 6.

Zachary, G. Pascal. "Nursing Homes Are Often Hotbeds of Injury for Aides." *The Wall Street Journal,* March 20, 1995, Sec. B, p. 1.

Nutrition

American Cancer Society. *Eat Smart.* 1989.

———. *Eat to Live!* 1986.

———. *Taking Control.* 1985.

American College of Obstetricians and Gynecologists. *Cholesterol and Your Health.* 1993.

———. *Weight Control: Eating Right and Keeping Fit.* 1993.

American Institute for Cancer Research. *Dietary Guidelines to Lower Cancer Risk.* 1990.

Cahill, Matthew, ed. *Nurse's Reference Library.* Springhouse, PA: Springhouse Corp., 1987.

Clayman, C.B., ed. *The American Medical Association Encyclopedia of Medicine.* New York: Random House, 1989.

Cooking with Less Fat. Parlay International. 1990.

Delaware Assistive Technology Initiative and Maryland Technology Assistance Program. *"What's for Dinner?"* n.p., n.d.

"Eating Well: An Important Part of Cancer Treatment." *Inova Health System.* Spring 1995, p. 3.

Fat Percentage Calculator. Parlay International. 1990.

"Good Nutrition: Good for Your Health at Any Age." *Perspectives in Health Promotion and Aging,* 6, No. 1 (1991), p. 1.

Hurley, Jane, and Schmidt, Stephen. "Salty Snacks—Letting the Chips Fall." *Nutrition Action Healthletter,* Nov. 1993, p. 8.

Kozier, Barbara, et al. *Techniques in Clinical Nursing.* Redwood City, CA: Benjamin/ Cummings Publishing Co., Inc., 1993.

National Center for Nutrition and Dietetics. *The ABCs of Fats, Oils and Cholesterol.* 1994.

National Dairy Council. *How Significant are Your "Others"?* 1992.

Nowlan, Mary H., and Hiser, Elizabeth. "The Hungry Mind." *Eating Well,* May-June 1995, p. 28.

"Nutrition Facts." *Food Technology,* Feb. 1993, p. 83.

Osman, J.D. *Hints to Decrease Total Caloric Intake—Thin from Within.* 1988.

Squires, Sally. "A Picnic's Toxic Punch—Food Poisoning is a Hot Weather Hazard." *The Washington Post,* July 4, 1995, Sec. Health, p. 9.

———. "Is Mayonnaise Really So Bad?" *The Washington Post,* July 4, 1995, Sec. Health, p. 9.

U.S. Dept. of Agriculture. Human Nutrition Information Service. *Food Facts for Older Adults.* 1993.

———. *The Food Guide Pyramid.* 1992.

U.S. Dept. of Health and Human Services. National Institute on Aging. *Be Sensible About Salt.* 1991.

———. *Dietary Supplements: More Is Not Always Better.* 1993.

———. *Hints for Shopping, Cooking, and Enjoying Meals.* 1993.

———. *Nutrition: A Lifelong Concern.* 1991.

———. Public Health Service. *Diet, Nutrition & Cancer Prevention: The Good News.* 1986.

———. Public Health Service. *Progress Report for: Nutrition.* 1994.

Wootan, Margo, and Liebman, Bonnie. "The Great *Trans* Wreck." *Nutrition Action Newsletter,* Nov. 1993, p. 10.

Osteoporosis

American College of Obstetricians and Gynecologists. *Preventing Osteoporosis.* 1993.

Berkow, Robert, ed. *The Merck Manual.* Rahway, NJ: Merck Research Laboratories, 1992.

Cahill, Matthew, ed. *Nurse's Reference Library.* Springhouse, PA: Springhouse Corp., 1987.

Clayman, C.B., ed. *The American Medical Association Encyclopedia of Medicine.* New York: Random House, 1989.

Franklin, Mary B. "'It's Not Your Grandmother's Disease.'" *The Washington Post,* April. 25, 1995, Sec. Health, p. 9.

————. "New Hope for Osteoporosis Sufferers? *The Washington Post*, April. 25, 1995, Sec. Health, p. 8.

National Dairy Board. *Dairy Calcium for Women of All Ages.* 1990.

U.S. Dept. of Health and Human Services. National Institute on Aging. *Osteoporosis: The Bone Thinner.* 1992.

What Women Should Know About . . . Osteoporosis. Parlay International. 1989.

Pain

Batten, Mary. "Take Charge of Your Pain." *Modern Maturity,* Jan.-Feb. 1995, p. 35.

Berkow, Robert, ed. *The Merck Manual.* Rahway, NJ: Merck Research Laboratories, 1992.

Bigos, Stanley J., et al. *Acute Low Back Problems in Adults.* Clinical Practice Guideline. Quick Reference Guide No. 14. AHCPR Pub. No. 95-0643. Rockville, MD: U.S. Dept. of Health and Human Services, Public Health Service, Agency for Health Care Policy and Research. 1994.

————. *Acute Low Back Problems in Adults. Understanding Acute Low Back Problems.* Clinical Practice Guideline. Consumer Version No. 14. AHCPR Pub. No. 95-0644. Rockville, MD: Agency for Health Care Policy and Research, Public Health Service. 1993.

Cahill, Matthew, ed. *Nurse's Reference Library.* Springhouse, PA: Springhouse Corp., 1987.

Carr, Daniel B., et al. *Acute Pain Management: Operative or Medical Procedures and Trauma. Clinical Practice Guideline No. 1.* AHCPR Pub. No. 92-0032. Rockville, MD: Agency for Health Care Policy and Research, Public Health Service, U.S. Dept. of Health and Human Services. 1992.

Clayman, C.B., ed. *The American Medical Association Encyclopedia of Medicine.* New York: Random House, 1989.

Disc Facts and Fallacies. Parlay International. 1990.

Kozier, Barbara, et al. *Techniques in Clinical Nursing.* Redwood City, CA: Benjamin/ Cummings Publishing Co., Inc., 1993.

Low Back Pain—A Modern Epidemic. Parlay International. 1990.

U.S. Dept. of Health and Human Services. Acute Pain Management Guideline Panel. *Acute Pain Management in Adults: Operative Procedures. Quick Reference Guide for Clinicians.* AHCPR Pub. No. 92-0019. Rockville, MD: Agency for Health Care Policy and Research, Public Health Service. 1993.

————. *Pain Management in Infants, Children, and Adolescents: Operative and Medical Procedures. Quick Reference Guide for Clinicians.* AHCPR Pub. No. 92-0020. Rockville, MD: Agency for Health Care Policy and Research, Public Health Service. 1993.

————. *Pain Control After Surgery. A Patient's Guide.* AHCPR Pub. No. 92-0021. Rockville, MD: Agency for Health Care Policy and Research, Public Health Service. 1992.

————. National Institute of Nursing Research. *Symptom Management: Acute Pain. A Report of the NINR Priority Expert Panel on Symptom Management: Acute Pain.* Bethesda, MD: National Institutes of Health. 1994.

Parkinson's Disease

Berkow, Robert, ed. *The Merck Manual.* Rahway, NJ: Merck Research Laboratories, 1992.

Cahill, Matthew, ed. *Nurse's Reference Library.* Springhouse, PA: Springhouse Corp., 1987.

Clayman, C.B., ed. *The American Medical Association Encyclopedia of Medicine.* New York: Random House, 1989.

The Parkinson's Patient: What you and your family should know. National Parkinson Foundation. n.d.

U.S. Dept. of Health and Human Services. National Institute on Aging. *Don't Take It Easy— Exercise!* 1992.

Personal Data

Allee, Virginia. "A Family History Questionnaire." *Family Heritage,* Oct. 1978, p. 152.

American Association of Retired Persons. *A Checklist of Concerns/Resources for Caregivers.* 1987.

————. *Miles Away & Still Caring.* 1994.

Anders, George, and Winslow, Ron. "The HMO Trend: Big, Bigger, Biggest." *The Wall Street Journal,* March 30, 1995, Sec. B, p. 1.

Dickerson, John F. "Never Too Old." *Time,* Spring 1995, p. 41.

Maximizing Deductions For Business Travel, Entertainment, Meals, and Automobiles. Swartz Retson. 1994.

Pills & Shots

Boodman, Sandra G. "Bad Reactions to Drugs Linked to Human Error." *The Washington Post,* July 11, 1995, Sec. Health, p. 7.

Cahill, Matthew, ed. *Nurse's Reference Library.* Springhouse, PA: Springhouse Corp., 1987.

Kozier, Barbara, et al. *Techniques in Clinical Nursing.* Redwood City, CA: Benjamin/ Cummings Publishing Co., Inc., 1993.

"Over-the-Counter Medication Basics." *Perspectives in Health Promotion and Aging,* 5, No. 1 (1990), p. 5.

"Safe Use of Medications: A Consumer Issue." *Perspectives in Health Promotion and Aging,* 5, No. 1 (1990), p. 1.

"10 Questions to Ask About All Medications." *Medizine Guidebook for Mature Adults.* 1995, p. 17.

U.S. Dept. of Health and Human Services. National Institute on Aging. *The Pneumonia Vaccine—It's a One-Shot Deal.* 1993.

————. *Safe Use of Medicines by Older People.* 1982.

————. *"Shots" for Safety.* 1988.

"Update: Current Issues in the Safe Use of Medications—How Safe Are Generic Drugs?"

Healthy Older People, 2, No. 2, p. 5.

Prostate

American Institute for Cancer Research. *Reducing Your Risk of Prostate Cancer.* 1994.

Boodman, Sandra G. "Self-Interest Yields High Profile on Hill." *The Washington Post,* May 23, 1995, Sec. Health, p. 20.

Campbell, John C. "Treatment 'Is as Personal as It Is Medical.'" *The Washington Post,* May 23, 1995, Sec. Health, p. 24.

Colburn, Don. "Cancer More Common, Virulent Among Blacks." *The Washington Post,* May 23, 1995, Sec. Health, p. 21.

————. "Prostate Woes Demand Educated Guesswork." *The Washington Post,* May 23, 1995, Sec. Health, p. 5.

————. "The PSA Test: Too Much of a Good Thing?" *The Washington Post,* May 23, 1995, Sec. Health, p. 8.

Harkin, J.W. "'I Had the Classic Symptoms.'" *The Washington Post,* May 23, 1995, Sec. Health, p. 25.

Herman, Robin. "Benign Growth Is a Price of Longevity." *The Washington Post,* May 23, 1995, Sec. Health, p. 22.

McConnell, John D., et al. *Benign Prostatic Hyperplasia: Diagnosis and Treatment. Clinical Practice Guideline, No. 8.* AHCPR Pub. No. 94-0582. Rockville, MD: Agency for Health Care Policy and Research, Public Health Service, U.S. Dept. of Health and Human Services. 1994.

————. *Benign Prostatic Hyperplasia: Diagnosis and Treatment. Quick Reference Guide for Clinicians.* AHCPR Pub. No. 94-0583. Rockville, MD: Agency for Health Care Policy and Research, Public Health Service, U.S. Dept. of Health and Human Services. 1994.

"Prostate Cancer: Prevention, Treatment, Support." *Inova Regarding Health,* Summer 1995, p. 10.

Squires, Sally. "How Wives Are Affected by Spouse's Cancer." *The Washington Post,* May 23, 1995, Sec. Health, p. 19.

Trafford, Abigail. "A Symbol of Evolution In Our Views on Illness." *The Washington Post,* May 23, 1995, Sec. Health, p. 18.

U.S. Dept. of Health and Human Services. National Institute on Aging. *Prostate Problems.*

Weiss, Rick. "After a Diagnosis of Cancer, Then What?" *The Washington Post,* May 23, 1995, Sec. Health, p. 11.

————. "Controversy Surrounds Marketing of PSA Test." *The Washington Post,* May 23, 1995, Sec. Health, p. 9.

————. "Little Is Known About Causes." *The Washington Post,* May 23, 1995, Sec. Health, p. 17.

————. "Sex Problems Can Be Treated." *The Washington Post,* May 23, 1995, Sec. Health, p. 17.

Respite Care

American Association of Retired Persons. *A Profile of Older Americans.* 1994.

Davis, Patricia. "Seeking a Carefree Vacation." *The Washington Post,* Sec. B, p. 1.

U.S. Dept. of Health and Human Services. National Institute on Aging. *Aging Research: Practice, Promise & Priorities.* NIH Pub. No. 94-3696. 1994.

————. *Health Quackery.* 1994.

————. *In Search of the Secrets of Aging.* NIH Pub. No. 93-2756. 1993.

————. *Life Extension: Science or Science Fiction?* 1994.

Sickle Cell Anemia

Berkow, Robert, ed. *The Merck Manual.* Rahway, NJ: Merck Research Laboratories, 1992.

Cahill, Matthew, ed. *Nurse's Reference Library.* Springhouse, PA: Springhouse Corp., 1987.

Clayman, C.B., ed. *The American Medical Association Encyclopedia of Medicine.* New York: Random House, 1989.

Sickle Cell Disease Guideline Panel. *Sickle Cell Disease. Comprehensive Screening and Management in Newborns and Infants. Clinical Practice Guideline No. 6.* AHCPR Pub. No. 93-0563. Rockville, MD: Agency for Health Care Policy and Research, Public Health Service, U.S. Dept. of Health and Human Services. 1993.

———. *Sickle Cell Disease in Newborns and Infants. A Guide for Parents.* AHCPR Pub. No. 93-0564. Rockville, MD: Agency for Health Care Policy and Research, Public Health Service, U.S. Dept. of Health and Human Services. 1993.

———. *Sickle Cell Disease: Screening, Diagnosis, Management, and Counseling in Newborns and Infants. Clinical Practice Guideline No. 6.* AHCPR Pub. No. 93-0562. Rockville, MD: Agency for Health Care Policy and Research, Public Health Service, U.S. Dept. of Health and Human Services. 1993.

Sleep Disorders

"Life-Threatening Sleep Apnea Treatable." *Health Focus,* Winter 1994.

Report of the National Commission on Sleep Disorders Research. *Wake Up America: A National Sleep Alert.* 1993.

U.S. Dept. of Health and Human Services. National Institute on Aging. *A Good Night's Sleep.* 1990.

When You Can't Sleep—ABCs of ZZZs. Washington, D.C.: National Sleep Foundation. 1994.

Why We Should Care About Sleep. Alexandria Hospital. n.d.

Social Security

U.S. Dept. of Health and Human Services. Social Security Administration. *Household Workers.* SSA Pub. No. 05-10021. 1995.

———. *How Your Retirement Benefit Is Figured.* SSA Pub. No. 05-10070. 1995.

———. *Request for Earnings and Benefit Estimate Statement.* SSA Form No. SSA-7004-SM-OP1. 1995.

———. *Reviewing Your Disability.* SSA Pub. No. 05-10068. 1995.

———. *Social Security and SSI Benefits for Children with Disabilities.* SSA Pub. No. 05-10026. 1993.

———. *Social Security and Your Right to Representation.* SSA Pub. No. 05-10075. 1992.

———. *When You Get Social Security Disability Benefits.* SSA Pub. No. 05-10153. 1994.

———. *Your Social Security Number.* SSA Pub. No. 05-10002. 1993.

U.S. GAO. *Report to the Chairman, Committee on Finance, U.S. Senate, and the Chairman, Committee on Ways and Means, House of Representatives. Supplemental Security Income. Growth and Changes in Recipient Population Call for Reexamining Program.* GAO/HEHS-95-137. Washington, D.C.: GAO, 1995.

Stress

Clayman, C.B., ed. *The American Medical Association Encyclopedia of Medicine.* New York: Random House, 1989.

Coping with a Serious Loss. Parlay International. 1992.

Getting Past Anger. Parlay International. 1992.

Kozier, Barbara, et al. *Techniques in Clinical Nursing.* Redwood City, CA: Benjamin/Cummings Publishing Co., Inc., 1993.

Laugh—It's Good for You. Parlay International. 1992.

Letting Go of Worry and Anxiety. Parlay International. 1992.

Sheridan, Pat. "Financial Stress Linked to Periodontal Disease." *NIDR Research Digest,* July 1995, p. 2.

U.S. Dept. of Health and Human Services. *Safe Use of Tranquilizers.* 1989.

Stroke

American Heart Association. *Facts About Stroke.* 1992.

Berkow, Robert, ed. *The Merck Manual.* Rahway, NJ: Merck Research Laboratories, 1992.

Neurath, Otto, et al. "Stroke and the Older Adult." In *Our Aging Parents.* Ed. Colette Brown and Roberta-Onzuka-Anderson. Honolulu, HA: Univ. of Hawaii Press, 1985, p. 118.

Stroke. National Rehabilitation Information Center. March 1994.

U.S. Dept. of Health and Human Services. National Institute on Aging. National Heart, Lung, and Blood Institute. *Stroke: Prevention and Treatment.* 1991.

Transportation & Travel

American Automobile Association. *Disabled Driver's Mobility Guide.* 1995.

Americans with Disabilities Act of 1990 (42 USC §§12101 et seq.)

Kaye, Ira. "Transportation Problems of the Older American." In *The Neglected Older American.* Ed. Charles C. Thomas. Springfield, IL, 1973.

National Restaurant Association. *Americans with Disabilities Act. Answers for Foodservice Operators.* 1992.

Nelson, Beverly. "Tips for the Disabled Traveler." *AAA World,* Sept.-Oct. 1992, p. 26.

Packing Smart. Southwest Airlines. 1994.

U.S. Equal Employment Opportunity Commission and U.S. Dept. of Justice, Civil Rights Division. *The Americans with Disabilities Act—Questions and Answers.* 1992.

Wheelchairs

American Association of Retired Persons. *Product Report: Wheelchair.* 1990.

Belknap, Katherine. "Wheelchairs for Children." *ABLEDATA Database of Assistive Technology,* Fact Sheet No. 22, April 1994, p. 1.

Bryant, Lynn, and Belknap, Katherine. "Informed Consumer Guide to Wheelchair Selection." *ABLEDATA Database of Assistive Technology,* May 1994, p. 1.

———. "Manual Wheelchairs." *ABLEDATA Database of Assistive Technology,* Fact Sheet No. 23, July 1994, p. 1.

———. "Powered Wheelchairs." *ABLEDATA Database of Assistive Technology,* Fact Sheet No. 24, July 1994, p. 1

Cahill, Matthew, ed. *Nurse's Reference Library.* Springhouse, PA: Springhouse Corp., 1987.

Kaplan, Richard S. "Physicians and Assistive Technology: A Practical Spectrum from 'Low Tech' to 'High Tech.'" *Tapping Technology,* Sept. 1995, p. 2.

Kozier, Barbara, et al. *Techniques in Clinical Nursing.* Redwood City, CA: Benjamin/Cummings Publishing Co., Inc., 1993.

"Patient Lifts." *ABLEDATA,* Fact Sheet No. 9, April 1990, p. 1.

Sources for Health Information

	Telephone
AIDS	
Centers for Disease Control and Prevention	
National AIDS Clearinghouse	1-800-458-5231
English Hotline	1-800-342-2437
TTY	1-800-243-7012
Spanish Hotline	1-800-344-7432
Names Project Foundation	1-415-882-5500
National Gay and Lesbian Task Force	1-202-332-6483
National Native American AIDS Prevention Center	1-800-283-2437
ALCOHOL	
American Council for Drug Education	1-800-488-3784
Al-Anon Family Group Headquarters	1-800-356-9996
National Council on Alcoholism	1-800-622-2255
ALZHEIMER S DISEASE	
Alzheimer's Association	1-800-272-3900
Alzheimer's Disease Education and Referral Center	1-800-438-4380
Alzheimer's Disease and Related Disorders Association, Inc.	1-312-335-8700
TTY	1-312-335-8882
Alzheimer's Safe Return Program	1-800-272-3900
ARTHRITIS	
Arthritis Foundation	1-800-283-7800
National Institute of Aging	1-800-222-2225
BRAIN TUMORS	
American Brain Tumor Association	1-800-886-2282
National Brain Tumor Foundation	1-800-934-2873
Wellness Community Headquarters	1-310-314-2555
National Neurofibromatosis Foundation	1-800-323-7938
National Familial Brain Tumor Registry, The Johns Hopkins Oncology Center	1-410-955-0227
CANCER	
The American Cancer Society	1-800-227-2345
American Cancer Institute	1-800-422-6237
American Institute for Cancer Research	1-800-843-8114
National Association of Professional Geriatric Care Managers	1-520-881-8008
CATARACTS	
National EyeCare Project Helpline	1-800-222-3937

	Telephone
DENTAL	
National Oral Health Information Clearing House	1-301-402-7364
National Institute of Dental Research . . .	1-301-496-4261
National Dental Association	1-202-244-7555
DEPRESSION	
National Depressive and Manic-Depressive Association	1-800-826-3632
National Alliance for the Mentally Ill . . .	1-800-950-6264
National Mental Health Association	1-800-969-6642
DIABETES	
National Diabetes Information Clearing House	1-301-654-3327
The American Diabetes Association	1-800-232-3472
DOCTORS	
American Medical Association	1-312-464-5000
Medicare Hotline	1-800-638-6833
ELDERCARE	
Eldercare Locator	1-800-677-1116
HEART	
American Heart Association	1-800-242-8721
The Coronary Club, Inc.	1-216-444-3690
National Heart, Lung and Blood Institute Information Center	1-301-251-1222
National Institute on Aging	1-800-222-2225
The Mended Hearts, Inc.	1-214-373-6300
International Society on Hypertension in Blacks, Inc.	1-404-875-6263
HEARING	
American Academy of Otolaryngology Head & Neck Surgery	1-703-836-4444
National Information Center on Deafness, Gallaudet University	1-202-651-5051
TTY	1-202-651-5052
Self Help for Hard of Hearing People . . .	1-301-657-2248
HEAT STROKE & HYPOTHERMIA	
National Institute on Aging	1-800-222-3937
HOSPICE	
Hospice Association of America	1-800-658-8898
Hospice Alliance	1-800-545-0522
National Hospice Organization	1-800-338-8619
HOSPITAL	
Joint Commission on Accreditation of Health Care Organization	1-708-916-5800
National Association of Professional Geriatric Care Managers	1-520-881-8008

INCONTINENCE

	Telephone
Help for Incontinent People	1-800-252-3337
National Association of Professional Geriatric Care Managers	1-520-881-8008

KIDNEY

National Kidney Foundation	1-800-622-9010

LUNGS

Allergy and Asthma Association	1-800-727-8462
American Lung Association	1-800-586-4872
National Association of Professional Geriatric Care Managers	1-520-881-8008

MENOPAUSE

National Institute on Aging	1-800-222-2225
The American College of Obstetricians and Gynecologists	1-202-638-5577

MENTAL ILLNESS

National Alliance for the Mentally Ill . . .	1-800-950-6264
American Mental Health Fund	1-800-433-5959

MULTIPLE SCLEROSIS

Multiple Sclerosis Association of America	1-800-833-4672
National Association of Professional Geriatric Care Managers	1-520-881-8008

NURSING

American Nurses Association	1-800-274-4262

NURSING HOMES

National Citizens Coalition for Nursing Home Reform	1-202-332-2275
American Association of Retired Persons	1-202-434-2277
National Council of Senior Citizens	1-202-347-8800

NUTRITION

Human Nutrition Information Service . . .	1-301-436-5724
National Institute on Aging	1-800-222-2225

OSTEOPOROSIS

National Osteoporosis Foundation	1-202-223-2226
American Society for Bone and Mineral Research	1-202-857-1161
Older Women s League	1-800-825-3695
National Institute on Aging	1-800-222-2225

PARKINSON S DISEASE

National Parkinson's Foundation Hotline	1-800-327-4545

PILLS & SHOTS

National Institute on Drug Abuse	1-800-662-4357

PROSTATE

American Cancer Society	1-800-227-2345
National Cancer Institute	1-800-422-6237

SICKLE CELL ANEMIA

	Telephone
American Medical Association	1-312-464-5000
U.S. Department of Health and Human Services	1-301-443-2403

SLEEP DISORDERS

Sleep Disorders Center	1-703-504-3220
National Sleep Foundation	1-202-785-2300

SOCIAL SECURITY

Social Security Office	1-202-347-8800

STRESS & HEADACHES

National Headache Foundation	1-800-843-2256

STROKE

The National Institute of Neurological Disorders and Stroke	1-800-352-9424
The National Stroke Association	1-800-787-6537
National Rehabilitation Information Center	1-800-347-2742

TRANSPORTATION & TRAVEL

Chrysler's Automobility Program	1-800-255-9877
Ford Motor Mobility Motoring	1-800-952-2248
Greyhound Lines, Inc.	1-800-231-2222
TTY	1-800-345-3109
Amtrak	1-800-872-7245
TTY	1-800-523-6590
National Mobility Equipment Dealers Association	1-800-833-0427
General Motors Corp. GM Mobility Assistance Center	1-800-323-9935

VISION

American Foundation for the Blind	1-800-232-5463
National Society to Prevent Blindness . . .	1-800-221-3004
Library of Congress, National Library Services for the Blind and Physically Handicapped	1-800-424-8567
TTY	1-800-523-6590

Index

Order Form

LeBoeuf's
The only source you need to be a caregiver in the home

768 Walker Road, Suite 266 • Great Falls, VA 22066
1-800-546-5559 VOICE
1-800-855-2880 TTY   **1-800-233-9692** FAX

Order Date	Customer Number

Ordered by / Bill to:

Name

Address

City

State   Zip Code

DAYTIME
Phone   (   )   n Voice n TTY

EVENING
Phone   (   )   n Voice n TTY

Fax   (   )

Shipping Address (if different from mailing address):

Name

Address

City

State   Zip Code

Phone   (   )   n Voice n TTY

Note: UPS does not deliver to Post Office Box addresses.

Quantity	Item Number	Page #	Description	Size	Color	Unit Cost	Total
	LE-65EE	—	*LeBoeuf's Home Healthcare Handbook* **Eldercare Edition** 544 pages, softcover	—	—	24.95	
	LE-65TR	—	Same as above except pages are in a convenient looseleaf three-ring binder	—	—	29.95	

LeBoeuf's will present Caregiving Workshops for groups of 20 or more people. Workshop fee of $35.00 person includes *LeBoeuf's Home Healthcare Handbook* for each participant. Call 1-800-546-5559 for information.

Subtotal $	
State Sales Tax	
Shipping (see chart at left)	
GRAND TOTAL $	

Shipping & Handling

Shipping and handling costs are for continental U.S. (48 states) only. Call for quote if items are to be shipped to Alaska, Hawaii, Puerto Rico, Canada or international destinations. Items too bulky or heavy to be shipped by U.S. Mail or UPS do not qualify for regular shipping and handling costs. Call for quote.

If your order total is   *Add*
Up to $5.00 . . . . $4.00
$5.01 – $10.00 . . . . $4.75
$10.01 – $25.00 . . . . $5.25
$25.01 – $50.00 . . . . $6.00
$50.01 – $100.00 . . . . $7.00
$100.01 – $200.00 . . . . $8.75
$200.01 – $300.00 . . . . $10.50
$300.01 – $400.00 . . . . $12.25
$400.01 – $500.00 . . . . $14.00
$500.01 – $750.00 . . . . $15.75
$750.01 – $1,000.00 . . . . . . $17.50
Over $1,000.00 . . . . . will be billed

METHOD OF PAYMENT

n Check or Money Order enclosed (make payable to "LeBoeuf's")

Charge my   n VISA   n MasterCard   n Discover

CREDIT CARD NUMBER   EXP. DATE

SIGNATURE (required for credit card orders)

LeBoeuf's Ordering Information

Convenient Personal Service

Enjoy the convenience of shopping without leaving home. If you have any questions — even for information about products not shown in this Healthcare Handbook — just give us a call. Our knowledgeable customer representatives understand your special needs. Call toll free 1-800-546-5559 from 9 a.m. to 5 p.m., Monday through Friday.

How to Order

By Phone   1-800-546-5559 Voice
              1-800-855-2880 TTY

Credit card customers can order by phone 24 hours a day, seven days a week. MasterCard, Visa and Discover accepted.

By Fax   1-800-233-9692

Fill out order form completely and type or print clearly. Remember to include your credit card number, expiration date, daytime phone number, and your signature.

By Mail

Fill out order form completely and type or print clearly. **Your daytime phone number is required.** We will call you only if we have questions regarding your order.

If you prefer to charge your order to a credit card, please include the credit card number, expiration date and signature. Checks, money orders and cashiers checks should be made payable to **LeBoeuf's** (in U.S. funds only) and mailed with your order to:

> Order Department
> **LeBoeuf's**
> 768 Walker Road, Suite 266
> Great Falls, VA 22066

Foreign Orders

Payment for orders from outside the United States must be in U.S. funds only and made payable to **LeBoeuf's.** For shipping and handling costs, call for a quote.

Delivery

Whenever possible, merchandise will be shipped by UPS Ground. LeBoeuf's will send all items that can be shipped by UPS to your home, workplace, or anywhere you tell us when you place your order (see shipping/handling cost for 48 contiguous United States on order form). Call for quote if items are to be shipped to Alaska, Hawaii, Puerto Rico, Canada or international destinations.

Orders must be prepaid with credit card, pre-paid check or money order. Please include delivery charges plus appropriate sales tax based on the destination of your order.

Non-Mailable Items. Items too heavy or too bulky to be shipped by U.S. Mail or UPS (odd shapes or items weighing over 70 lbs) do not qualify for regular shipping and handling costs. These items will be delivered to you for an additional charge. Delivery charges and service vary by area. We'll provide details

when you place your order. Some items are available only within the 48 contiguous United States, and cannot be shipped to Alaska, Hawaii or Puerto Rico.

Damaged Goods

If you receive an item that was damaged in shipping, please do the following:

- Keep all packaging materials in the same condition as you received them. Claims cannot be made if packing materials are missing.
- Report the damage immediately to the carrier (UPS, U.S. Postal Service, etc.)
- Do not ship the package back to LeBoeuf's. Wait for the carrier to inspect and pick up the package.
- Call LeBoeuf's to report the damage so that we can process a replacement order.

Shipping Errors

Shipping errors must be reported within five business days of receipt of order.

Returns or Exchanges

For returns or exchanges, please call our Customer Service Department ☎ 1-800-546-5559 for a Return Authorization Number (R.A.N.). Then repack the merchandise carefully in its original packaging. Include any instruction manuals, warranty card, etc. Send the merchandise, packing slip and the completed returns form prepaid and insured to:

> Customer Service
> **LeBoeuf's**
> 768 Walker Road, Suite 266
> Great Falls, VA 22066

To return non-mailable items, just call 1-800-546-5559 to arrange for pickup. LeBoeuf's will give you full credit on your merchandise. Delivery charges, however, are not refundable. *Videotapes, audiotapes and computer software are not returnable unless defective.*

Out-of-Stock Items

If an item is out of stock we'll notify you as soon as possible. If we don't think we can fill the order within 30 days, we'll ask if you still want the item when it becomes available.

In some cases, we may send a substitute of equal or greater value at the same price as your original order. If a substitute is not available and additional stock cannot be obtained, we will cancel your order and issue a full refund.

We reserve the right to limit quantities to properly service all of our customers.

Mailing Lists

We occasionally make our customer list of names and addresses available to carefully screened companies and organizations whose products and activities might be of interest to you. If you prefer not to receive such mailings, just let us know.

Product Pricing

Prices in *LeBoeuf's Home Healthcare Handbook* are effective June 1, 1996. All prices are subject to change without notice. Orders will be billed at the prices in effect at the time the order is received.

Your Satisfaction is Always Guaranteed

You must be satisfied with the performance and quality of any item you purchase from *LeBoeuf's Home Healthcare Handbook.* If you are not satisfied with your purchase for any reason, return the item to LeBoeuf's within 30 days for a full merchandise refund, credit or exchange. You pay only shipping and handling. *Videotapes, audiotapes and computer software are not returnable unless defective.*

Medicare Claims Filing

LeBoeuf's is a non-assigned Medicare provider. When you place an order, simply mention that you are a Medicare beneficiary. LeBoeuf's will file your claim to the appropriate office and Medicare will reimburse you directly.

You need to provide the following information about the Medicare recipient:

- Name and Address
- Date of Birth
- Medicare Number
- Doctor's prescription for the item (dated on or before the date of your order)
- Doctor's UPIN Number
- Diagnosis code and description

Mail the necessary papers to:

> Claims Department
> **LeBoeuf's**
> 768 Walker Road, Suite 266
> Great Falls, VA 22066

Inquiries about reimbursement should be made through your Medicare office. *Allow 10 to 12 weeks for reimbursement.*

Please note that:

- LeBoeuf's does not guarantee Medicare reimbursement. Reimbursement is based on Medicare's assessment of the patient's need.
- Payment must be received in full before a claim will be filed. Medicare will send the Explanation of Benefits and any payment awards directly to the patient or beneficiary.
- Certain items in LeBoeuf's Handbook require a Certificate of Medical Necessity (CMN) to be completed by the patient's doctor. LeBoeuf's will send the appropriate CMN to the doctor once we have received the prescription. Please note that claims requiring a CMN take longer to process.
- Medicare will only pay up to 80% of the lift mechanism in a lift recliner chair.